emergency care

emergency care:

A TEXTBOOK FOR PARAMEDICS

Edited by

Ian Greaves
MB ChB MRCP(UK) DTM&H DipIMC RCS(Ed)
Specialist Registrar in Accident & Emergency Medicine, St James's University Hospital, Leeds

Tim Hodgetts
MB BS(Hons) MRCP(UK) FFAEM DipIMC RCSEd RAMC
Consultant in Accident & Emergency Medicine, British Army

and
Keith Porter
MB BS FRCS DipIMC RCS(Ed)
Consultant Trauma Surgeon, Selly Oak Hospital, Birmingham

Paramedic Advisor
Malcolm Woollard
RN AASI DipMgmt FAETC LicIPD
Director of Emergency Medical Services
South and East Wales Ambulance Service

WB Saunders Company Ltd

LONDON PHILADELPHIA TORONTO SYDNEY TOKYO

W B SAUNDERS
A Division of Harcourt Publishers Limited

British Library Cataloguing in Publication Data
A catalogue record for this book is available from the British Library

Library of Congress Cataloging in Publication Data
A catalog record for this book is available from the Library of Congress

Medical knowledge is constantly changing. As new information
becomes available, changes in treatment, procedures, equipment
and the use of drugs become necessary. The authors and Publishers
have, as far as it is possible, taken care to ensure that the information
given in the text is accurate and up to date. However, readers are
strongly advised to confirm that the information, especially with
regard to drug usage, complies with latest legislation and standards
of practice.

The Publishers and authors have made every effort to trace the
copyright holders for borrowed material. If they have inadvertently
overlooked any, they will be pleased to rectify the matter at the
first opportunity.

ISBN 0-7020-1975-5

Typeset by Selwood Systems, Midsomer Norton
Printed in Great Britain by The Bath Press, Bath

PREFACE

The role of the ambulance service paramedic in the pre-hospital management of the acutely ill and injured has been increasingly recognized during the last few years. Along with the development of this role has come a general acceptance of the need for consistent and rational education for the paramedical profession. As this book goes to press, the first degree courses for paramedics in the UK are in preparation.

The time is right for a paramedic textbook that offers guidelines for safe practice against a background of sound scientific information. We hope that this book will fill this role. *Emergency Care: A Textbook for Paramedics* is the first comprehensive British textbook for paramedics – and importantly, the first book based on British practice.

As there are variations in practice between ambulance services in different parts of the UK, there may be occasional discrepancies between the text and readers' local guidelines. An editorial path has been taken which corresponds (we hope) with the practice in a majority of services. Additionally, we have described a number of procedures which we believe are likely to be added to the paramedic role in the not too distant future.

This book is intended to be a comprehensive textbook for paramedics from basic training to an advanced level of practice, and we have not therefore provided extensive references.

Suggestions for further reading are given at the end of individual chapters for those who wish to study particular subjects in greater detail.

Because of the size of the book, we suspect that most readers will read individual chapters as the need arises. For this reason, chapters need to be able to stand alone and we make no apology for any repetition of important material that this entails.

Those who wish to assess their knowledge may find the companion book *Emergency Care: A Self-assessment Guide* useful.

This book is written primarily for ambulance service paramedics, but we believe that it will also be useful to doctors (especially those involved in immediate care), members of the emergency and rescue services, first-aiders, and medical students.

We hope that this text will prove popular with paramedics, and will go some way to establishing a consistent national standard for practice. We would welcome any comments, suggestions or criticisms from readers.

Ian Greaves
Tim Hodgetts
Keith Porter

CONTENTS

Preface v
Acknowledgements x
Contributors xi

section 1 **SETTING THE SCENE** 1

Chapter 1	Scene approach and assessment	3
Chapter 2	Approach to the patient	10

section 2 **RESUSCITATION SKILLS** 15

Chapter 3	Basic life support	17
Chapter 4	Simple management of the airway and ventilation	27
Chapter 5	Advanced management of the airway and ventilation	42
Chapter 6	Intravenous access	60

section 3 **MEDICINE** 69

Chapter 7	Taking a medical history	71
Chapter 8	Introduction to pharmacology	74
Chapter 9	Respiratory emergencies	81
Chapter 10	The heart: anatomy, physiology and the ECG	88
Chapter 11	Monitoring and defibrillation	115
Chapter 12	Cardiac arrest in adults: advanced life support	122
Chapter 13	Cardiovascular emergencies	131
Chapter 14	The unconscious patient	139
Chapter 15	The acute abdomen	149
Chapter 16	Poisoning	156
Chapter 17	Risk of infection	162

section 4 **TRAUMA** 169

Chapter 18	Obtaining a trauma history	171
Chapter 19	The primary and secondary survey	175
Chapter 20	Shock	181
Chapter 21	Head injuries	187
Chapter 22	Facial injuries	196
Chapter 23	Chest injuries	201
Chapter 24	Abdominal and genitourinary trauma	209
Chapter 25	Bone and joint injuries	213
Chapter 26	Spinal injuries	236
Chapter 27	Patient immobilization and extrication	249
Chapter 28	Blast and gunshot injuries	266
Chapter 29	Burns	270
Chapter 30	Wound management	279
Chapter 31	Overview of trauma resuscitation	286

ACKNOWLEDGEMENTS

Our greatest thanks are due to Ian and Gill Oxley who have laboured through the drafts of this book to produce an immaculate final manuscript. We look forward to further collaborations. Our thanks are also extended to the many people (often unknown by name to the editors) who took the trouble to read and comment on the chapters in manuscript.

This book would never have happened if Georgina Bentliff (formerly of Baillière Tindall) had not recognized the need for it and acted as its enthusiastic advocate: once again our sincere thanks to her, and to Tim Kimber of W. B. Saunders. We are grateful to the following for allowing us to reproduce copyright material: Churchill Livingstone, Gower Medical Publishing, Little, Brown and Co. and Smith and Nephew Pharmaceuticals.

Finally we should like to thank our families for their continuing patience and support.

CONTRIBUTORS

Bruce Armstrong RGN, RMN
Staff Nurse, Accident & Emergency Department,
Southampton General Hospital, Southampton

Harry Baker BSc, MRCP(UK)
Consultant in Rehabilitation Medicine and Spinal Injuries,
Welsh Regional Spine Injuries Centre, Rookwood Hospital,
Cardiff

Peter Baskett FRCA, MRCP
Consultant Anaesthetist, Frenchay Hospital, Bristol

James Briscoe MRCPsych
Honorary Clinical Lecturer, Department of Psychiatry,
University of Birmingham, Birmingham

Terry Brown FRCS(Ed), DA
Consultant in Accident & Emergency Medicine, Whiston
Hospital, Merseyside

Christopher Carney DipIMC.RCS(Ed)
Director of Operations, Staffordshire Ambulance Service
Headquarters, Stoke-on-Trent

Timothy Coats FRCS
Senior Registrar in Accident & Emergency Medicine, Royal
London Hospital, London

Michael Colquhoun MRCP(UK), MRCGP
General Practitioner, Great Malvern, Worcestershire

Gareth Davies MRCP(UK)
Consultant in Accident & Emergency Medicine and
Prehospital Care, Royal London Hospital, London

Corah Dempsey
Field Training Officer, Staffordshire Ambulance Service NHS
Trust, Stafford

Peter Driscoll MD, FRCS, FFAEM
Consultant and Senior Lecturer, Department of Emergency
Medicine, Hope Hospital, Salford

Peter Dyer FRCS(Ed), FFD.RCSI
Senior Registrar in Maxillofacial Surgery, Royal London
Hospital, London

Judith Fisher FRCGP
Consultant in Primary Care, Royal London Hospital, London

Alasdair Gray FRCS(Ed)
Specialist Registrar in Accident & Emergency Medicine, Hull
Royal Infirmary, Kingston upon Hull

Ian Greaves MB ChB, MRCP(UK), DTM&H,
DipIMC.RCS(Ed)
Specialist Registrar in Accident & Emergency Medicine, St
James's University Hospital, Leeds

Marcus Green BSc, FRCS, DipIMC.RCS(Ed)
Specialist Registrar in Trauma and Orthopaedic Surgery,
University Hospital, Birmingham

Paul Grout DA, DCH, FRCS(Ed)
Consultant in Accident & Emergency Medicine, Hull Royal
Infirmary, Kingston upon Hull

Carl Gwinnutt FRCA
Consultant Anaesthetist, Hope Hospital, Salford

Jacqueline Hanson FRCS, FFAEM
Consultant in Accident & Emergency Medicine, Preston
Royal Infirmary, Preston

Kenneth Hines
General Practitioner, London

Tim Hodgetts MB BS(Hons), MRCP(UK), FFAEM,
DipIMC.RCS(Ed), RAMC
Consultant in Accident & Emergency Medicine, British Army

Peter Holden DRCOG, DipIMC.RCS(Ed)
General Practitioner, Matlock, Derbyshire

John Hopper FRCS(Ed), DipIMC.RCS(Ed)
Senior Registrar in Trauma and Orthopaedics, West Midlands
Training Programme

Phil Hormbrey FRCS(Ed), MRCP(UK), DA,
DipIMC.RCS(Ed)
Consultant in Accident & Emergency Medicine, John
Radcliffe Hospital, Oxford

Jason Kendall MRCP(UK), DipIMC.RCS(Ed)
Senior Registrar in Accident & Emergency Medicine,
Frenchay Hospital, Bristol

Juergen Klein DipIMC.RCS(Ed), DA
Specialist Registrar in Anaesthesia and Intensive Care
Leicester Royal Infirmary, Leicester

Colville Laird DipIMC.RCS(Ed)
General Practitioner, Maesteg, Mid-Glamorgan

Richard Lewis MRCGP, DipIMC.RCS(Ed)
Medical Director, Mid-Glamorgan Ambulance Service
General Practitioner, Maesteg, Mid-Glamorgan

Kevin Mackway-Jones MRCP(UK), FRCS(Ed), FFAEM
Consultant in Accident & Emergency Medicine, Manchester
Royal Infirmary, Manchester

Alastair Main MD, FRCP
Consultant in Geriatric Medicine, Queen Elizabeth Hospital,
Birmingham

Alastair McGowan FRCP, FFAEM
Consultant in Accident & Emergency Medicine, St James
University Hospital, Leeds

Ian McNeil DipIMC.RCS(Ed), DRCOG
General Practitioner, Horsham, Sussex

Gordon J A Morris MRCGP, AFOM, DRCOG
Senior Medical Officer, Occupational Health Care Services,
Glasgow

Chris Moulton DRCOG, MRCGP, FRCA, FFAEM
Senior Lecturer in Emergency Medicine, Bolton Royal
Infirmary, Bolton

Julie Nancarrow FRCS, MRCGP, DRCOG, DA,
DipIMC.RCS(Ed)
Senior Registrar in Emergency Medicine, Hope Hospital,
Salford

Jerry Nolan FRCA
Department of Anaesthesia, Royal United Hospital, Bath

Mike Parr FRCA
Intensive Care Unit, Royal North Shore Hospital, Sydney,
Australia

Keith Porter MB BS, FRCS, DipIMC.RCS(Ed)
Consultant Surgeon, Selly Oak Hospital, Birmingham

Brian Robertson OStJ TD
General Practitioner, Aldershot, Hampshire

Colin Robertson FRCS(Ed), FRCP, FFAEM, FSA(Scot)
Consultant in Accident & Emergency Medicine, Edinburgh
Royal Infirmary, Edinburgh

Jim Ryan Mch, FRCS
Leonard Cheshire Professor of Post Conflict Recovery,
University College London

John Scott DipIMC.RCS(Ed), DA
General Practitioner, Cambridge

Howard Sherriff FRCS, MA, FFAEM
Consultant in Accident & Emergency Medicine,
Addenbrookes Hospital, Cambridge

Andrew H Swain BSc PhD FRCS FFAEM
Consultant, Accident & Emergency Department, General
Hospital, Weston-Super-Mare; National Convenor,
Advanced Life Support Courses, Resuscitation Council, UK
Services and Senior Clinical Lecturer in Accident &
Emergency Medicine, University of Bristol

Sean Walsh MRCPI, DCH, DRCOG
Consultant in Paediatric Accident & Emergency Medicine,
Leeds General Infirmary, Leeds

Alastair Wilson FRCS
Consultant in Accident & Emergency Medicine, Royal
London Hospital, London

Malcolm Woollard RN, AASI, DipMgmt, FAETC, LicIPD
Director of Emergency Medical Services, South and East
Wales Ambulance Service

to
Margaret and Robert Greaves
Mags and Jack Hodgetts
and
Sally, Matthew, James
and Sarah Porter

DRUG DOSES

We believe the drug doses and regimens in this book to be correct. However, we recommend that if you are using a drug with which you are not familiar you should consult the *British National Formulary* first.

1

SETTING
THE
SCENE

chapter one:

SCENE APPROACH AND ASSESSMENT

APPROACHING THE SCENE

Driving to the Scene

When driving an emergency vehicle to the scene of an accident or medical emergency the priority is safety, not speed – safety of yourself and of other road users. If expeditious transport is required from the scene to the hospital, then the safety of the patient is an additional concern.

> When driving an emergency vehicle the priority is safety, not speed

Consider this: a vehicle driven 3 miles on urban roads at an average of 60 miles per hour will take 3 minutes to travel the distance, whereas a vehicle driven at an average of 40 miles per hour will take $4\frac{1}{2}$ minutes. It can be argued that such a time saving may be critical if the patient is in ventricular fibrillation following myocardial infarction, or has an obstructed airway following head injury, but this will not be true in the majority of cases. The likelihood of an accident *en route* (of the emergency vehicle or road users trying to avoid the emergency vehicle) will increase as the driving speed increases. The driver of an emergency vehicle therefore has a responsibility to balance safe driving with an acceptable response time.

> An emergency vehicle driver must balance safe driving with an acceptable response time

The quality of the despatch information may influence, consciously or subconsciously, how the emergency vehicle driver responds to the scene. The following are three examples of despatch information to the same incident, which illustrate the importance of high-quality information. How would you respond in each case?

1. *Seventy-year-old woman collapsed in East Street outside Lloyds Bank.*
2. *Seventy-year-old woman collapsed, not breathing, no pulse* in East Street outside Lloyds Bank.*
3. *Seventy-year-old woman collapsed, now fully alert but injured right wrist in fall, in East Street outside Lloyds Bank.*

The advanced driving techniques taught to emergency service personnel are often referred to as *defensive driving*. These techniques are described in detail in *Roadcraft, The Police Driver's Handbook* (see Further reading). The fundamental principle is to provide an appropriate attitude to driving, particularly towards speed and risk-taking. In the heat of battle soldiers may become blind to everything other than their immediate objective: this 'red mist' may also engulf the emergency service driver, who will ignore road conditions and threaten the safety of other road users in an attempt to reach the scene as quickly as possible. This 'red mist' can be minimized by concentration on the driving, rather than concentration on anticipated problems and tasks at the scene.

In the UK an emergency service vehicle has no legal right of way when using visual and audible warnings: the ambulance driver must rely on the courtesy of other road users to give way. Defensive driving techniques recognize the need for continuous caution in case other vehicles do not give way, while teaching the driver how best to use the available road. Figure 1.1 shows how an ambulance can position itself on a rural road to get the best view of oncoming traffic and to anticipate oncoming hazards; Figure 1.2 explains the 'arrowhead' principle.

The public road user may react in a variety of ways to an approaching ambulance:

sudden braking
sudden changing of lane
failure to give way

It is important that the emergency vehicle is not driven aggressively. If the ambulance is too close to the vehicle in front there may be a collision if the vehicle suddenly brakes. Alternatively,

---

*Ambulance services commonly assign a radio code for key conditions such as cardiac arrest.

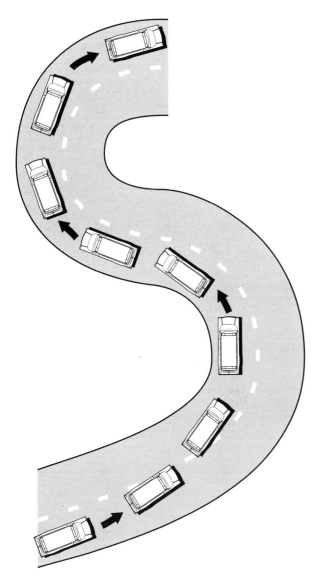

Fig. 1.1 Driving on a rural road: position the vehicle to get the best view of the road ahead

other vehicle drivers may be panicked into an erratic move which is dangerous to themselves or to others. Where a driver makes a special effort to give way this should be acknowledged: the same driver will then be disposed to give way the next time. There should be a 2-second gap between your vehicle and the vehicle in front. Identify a roadside marker such as a lamp-post, and as the vehicle in front passes the marker say:

> 'Only a fool breaks the two-second rule'

You should be able to complete this sentence before passing the marker yourself.

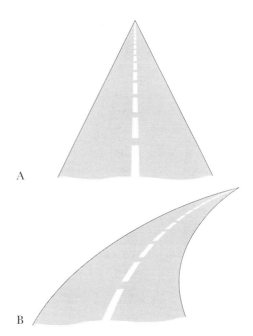

Fig. 1.2 The arrowhead principle. The verges of the road form an 'arrowhead' on the horizon; when the arrowhead is moving (A), accelerate; when the arrowhead is stationary (B), maintain speed or decelerate until it starts to move again

The ambulance driver should be aware of the limitations of the ambulance's visual and audible warnings. Stroboscopic lights are generally of higher intensity than rotating halogen lights, but tend to be unidirectional: additional stroboscopic lights must be mounted on the side of the vehicle or on the end of a light-bar for all-round visibility. Roof-mounted lights may not be seen if the ambulance is very close to the vehicle in front, and its driver may simply think he or she is being followed by an angry van driver. Stroboscopic lights mounted on the ambulance's grille or dashboard will identify the vehicle in this situation.

Sirens also tend to be directional, and vehicles approaching a junction at right angles to the ambulance may not hear the ambulance's siren. Even when the siren is heard it can be difficult to determine from which direction the ambulance is coming. When travelling at high speed, as on a motorway, a siren will provide very little advance warning: far more effective here is the use of alternating dipped and full-beam headlights.

The biggest limitation of lights and sirens is that they provide no legal protection in the event of an accident. An ambulance driver who causes an accident can expect to be charged with dangerous driving at the least.

> Lights and sirens provide no legal protection in the event of an accident

It has been popular to request a police escort for an ambulance, especially for the seriously ill or injured patient who is trans-ferred between hospitals. Such a decision should be considered carefully. A police escort is effective if the police vehicle moves ahead of the ambulance to clear a route (for example to stop traffic at a junction) and then allows the ambulance to pass. This would be useful in city traffic and may best be performed by two police cars or motorcyclists alternately moving ahead of the ambulance. The danger of a police escort is that it may become a race to keep up with the more powerful car; worse, other road users may only identify the first emergency vehicle and turn back into the path of the ambulance (the incidence of ambulance accidents is increased when a police escort is used).

Advanced safe driving tips

- Devote your concentration to driving, not to how you will respond on arrival at the scene (beware of 'red mist')
- Always ensure you can stop within the distance you can see
- Keep a safe distance between the vehicle in front (remember the 2-second rule)

Parking at the Scene

On a residential street it may be possible to extinguish all warn-ing lights; on a commercial street in the day double-parking may be unavoidable, which may obstruct the flow of traffic – hazard lights or beacons are then used at the driver's discretion. When an ambulance is the first or only emergency vehicle to arrive at the scene of a road traffic accident the vehicle is parked in the *fend-off* or *on-line* position (Figure 1.3) to protect the incident. In the fend-off position beacons may be less visi-ble to approaching traffic, and headlights may distract traffic in the opposite carriageway; but if a vehicle shunts an ambulance in the on-line position the ambulance may be pushed forward onto the casualties and rescuers. The parking position for a combined emergency service response to a road traffic accident entrapment is shown in Figure 1.4.

If the ambulance is left unattended it should be locked. Although

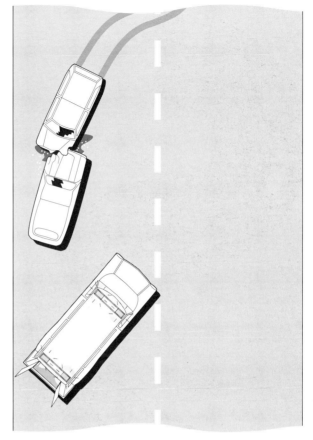

Fig. 1.3 *The fend-off position*

ambulances in the UK do not routinely carry controlled drugs (unlike services in Australia where morphine is carried for use by ambulance personnel), opportunist thieves may look for such drugs or take other items of valuable equipment. If the police are controlling an incident the keys should be left in the ignition so that a vehicle can be moved if necessary.

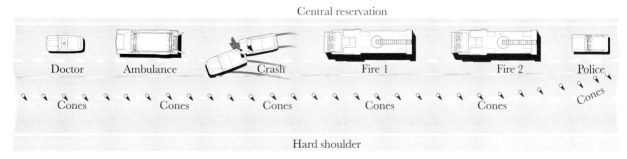

Fig. 1.4 *Combined emergency services parking at a motorway accident*

Approach for Immediate Care Doctors

Immediate care doctors may be requested to attend the scene by the ambulance service, where a British Association for Immediate Care (BASICS) scheme exists.

Driving to the scene
  a green beacon identifies a registered medical practitioner
  sirens can only be used with the approval of the county's chief police officer

Parking at the scene
  the doctor will be directed by the police
  the accepted position is in front of the ambulance
  beacons are extinguished and keys should be left in the ignition

PRIORITIES AT THE SCENE

Setting the Scene

It is 1600 hours on Monday and you have arrived at the scene of a pedestrian road traffic accident. A member of the public dialled 999, asked for the ambulance service and simply said a child had been hit by a car when crossing the road at the busy corner of North and East Streets in Townsville. There is a crowd of 15 people. Traffic is at a standstill behind the incident, and is moving very slowly in the opposite direction, which is the direction from which you approach. The child is lying unconscious, but breathing on the road. A woman is cradling the child's head. What do you do?

The priorities at the scene can be remembered as CONTROL then 'ACT':

  A > ASSESS
  C > COMMUNICATE
  T > TRIAGE, TREAT and TRANSPORT

Scene Control

The first priority is to control the scene. You approach and park in the carriageway that is free beyond the incident. The incident is now protected in both directions. You leave your beacons switched on. Members of the public should be cleared from obstructing the road and the engine of the vehicle involved in the accident turned off.

Scene control is a responsibility of the police, who will be required at this incident for traffic control. In a protracted incident, such as a vehicle entrapment, the police will establish and maintain a cordon to protect the rescuers and will determine the approach routes for emergency service vehicles.

Safety is of paramount concern. Always think of your own safety first, then the safety of other rescuers and bystanders, and finally the safety of the casualties. This is the 1-2-3 of safety.

The 1-2-3 of safety

  1 > Yourself
  2 > The scene (bystanders, rescuers)
  3 > The casualties

Protecting yourself

Individual emergency service personnel must be responsible for their own safety. In this situation at least a high-visibility vest marked with the level of training ('Ambulance' for general duties personnel, or 'Paramedic') must be worn. Where there is a hazard from glass or sharp metal a jacket with full-length sleeves should be worn, again appropriately marked, together with a helmet with integral visor. Helmets must be fitted with a secure chin-strap, otherwise the temptation will be to discard one that falls off when the officer bends forward to treat a patient. A high-visibility jacket is mandatory at a motorway incident. All patients should be assumed to be infectious in terms of communicable diseases such as acquired immune deficiency syndrome (AIDS), hepatitis B or hepatitis C. Protective gloves must be worn when treating patients, and where there is contact with blood, eye protection is also recommended – this may be the visor of a helmet, goggles or protective glasses (the latter being the most suitable for general daily use).

Ambulance officer's personal protective equipment

- Hard hat with chin-strap
- Eye protection (goggles, glasses or visor)
- Ear protection
- High-visibility jacket, with identifying markings
- Heavy-duty gloves
- Patient treatment gloves
- Robust footwear

If a chemical hazard is identified, the scene must not be entered until it is declared safe to do so by the fire service. It is the fire service's responsibility to identify the nature of a chemical hazard, which is done from the United Nations product number displayed on the hazard plate (see Chapter 42). The fire service control centre will have computerized access to information on the chemical, including first-aid action and specific antidotes, and this information can be made available through the CHEMDATA system on the pumping appliances. Extreme caution must also be exercised when attending other specific incidents, as described below.

Shooting Is there still a threat from the assailant? Is the patient also carrying a weapon?

Do you require police support before proceeding?

Bomb *Unexploded bomb:* can you see the suspect device? You are in the wrong place!

Exploded bomb: have the police searched for secondary devices? Do not use your radio until this search has been made (it may detonate a radio-controlled device).

Electric cable down Power may be restored without investigation of the cause. Notify the power company.

Rail Has power to overhead cables or the live rail been isolated? Diesel trains can still run.

Protecting bystanders

Bystanders must be protected from becoming part of the incident, and approaching vehicles (for example on a motorway) must have adequate warning to slow down safely.

Protecting casualties

The safety of the casualties is ensured by protecting the scene with the emergency service vehicles and a cordon. A *snatch rescue* may be appropriate when the patient's life is in immediate danger, for example from fire or toxic chemical. In the UK it is the responsibility of the fire service to rescue casualties from a hazardous environment. It would be unwise for an ambulance officer to attempt such a rescue without adequate personal protective equipment. During a snatch rescue every reasonable attempt will be made to extricate the patient safely, but spinal immobilization in particular may have to be compromised to save life.

Scene Assessment

After taking control of an incident the next priority is to assess the scene. There are three important elements to the scene assessment:

    assessment of hazards, both present and potential
    reading the scene
    rapid assessment of the number and severity of casualties

An *assessment of hazards* will be made during the approach to the incident, but further hazards, which may not have been initially evident, are evaluated during the scene assessment. Hazards at a road traffic accident can be actual (fire, chemical spillage), or potential (petrol on road). Electricity supply through overhead cables is commonly interrupted as a result of 'bird strike', and it is therefore usual for power to be restored without the reason being investigated. Emergency service personnel should not approach an incident involving a downed electricity cable, unless the power company has been contacted and the supply isolated. You do not have to touch a cable to be electrocuted – electricity can arc several metres.

An assessment of hazards is not restricted to the scene of a road traffic accident. For example, electricity could also be a hazard when a gardener has run over a lawnmower cable, or a child is still holding a fork that was pushed into a mains adaptor.
It is important to take time to *read the scene*. At a road traffic accident this involves 'reading the wreckage' – where observation of the nature of deformation of a vehicle and its position may help to identify the injuries the patient has sustained. This is discussed in detail later in this chapter. Additionally, reading the scene may give vital clues to the nature of a medical illness: a young woman found unconscious at home with an empty bottle of pills will be assumed to have taken an overdose, and a sweaty, unresponsive man with a Medic-Alert bracelet which says 'I am an insulin dependent diabetic' has a high probability of being unresponsive because of hypoglycaemia.

> **Read the scene for clues to injuries following trauma, or to the reason for medical illness**

Assessment of the scene also involves an assessment of the *number and severity of casualties*. At this stage the need is to establish what resources are immediately required at the scene. A detailed examination of each patient is not necessary, but a rapid assessment of each patient's airway, breathing and circulation should be done (see Chapter 2).

Communication

Pre-hospital care requires teamwork, and good teamwork demands good communication. There are several levels of communication to consider:

- Communication between ambulance crew members
- Communication with ambulance control
- Communication with other emergency services at the scene
- Communication with the hospital

> **Good communication is central to effective emergency service teamwork**

When assistance is required at an incident scene it is useful to remember the mnemonic 'ETHANE' when communicating with ambulance control:

E	>	EXACT LOCATION
T	>	TYPE OF INCIDENT
H	>	HAZARDS, PRESENT AND POTENTIAL
A	>	ACCESS
N	>	NUMBER, SEVERITY AND TYPE OF CASUALTIES
E	>	EMERGENCY SERVICES, PRESENT AND REQUIRED

'CHALET' is also used as a mnemonic by some services, and is described in Chapter 55.

Information is usually passed to the hospital indirectly via the ambulance control. Some ambulance services allow direct radio communication between hospital and the crew, but this 'talk through' must be requested through ambulance control. The value of advance warning is that appropriate staff can be summoned to assemble in the accident and emergency department to receive the patient, which is particularly important in cases of severe trauma and cardiac arrest.

The essential information the hospital will require to be able to assemble the appropriate staff and prepare equipment is:

- *Age of the patient* (adult or child is adequate, but knowing the age of a child allows the preparation of equipment such as endotracheal tubes, and the calculation of drug doses)
- *Nature of the priority call* (trauma, or cardiac arrest)
- *Abnormal vital signs* (a head-injured patient with a Glasgow Coma Scale score below 9 requires intubation, if not already performed; the senior duty surgeon should be informed if there is an adult with hypotension of below 90 mmHg following trauma)

Triage, Treatment and Transport

Triage is the sorting of patients into priorities for treatment and is discussed in detail in Chapter 56. Where there is only one injured victim, then the patient's injuries are prioritized. The systematic approach to the individual patient assessment and treatment is discussed in Chapter 2. This is the 'ABC' system:

A > AIRWAY (with control of the cervical spine)
B > BREATHING (with oxygen)
C > CIRCULATION (with control of external bleeding)

Transport to hospital should not be delayed for treatment that is not essential to saving life, reducing suffering or reducing long-term morbidity. The *'golden hour'* is the time from injury to the time of definitive treatment (emergency operation), and following trauma every attempt should be made to deliver the patient well inside this golden hour. If the patient is trapped in a vehicle, this hour can easily slip by at the scene. Every 10 minutes you spend at the scene, ask yourself, 'Why am I still here?' It is more appropriate in pre-hospital care, therefore, to think in terms of a *'platinum 10 minutes'* to rapidly assess and stabilize the patient before transport.

Packaging for transport (treatment and monitoring) and the selection of the best method of transport are discussed later in this book.

READING THE WRECKAGE

Relating the deformation of a vehicle involved in an accident to the occupants' potential injuries is known as *reading the wreckage*. Metal is stronger than tissue and bone – so if there is significant deformation of the vehicle involving the passenger compartment, the ambulance officer should anticipate a greater deformity of the human body, even if this was only temporary at the time of impact. Reading the wreckage enables the ambulance officer to actively seek a pattern of injuries, even if the patient is unaware of them all (pain in one body region can distract the patient from injuries elsewhere).

> Reading the wreckage allows the ambulance officer to anticipate a pattern of injuries

The pattern of injuries will depend on the type of impact. Table 1.1 lists the injuries that should be anticipated from a front or side impact.

Entrapment may be relative or absolute. *Relative entrapment* is

Table 1.1 Patterns of injury with front and side vehicle impact

Front Impact	Side Impact
Facial injuries/airway compromise (windscreen)	Lateral flexion injury of cervical spine
Head injury (facial impact)	Ipsilateral chest injury
Cervical spine injury (flexion on deceleration; extension on facial impact)	Ipsilateral pelvis injury; central dislocation of the hip
Clavicle, sternum and rib fractures (and underlying organ injury) from seat-belt	Ipsilateral limb injuries
Chest injury (steering wheel)	Ipsilateral abdominal visceral injury
Abdominal visceral injury (seat-belt/steering wheel)	
Patella and femoral fracture, posterior dislocation of hip (dashboard intrusion)	
Lower leg fractures and dislocations (engine intrusion/pedals)	

when the occupant is unable to get out of the vehicle unassisted, for example is unable to open the car door because of a broken arm. An *absolute entrapment* is when the occupant is physically restrained by the deformed wreckage.

Vehicle entrapment may be relative or absolute

FURTHER READING

Hodgetts T & Mackway-Jones K, eds (1995) *Major Incident Medical Management and Support.* London: BMJ Publications.
Roadcraft, The Police Driver's Handbook. (1994) London: HMSO.

chapter two:

APPROACH TO THE PATIENT

The approach to the patient follows scene safety and scene assessment. In trauma cases you will already have information about the patient's likely injuries after 'reading the wreckage' or understanding the nature of the accident. In medical cases important clues will be gained on approach – the salbutamol inhaler by the bedside, the oxygen cylinder in the corner of the room, or the box of assorted medications on the table. Assessment of the scene and assessment of the patient are vital and complementary parts of the same process.

Remember when dealing with a trauma case that certain mechanisms predict serious injuries whatever the apparent state of the patient:

- Patient falling from a height greater than 5 metres
- Road traffic accident (Figure 2.1) with an extrication time greater than 20 minutes
- Patient ejected from a vehicle
- Loss of life in the same vehicle
- Child (less than 12 years old) pedestrian or cyclist struck by a vehicle

- Pedestrian struck by a vehicle and thrown
- Vehicle intrusion greater than 30 cm

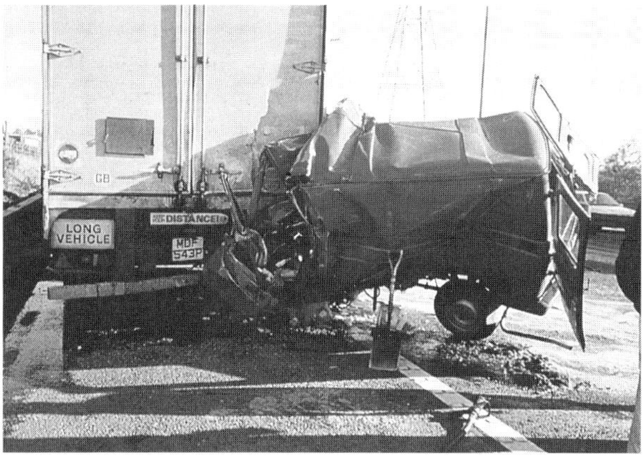

All such patients must be taken to hospital whatever their apparent injuries.

When dealing with an incident involving multiple casualties it will be necessary to carry out the process of triage; that is, to sort casualties into priorities for treatment and to 'do the most for the most' (Chapter 56).

During the course of examining a patient, any Medic-Alert bracelet or card (Figure 2.2) should be identified. Wherever possible relevant medical history, current medication and

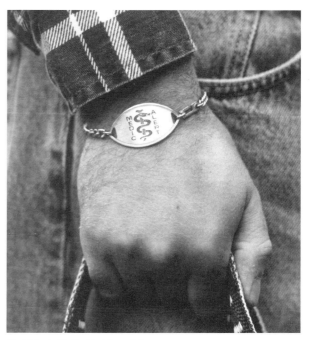

Fig. 2.1 *A road traffic accident*

Fig. 2.2 *A Medic-Alert bracelet*

allergies should be established. These points can be remembered using the mnemonic 'AMPLE':

A	>	ALLERGIES
M	>	MEDICATION
P	>	PAST HISTORY
L	>	LAST MEAL
E	>	EVENT (I.E. CURRENT PROBLEM)

This information is just as important in a trauma case as in a medical case: why did the patient crash the car on a straight road in good visibility? Does the patient suffer from diabetes mellitus or epilepsy, i.e. did a hypoglycaemic episode or a fit *cause* the accident?

PRIMARY AND SECONDARY SURVEYS

The patients seen by ambulance personnel may be divided broadly into two groups:

medical patients
trauma patients

The initial approach to these two groups *is identical*. The components of the systematic approach are:

- Primary survey   *Life threatening*
- Resuscitation
- Secondary survey
- Definitive care

The role of the *primary survey* is to identify any life-threatening problems or injuries.

> The primary survey identifies life-threatening problems

Whenever possible, treatment of any life-threatening problem is carried out as soon as that problem is identified.

> Primary survey and resuscitation take place simultaneously

The primary survey is a rapid process taking ideally only a minute or two. In critical trauma (and in some medical conditions) only the primary survey and resuscitation should be undertaken by the paramedic. The secondary survey (which identifies non-life-threatening problems) and definitive treatment are most appropriately carried out in hospital.

> The secondary survey identifies non-life-threatening problems

THE PRIMARY SURVEY

The primary survey follows the simple system of 'ABCDE':

A	>	**A**IRWAY WITH CERVICAL SPINE CONTROL
B	>	**B**REATHING WITH ADEQUATE VENTILATION/OXYGENATION
C	>	**C**IRCULATION WITH CONTROL OF EXTERNAL HAEMORRHAGE
D	>	**D**ISABILITY AND NEUROLOGICAL EXAMINATION
E	>	**E**XPOSURE AND EVALUATION

The philosophy of this approach is to deal with life-threatening problems in order of priority. Rigorous application of this approach is the basis of good paramedical practice.
Importantly, if the patient's condition deteriorates one must *always* revert to the ABCs. It can be said that *the most important examination is the re-examination*.
In time-critical trauma cases (where the patient is not entrapped) the principle should be establishment of airway and breathing on scene, with consideration of vascular access *en route* to hospital. Unnecessary delay at the scene may well jeopardize patient outcome. Although this system was originally designed for use in trauma, it is equally relevant to the management of medical conditions.

> Unnecessary delay at the scene may well jeopardize patient outcome

'A' – Airway with Cervical Spine Control

A clear airway free from obstruction or potential obstruction is essential. Causes of obstruction include the tongue, blood, vomitus, broken dentures, teeth and debris, foreign bodies, laryngotracheal injuries, and swelling from burns or allergies.
In medical emergencies a clear airway is obtained by using a combination of head tilt and chin lift. In trauma patients, however, it is important to prevent cervical movement – so *only* use a chin lift or a jaw thrust manoeuvre. In-line cervical immobilization should be maintained during all airway manoeuvres. Cervical immobilization means in-line stabilization, *not* traction which may produce or exacerbate spinal cord injury.
Well-fitting dentures should be retained. Foreign bodies and debris should be removed using a finger sweep (though this should be avoided in infants and very young children) or suction. A blind finger sweep is not recommended, as this may further impact a foreign body.
The airway once opened and cleared should be secured; this may involve the use of an appropriately sized oropharyngeal or nasopharyngeal airway, and in some cases orotracheal intubation. It is important to remember that opening an airway has priority over cervical spine protection, and in a difficult

situation it may be necessary to accept some cervical spine movement.

Approximately 5% of unconscious trauma patients have a cervical spine injury. It is imperative to have a high index of suspicion, and anyone who is unconscious, who has an altered level of consciousness or who has evidence of blunt injury above the clavicle should be regarded as having a cervical spinal injury until it is proved otherwise. Once the airway has been opened, cleared and secured, an appropriately sized semi-rigid collar is fitted and manual immobilization is maintained. Failure to obtain a clear airway may demand specialized interventions with appropriate advice and assistance (Chapter 5). It may be possible to achieve some assisted ventilation in the case of partial airway obstruction, in which case the patient should be transferred to hospital urgently. Where the patient is trapped, skilled medical assistance may be available from a hospital 'flying squad' or an immediate care (BASICS) doctor.

Cervical spine injury may also complicate medical problems if, for example, a fit has caused a fall, or a patient with severe rheumatoid arthritis has a relatively minor car accident.

'B' – Breathing

Look, feel and listen for 5 seconds to ascertain whether the patient is breathing. It is important to recognize patients in whom there is *no* spontaneous respiration, or who are hypoventilating (Greek *hypo*, under), as hypoxia is rapidly life-threatening.

The respiratory rate should be determined by counting for 15 seconds and multiplying by 4 to give an approximate minute rate. During the secondary survey a more accurate rate may be determined, by counting for a whole minute.

The normal respiratory rate in adults is between 12 and 18 breaths per minute. In patients with a respiratory rate between 10 and 12, or between 18 and 29, oxygen therapy should be given, but if the rate is below 10 or above 29 breaths per minute assisted ventilation may be necessary.

It is important to recognize that hypoventilation may lead to carbon dioxide (CO_2) retention, which itself will alter the level of consciousness and result in brain injury.

During the primary survey life-threatening chest conditions should be identified – these are open chest wounds, flail chest and tension pneumothorax. The chest wall should be observed for symmetry and normal pattern of movement (there is 'paradoxical movement' with a flail segment). A deviated trachea suggests a tension pneumothorax on the side *away* from the deviation, and requires urgent medical intervention (see Chapter 23).

Mouth-to-mask ventilation, ventilation using a bag–valve–mask with reservoir, or mechanical ventilation, may be necessary to assist or replace ventilation if it is inadequate or absent. In all spontaneously breathy trauma cases oxygen at 15 litres per minute through a Hudson mask with an attached reservoir (giving an inspired concentration of about 90%) should be given.

'C' – Circulation and Control of External Haemorrhage

It is first essential to determine if the patient has a cardiac output, and to start basic life support if this is absent.

External haemorrhage should be controlled where possible by direct pressure and elevation. Rarely, it is necessary to apply pressure over a pressure point or to use a tourniquet. The latter, if applied, should be released for 2 minutes in every 15 minutes during an entrapment and should be left on if the total time exceeds 2 hours.

Circulatory status can be assessed by the pulse volume and pulse rate. Peripheral perfusion can be estimated by observing the capillary refill time: this is the time taken for the normal pink colour of the nail beds to return after 5 seconds of compression, and is normally less than 2 seconds. This test is unreliable in the dark and in very cold conditions.

An early assessment of blood pressure is important. As a rough guide the presence of a:

- Carotid pulse indicates a minimum blood pressure of 60 mmHg
- Femoral pulse indicates a minimum blood pressure of 70 mmHg
- Radial pulse indicates a minimum blood pressure of 80 mmHg

Traumatic blood loss is corrected by placing two large-bore cannulae (if possible 14–16 gauge) and giving 2 litres of Hartmann's solution. If the patient is not trapped and has critical injuries the infusion should be started *en route* to hospital, rather than delaying at the scene.

Other, usually medical, causes of low blood pressure will normally simply require rapid evacuation to hospital.

'D' – Disability

The objective of assessing the neurological status is to provide a baseline for further observations. In the primary survey the 'AVPU' scale is used:

A	>	ALERT
V	>	RESPONDS TO VERBAL STIMULI
P	>	RESPONDS TO PAINFUL STIMULI
U	>	UNRESPONSIVE

In addition, pupillary size and reaction should be recorded.

'E' – Exposure and Environment

The patient needs to be exposed to allow clinical examination to exclude any obvious life-threatening conditions. In particular, exposure to inspect the chest is vital. It is important not to miss blood loss concealed by clothes, or under the patient. Exposure should preserve the patient's dignity where possible, and should protect from the extremes of temperature.

Summary of the Primary Survey

Life-threatening problems are identified and treated (wherever possible) during the *primary survey*. These problems may include maxillofacial trauma, for example (A), airway obstruction due to vomit in diabetic hypoglycaemia (A), severe pulmonary oedema following a heart attack (B), penetrating chest trauma (B) or blood loss due to trauma or bleeding duodenal ulcer (C). Whether the emergency is medical or traumatic, the approach remains the same. Sometimes a problem will be identified which the paramedic cannot remedy on scene. The emphasis must then be on transferring the patient to hospital as rapidly as possible.

Assessment of the conscious level (using 'AVPU') and the pupils will give information about the primary problem (head injury or stroke), or about neurological complications that have ensued (e.g. deteriorating conscious level in untreated hypoglycaemia). Exposure ('E') will prevent the missing of other significant injuries or useful clues (e.g. drug injection sites in comatose patient, or purpuric rash in unwell child indicating meningococcal septicaemia).

Prior to or during transport of all critical or seriously injured patients, radio communication either direct or through ambulance control should be made to the receiving hospital, giving a status report and requesting an appropriate response to meet the patient.

Resuscitation should be maintained *en route* to hospital. Monitoring should ideally include pulse, respiratory rate, blood pressure, level of consciousness, electrocardiogram (ECG) and pulse oximetry. It is still common practice in the UK to transport to the nearest hospital. It would be to the patient's advantage to transport directly to the *most appropriate* hospital.

A patient report form should be completed as soon as possible after arriving at hospital and should follow a clear hand-over of the patient. It is reasonable to allow the ambulance crew *45 seconds* to hand over the patient, unless *all* members of the receiving medical team listen – unles there is a problem with the airway or cardiopulmonary resuscitation is in progress.

Only key information needs to be given at this stage – the mechanism of injury, the apparent and suspected injuries, the vital signs and the treatment given. This can be remembered by the acronym 'MIST':

M	>	MECHANISM OF INJURY
I	>	INJURIES – APPARENT AND SUSPECTED
S	>	SIGNS – ABNORMAL VITAL SIGNS
T	>	TREATMENT GIVEN

> **Remember in critical trauma:**
> **A + B on scene**
> **C *en route***
> **Do not allow the placing of intravenous lines to delay transfer**

SECONDARY SURVEY

The secondary survey will identify non-life-threatening injuries. In medical emergencies a similar approach to the patient may uncover vital clues to the patient's condition – injection marks, bruises, rashes, scars, or informative tattoos.

If the patient's injuries are non-critical then a secondary survey may be undertaken. Depending on circumstances this may best be done in the shelter and protection of the ambulance. The secondary survey should begin with reassessing the airway. In burns patients, for example, it is important to check for evidence of soot in the nose and on the lips, or evidence of oedema of the upper airway.

> **The secondary survey must never delay transfer to definitive care**

Head

Pupil size and reaction are assessed. Evidence of bruising, lacerations, tenderness, and other signs of fractures involving the skull or face should be identified. The nose and ears should be specifically inspected for blood and cerebrospinal fluid leakage (see Chapter 21).

Neck

The neck is assessed for signs of trauma, although in-line stabilization *must* be maintained. The larynx and trachea are palpated for evidence of injury, and the latter for tracheal deviation. Assessment of the neck veins (distended in tension pneumothorax and cardiac tamponade) and carotid pulse should be made. The collar may need to be removed while retaining stabilization to permit adequate examination.

Chest

The chest is inspected for open wounds, contusion (bruising), seat-belt markings, a flail segment, and respiratory rate and effort. Palpation may reveal local tenderness indicative of rib fractures; chest wall instability with a flail segment; or surgical emphysema following a pneumothorax. The chest wall is auscultated for air entry and added sounds (e.g. wheeze), and percussion used to determine a haemothorax (dull, like a full barrel) or pneumothorax (resonant, like an empty barrel). Often this can only be adequately performed in the back of an ambulance because of the ambient noise at the scene.

Abdomen

The abdomen is inspected for open wounds, seat-belt markings and contusion. It is palpated for tenderness in all four quadrants. Swelling and tenderness can be seen in non-traumatic cases (e.g. bowel obstruction or ruptured abdominal aortic aneurysm).

Pelvis

In trauma cases the pelvis is 'sprung' to determine tenderness and any instability; this involves pressing firmly on the front of each wing of the pelvis, but if a fracture is present this will be very painful and may exacerbate blood loss. Bleeding from the urethra (*per urethra*) may be noted, along with genital bruising which can be indicative of serious injury to the urethra, often following a pelvic fracture.

Upper and Lower Limbs

The limbs are inspected for swelling, deformity and wounds. They are palpated for fractures (a step in the cortex) or crepitus (broken ends grating together – very painful!).
The limb examination should include assessment of:

- Motor response – test for active movements
- Sensation – response to touch
- Circulation – pulse and skin temperature

Use the mnemonic 'MSC × 4':

M	>	MOTOR
S	>	SENSATION
C	>	CIRCULATION
× 4	>	ALL FOUR LIMBS

Limb injuries are treated as necessary, with dressings and splintage. Analgesia should be considered with suspected long-bone fractures, but following local ambulance service protocols (see Chapter 25). The choice may include:

- Reassurance
- Splintage (possibly with traction splint)
- Nitrous oxide inhalation (Entonox, Nitronox)
- Parenteral drugs, e.g. nalbuphine

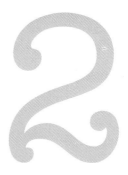

RESUSCITATION SKILLS

chapter three

BASIC LIFE SUPPORT

Cardiopulmonary resuscitation is not new. In the sixteenth century, Versalius reported how he had blown air into a patient via a reed, to try to revive the heart. In the eighteenth century, mouth-to-mouth breathing was described, and by the nineteenth century descriptions of ventilation included chest compression and the arm lift method. It was not until the 1950s that expired air ventilation was proved to be both physiologically sound and superior to other mechanical methods.

Closed chest cardiac compression was first reported in 1878, but this was rapidly abandoned in favour of direct compression of the heart, usually via the abdominal route. By the 1950s, 'open cardiac massage' was most commonly achieved via a thoracotomy, but this was abandoned following the rediscovery and development of 'closed cardiac massage' by Kowenhoven and colleagues in 1960.

By 1961, expired air ventilation and closed chest cardiac compression were combined, and Safar described the feasibility of teaching the public cardiopulmonary resuscitation (CPR), without the use of any equipment or surgical skills. The 1960s therefore can be regarded as the starting point of modern cardiopulmonary resuscitation.

WHAT IS BASIC LIFE SUPPORT?

Collapsed patients may require assistance to maintain their airway, breathing and circulation in order to prevent deterioration in their condition. When this is achieved without the use of equipment it is termed *basic life support* (BLS). More recently this definition has been expanded to include the use of simple protective shields interposed between the mouth of the rescuer and patient, e.g. Ambu face shield and the Laerdal pocket mask (Figure 3.1).

A patient's best chance of survival occurs when the collapse is witnessed and a bystander starts basic life support immediately, as the brain is irreversibly damaged within 3–4 minutes of being deprived of oxygen. Therefore, BLS must be started in all patients who have collapsed suddenly, who are unresponsive,

and who are not breathing or have no major pulse palpable (or both).

Although paramedical staff will have access to – and the skill to use – equipment for advanced life support during working hours, the importance of BLS cannot be overstated. Cardiac arrests do not only happen when you are at work!

How is BLS Performed?

In order that the rescuer suffers no harm and BLS is carried out effectively and in the most efficient manner, the following sequence of actions should be performed.

- Safety check: to avoid danger to the rescuer and patient
- Evaluation: to identify whether the patient has any spontaneous ventilation or a palpable pulse
- Airway control: to obtain and maintain a patent airway

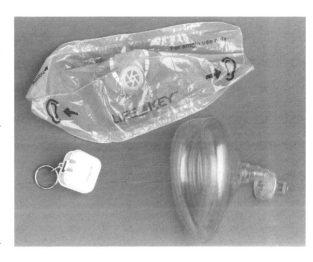

Fig. 3.1 *The Ambu face shield and Laerdal pocket mask*

- Ventilatory support: to establish artificial ventilation using expired air
- Circulatory support: to establish an artificial circulation by external cardiac compression

The SAFE Approach

On discovering or being asked to attend to a collapsed patient, the first response must be to *shout* for help. Basic life support techniques are physically demanding and are more effective if performed by two rescuers. Furthermore, the arrival of help will allow the performance of other simple tasks.

People collapse anywhere, at any time, and from many different causes. Rescuers should therefore *approach* a collapsed person with care, never putting themselves (or others) at risk. This is clearly important when the collapse occurs outside a hospital environment, where there may be gas, toxic fumes, traffic, electricity or fire endangering the rescuer.

If it is perceived that there are risks either to the victim or rescuer, then the patient must be moved to a place of greater safety which is *free from danger* before starting resuscitation.

Finally, the rescuer must *evaluate* the patient's 'ABC' (airway, breathing and circulation). Not all collapsed patients will need artificial ventilation and external cardiac compressions.

In summary:

S	>	SHOUT FOR HELP
A	>	APPROACH WITH CARE
F	>	FREE FROM DANGER
E	>	EVALUATE THE ABC

Patient Evaluation

The first step is to see if the patient is responsive. This is achieved by placing one hand on the patient's forehead and shaking the shoulder gently with the other hand. At the same time the rescuer asks loudly, 'Are you all right?' (Figure 3.2). One of two things may now happen and will determine further action.

The patient responds by either talking or moving

If it is safe to do so, leave the patient in the position in which he or she was found and summon medical assistance or prepare for transfer. However, remember that the patient may deteriorate before help arrives, so reassessment is mandatory.

Points to note

- The head is held stable during the assessment to guard against the possibility of aggravating an injury to the cervical spine
- Always remember that the patient may be deaf, therefore ensure he or she can see your lips moving when assessing responsiveness
- In the responsive patient, where there is obvious trauma, immobilize the cervical spine by manual in-line stabilization and a semirigid collar (Figure 3.3)

There is no response to voice or touch

Evaluate the state of the patient's airway, breathing and circulation.

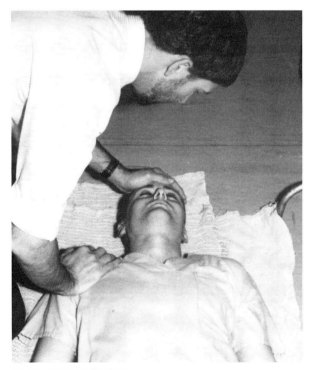

Fig. 3.2 'Are you all right?'

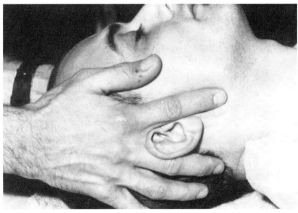

Fig. 3.3 In-line cervical stabilization

Airway Control

In most unconscious patients the airway will become obstructed. This occurs at the level of the hypopharynx as the reduced tone in the muscles of the tongue, jaw and neck allow the tongue to fall against the posterior pharyngeal wall (Figure 3.4). The following manoeuvres are designed to achieve a clear airway.

Head tilt plus chin lift

The rescuer's hand nearest the head is placed on the forehead, gently tilting (extending) the head backwards. The chin is then lifted using the index and middle finger of the rescuer's other hand (Figure 3.5). If this causes the mouth to close, the lower lip should be retracted downwards by the thumb. This is the 'triple airway manoeuvre' – head tilt, chin lift, mouth open.

Jaw thrust

If the above technique fails to open the airway, or there is a suspicion that the cervical spine may have been injured, then the jaw thrust alone is used. The patient's jaw is thrust upwards (forwards) by applying pressure behind the angles of the mandible. The rescuer uses the fingertips, with the base of the thumbs resting on the patient's cheeks (Figure 3.6).

Finger sweep

If there is any evidence that foreign material may be contributing to airway obstruction, the mouth must be opened and inspected. Obvious material may be removed by placing a finger in the mouth and gently sweeping from side to side, hooking out loose material (Figure 3.7). At the same time, broken, loose or partial dentures should be removed, but well-fitting dentures may be left in place (see below). A

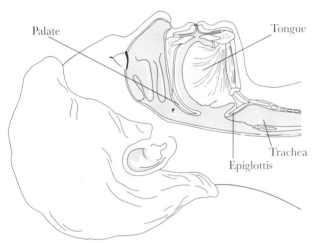

Fig. 3.4 Vertical section through the airway

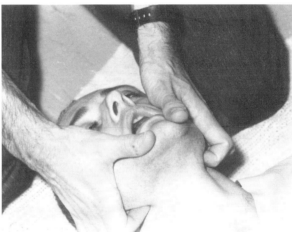

Fig. 3.6 The jaw thrust

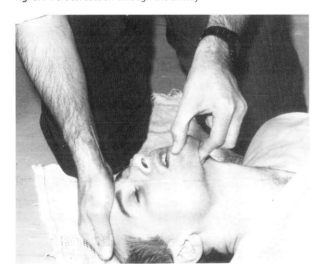

Fig. 3.5 Head tilt, chin lift

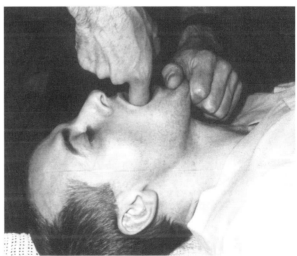

Fig. 3.7 The finger sweep

blind finger sweep is not recommended, as this may further impact a foreign body.

Breathing

As soon as an airway has been created using one of the above techniques, the patient's breathing must now be rapidly evaluated in the following manner:

- *Look* down the line of the chest to see if it is rising and falling.
- *Listen* at the mouth and nose for breath sounds, gurgling or snoring sounds.
- *Feel* for expired air at the patient's mouth and nose with the side of one's cheek.

Look, listen and feel for 10 seconds before deciding whether breathing is absent (Figure 3.8).

The patient is breathing

Place the patient in the recovery position (see later) unless it is unsafe to do so because of other injuries (for example to the cervical spine). The majority of these patients will require urgent hospital transfer, but occasionally a request for medical assistance at the scene may be more appropriate.

The patient is not breathing

Help must be sought immediately, either by sending someone else or going yourself, even if this means temporarily leaving the patient. On return give 2 breaths of expired air (see below) and then assess the circulation.

Circulation

A check must now be made for evidence of the patient's circulation by feeling for a pulse. In an emergency, central arteries are more reliable and the carotid artery is usually the most accessible and acceptable. The carotid arteries are found on either side of the neck in the 'gutter' between the larynx and sternomastoid muscles (Figure 3.9).

> It is important to feel for 10 seconds before deciding that a pulse is absent

If a pulse is present, continue with ventilation, reassessing approximately every minute. If a pulse is no longer palpable, chest compressions must be started (see below).

The patient is not breathing and does not have a pulse

Often referred to as a 'cardiac arrest', this condition requires cardiopulmonary resuscitation (CPR) to be commenced immediately. CPR consists of expired air ventilation plus external cardiac compressions – see below.

> Before starting CPR call for help and a defibrillator if you are just a bystander, and not responding on duty

The only exceptions to this sequence of events are cases of trauma, drowning or infants and children, when a single rescuer should perform resuscitation for one minute before going for help.

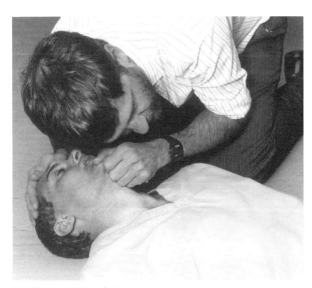

Fig. 3.8 *Look, listen, feel*

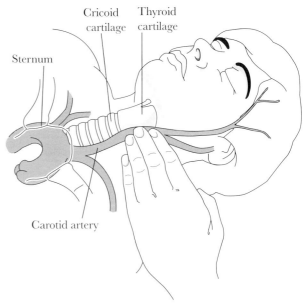

Fig. 3.9 *Feeling for the carotid pulse*

TECHNIQUES OF EXPIRED AIR VENTILATION

To successfully ventilate a patient with expired air there must be a clear path, with no leaks, between the rescuer's lungs and the patient's lungs.

Mouth-to-Mouth Ventilation

1. The patient's airway is kept patent by the rescuer using the palm of the uppermost hand to perform a head tilt, leaving the index finger and thumb free to pinch the patient's nose to prevent leaks. The fingers of the lower hand are then used to perform a chin lift, and if necessary the thumb is used to open the mouth (Figure 3.10).

A

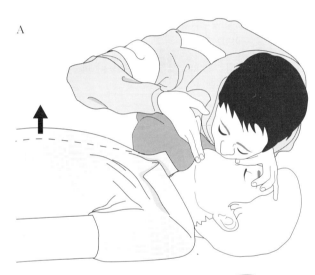

B

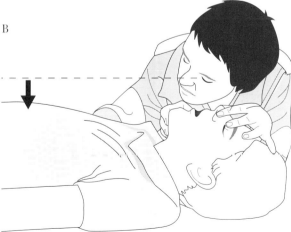

Fig. 3.10 Mouth-to-mouth (expired air) ventilation

2. The rescuer takes a deep breath in and makes a seal with his or her lips around the patient's mouth. Well-fitting dentures should be left in the patient's mouth as they help maintain the contour of the mouth and make it easier to create a good seal. Poorly fitting false teeth or dental plates should be removed, as they may obstruct the airway.
3. The rescuer blows gently into the patient's mouth for 1½–2 seconds, at the same time listening for leaks and looking down the patient's chest to ensure that it rises (Figure 3.10A).
4. While maintaining the head tilt and chin lift, the rescuer moves away from the patient's mouth to allow passive exhalation for 2 seconds, watching to make sure the chest falls (Figure 3.10B).

Mouth-to-Nose Ventilation

Mouth-to-nose ventilation is used where mouth-to-mouth ventilation is unsuccessful, e.g. if an obstruction in the mouth cannot be relieved, or when the rescuer is a child (child's mouth would not completely cover adult's mouth). The airway is maintained as already described, but the mouth is closed with the fingers of the lower hand. The seal is made with the rescuer's lips around the base of the patient's nose. Inflation is as above, checking to ensure that the chest rises. The mouth is opened to assist expiration, with the rescuer watching to ensure that the chest falls.

Each complete cycle of expired air ventilation should take approximately 4 seconds, thereby allowing 15 breaths per minute.

Common causes of inadequate ventilation

- Obstruction – failing to maintain head tilt or chin lift
- Leaks – inadequate seal around the mouth or failure to occlude the patient's nose
- Inflating too hard – trying to overcome an obstructed airway, resulting in gastric distension and regurgitation
- Foreign body – unrecognized in the patient's airway

TECHNIQUE OF CARDIOPULMONARY RESUSCITATION

A patient who is not breathing and has no pulse should be placed in the supine position on a firm surface and CPR commenced immediately.

Using the technique described above, two expired air ventilations are given followed immediately by 15 external cardiac compressions (see below). This cycle (2:15) is performed continuously, each time remembering to tilt the head and lift the chin to create a patent airway, and checking the correct position of the hands before commencing chest compressions. If a second rescuer is available, quickly decide who is to perform which function. With two rescuers the cycle used is one breath followed by five compressions. This cycle (1:5) is performed continually and each breath should again last for approximately 1½–2 seconds. External cardiac compression should stop momentarily to allow ventilation then recommence without waiting for exhalation to occur. The person performing external cardiac compressions can leave the hands on the sternum between each series of compressions, but in doing so the pressure must be *totally* released so as not to interfere with the efficacy of ventilation.

Once started, CPR must not be interrupted unless the patient shows signs of spontaneous ventilation or movement. If this does happen, then the carotid pulse should be reassessed for 5 seconds before deciding how to continue. However, such an occurrence is *extremely rare*.

External Cardiac (Closed Chest) Compression

The exact mechanism by which external cardiac compression results in blood flow is unclear. It is probably a combination of direct compression of the heart between the sternum and the spine, along with a sudden rise in the intrathoracic pressure during compression generating forward flow in the arteries. Whatever the mechanisms, at its best it can achieve a maximum flow 30% of normal. The position of the hands is critical for maximal effect.

1. The rescuer takes up a position on one side of the patient.
2. The patient's chest is exposed and the xiphisternum identified (this is the bony prominence in the midline at the junction of the lower borders of the ribs).
3. The index and middle fingers of the rescuer's lower hand are placed on the xiphisternum and without removing them, the heel of the other hand is placed adjacent to the index finger on the sternum (Figure 3.11).
4. The lower hand is removed and placed on the back of the hand resting on the sternum, interlocking the fingers.
5. The sternum is alternately depressed 4–5 cm, and released. This is repeated at a rate of 80 per minute, with compression and relaxation each taking the same length of time.
6. External cardiac compressions are best performed with the rescuer leaning well forward over the patient, with straight arms. This allows the rescuer to use upper body weight to achieve compression rather than using the arm muscles, which will rapidly tire and reduce efficiency (Figure 3.12).

Common causes of ineffective external chest compressions

- Wrong hand position
  too high – the heart is not compressed
  too low – the stomach is compressed and the risk of aspiration increased
  too far laterally – will injure underlying organs
- Overenthusiastic effort
  causes cardiac damage
  fractures ribs causing damage to underlying organs, particularly lungs and liver

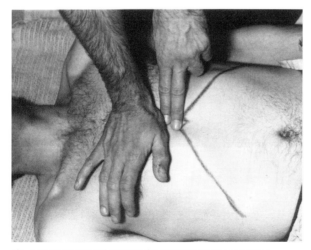

Fig. 3.11 Correct hand position for external cardiac compression

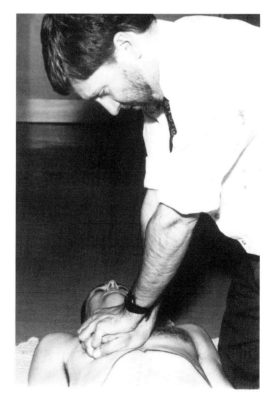

Fig. 3.12 External cardiac compression

- Inadequate effort
  the rescuer is not high enough above the patient to use his or her body weight
  fatigue during prolonged resuscitation or poor technique
- Failure to release between compressions
  prevents venous return and filling of the heart
- Inadequate or excessive rate

Summary of Basic Life Support

Basic life support procedures are summarized in Figure 3.13.

THE RECOVERY POSITION

In the unconscious patient who is breathing and has a pulse, the airway is best maintained and the risk of aspiration of gastric contents minimized by placing the patient in the *recovery position*. There is more than one method that a single rescuer can use.

The following is an adaptation of the method supported by the European Resuscitation Council.

1. Place the patient supine, with legs extended, and ensure the airway is open (head tilt, chin lift) (Figure 3.14A).
2. Kneeling against the patient's chest, move the patient's closest arm away from the body so that it lies at 90 degrees, then flex the elbow to 90 degrees so that the palm lies facing upwards.
3. Bring the patient's far arm to lie across the chest, so that the back of the hand lies against the cheek (Figure 3.14B).
4. Flex the far leg at the hip and knee, keeping the foot on the ground. Grasp the far shoulder.
5. Roll the patient by pulling the shoulders towards you, while using the bent leg as a lever – this is achieved by gently pulling the flexed knee towards you and pressing down (Figure 3.14C).
6. Adjust the upper leg so that both the hip and the knee are flexed to 90 degrees. Adjust the hand under the cheek to help maintain the head tilt (Figure 3.14D).
7. Finally, the airway, breathing and pulse are checked regularly.

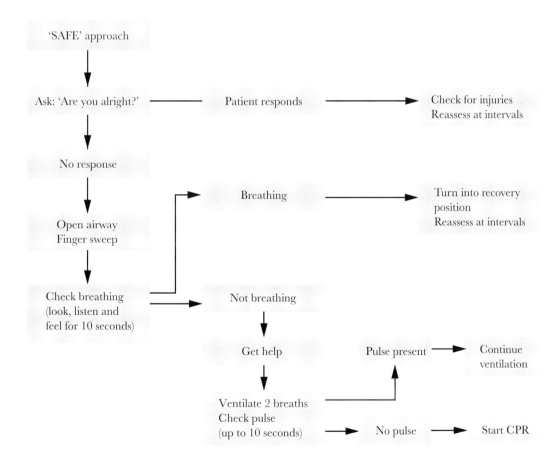

Fig. 3.13 *Summary of basic life support procedures*

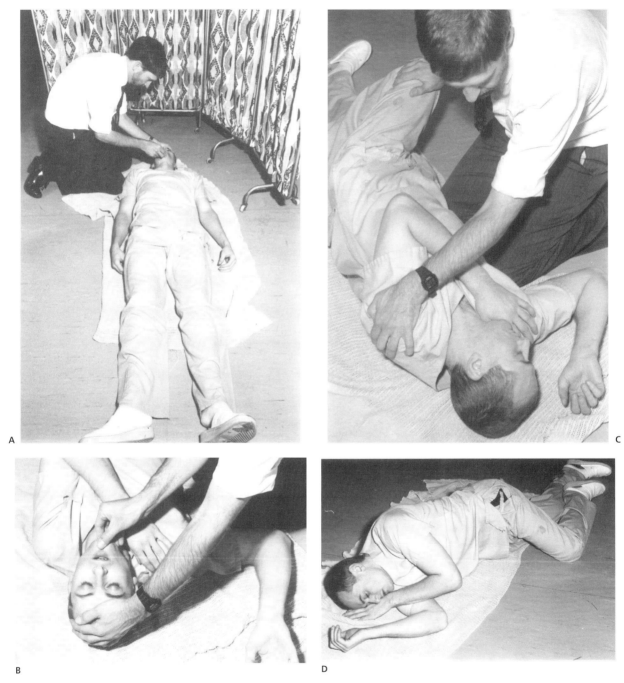

Fig. 3.14 *The recovery position*

In the recovery position, gravity helps keep the tongue away from the posterior pharyngeal wall, thereby preventing airway obstruction while at the same time allowing any vomit or secretions to drain out of the patient's mouth.

If there is *any* suspicion of a spinal injury, then the recovery position should not be used. Instead, the airway is maintained and continually supervised, and the patient only turned when there are sufficient people available to perform a 'log roll' (see Chapter 27).

THE CHOKING PATIENT

Although almost any foreign body can cause airway obstruction, in adults it is usually food, as a result of trying to eat, talk and breathe simultaneously. This has been misleadingly termed the 'café coronary'. In these circumstances adults show signs of acute airway obstruction, with extreme distress and activity to try to dislodge an obstruction. If the obstruction is incomplete, there may be severe coughing and inspiratory stridor.

If the patient is still conscious, then back blows should be used initially. Standing to one side of the patient, the rescuer should encourage the patient to lean forwards. While supporting the chest with one hand, five firm blows are delivered between the scapulae. If the obstruction is relieved quickly, all five blows need not be delivered.

If this fails then proceed rapidly to the Heimlich manoeuvre.

The Heimlich Manoeuvre

The Heimlich manoeuvre can be performed with the patient standing, sitting or kneeling down. The aim is to produce a rapid rise in the intrathoracic pressure (by forcing the diaphragm into the chest) which will expel the foreign body.

If the patient is standing, the rescuer should move behind the patient and pass both arms around the body at the level of the upper abdomen. The rescuer makes one hand into a fist and places it firmly in the patient's epigastrium. The rescuer's other hand is then placed over the fist and both together forced vigorously upwards and backwards into the epigastrium (Figure 3.15); this should be repeated up to five times. With luck this will force the object into a position where the patient can remove it by coughing or it can be hooked out with a finger. If this fails to dislodge the foreign body, the sequence of five back blows and five Heimlich manoeuvres should be repeated until the patient recovers, or becomes unconscious.

When the patient is unconscious, he or she should be placed supine and a finger sweep quickly attempted. The rescuer should then kneel astride the patient facing the patient's head. The rescuer's hands are placed in the epigastrium in the same way as described above, and a series of vigorous thrusts applied upwards and backwards, taking care to apply the pressure in the midline (Figure 3.16). Up to ten thrusts can be applied, after which the airway should be inspected and a finger sweep performed to check for any dislodged objects.

If this fails to remove the obstruction, two further series of ten thrusts can be applied, or alternatively chest thrusts in the style of external cardiac compressions as used during CPR may be tried.

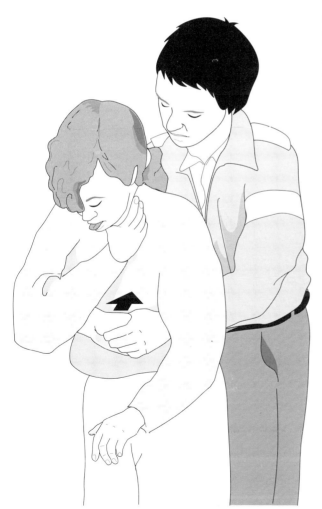

Fig. 3.15 *The Heimlich manoeuvre*

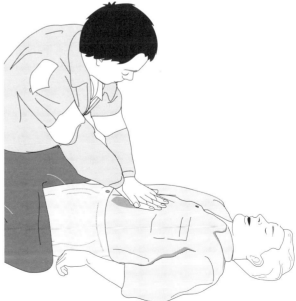

Fig. 3.16 *Supine abdominal thrusts*

If all these efforts fail to clear the obstruction, little else can be done without the equipment for either laryngoscopy and intubation, or the creation of a surgical airway (cricothyroidotomy).

FURTHER READING

Driscoll PA, Gwinnutt CL, Mackway-Jones K & Wieteska S, eds (1997) *Advanced Cardiac Life Support – The Practical Approach*, 2nd edn. London: Chapman & Hall (in press).

European Resuscitation Council (1992) Guidelines for Basic Life Support. *Resuscitation* **24**: 103–110.

Hanley AJ & Swain A, eds (1994) *Advanced Life Support Manual*. 2nd edn. Resuscitation Council.

chapter four

SIMPLE MANAGEMENT OF THE AIRWAY AND VENTILATION

INTRODUCTION

The airway is the first priority during resuscitation, and airway management skills are essential for those involved in emergency care. In the presence of airway obstruction, hypoxia leading to circulatory arrest and irreversible central nervous system damage can be expected to occur within 4 minutes. Basic airway management requires relatively simple skills, but emergency conditions are often difficult and add to the stress of the situation. Advanced airway management demands much more skill and experience. To be effective, airway management requires an understanding of functional airway anatomy and physiology, and the possession of skills to assess and intervene rapidly. The basic skills of maintaining an open airway cannot be overemphasized, and should be mastered before embarking upon advanced airway management techniques.

ANATOMY OF THE RESPIRATORY SYSTEM

The anatomy of the respiratory tract is illustrated in Figures 4.1–4.3.

The Upper Airway

The upper airway extends from the mouth and nose to just below the larynx (Figure 4.1).

The nose

The nasal cavity extends from the nostrils to the nasopharynx. The roof of the nasal cavity contains the receptors for the sense of smell and lies below the anterior aspect of the base of the skull, which is quite thin. Thus, nasal tubes inserted when the base of the skull is fractured may enter the cranial cavity. The floor of the nasal cavity is formed from the hard and the soft palate. Inside, the nose is lined with a thick, vascular mucous membrane. The conchae (or turbinates) project into the nasal cavity from the side and may be damaged during nasal intubation, causing haemorrhage. The paranasal sinuses open into the nasal cavity below the conchae. The nasolacrimal duct and the eustachian (pharyngotympanic) tube also drain into the nasal cavity.

The nasal cavity is divided by the nasal septum, which in older children and adults is often deviated to one side, making one nostril narrower than the other. The main nasal air passage lies in the floor of the nasal cavity; correctly placed nasal tubes will be directed backwards along the upper aspect of the palate. The nasal cavity continues as the nasopharynx, starting above

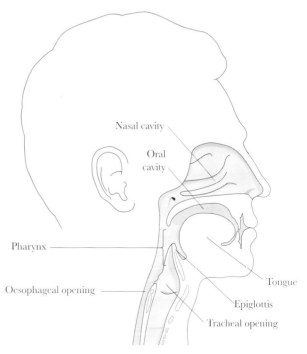

Fig. 4.1 The upper airway

Labels: Nasal cavity, Oral cavity, Pharynx, Oesophageal opening, Tongue, Epiglottis, Tracheal opening

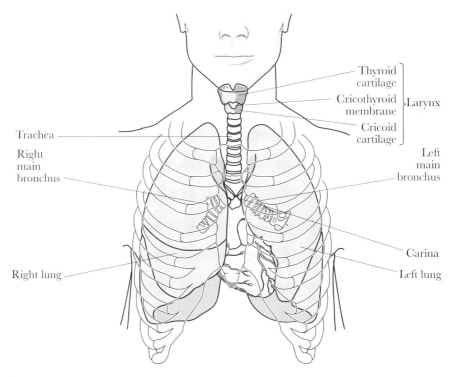

Fig. 4.2 *The lower airway*

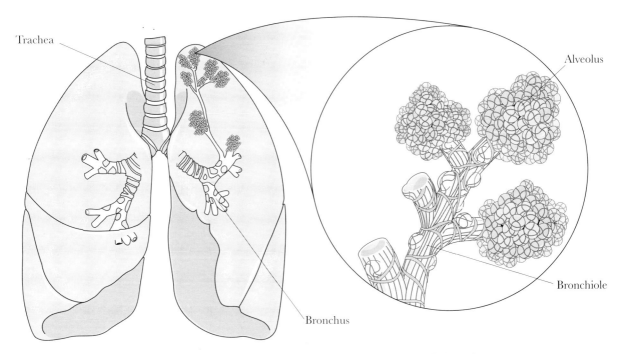

Fig. 4.3 *The lower airway: the bronchi subdivide into smaller bronchioles, terminating in air sacs called alveoli*

and behind the soft palate. Above the nasopharynx lies the base of the skull and behind it the first cervical vertebra. The lateral walls are made up of the superior constrictor muscle and the pharyngobasilar membrane.

The nasal blood supply is from the ophthalmic, maxillary and facial arteries. Most nose bleeds arise from the front lower part of the nasal septum which receives a blood supply from branches of the maxillary and facial arteries. The nerve supply of the nasal cavity originates from the olfactory nerve which supplies the smell receptors and from branches of the trigeminal nerve which supply sensation.

At the back of the nasopharynx there is a collection of lymphoid tissue, the adenoid or nasopharyngeal tonsil. In children, adenoids may enlarge and obstruct the airway and the pharyngotympanic tube. Enlarged adenoids are likely to bleed if damaged by a nasal tube.

The functions of the nasal cavity include providing the respiratory airway, the sense of smell, humidification, heat exchange, filtering of particulate matter and speech enunciation.

The mouth

The oral cavity is bound by the lips, cheeks and teeth in the front and at the side, the hard and soft palates above, the tongue below, and the oropharyngeal isthmus behind.

The soft palate contains muscles which act in a coordinated manner to close off the mouth from the nasopharynx during speech and swallowing.

The oropharynx

The oropharynx communicates with the oral cavity and the nasopharynx and extends from the soft palate to the tip of the epiglottis. The tonsils are situated at the sides. In children, tonsillar enlargement and infection (tonsillitis or tonsillar abscess – quinsy) may cause airway obstruction.

The laryngopharynx

The laryngopharynx is the continuation of the oropharynx and extends from the tip of the epiglottis to the lower border of the cricoid cartilage at the level of the sixth vertebral body. The laryngeal inlet is normally protected from aspiration during swallowing. When swallowing occurs, breathing is temporarily interrupted, contraction of the pharyngeal constrictor muscles forces the bolus into the oesophagus and elevation of the larynx assists in closing the laryngeal inlet. The inlet is also protected by tilting of the epiglottis backwards and downwards. Nerve damage or intoxication with alcohol or drugs, causing a depressed level of consciousness, impairs these mechanisms and depress these protective reflexes. In these situations there is a great risk that vomiting or regurgitation will result in aspiration of foreign material into the lower airway and lungs.

The larynx

The larynx lies between the laryngopharynx and the trachea and is made up of cartilages, membranes and ligaments. The principal cartilages are the thyroid, cricoid and arytenoids. The cricothyroid membrane joins the cricoid cartilage to the thyroid cartilage. The free upper border forms the vocal cords at the level of the thyroid cartilage notch behind the laryngeal prominence (Adam's apple). When separated, the vocal cords form the narrowest part of the adult airway. The larynx is supplied from the vagus nerve via its superior and recurrent laryngeal branches.

The Lower Airway

The lower airway continues as the trachea and bronchi (Figure 4.2). The adult trachea is 10–12 cm long, 2.5 cm in diameter and has 16–20 C-shaped cartilages. It divides at the carina, at the level of the sternal angle and the fourth or fifth thoracic vertebra. The right main bronchus continues more vertically than the left, accounting for the tendency for aspiration or intubation with a long tracheal tube to enter the right rather than the left side. The left main bronchus is usually about 5 cm long. The nerve supply is via the recurrent laryngeal nerve.

Anatomy and Physiology of the Paediatric Airway

Neonates breathe principally through their noses, so nasal obstruction may be immediately life-threatening. The infant head compared with adults is relatively large so in the supine position the neck tends to be flexed; placing a pillow under the head may actually obscure the view of the larynx and increase obstruction. The tongue, tonsils and adenoids are relatively large in children, increasing the risk of upper airway obstruction, and may interfere with laryngoscopy. At laryngoscopy, the larynx is more anterior. The epiglottis tends to be a large, floppy structure which may need to be lifted directly with the laryngoscope blade to obtain a view of the larynx.

The neonatal trachea is narrow (3–4 mm) and short (4–5 cm), increasing the risks of bronchial intubation. Up to the age of 10 years, the cricoid cartilage represents the narrowest part of the upper airway. Damage at this level is associated with scarring and narrowing; the risk is reduced by using uncuffed tracheal tubes. In adults, the narrowest part of the airway is at the level of the vocal cords.

Reflexes are sensitive in children, and instrumentation of the airway in those not profoundly unconscious can result in laryngospasm, bronchospasm, bradycardia and even cardiac arrest. Oxygen consumption is relatively much higher in the child because of the raised metabolic rate. This results in a high respiratory rate. The increased oxygen consumption results in rapid cyanosis in the presence of upper airway obstruction or apnoea.

Airway Anatomy and Physiology During Pregnancy

In pregnancy (see Chapter 47) capillary engorgement may cause significant swelling of the upper airway and this may be exacerbated by the oedema of pre-eclamptic toxaemia (PET) and upper respiratory tract infections. This swelling, together with the weight gain and breast enlargement associated with pregnancy, can make intubation more difficult. The increased oxygen consumption coupled with a reduced oxygen reserve results in rapid cyanosis in the presence of upper airway obstruction or apnoea.

RESPIRATORY CONTROL

Central Control

Central nervous system control of respiration is mediated through respiratory centres in the brain stem. These centres receive input from other areas of the brain and from the contents of the blood perfusing them. Sleep, sedatives, alcohol, many analgesic drugs and injury to the respiratory centres result in a reduction in ventilation (hypoventilation) (Table 4.1). This reduction in ventilation may result from a fall in respiratory rate or tidal volume (the volume of air shifted with each breath), or from a fall in both.

Table 4.1 Causes of hypoventilation

Mechanism	Cause
Thoracic cavity disruption	Penetrating trauma
	Flail chest
Respiratory muscle failure	Drugs and poisons
	Muscular dystrophy
	Myasthenia gravis
Respiratory nerve failure	Spinal cord injury
	Neurological disease
Respiratory centre depression	Hypoxia
	Hypercarbia
	Hypotension
	Head injury
	Electrocution
	Poisoning
	Brain haemorrhage
	Brain infarction
	Brain thrombosis
	Brain infection
Lung failure	Lung contusion
	Lung disease
	Pneumothorax
	Haemothorax
	Obesity
	Pregnancy

Ventilation is stimulated by a rise in arterial carbon dioxide or a fall in arterial oxygen. However, very high levels of carbon dioxide and very low levels of oxygen *depress* ventilation.

Ventilation is also stimulated by a fall in blood pH (rise in level of blood acidity) which may occur, for example, in a hyperglycaemic diabetic coma.

Breathing is normally controlled by the partial pressure of carbon dioxide in arterial blood (Pa_{CO_2}). In some patients with chronic obstructive pulmonary disease (COPD), previously termed chronic bronchitis, who have grown accustomed to a high Pa_{CO_2}, this drive has been replaced by a hypoxic drive dependent on low partial pressures of oxygen in arterial blood (Pa_{O_2}). *In other words, low levels of blood oxygen rather than high levels of blood carbon dioxide act as a stimulus to breathing.* If high inspired concentrations of oxygen are given to these patients, this drive is lost and a reduction of ventilation with further carbon dioxide retention and decreasing consciousness may occur. However, it is important to remember that a high carbon dioxide content kills slowly, but a low oxygen content kills quickly. *The need to provide immediate adequate oxygenation takes precedence.* Cyanotic patients should always be treated with high oxygen concentrations.

Peripheral Control

Adequate ventilation also requires an intact chest wall and intrapulmonary mechanics. Peripheral causes of impaired ventilation (see Table 4.1) include obstruction to the upper airway, most commonly due to the tongue. Peripheral nerve damage or blockade involving the phrenic and intercostal nerves may be seen with spinal cord damage. The phrenic nerves originate from cervical spinal roots C3–C5, therefore diaphragmatic function will be maintained with cord lesions below this level.

AIRWAY AND VENTILATION ASSESSMENT

Airway obstruction arises from a variety of causes at a variety of levels in the respiratory tract. These are listed in Table 4.2. The history should include the circumstances of the immediate event and any pre-existing conditions of relevance such as asthma, congenital anatomical deformity and previous injury to the spine or craniofacial region.

Airway and ventilation problems may be delayed in onset. The effects of smoke or chemical inhalation may not develop until hours after the event.

Physical assessment of the airway and ventilation involves looking, listening and feeling for chest movement and air flow. During the examination, attention should be directed to the respiratory rate, the presence of cyanosis (a blue discolouration due to lack of oxygen in the blood) and/or agitation and the use of the accessory muscles of respiration (Figure 4.4) and abnormal movement of the abdominal muscles.

Table 4.2 Causes of airway obstruction

Cause	Leads to
Coma Mandible trauma	Tongue displacement
Anaphylaxis	Tongue oedema
Foreign body	Oropharynx obstruction
Irritants	Laryngeal spasm
Foreign body	Laryngeal obstruction
Larynx trauma	Laryngeal oedema/obstruction
Infection Anaphylaxis	Laryngeal oedema
Foreign body	Tracheal or bronchial obstruction
Irritants Anaphylaxis Infection Near-drowning Neurogenic shock Cardiac failure	Pulmonary oedema

Noisy breathing during inspiration generally indicates obstruction *above* the level of the larynx, whereas an expiratory wheeze usually indicates that the problem lies *at or below* the larynx. Characteristically, the patients who are choking indicate their predicament by clasping their neck or pointing to their larynx. The examination steps to assess airway and ventilation are set out in Table 4.3.

SIMPLE AIRWAY MANAGEMENT

Upper airway patency can generally be re-established by simple manual and positional manoeuvres involving correct alignment of the head, neck and mandible. Simple adjuncts may further improve the situation.

Head Tilt

Backward tilt of the head overcomes obstruction from the relaxed tongue in the majority of cases. The manoeuvre stretches the muscles in the front of the neck and lifts the base of the tongue away from the posterior pharyngeal wall (Figure 4.5). Ideally, the patient's head should be placed on a small pillow.

Chin Lift

The tongue is a muscle which is attached to the mandible, and relief of the obstruction may be provided by lifting the chin (Figure 4.6).

Jaw Thrust

Jaw thrust provides an amplified effect of chin lift. The technique involves lifting the mandible upwards and forward with the index, middle and ring fingers, and depressing the point of the chin slightly with the thumbs in order to open the mouth to allow air entry (Figure 4.7).

Positional Methods of Airway Alignment in Patients with Suspected Cervical Spine Injury

Great care should be taken with airway alignment in patients with suspected cervical spine injury. Flexion and rotation of the neck are the most dangerous movements. At all times manual in-line stabilization should be applied by an assistant.

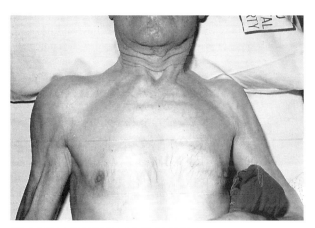

Fig. 4.4 *The accessory muscles of respiration*

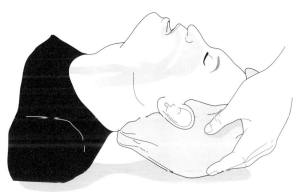

Fig. 4.5 *Head tilt*

Table 4.3 Assessment of the airway and ventilation

	Airway	Ventilation
Check for	Unconsciousness	
Look for	Cyanosis	Penetrating injury
	Pallor	Cyanosis
	Blood	Pallor
	Excessive salivation	Respiratory rate
	Stomach contents	Chest movements (adequate; flail; equal)
	Foreign body	Use of accessory muscles
	Maxillofacial injury	Use of abdominal muscles
	Neck trauma	Chest wall bruising
	Broken dentures	
Listen for	Voice quality	Voice quality
	Air entry	Air entry
	Wheeze — inspiratory/expiratory	Wheeze — inspiratory/expiratory
	Abnormal sounds (stridor)	Adventitious sounds (crackles)
Feel for	Air flow on your cheek	Chest movement
		Subcutaneous emphysema

> **The safest way to achieve airway patency in patients with suspected cervical spine injury is by jaw thrust**

Extension of the head on the neck should be minimized to that just necessary to establish an airway. Remember, however, that

airway obstruction is immediately lethal and airway management takes precedence.

Recovery Position

Once airway patency and adequate spontaneous ventilation are assured, the patient should be turned into the recovery position (Figure 4.8). In cases with suspected spinal injury this manoeuvre should be accomplished by a team consisting of a minimum of four people with the patient's head and neck sup-

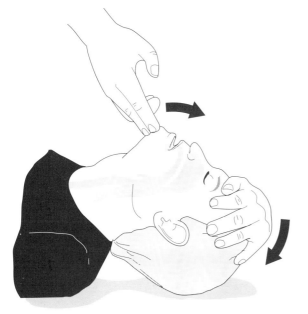

Fig. 4.6 Chin lift

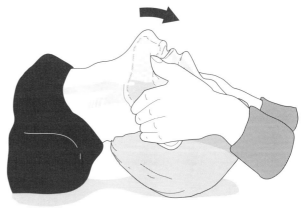

Fig. 4.7 Jaw thrust

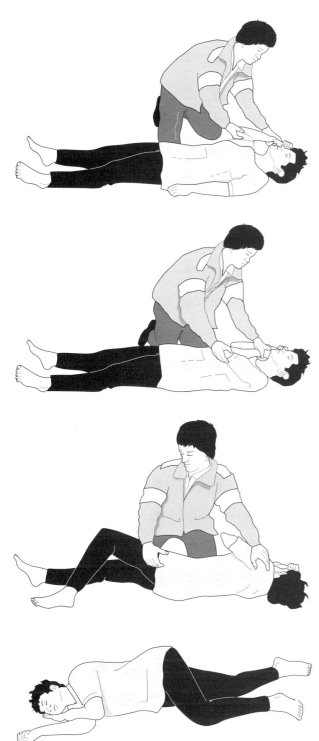

Fig. 4.8 *The recovery position. Adapted from Baskett, PJF (1993)* Resuscitation Handbook, *2nd edn, with permission from Gower Medical Publishing*

ported in neutral alignment at all times (Figure 4.9). The attendant supporting the head and neck should call the commands.

Clearance of the Airway Obstructed by Foreign Material

In conscious patients airway obstruction from a foreign body which is not relieved by spontaneous coughing must be cleared by back blows (Figure 4.10). In adults, the usual obstruction is a bolus of unchewed food – in children and the mentally deranged it can be a variety of objects.

The manoeuvre can be carried out with patients lying on their side, or in the sitting or standing position leaning forward. Children can be placed head down lying along the rescuer's thigh or arm (Figure 4.11).

Abdominal thrusts (the Heimlich manoeuvre) may expel an impacted foreign body from the upper airway in a conscious patient when back blows have failed. The rescuer stands behind the patient with hands clasped together in a fist just below the patient's rib-cage margin. A series of sharp upward thrusts raise the intrathoracic pressure and the object may be forcibly dislodged (Figure 4.12). This manoeuvre is not without danger of causing visceral injury to the stomach, spleen and liver, and it is *not* recommended for infants and small children. While the patient remains conscious, cycles of five back blows and five abdominal thrusts can be repeated.

In unconscious patients with foreign body obstruction of the airway, clearance may be attempted by finger sweeps. When solid material is involved the mouth should be opened, the jaw depressed, and with gloved fingers wrapped in gauze the obstruction hooked and swept out of the mouth (Figure 4.13). The technique is not recommended in infants and small children unless the object is directly visible, for there is a danger of pushing the object further into the airway.

Back blows and modified abdominal thrusts may also be used in unconscious patients. The standard sequence to follow in an unconscious patient is

1. Open the airway
2. Finger sweep
3. Attempt to inflate
4. Five back blows
5. Five abdominal thrusts
6. Repeat steps 1–6

When liquid material such as blood or stomach contents contaminates the airway, the patient should be placed head down in the recovery position. Back blows and finger sweeps should be performed.

The best way of removing liquid material from the oropharynx is by direct suction using a Yankauer suction catheter, which is a stiff, angled catheter. Ideally the suction end should be manipulated under direct vision using a laryngoscope (Figure 4.14). A flexible catheter can be used to clear the lumen of an airway adjunct, such as a nasopharyngeal airway, tracheal tube or laryngeal mask.

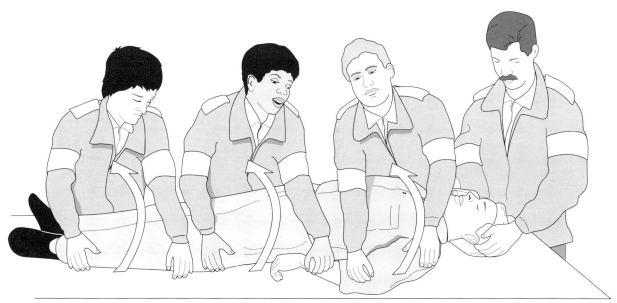

Fig. 4.9 *The 'log roll'*

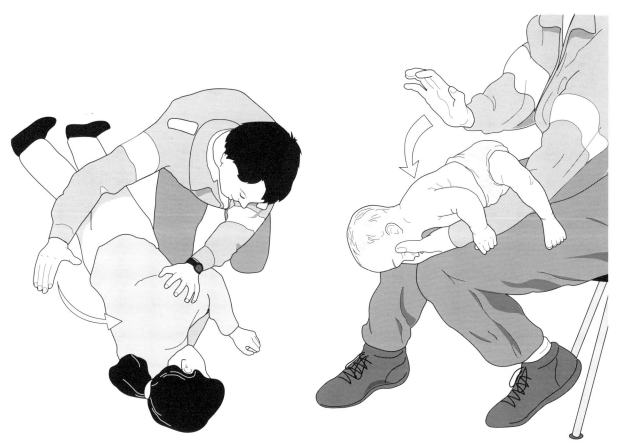

Fig. 4.10 *Back blows*   **Fig. 4.11** *Back blows in children*

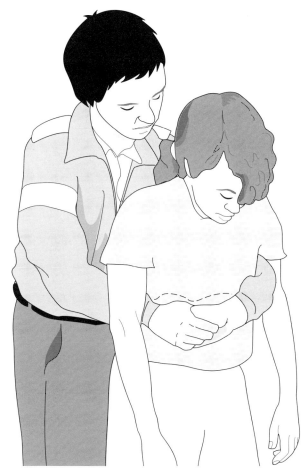

Fig. 4.12 *Abdominal thrusts (Heimlich manoeuvre)*

Portable suction apparatus

Several manufacturers produce portable suction apparatus which may be powered electrically, by hand, or by foot. The following points should be considered when choosing a particular model.

- Performance — generation of sufficient vacuum (600 mmHg), and flow rate (35 l/min) of free air
- Suitable fitments for Yankauer flexible catheter and suction booster
- Suitable power options of mains, rechargeable battery or 12-volt supply, or hand or foot power where appropriate
- Compact size and height for portability
- Adequate-sized container for aspirated material
- Ease of disassembly, cleaning and reassembly without error
- Reliability and robust manufacture

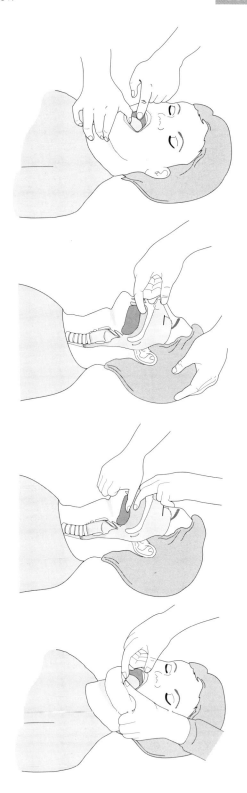

Fig. 4.13 *The use of the finger sweep to remove a foreign body*

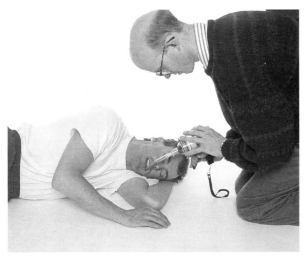

Fig. 4.14 *Clearance of the airway using suction*

The neonatal aspirator is used to clear mucus from the mouth and nose of the newborn. It consists of a soft, flexible catheter attached to a small collecting chamber. A suction tube is also attached to the chamber which is placed in the mouth of the operator. Suction is generated in the operator's mouth and mucus is aspirated from the baby via the catheter into the collecting chamber.

Simple Airway Adjuncts

In some patients it is difficult to establish and maintain a clear airway using manual methods alone. Simple airway adjuncts may improve the position considerably. Two airway adjuncts, the oropharyngeal airway and the nasopharyngeal airway, are considered here. More advanced airways are considered in Chapter 5.

Oropharyngeal airway

The oropharyngeal airway controls backward displacement of the tongue and provides a free air passage from the mouth to the hypopharynx. It reduces the need for prolonged application of jaw thrust.

The airway is introduced through the mouth in an inverted position and rotated through 180 degrees as it passes the edge of the palate. The distal end locates in the oropharynx (Figure 4.15). The airway may also be introduced directly using a tongue spatula or laryngoscope. This method is recommended in infants and small children. The oropharyngeal airway comes in a range of six sizes suitable for an infant (size 000) to a large adult (size 4). The correct size for any individual equates to the distance from the corner of the mouth to the angle of the mandible.

In patients with active protective reflexes insertion of the airway may provoke vomiting, retching or laryngeal spasm. The airway should be removed at the first sign of such intolerance.

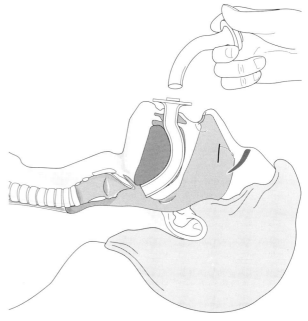

Fig. 4.15 *Inserting the oropharyngeal airway*

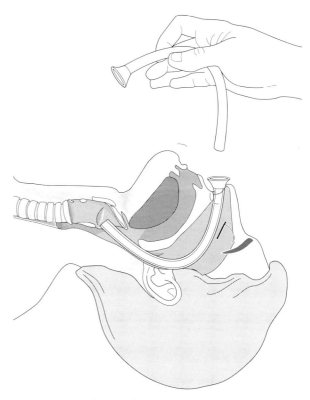

Fig. 4.16 *The nasopharyngeal airway*

Nasopharyngeal airway

The nasopharyngeal airway consists of a bevelled tube with a flange at the proximal end. It should be made of soft material to minimize intranasal damage.

The airway is introduced, well lubricated, into either nostril (generally the right is attempted first). It should be directed backwards (*not* upwards) along the roof of the palate so that the tip lies in the hypopharynx, just above the larynx (Figure 4.16). If resistance to the passage of the airway is encountered it should be withdrawn and an attempt made through the other nostril. Suction should be on hand to control bleeding.

The correct size of airway equates approximately with the diameter of the patient's little finger – an airway of 6.0 or 6.5 mm internal diameter will be suitable for the majority of adults.

The nasopharyngeal airway is particularly valuable in patients with maxillofacial injuries and a clenched jaw. Once in place it is better tolerated than an oropharyngeal airway. Even given these advantages, this simple airway adjunct is not commonly used by ambulance services in the UK.

SIMPLE VENTILATION TECHNIQUES

Techniques of expired air ventilation without adjuncts were discussed in Chapter 3. This chapter deals with simple adjuncts for artificial ventilation. More advanced equipment is discussed in Chapter 5. The following devices are described in this chapter:

- the simple foil type
- the tube flange type
- the mask type
- the self-inflating bag–valve device

The Simple Foil

Foil devices were introduced for use by members of the public in an effort to minimize direct contact with the patient during expired air ventilation.

These foils consist of a plastic film which is applied to the oronasal region. There is a central orifice with a textile filter or one-way valve which is aligned with the patient's mouth. Expired air ventilation is applied in the usual way (see Chapter 3) with the patient's nostrils occluded with the fingers of one hand, while the other hand applies chin lift and seals the foil to the face (Figure 4.17). On occasion the foil may tear when in contact with the patient's or rescuer's teeth.

The Tube Flange Device

This type consists of a flange to provide a seal around the lips, a short oropharyngeal airway and an inflation tube. Some

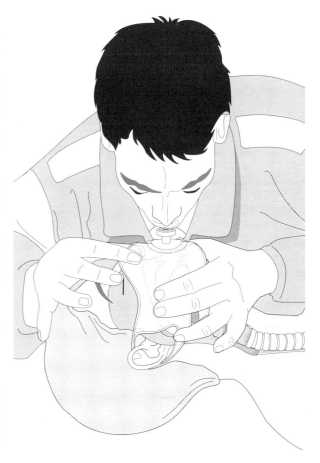

Fig. 4.17 *The foil device used for expired air ventilation. From Baskett, PJF (1993)* Resuscitation Handbook, *2nd edn, with permission from Gower Medical Publishing*

devices have a unidirectional valve incorporated in the inflation tube to direct the patient's exhaled air away from the rescuer. Some come with a nose clip.

The device is introduced into the mouth and a seal maintained by the fingers holding the head and neck to achieve clear airway alignment, and the thumbs applying the flange to the circumoral region (Figure 4.18). Expired air ventilation is provided via the inflation tube in the usual manner. This is a poor ventilation device and its adoption by ambulance services is not recommended.

The Mask Device

A moulded face mask, made from transparent material, is fitted with an inflation port incorporating a one-way valve which directs the patient's exhaled air away from the rescuer and traps macroscopic particles. Some models incorporate an additional port for supplemental oxygen. The oxygen flow rate should be set at the maximum available.

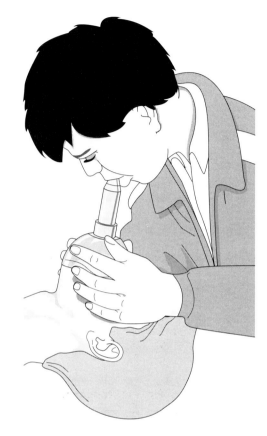

Fig. 4.18 *The tube flange device*

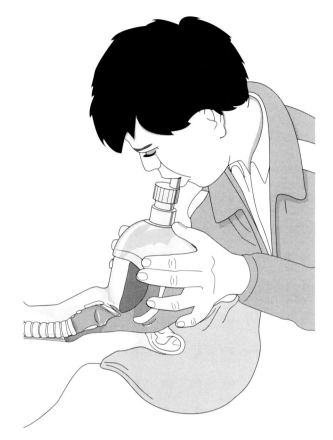

Fig. 4.19 *Mouth-to-mask ventilation*

The mask is applied over the mouth and nose with both hands, applying jaw thrust and head tilt to draw the face into the mask. The mask is sealed to the face with the index fingers and thumb of each hand (Figure 4.19).

The Self-inflating Bag–Valve Device

The self-inflating bag–valve device is designed to inflate the patient's lungs with air or an air and oxygen mixture.

Inflation of the lungs is provided through a valve which directs the air/oxygen to the patient, and vents exhaled air to the atmosphere. Oxygen enrichment (only achieving an inspired concentration of up to 50% – Fio_2 0.5) can be provided through a port adjacent to the unidirectional air inlet valve. Much better inspired concentrations can be achieved (Fio_2 0.9, i.e. an inspired oxygen concentration of 90%) when an oxygen reservoir bag is attached to the air inlet valve, and the flow rate adjusted to 10–15 l/min (Figure 4.20). The aim is to adjust the flow rate to ensure that the reservoir bag remains at least partially inflated at all times. If this is achievable with a flow rate of 10 l/min then a valuable resource can be conserved.

The self-inflating bag may be used with a face mask, or may be attached to a tracheal tube or laryngeal mask airway (see Chapter 5). Use of the bag and mask by one operator requires significant skill – the mask must be applied to the face with an airtight seal and the airway maintained in correct alignment, all with one hand. Expertise only comes with considerable practice. Importantly, operators may not be aware of their ineptitude, and incorrect technique may result in hypoventilation due to a leak between the face and mask, or inflation of the oesophagus due to imperfect airway alignment. For these reasons the two-person technique is advocated – one person using two hands to hold the mask with the airway aligned, and the other inflating the patient's lungs by squeezing the bag.

A modified patient valve can permit positive end-expiratory pressure (PEEP) to be applied when the bag is used with a tracheal tube. The use of PEEP may be particularly valuable in patients with pulmonary oedema following exposure to irritants, smoke inhalation, near-drowning, aspiration and cardiac failure. Some bag–valve devices can also be fitted with a filter on the intake valve to permit operation in contaminated atmospheres. The effect of PEEP is to maintain some pressure

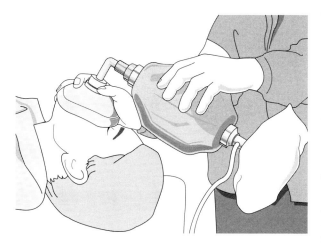

Fig. 4.20 *The self-inflating bag–valve–mask with oxygen reservoir*

in the airways, even at the end of expiration, which reduces and even reverses the leakage of fluid into the alveoli (as occurs in pulmonary oedema). The 'downside' is that the positive intrathoracic pressure reduces cardiac filling, and may lead to a reduction in blood pressure.

Points to look for when choosing a self-inflating bag–valve device

- The bag should be made of suitable material which provides adequate 'feel' during inflation and sufficient recoil to draw in air or gases in the reservoir bag. Foam-filled units should not be capable of undetected disintegration. The material should not absorb noxious gases or anaesthetic agents
- The patient valve should be easy to take apart for cleaning, and incorrect reassembly should be impossible
- The inlet valve should be capable of accommodating an oxygen reservoir bag and/or a noxious gas filter
- The bag should have International Standards Organization (ISO) fittings

Ventilation Volumes

For many years the American Heart Association has advocated a tidal volume of 800–1200 ml in patients with cardiac arrest. It is likely that such volumes are excessive, particularly in patients with cardiac arrest who produce relatively little carbon dioxide. Inflation with such high volumes in the patient with an unprotected and unsecured airway is likely to produce high inflation pressures with oesophageal and gastric inflation, and hypoventilation of the lungs owing to leakage between the face and mask. Inflation pressures in these circumstances can only

be minimized by a prolonged inspiratory period, which encroaches on the time for chest compressions.

Pending definitive information arising from specific research in this field, the best advice is to inflate the lungs sufficiently to resemble a normal breath. This is of the order of 400–500 ml, and is probably what is actually used with patients, as opposed to when practising with manikins (with lights and indicators that appear only at tidal volumes of 800 ml or more).

Cricoid Pressure

The unconscious patient with the insecure airway is continually at risk of regurgitation of gastric contents and pulmonary aspiration. True security of the airway can only be provided by tracheal intubation or use of other advanced airway adjuncts including the surgical airway.

Cricoid pressure (Sellick's manoeuvre) during artificial ventilation in the patient with the unsecured airway substantially reduces the risk of gastric regurgitation. The technique should always be used in this situation when sufficient personnel are available. Cricoid pressure is applied to either side of the cricoid cartilage using the thumb and forefinger of one hand. The other hand may provide counterpressure at the back of the neck (Figure 4.21).

Oxygen Therapy in the Spontaneously Breathing Patient

All patients with airway or ventilatory compromise, major trauma or cardiac disease should be given oxygen. High inspired concentrations can only be achieved with a mask that incorporates an oxygen reservoir bag. This is recommended in all of

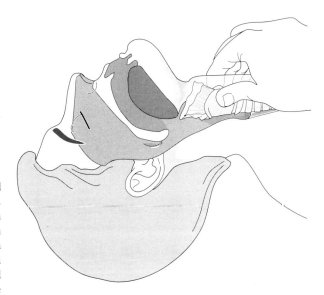

Fig. 4.21 *Cricoid pressure*

the above examples, and the oxygen flow rate should be set at 10–15 l/min, to ensure the reservoir bag remains inflated. Patients with severe chronic obstructive pulmonary disease (COPD) depend, to some extent, on a hypoxic drive to stimulate their respiratory centre. In these patients a high inspired oxygen concentration may *reduce* the respiratory drive and lead to hypoventilation and an accumulation of carbon dioxide

which has deleterious effects on the circulation and intracranial pressure. In such patients oxygen should be administered at a concentration of 24–28% using a Venturi mask. However, if cyanosis develops the attendant should not hesitate to assist ventilation with a high inspired oxygen concentration (see Chapter 5).

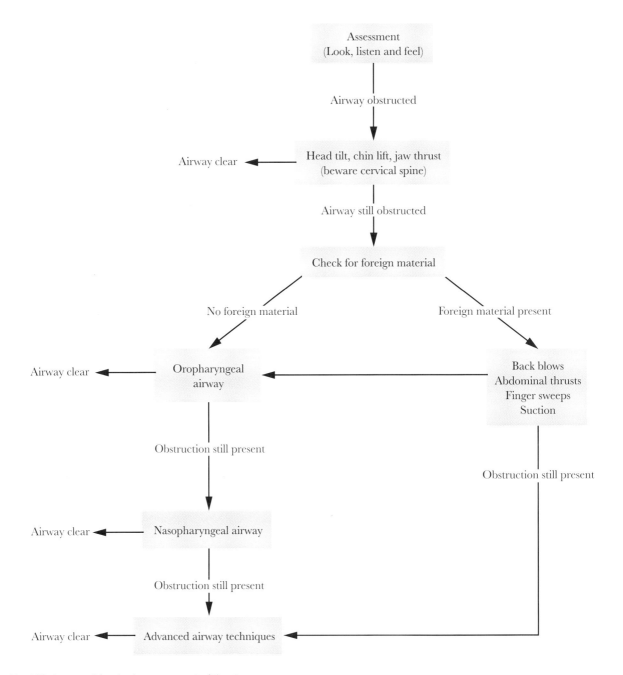

Fig. 4.22 A protocol for simple management of the airway

MANAGEMENT PROTOCOLS

Management protocols are useful in pre-hospital care. 'Decision tree' algorithms for management of the airway and ventilation are given in Figures 4.22 and 4.23.

FURTHER READING

American Heart Association (1992) National Consensus Conference Standards and Guidelines for Cardiopulmonary Resuscitation (CPR) and Emergency Cardiac Care (ECC). *Journal of the American Medical Association* **268**: 2171–2307.
Baskett PJF (1993) *Resuscitation Handbook*, 2nd edn. London: Mosby.
Baskett PJF, Daw AAC & Nolan JP (1994) *Practical Procedures in Anaesthesia and Critical Care*. London: Gower Medical Publishing.
Committee on Trauma of the American College of Surgeons (1993) *Advanced Trauma Life Support Instructor Manual*. Chicago: American College of Surgeons.

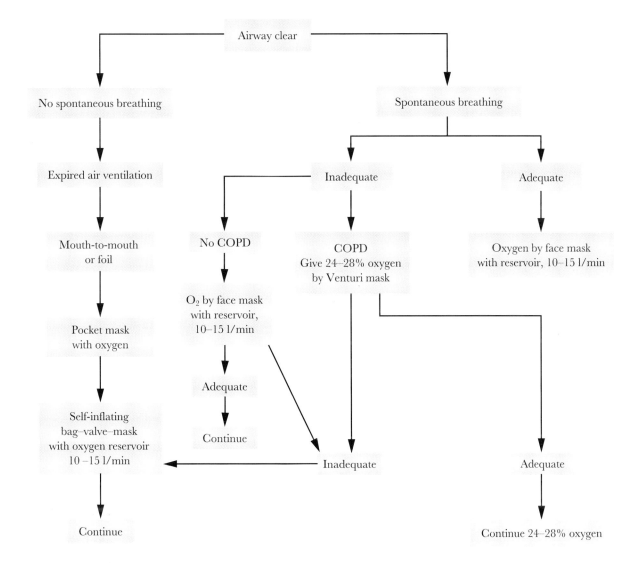

Fig. 4.23 A protocol for simple management of ventilation

chapter five:

ADVANCED MANAGEMENT OF THE AIRWAY AND VENTILATION

Management of the airway and ventilation using advanced techniques complements the basic methods but does not in any way replace them.

Advanced airway techniques are designed to secure the airway from aspiration of foreign material, and to allow positive pressure ventilation without danger of inflation of the stomach or leak at the mouth/mask interface.

The 'gold standard' for airway control in pre-hospital care is tracheal intubation using a cuffed endotracheal tube. However, the technique of placement of the tube under direct vision using a laryngoscope requires extensive and prolonged training and regular practice to maintain the skill. Excessive movement of the head and neck during laryngoscopy and intubation may aggravate a cervical spine injury.

For these reasons other techniques have been introduced to aid tracheal intubation and alternative devices have been developed which may be introduced blindly without the need for direct laryngoscopy.

CONVENTIONAL TRACHEAL INTUBATION

Conventionally the tracheal tube is passed through the mouth using a laryngoscope to visualize the vocal cords which form the gateway to the trachea. The tube may also be passed through the nose and directed into the trachea blindly, or with the aid of a laryngoscope.

Tracheal intubation can be used for any age group, and a range of tube sizes is available to accommodate neonates to large adults. Tubes of internal diameter greater than 6.5 mm are available with a cuff to seal the airway, permitting leak-proof positive pressure ventilation and preventing aspiration of foreign material into the lungs. In children and babies a good seal usually occurs without a cuff as the larynx and cricoid ring grip the tube sufficiently.

Size of Tube

Tubes of size 7.5–9.0 mm will fit most adults. An 8.0 mm tube is a useful size to carry for all-purpose emergency use. Tubes are made longer than is generally needed and should be cut to a length of 21–25 cm. The length required in any individual will be twice the distance from the corner of the mouth to the angle of the jaw (2 cm longer if the nasal route is to be used). For children the correct size can be calculated using the following formulae:

$$\text{correct internal diameter (mm)} \quad \frac{(\text{age of child in years})}{4} + 4$$

$$\text{correct length (cm)} \quad \frac{(\text{age of child in years})}{2} + 12$$

The length should be increased by up to 2 cm if the nasal route is to be used.

Equipment for Conventional Tracheal Intubation

The following equipment is required (Figure 5.1):

- Appropriate sized laryngoscope in working order
- Appropriate range of tubes cut to correct length with connections (15 mm) to fit the ventilating apparatus
- Scissors
- Suction apparatus
- Lubricant on a gauze swab
- 20 ml syringe for cuff inflation
- Clamp to secure the cuff inflation port
- Flexible bougie and stylet
- Magill's forceps
- Tape or tie to secure tube in place
- Apparatus to inflate the lungs (bag–valve or mechanical ventilator)

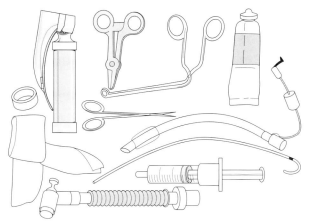

Fig. 5.1 *Intubation equipment. Adapted from Baskett, PJF (1993)* Resuscitation Handbook, *2nd edn, with permission from Gower Medical Publishing*

- Pulse oximeter to monitor patient during and after intubation attempt (optional)
- End-tidal CO_2 apparatus to detect correct tube placement (optional) (described later in this chapter)

Indications

The indications for conventional tracheal intubation in the pre-hospital setting are as follows.

Indications for tracheal intubation

- Airway obstruction or potential airway obstruction in the profoundly unconscious patient
- Patient at risk of aspiration of foreign material (e.g. gastric contents, blood from maxillofacial trauma)
- Patient requiring positive pressure ventilation, e.g. in cardiorespiratory arrest
- To gain access to the lower respiratory tract to aspirate secretions or foreign material

Contraindications

Tracheal intubation is contraindicated in the absence of a skilled operator and the necessary equipment. It is also contra-indicated in patients who are not profoundly unconscious. Forced intubation in, for instance, the lightly unconscious patient with a head injury will do more harm than good by raising the intracranial pressure and reducing the perfusion of the brain. In such circumstances simpler methods of airway management, such as insertion of a nasopharyngeal or oropharyngeal airway, will be adequate.

Relative contraindications include immobility of the head and neck, or distorted anatomy due to tumour, infection or oedema

– all of which impair the view of the larynx and the glottis opening.

On no account should attempts be made to intubate children with croup or infections such as acute epiglottitis, except in hospital. Intervention with a laryngoscope in such patients may provoke bleeding or further oedema, and convert a partial airway obstruction to a complete airway obstruction.

Contraindications to tracheal intubation

- Insufficient operator skill or experience
- Conscious or semiconscious patient
- Immobility of the head and neck (relative)
- Distorted anatomy (relative)
- In children
  - croup
  - epiglottitis

Technique for Orotracheal Intubation using Laryngoscopy

The technique is illustrated in Figure 5.2.

1. Ensure that all equipment functions correctly and that tubes and bougies are well lubricated.
2. The patient, if possible, should be supine with the head and neck aligned in the clear airway position (preferably with the head on a small pillow or rolled-up blanket).
3. Holding the laryngoscope in your left hand, insert the curved blade into the right-hand corner of the patient's mouth, ensuring that the lip is not caught between the blade and lower teeth (Figure 5.2A).
4. Advance the blade, aiming for the larynx in the midline, and displacing the tongue towards the left-hand side of the mouth to leave a clear view.
5. When the tip of the blade reaches laryngeal level, lift the handle forwards and upwards. Slide the tip of the blade into the recess between the epiglottis and the base of the tongue.
6. Maintain the backwards tilt of the head by pressing on the occiput with your other hand and against the tip of the blade to get the best view of the glottic opening (Figure 5.2). Cricoid pressure will generally improve the view and should be used in all patients in the field.
7. Pass the tracheal tube through the glottic opening, rotating it 90 degrees counter-clockwise if necessary to ease entry between the vocal cords.
8. If a full view of the glottis is not possible a bougie may be passed under direct vision through the cords and the tube reintroduced over the bougie into the trachea. The bougie is then withdrawn. Alternatively, a malleable stylet may be placed inside the lumen of the tube and bent to a

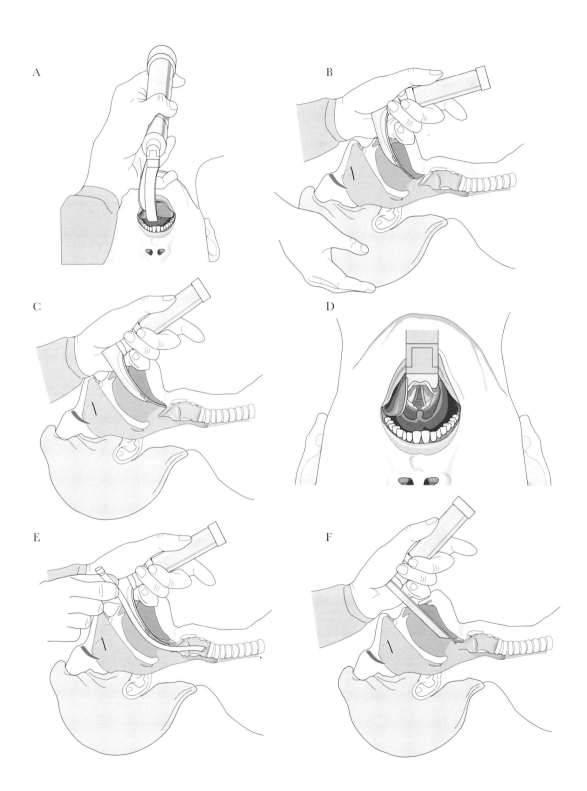

Fig. 5.2 Orotracheal intubation. A–E, adult intubation; F, use of straight bladed laryngoscope in infants. From Baskett, PJF (1993) Resuscitation Handbook, 2nd edn, with permission from Gower Medical Publishing

curve suitable for introduction of the tube through the glottis.

9. Once the tube has passed between the vocal cords it should be advanced so that the cuff lies below the larynx.

10. The cuff should be inflated with air (or water if the patient is to be transported at altitude, or in a decompression chamber). Sufficient air should be introduced to eliminate any leak at the peak of positive pressure ventilation. Cuff inflation volumes requiring more than 15 ml should lead to a suspicion that the tube is misplaced in the oesophagus or that the cuff itself has developed a leak.

11. Check that the tube is in the trachea by observing bilateral chest movement and listening for air entry over both upper lobes. Unilateral chest movement (generally on the right) may indicate that the tube has gone down too far and has entered the main bronchus. A check should also be made that air entry is not heard in the epigastric area. Other methods of checking correct tube placement are described later in this chapter.

12. Secure the tube in place with a tie or tape.

The entire process of intubation should be accomplished in 30–40 seconds (current National Health Service Training Directorate recommendations are to achieve intubation within 15 seconds, although other advanced life support teaching is more generous). If the attempt is taking longer then it should be temporarily abandoned and the patient ventilated with a face mask for 1–2 minutes before trying again. No more than three attempts should be made.

Problems and Hazards Associated with Orotracheal Intubation

Tracheal intubation attempts using direct laryngoscopy are not without hazards. These include:

- Trauma to lips, teeth, tongue and structures in the pharynx and larynx (a common problem is to use the teeth as a fulcrum, causing damage to crowns particularly)
- Oesophageal intubation (this in itself is not a major problem unless it is undetected; however, undetected oesophageal intubation generally leads to serious hypoxic brain damage or death, and represents probably the most serious technical error a paramedic can make)
- Intubation of a single bronchus will lead to hypoxia and collapse of the opposite lung
- Aspiration of foreign material such as stomach contents or blood during the intubation attempt
- Kinking of the tracheal tube
- Overinflation of the cuff leading to pressure damage of the tracheal mucous membrane, or ballooning of the cuff over the lumen of the tube

- Exacerbation of cervical spine injury (see Chapter 26)
- Trauma from the tip of a stylet protruding from the end of the tube (stylet used to stiffen or shape the tube during a difficult intubation)

NASOTRACHEAL INTUBATION

Nasotracheal intubation is sometimes used when the oral route has failed and is preferred by some authorities in patients with suspected cervical spine injury because it may be accomplished with the head and neck in the neutral position (see Chapter 27). However, it is generally agreed that the nasal route requires more technical skill and may take longer. There is also a risk of bleeding from the nose. *It is not a technique recommended for use by paramedics, and is included here for completeness only.*

Nasal tubes are available with a flexible tip which allow the curve to be varied by traction on a ring pull to negotiate the curve from the nasopharynx towards the glottic opening (Figure 5.3).

Two methods of nasal intubation may be used in pre-hospital care:

Blind nasal intubation (Figure 5.4)
Nasal intubation assisted by direct laryngoscopy and Magill's forceps (Figure 5.5).

Technique of Blind Nasotracheal Intubation

1. The patient is positioned as for orotracheal intubation. The head and neck may be placed in the neutral position, avoiding hyperextension.

2. The tube should be sized for the patient and well lubricated. A suitable tube will have a similar diameter to the patient's own little finger (7.0–8.0 mm for an adult).

3. The tube is introduced through the most patent nostril (generally the right side is attempted first) and passed directly backwards (*not* upwards) through the nasal cavity along the floor of the nose to enter the nasopharynx.

4. In patients who are breathing spontaneously the mouth and

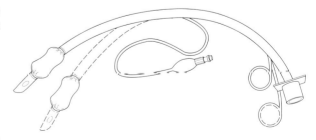

Fig. 5.3 *A nasotracheal tube. From Baskett, PJF (1993)* Resuscitation Handbook, *2nd edn, with permission from Gower Medical Publishing*

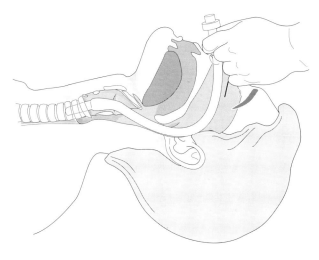

Fig. 5.4 Blind nasal intubation. Adapted from Baskett, PJF (1993) Resuscitation Handbook, *2nd edn, with permission from Gower Medical Publishing*

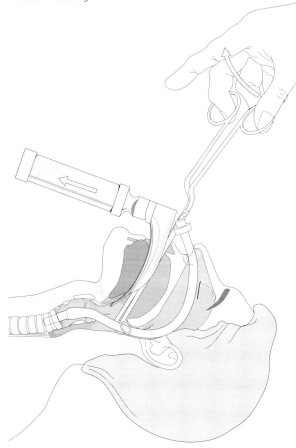

Fig. 5.5 Nasal intubation by direct laryngoscopy. Adapted from Baskett, PJF (1993) Resuscitation Handbook, *2nd edn, with permission from Gower Medical Publishing*

opposite nostril should be occluded manually and breath sounds should be listened for as the tube is steered towards the larynx and onwards through the glottis into the trachea. Generally a cough heralds successful passage through the cords.

5. The technique may also be used in the apnoeic patient, although it is more difficult. Considerable skill and practice, and optimal head and neck positioning, are required to steer the tube through the glottic opening.

6. Secure the tube and check for correct positioning as in orotracheal intubation.

Technique of Nasotracheal Intubation using Direct Laryngoscopy and Magill's Forceps

1. Proceed as with blind nasal intubation until the tip of the tube lies just above the glottis.

2. Introduce the laryngoscope as for orotracheal intubation and view the glottis.

3. Grasp the tube with Magill's forceps 1–2 cm from its tip and steer it through the glottic opening.

4. Secure the tube and check for correct positioning as in orotracheal intubation.

Hazards of Nasotracheal Intubation

Nasal intubation is associated with the same hazards as orotracheal intubation. Additionally, the nasal passage and adenoids may be damaged with associated bleeding, which may obscure the view at direct laryngoscopy. The tube may enter a false passage beneath the mucous membrane of the nasopharynx. In patients with a fracture of the base of the skull, a tube directed upwards instead of backwards may penetrate the cribriform plate and enter the cranial cavity.

> **NASAL INTUBATION IS NOT GENERALLY RECOMMENDED IN THE PRE-HOSPITAL ENVIRONMENT**

AIDS TO OROTRACHEAL INTUBATION AVOIDING DIRECT LARYNGOSCOPY

Certain techniques have been introduced in an effort to avoid the difficulties and hazards associated with direct laryngoscopy at intubation and to enable the tracheal tube to be introduced blindly via the mouth.

Two of these techniques are suitable for use in pre-hospital care:

- The Augustine guide
- The lighted stylet

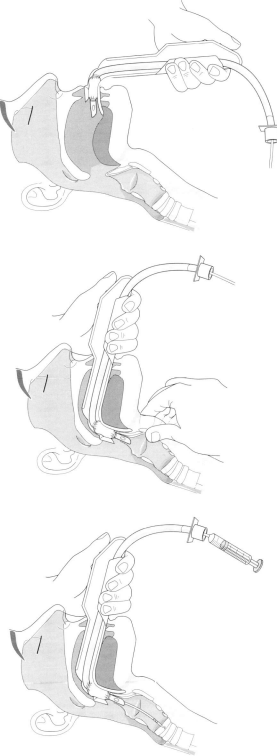

Both have the advantage that they can be used with the head and neck aligned in the neutral position. However, neither have yet found acceptance in UK ambulance service practice.

The Augustine Guide

The Augustine guide (Augustine Medical) is a rigid, right-angled guide designed to be passed blindly through the mouth so that the tip locates between the base of the tongue and the epiglottis (Figure 5.6). The lubricated tracheal tube and hollow stylet are mounted in the guide, and once the device is properly located may be passed through the glottis into the trachea. A syringe to detect correct placement by aspiration of air through the hollow stylet is provided as part of the kit.

The technique requires practice on a manikin and patients for expertise to be achieved. Use of the device has shown considerable initial promise, but the results of extensive experience in pre-hospital care are still awaited.

Technique
1. The guide stylet and tracheal tube are lubricated.
2. The stylet is inserted into the tracheal tube so that its tip just protrudes from the distal end.
3. The stylet and tube are bent at right angles and mounted in the slot provided in the guide.
4. A bite block is inserted between the molar teeth.

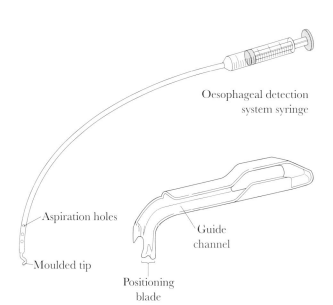

Oesophageal detection system syringe

Aspiration holes

Moulded tip

Guide channel

Positioning blade

Fig. 5.6 *The Augustine guide. Adapted from Baskett, PJF (1993)* Resuscitation Handbook, *2nd edn, with permission from Gower Medical Publishing*

5. With the patient's head and neck aligned in the neutral position and the tongue pulled forward wrapped in a gauze swab, the guide is introduced into the mouth and passed back over the tongue to reach the hypopharynx. Introduction into the mouth may be directly in the midline or via the corner of the mouth, rotating the device into the midline as it reaches the entrance to the pharynx.

6. The guide is lifted upwards to locate in the pit between the base of the tongue and the epiglottis (the vallecula). Correct placement is confirmed if short rotational movements are transmitted to the hyoid bone. The movements of the hyoid bone can be observed directly and felt with the other hand.

7. Once the correct position is confirmed the guide handle is lifted slightly upwards and backwards and the stylet and then the tube advanced through the glottic opening into the trachea.

8. Correct tube placement is confirmed by aspiration of 30 ml of air into the syringe attached to the hollow stylet. The guide and stylet are then removed after dislocating the tube from the slot.

9. The tube is secured in place in the usual way.

Problems and hazards

- Inability to introduce and locate the guide correctly
- The stylet and tube will not pass cleanly into the trachea
- Local trauma to the pharyngeal and laryngeal structures
- Oesophageal intubation

The Lighted Stylet

Another intubation method uses a malleable lighted stylet (Laerdal Medical) passed through the lumen of the tracheal tube so that the light at the end just emerges from the distal end of the tube (Figure 5.7). Bent to a 'J' shape, the tube is introduced directly through the glottis into the trachea. Correct positioning just above the glottic opening is confirmed by maximal transillumination in the midline.

Technique

1. The tracheal tube and lighted stylet are lubricated and confirmed to be in working order.

2. The lighted stylet is introduced into the tube so that the lighted end just emerges from the distal end of the tube.

3. The tube and wand are bent into a 'J' shape so that the base of the 'J' is equal in length to the distance from the tip of the chin to the thyroid cartilage (Adam's apple). The proximal end of the tube is clipped to the wand handle.

4. With the patient's head and neck in the neutral position and the tongue pulled forward wrapped in a gauze swab, the tube is introduced into the mouth and passed backwards over the tongue aiming for the larynx in the midline.

5. As the tube enters the hypopharynx transillumination will be observed. The position of the tube should be adjusted so that the transillumination is in the midline.

6. Advance the tube. If it passes easily and transillumination intensifies it has passed into the trachea. If the light intensity dims the tube is lying in the oesophagus.

7. Transillumination on either side of the midline with difficulty in tube advancement means that the tip is in the piriform fossa to the side of the larynx. The tip of the tube should be repositioned in the midline.

8. Once the tube is correctly placed the lighted stylet should be unclipped from the proximal end and withdrawn from the tube.

9. Correct placement in the trachea should be confirmed using the usual methods and the tube should be secured in place with a tie or tape.

Problems and hazards

- Inability to introduce and locate the tube correctly, resulting in persistent lodging in the piriform fossa or in front of the epiglottis
- Local trauma to the pharyngeal and laryngeal structures
- Oesophageal intubation
- Difficulty in detecting maximal transillumination in ambient bright light

ALTERNATIVES TO TRACHEAL INTUBATION

Alternatives to tracheal intubation have been introduced to circumvent some of the problems associated with direct laryngoscopy and intubation. These problems include the considerable technical skill required, the need for extensive training on human patients, the need for regular practice, the potential for patient injury during the procedure and the risk of unrecognized oesophageal intubation.

Three devices have potential for use in pre-hospital care. These are:

- The laryngeal mask airway
- The Combitube
- The pharyngotracheal lumen airway

None, however, has as yet undergone extensive trials in the hands of paramedics, and reports of further clinical experience are required before the place of any or all of the devices in pre-hospital care can be determined and firm recommendations made.

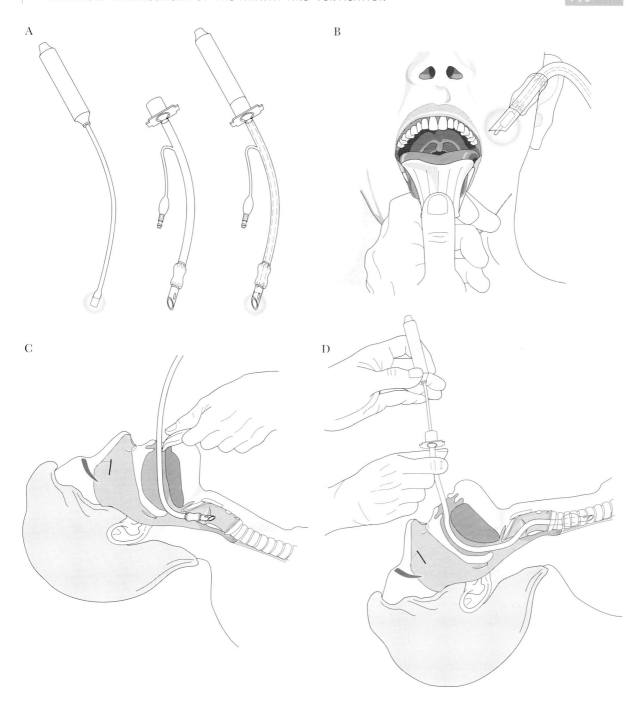

A

B

C

D

Fig. 5.7 *The lighted stylet. From Baskett, PJF (1993)* Resuscitation Handbook, *2nd edn, with permission from Churchill Livingstone*

The Laryngeal Mask Airway

The laryngeal mask airway (LMA or Brain airway) has found a niche in airway management during anaesthesia since its introduction into clinical practice in the mid-1980s (Figure 5.8).

The advantage of the LMA is that it can provide a secure airway without the training and skill required for laryngoscopy and tracheal intubation. The incidence of trauma, sore throat and laryngeal spasm is considerably less than with tracheal intubation. The technique is easily learnt by nurses and

Table 5.1 Laryngeal mask sizes

Patient	Weight (kg)	Size	Cuff volume (ml)
Neonate/infant	up to 6.5	1	2–4
Infant/child	6.5–15	2	10
Child	15–30	2.5	15
Small adult/child	30–50	3	20
Adult	50–75	4	30
Large adult	>75	5	40

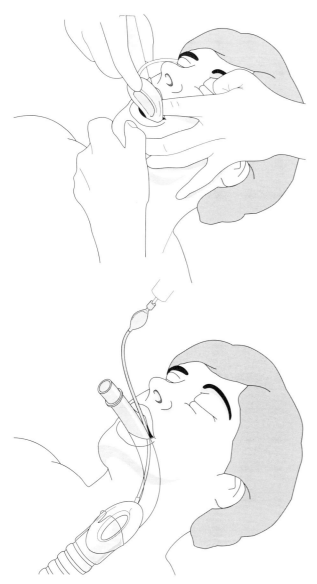

opening. The airway comes in a range of sizes suitable for an infant to a large adult (Table 5.1). It is not a single-use disposable item. After use it should be cleaned and autoclaved according to the manufacturer's instructions. It may be reused up to 40 times. If necessary, a 6.0–6.5 mm tracheal tube may be passed through the lumen of the size 4 and size 5 masks into the trachea.

Indications

The LMA is indicated when an airway is required in an unconscious patient and tracheal intubation is precluded by lack of available expertise or equipment, or has proved difficult or impossible.

Technique

1. Test cuff inflation for leaks and then lubricate the back and sides – but not the aperture – of the cuff and the distal part of the tube.
2. Deflate the cuff completely.
3. The patient should be supine with the head and neck in the clear airway position.
4. The mouth should be opened by an assistant depressing the chin.
5. The tube is held like a pen in the gloved hand and introduced into the mouth with the aperture facing the tongue. *As the LMA is advanced it should be applied to the roof of the palate.*
6. Once the hand cannot go further inside the mouth it should be moved to the proximal end of the tube and the mask pressed into position until resistance is felt as it locates in the hypopharynx. The coloured line on the tube should be aligned with the nasal septum.
7. The cuff is inflated with the correct amount of air for the size (see Table 5.1). As the cuff is inflated the tube rises out of the mouth by approximately 1 cm.
8. Confirm that a clear airway exists by listening for spontaneous breathing or check for chest movement and breath sounds during inflation with a bag attached to the tube.
9. Insert the bite block or oropharyngeal airway alongside the tube and secure it in place with a tie or tape.

Note: normally the operator will be positioned at the head of the patient to introduce the tube, but if access to this position is impossible the operator may stand or kneel in front of the patient and introduce the tube from below.

Fig. 5.8 *The laryngeal mask airway. Adapted from Baskett, PJF (1993)* Resuscitation Handbook, *2nd edn, with permission from Gower Medical Publishing*

paramedics. While not guaranteeing absolute protection of the airway in every case, the LMA does offer considerably greater security than most other airways except the endotracheal tube. The LMA has been reported to have been successful in the management of the airway by nurses during cardiopulmonary resuscitation and a similar study is in progress to assess the performance of paramedics and emergency medical technicians with the device in pre-hospital care.

The LMA consists of a wide-bore tube with a standard 15 mm connector at the proximal end. At the distal end is an elliptical cuff designed to seal the hypopharynx around the laryngeal

Problems and hazards

Laryngeal mask airways leak around the cuff if inflation pressures greater than 20 cmH$_2$O are generated. This can generally be overcome by careful attention to the ventilation pattern using slow flow rate inflation, but this may present difficulties in those with bronchospasm or chronic obstructive pulmonary disease.

Rejection of the LMA, straining, coughing and laryngeal spasm may occur in patients who are not profoundly unconscious and who retain active reflexes. Such limitations may confine the use of the LMA in pre-hospital care to cardio-respiratory arrest, near-drowning, drug overdose to the point of respiratory arrest, and in trauma except for the profoundly unconscious.

Oropharyngeal trauma may be aggravated by the LMA.

Incorrect placement may occur if the tip of the cuff folds back on itself, catches in the epiglottis or rotates during insertion. If this occurs withdraw the LMA, deflate the cuff completely and try again, adhering precisely to the manufacturer's recommended technique for insertion.

The LMA offers a method of establishing a clear airway in the unconscious patient before tracheal intubation skills and equipment are available, or if tracheal intubation proves difficult. It is not intended as a long-term airway and does not offer absolute protection against pulmonary aspiration.

The Combitube

The Combitube (Figure 5.9) is another device which has been introduced as an alternative to tracheal intubation. It is a pre-formed double-lumen tube which is passed blindly through the mouth avoiding the need for laryngoscopy. Ventilation of the lungs is possible whether the tube enters the trachea or the oesophagus.

The channels of the tube are designated 'tracheal' or 'oesophageal'. The tracheal tube has an open distal end and the oesophageal tube has a blind end with openings situated at the level just above the larynx. There is a small-volume (10–20 ml) cuff situated at the distal end of the oesophageal tube, and a large-volume (100 ml) cuff designed to occupy the hypopharynx. If the tube passes directly into the trachea the distal cuff is inflated and the ventilating apparatus is attached to the tracheal tube. The hypopharyngeal cuff is redundant. If the tube passes into the oesophagus (more usual), both distal and hypopharyngeal cuffs are inflated and the ventilating apparatus is connected to the oesophageal tube. Inflation of the lungs occurs through the openings at the laryngeal level, the inflating gas being prevented from passing into the oesophagus by the distal cuff and from leaking into the mouth and nose by the hypopharyngeal cuff.

The Combitube is not currently available in sizes suitable for children.

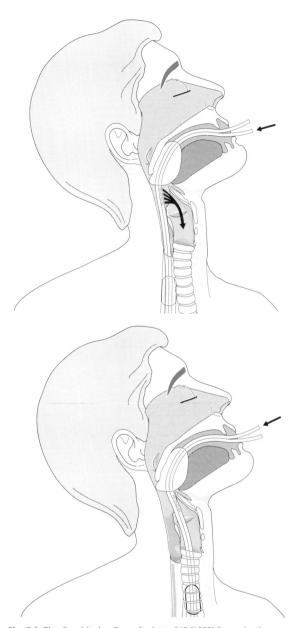

Fig. 5.9 *The Combitube. From Baskett, PJF (1993)* Resuscitation Handbook, *2nd edn, with permission from Gower Medical Publishing*

Technique

1. Lubricate the Combitube.
2. With the patient supine and the head and neck aligned in the clear airway position, introduce the tube through the mouth to a distance of approximately 24 cm.
3. Inflate the distal cuff and ventilate the patient through the tracheal tube port. If it is confirmed that the tube is located in the trachea (see below) continue ventilation by this route.

4. If the tube has passed into the oesophagus, then both cuffs should be inflated and the patient ventilated through the oesophageal tube port.
5. Confirm that the lungs are being ventilated (see below) and that gas is not entering the stomach.

Problems and hazards

Problems encountered with the Combitube include:

- The device is bulky and may be difficult to introduce into a small mouth. The cuffs may be damaged by sharp teeth
- Hypopharyngeal injuries may be aggravated
- There is a potential for ventilating the oesophagus and stomach if the tube position is incorrectly identified
- The tube may be rejected and coughing and straining may occur if the patient is not profoundly unconscious

The Combitube also offers a potential alternative to tracheal intubation in instances where expertise and equipment are not immediately available. There have as yet been no reports of large-scale trials of its use by ambulance personnel in pre-hospital care, and positive recommendations for use must await such clinical experience.

The Combitube is a single-use disposable item.

The Pharyngotracheal Lumen Airway

The pharyngotracheal lumen airway (PTLA) was introduced in the USA as a replacement for the oesophageal obturator airway (OOA). The OOA had been developed as a substitute for tracheal intubation in the early 1980s, but it lost popularity as a result of a number of shortcomings and complications.

The PTLA consists of two tubes: a longer one with a distal small-volume cuff and a shorter one incorporating a large (100 ml) cuff which envelopes both tubes (Figure 5.10). This large cuff is destined to lie in the hypopharynx above the larynx. Inflation of both cuffs is achieved through a common port.

The device, like the LMA and the Combitube, is introduced blindly through the mouth. Normally the longer tube enters the oesophagus. The distal cuff is inflated to prevent gastric contents being regurgitated into the hypopharynx and air from the short tube entering the stomach. The large-volume cuff is inflated and ventilation via the port of the short tube inflates the lungs through the larynx via the space below the hypopharynx.

If the long tube enters the trachea directly it acts as a tracheal tube and ventilation should be directed via the port of the long tube (after removal of the stylet).

The PTLA is not a single-use disposable item, and the manufacturers suggest it can be used up to five times.

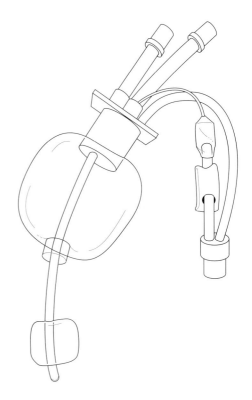

Fig. 5.10 *The pharyngotracheal lumen airway. From Baskett, PJF (1993)* Resuscitation Handbook, *2nd edn, with permission from Gower Medical Publishing*

Technique

1. Lubricate both tubes and cuffs.
2. Place the patient supine with the head and neck aligned in the clear airway position.
3. Introduce the long tube, following on with the short tube until the large cuff is judged to lie in the hypopharynx.
4. Blow in tube labelled '1' to inflate cuffs.
5. Blow in tube labelled '2' to ventilate.
6. If the chest does not rise, remove the stylet from tube labelled '3' and blow down this tube to ventilate.

Problems and hazards

Problems of using the PTLA are:

- The device is bulky and may be difficult to introduce in a small mouth. The large-volume cuff may by damaged by sharp teeth
- Further damage may occur in patients with injuries in the hypopharynx
- Incorrect identification of the location of the long tube may occur, and ventilation through the wrong port will cause hypoxia and massive inflation of the stomach

- The tube may be rejected and promote coughing and straining if the patient is not profoundly unconscious and has active protective reflexes

The PTLA has enjoyed some popularity in the USA as an alternative to tracheal intubation but there have been no reports of large-scale trials of its use by ambulance personnel. Its use in the UK and Europe has been scanty and it is likely to be subsumed by the LMA and the Combitube.

DETECTION OF CORRECT TUBE PLACEMENT

An undetected misplaced tracheal tube is the most serious complication of airway management. A protocol to check correct placement should follow each intubation attempt. If there is the slightest doubt that the tube is not in the trachea the rule is that it should be removed and the patient oxygenated by alternative methods.

> If there is any doubt about the correct placement of an endotracheal tube – remove it!

Four methods are available in the emergency setting for detecting that the tube is correctly placed in the trachea.

Clinical Methods

Clinical methods include:

- Visualizing the tube passing between the vocal cords during the intubation attempt
- Palpation of the tube as it passes through the larynx
- During positive pressure inflation applied to the tube, note
    absence of leak around the inflated cuff
    bilateral chest expansion
    breath sounds in both axillae
    absence of sounds in the epigastric area

These methods are generally effective in the majority of cases, but are not totally reliable. Fortunately, there are simple, inexpensive methods to supplement the clinical methods.

Transillumination

A lighted stylet passed down the lumen of the tube (see Figure 5.7) shows bright transillumination when the tube is in the trachea. A dull glow suggests that the tube is in the oesophagus. The method is subject to observer variation and is not reliable in bright light.

Detection of Carbon Dioxide

Detection of carbon dioxide emerging from the tube generally indicates that it is in the trachea. A simple, inexpensive colorimetric device is available and is a reliable carbon dioxide detector. Miniaturized electronic devices are also available which provide a capnograph trace and digital readings. However, carbon dioxide can also emerge from the oesophagus if the patient has recently imbibed a carbonated drink.

During cardiac arrest carbon dioxide is not produced and therefore will not be detected even in a correctly placed tube. Effective cardiopulmonary resuscitation results in some carbon dioxide production and indeed the amount of carbon dioxide detected provides some prediction of outcome.

The Oesophageal Detector

The oesophageal detector consists of a 50 ml syringe or self-inflating bulb joined by an airtight connection to the tracheal tube (Figure 5.11). If the tube is correctly placed, free aspiration of air into the syringe occurs. If the tube is located in the oesophagus aspiration attempts meet with resistance. This is a reliable and inexpensive method.

AIRWAY MANAGEMENT IN SUSPECTED CERVICAL SPINE INJURY

Special care must be taken during management of the airway in patients with suspected cervical spine injury. Aggravation of the injury must be avoided by the application of manual in-line stabilization of the head and neck in the neutral position during the attempt to secure the airway (Figure 5.12). However, the

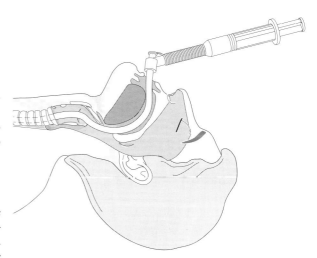

Fig. 5.11 *The oesophageal detector*

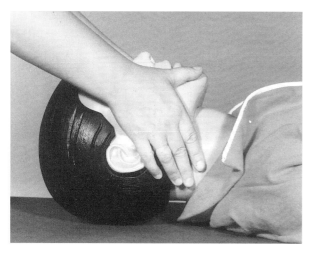

Fig. 5.12 *Airway management in suspected cervical spine injury*

importance of a clear airway is paramount, as a continuously obstructed airway is fatal.

Certain important principles should be borne in mind during management of such patients.

- Flexion and rotation of the head and neck are the most dangerous movements
- Oral intubation using direct laryngoscopy can be safely accomplished by a skilled operator in the vast majority of cases
- In cases of difficulty with intubation using direct laryngoscopy, the Augustine guide or lighted stylet may be used. The laryngeal mask airway or the Combitube may be used if tracheal intubation is not possible
- Patients with severe maxillofacial injury in whom the airway cannot be secured should be managed by needle cricothyrotomy and jet ventilation, or surgical cricothyrotomy and tracheal intubation

AIRWAY MANAGEMENT IN PATIENTS WITH PHARYNGEAL OR LARYNGEAL OEDEMA

Oedema in the pharyngeal or laryngeal region can be related to thermal injury, anaphylaxis or acute infection such as epiglottitis. Blind techniques such as use of the light wand, Augustine guide or alternatives to tracheal intubation (LMA, Combitube) are contraindicated. *Oral intubation should only be attempted by a skilled anaesthetist using deep inhalational anaesthesia.*

In the pre-hospital setting the airway should be managed by

basic positional methods and a high inspired oxygen concentration, with rapid transfer to a hospital. Life-threatening airway obstruction should be treated by needle cricothyroidotomy and jet ventilation or surgical cricothyrotomy (see below). Patients with inhalational thermal injury should be intubated early before serious oedema develops.

THE SURGICAL AIRWAY

The surgical airway is indicated in patients with life-threatening airway obstruction where basic positional methods and endotracheal intubation (or alternatives) have failed.

In pre-hospital care access to the trachea should be made through the cricothyroid membrane unless there is severe trauma in this region. Tracheostomy in the emergency situation is very difficult, and is usually hampered by severe bleeding from the thyroid vessels.

A number of methods of gaining access to the airway through the cricothyroid membrane have been developed. These include:

- Needle cricothyroidotomy
- Surgical cricothyroidotomy
- Blind stab techniques using specially designed equipment
- Percutaneous dilation methods

All of these methods are difficult and hazardous in the pre-hospital situation with a gasping patient. They should only be undertaken in extreme circumstances. In the first instance the recommended method is needle cricothyroidotomy.

Needle Cricothyroidotomy

The procedure is shown in Figure 5.13.

1. A 14 G intravenous cannula directed slightly towards the feet (caudally) is introduced through the cricothyroid membrane, while aspirating continually through an attached 20 ml syringe until a free flow of air is obtained.
2. The needle is withdrawn, leaving the cannula *in situ*.
3. Correct placement of the cannula is reconfirmed by free aspiration of air.
4. A 14 G cannula is of insufficient diameter to allow any significant spontaneous ventilation to occur. Positive pressure ventilation can be provided using a self-inflating bag attached to a 3.0 mm tracheal tube connector which will fit a Luer intravenous connection. *Ventilation provided by this method is marginal* and sufficient only to buy a few minutes time until an alternative is available.
5. Adequate ventilation *can* be provided using a high-pressure

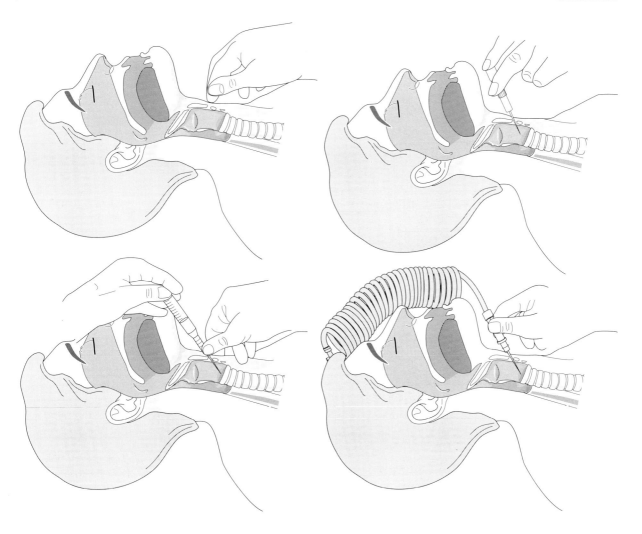

Fig. 5.13 *Needle cricothyroidotomy*

jet injector system. The cannula is connected by non-compliant tubing to an oxygen cylinder fitted with a regulator, which will produce a pressure in the region of 400 kPa.

6. Inflation is produced by a finger intermittently occluding a hole in the tubing, or by a specially designed system with a manually operated trigger which produces inflation when depressed. Alternatively, a 'Y' connector may be used to connect the tubing to the cannula, with the stem of the 'Y' towards the patient and one of the top ends attached via the tubing to the oxygen supply. The open branch can be intermittently occluded to produce insufflation. Each inflation must be very carefully observed and the trigger immediately released when normal chest expansion occurs, in order to avoid lung barotrauma.

7. Time must be left for lung deflation (1 second inflation: 4 seconds deflation). For the technique to be safe there must

be a clear route through the larynx and mouth for the expired gases, otherwise lung barotrauma will occur with gross, life-threatening subcutaneous and mediastinal emphysema.

Surgical Cricothyroidotomy

Surgical cricothyroidotomy (Figure 5.14) may occasionally be performed by a medical practitioner before the patient reaches hospital.

1. A 2–3 cm transverse incision is made in the skin over the cricothyroid membrane.
2. The subcutaneous tissues down to the membrane are dissected using blunt artery forceps and a self-retaining retractor is inserted to expose the membrane.

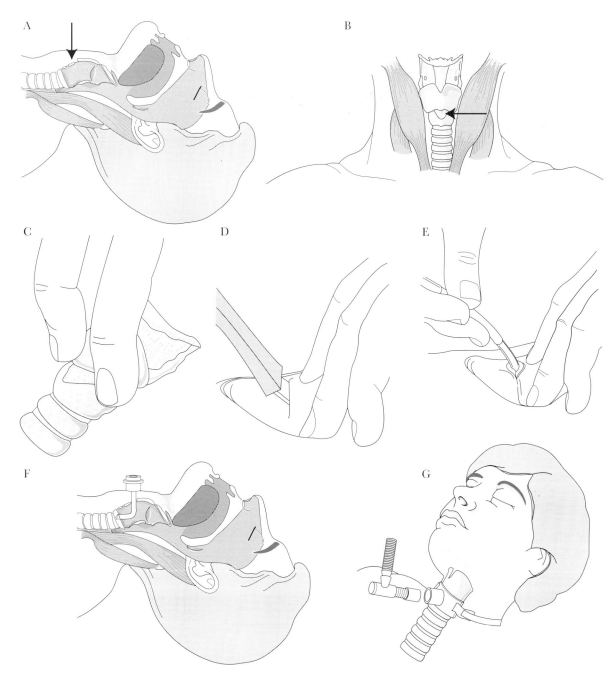

Fig. 5.14 *Surgical cricothyroidotomy*

3. The membrane is incised 1 cm transversely and a pair of forceps inserted into the wound to maintain the track.
4. A 6.0–7.0 mm lubricated tracheal tube (endotracheal/tracheotomy) is inserted through the incision and directed towards the lower trachea.
5. The cuff is inflated and the tube is secured with a tape and connected to the ventilating apparatus.

This method provides the optimum emergency surgical airway, but it is difficult in the pre-hospital environment and cannot be recommended except in experienced hands.

Blind Stab Techniques

Access to the trachea can be achieved with methods that use a blind stab through the skin, subcutaneous tissues and cricothyroid membrane. A bougie (Portex Mini-Trach II) (Figure 5.15) or expandable trochar system (Nu-Trach) is passed through the incision and directed into the trachea, and a tube inserted over the bougie or through the trochar. With the Mini-Trach system a 4.0 mm uncuffed tube is provided which is adequate for only about 1 hour. Using serial dilations, however, a tube of 6.5 mm can be inserted. With the Nu-Trach, tubes of 6.0–6.5 mm can be placed directly.

Blind stab techniques present considerable problems in the gasping patient in the emergency setting, and it can be very difficult to find the passage through the skin incision and into the trachea. This is because the larynx moves under the skin, with the result that the incision in the cricoid membrane is no longer directly beneath the skin incision.

Percutaneous Dilational Cricothyroidotomy

The Melker percutaneous dilational cricothyroidotomy kit is shown in Figure 5.16. The technique will only be performed by a medical practitioner.

1. A needle is inserted through the cricothyroid membrane into the trachea and correct placement is confirmed by aspiration of air. A guide wire is passed through the needle and the needle removed.
2. An incision is made in the skin alongside the guide wire and extended to pierce the cricothyroid membrane beneath.
3. A dilator is passed over the guide wire into the trachea and moved up and down to ensure a hole of sufficient size in the membrane.
4. A 6.0–6.5 mm lubricated tube is passed over the dilator into the trachea.
5. The dilator is removed and the tube is secured with a tie; the tube cuff is inflated and the tube connected to the ventilation apparatus.

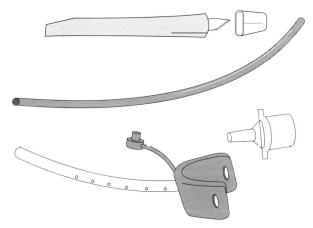

Fig. 5.15 *The Portex Mini-Trach system*

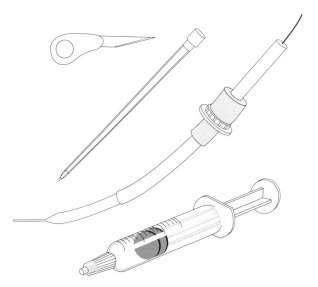

Fig. 5.16 *Percutaneous dilational cricothyroidotomy equipment*

For pre-hospital use the best methods of achieving a surgical airway are needle cricothyroidotomy or direct surgical cricothyroidotomy. *The percutaneous dilatation method is not appropriate for routine pre-hospital use.*

ADVANCED VENTILATION TECHNIQUES

Oxygen-Powered Resuscitators

Oxygen-powered resuscitators have been designed to take over from the self-inflating bag. They are driven from a high-pressure (400 kPa) oxygen source, so are valuable in contaminated atmospheres. The devices may be connected to a face mask, tracheal tube, laryngeal mask or Combitube.

The equipment should be designed to restrict the inspiratory flow rates to a maximum of 40 litres per minute and should incorporate a blow-off valve with automatic warning if the inflation pressure exceeds 60 cmH$_2$O in adults.

Two types are available:

Manually triggered resuscitators
Automatically triggered resuscitators

Manually triggered resuscitators

Manually triggered resuscitators (Figure 5.17) are triggered by pressing a lever or button at the patient valve. Both hands are used to ensure an airtight fit and to maintain airway alignment if a face mask is used, but there is a lack of direct 'feel', compared with a self-inflating bag, during the inspiratory phase. This may increase the risk of gastric inflation association with imperfect airway alignment.

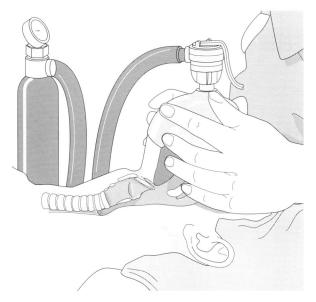

Fig. 5.17 A manually triggered resuscitator

Unlike the automatic resuscitator, one operator is committed to providing continuing ventilation, even when a tracheal tube is in place. Some models have a triggered demand valve to provide assisted ventilation in time with the patient's own inspiratory efforts.

Automatic resuscitators

Automatic resuscitators (Figure 5.18) cycle between inspiration and expiration using a fluid logic system or by electronic con-

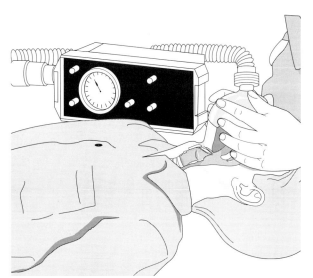

Fig. 5.18 An automatic resuscitator

trol. For pre-hospital work, cycling should be related to volume and time, not to pressure.

The automatic resuscitator provides consistent automatic ventilation at the pre-set tidal volume, rate and respiratory pattern. If a tracheal tube, Combitube or laryngeal mask is in place the rescuer is free to attend to other tasks, such as venous cannulation.

Automatic resuscitators vary in versatility in terms of variation of the inspiratory and expiratory pattern. Some models have the option of ventilation with air/oxygen mixtures to conserve oxygen supplies, and some incorporate a demand valve to synchronize with the patient's own inspiratory efforts.

Models with a low inspiratory flow rate and a blow-off valve with an audible warning signal (e.g. Pneupac) are most satisfactory. They are said to carry less danger of gastric inflation when used with a face mask than a self-inflating bag.

VENTILATION PATTERNS

Inspiratory Flow Rates

High inspiratory flow rates are associated with a higher incidence of gastric inflation in the unprotected airway owing to a raised inflation pressure. There is also reduced alveolar ventilation with a tendency to lung collapse.

In normal adult patients the inspiratory phase should occupy 1.5–2.0 seconds, and longer if there is an increased resistance to inspiration. Resuscitators should not generate inspiratory flow rates in excess of 40 litres per minute.

Expiratory Flow Rates

Generally the expiratory time should be about twice as long as the inspiratory time. It may need to be even longer in patients with increased expiratory resistance, e.g. bronchospasm due to asthma or chronic pulmonary disease.

Positive End-Expiratory Pressure

Valves are available which can be fitted to resuscitators or self-inflating bags which provide an obstruction to expiratory pressure above zero. Such valves can usually operate with a range of 0–10 cmH_2O positive end-expiratory pressure (PEEP). Usually 5 cmH_2O PEEP is sufficient.

Positive end-expiratory pressure allows recruitment of collapsed or oedematous alveoli and so increases the oxygen saturation in the systemic circulation. The technique is valuable in near-drowning and smoke inhalation. It may be associated with a fall in cardiac output and blood pressure, particularly in hypovolaemic patients. It is not a technique generally available in pre-hospital care.

NEBULIZERS

Nebulizers are increasingly used for the pre-hospital management of bronchospasm. Salbutamol is commonly available for paramedic and technician use and when given by nebulizer it is rapidly effective.

The most appropriate nebulizer for pre-hospital care is the gas-driven type. Oxygen, the carrier gas, is passed through a nozzle and generates an area of low pressure around it. The liquid drug placed beneath this area of low pressure is drawn up into the gas stream as droplets and carried forward to the face mask for inhalation. Although simple gas-driven nebulizers may not produce droplets of sufficiently small size to reach the extremes of the bronchial tree, in the main the droplets are small enough to be effective in the proximal areas.

The nebulizer (normally containing 2.5 ml) can be refilled and used several times in refractory cases.

chapter six

INTRAVENOUS ACCESS

The ability to gain access to the circulation is an essential skill that all those involved in the care of critically ill or injured patients must acquire. Intravenous access allows a number of therapeutic options:

- Fluid can be given to restore or maintain a patient's circulation
- Drugs can be administered, for example adrenaline during a cardiac arrest: this eliminates the delays and uncertainty following intramuscular or subcutaneous administration
- A blood sample can be taken: this can be sent ahead to the receiving hospital in order that cross-matched blood is available when the patient arrives

Intravenous access can be achieved in several ways. The most common is percutaneous puncture of a vein using a metal needle with subsequent introduction of a small-bore plastic tube or cannula into the vein. The alternative is to surgically expose a vein and insert a cannula under direct vision – the 'cut-down' technique. A third method, which is gaining popularity for use in children, is the insertion of a short metal needle into the marrow cavity of a long bone – the intraosseous route. This is described at the end of this chapter.

Venous cannulation is an invasive procedure and should not be treated with complacency. It is most likely to be successful and potential problems minimized if the person performing cannulation has:

- A knowledge of the local anatomy at the site chosen
- Familiarity with the equipment to be used
- An understanding of the technique to be used
- An awareness of the potential complications

Obtaining intravenous access is a skill, which is best learnt and maintained by practice. The following description is only intended as a guide and is not a substitute for practising under the guidance of an expert. It is a skill that once acquired will enhance patient care and help save lives.

ANATOMY

Veins used for Intravenous Access

The veins most commonly used are the superficial peripheral veins in the upper limbs. If for any reason these are not accessible then the saphenous vein at the ankle can be used. More recently, interest has been shown in using the superficial external jugular vein. Although it is possible to cannulate the deeper central veins, this technique is reserved for use by qualified medical staff.

The dorsum of the hand and forearm

The veins in the upper limb appear at first to be very variable in their layout, but certain common arrangements are found.
The veins draining the fingers unite to form three *dorsal metacarpal veins*. Laterally these are joined by veins from the thumb and continue up the radial border of the forearm as the *cephalic vein* (Figure 6.1).
Medially the metacarpal veins unite with the veins from the little finger and pass up the ulnar border or forearm as the *basilic vein*. There is often a large vein in the middle of the ventral (anterior) aspect of the forearm, the *median vein of the forearm* (Figure 6.2).

The antecubital fossa

Although the veins in this area are prominent and easily cannulated, there are many adjacent vital structures which can be easily damaged.
The cephalic vein passes through the antecubital fossa on the lateral side, and the basilic vein enters the antecubital fossa medially, just in front of the medial epicondyle of the elbow.

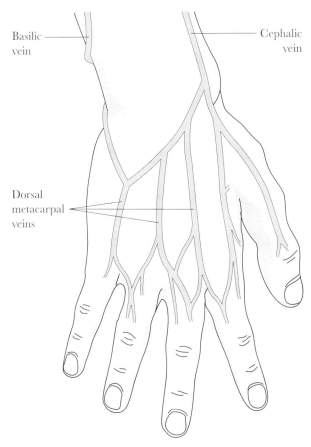

Basilic vein

Cephalic vein

Dorsal metacarpal veins

Fig. 6.1 *Veins of the hand and forearm*

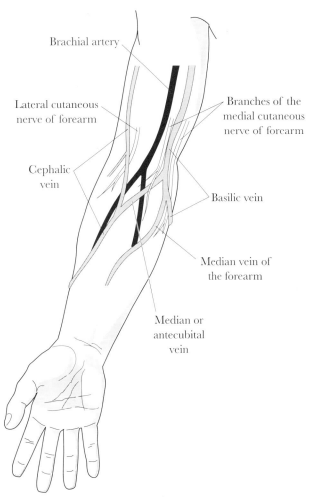

Brachial artery

Lateral cutaneous nerve of forearm

Cephalic vein

Branches of the medial cutaneous nerve of forearm

Basilic vein

Median vein of the forearm

Median or antecubital vein

Fig. 6.2 *Veins and other structures of the forearm and antecubital fossa*

These two large veins are joined by the *median cubital* or *antecubital vein*. The median vein of the forearm also drains into the basilic vein (Figure 6.2).

Other structures of importance

- The brachial artery lies beneath the median cubital vein, deep to the biceps tendon, and can be felt pulsating beneath this vein
- Medial to the brachial artery is the median nerve
- Branches of the medial cutaneous nerve of the forearm lie adjacent to the basilic vein and the lateral cutaneous nerve of forearm lies adjacent to the cephalic vein

The ankle

The most accessible vein in the ankle region is the long saphenous vein. It is consistent in its location, found 2 cm in front and 2 cm above the medial malleolus in adults (Figure 6.3). It is associated closely with the saphenous nerve.

The neck

Although there are many large veins in the neck, the most easily identified and accessible is the external jugular vein. This begins at the angle of the mandible and runs downwards and forwards to pass behind the middle of the clavicle (Figure 6.4). The vein is relatively superficial, covered only by a thin sheet of muscle (platysma), fascia and skin. Its use would be precluded by the application of a semi-rigid collar.

EQUIPMENT

A variety of devices of different lengths and diameters are used to secure venous access. The term 'cannula' is here used for those of 7 cm or less in length, and 'catheter' for those longer

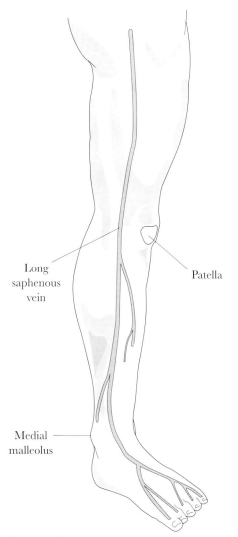

Fig. 6.3 *The long saphenous vein*

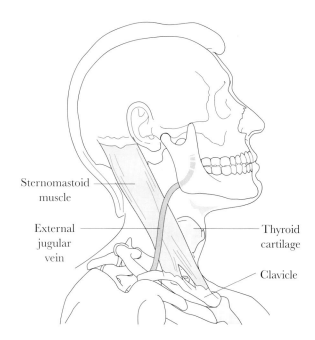

Fig. 6.4 *The right external jugular vein*

than 7 cm. The outside diameter of the device is often quoted in terms of its 'gauge'. Diameter increases with decreasing gauge. The external diameter is frequently quoted in millimetres.

Cannulae

Three types of cannulae are commonly used to secure venous access.

Metal needle (butterfly) cannula
The 'butterfly' cannula consists of a short metal needle with two flexible plastic wings attached (Figure 6.5A); a variety of diameters (19–25 G) is available. Although popular in the past, especially for use in small veins or for administering drugs, these

devices are no longer widely used. Because the cannula is entirely metal with a sharpened end to allow skin and vein puncture at insertion, it can tear the vein subsequently if it moves about, resulting in loss of access, haemorrhage and potential damage to surrounding structures.

Cannula over needle
The cannula over needle (e.g. Venflon) system is the most popular device in the UK for achieving intravenous access and is available in a wide variety of sizes, from 12 G to 27 G. It consists of a plastic (PTFE or similar material) cannula which is mounted on a smaller diameter metal needle, the bevel of which protrudes from the cannula. The other end of the needle is attached to a transparent 'flashback' chamber, which fills with blood indicating that the needle bevel lies within the vein (Figure 6.5B). Some devices have flanges or wings to facilitate attachment to the skin (Figure 6.5C). All cannulae have a standard Luer connector for attaching a giving set and some have a valved injection port through which drugs can be administered (Figure 6.5D).

Seldinger needle
The principle of the Seldinger technique is to puncture the skin with a small needle, then to introduce a blunt, flexible guide wire into the vein through the needle. Finally, a relatively large cannula is inserted over a dilator into the vein over the guide wire after the needle has been withdrawn. The technique can therefore be used to allow the insertion of a large-diameter catheter without having to use a large-diameter needle (Figure 6.5E).

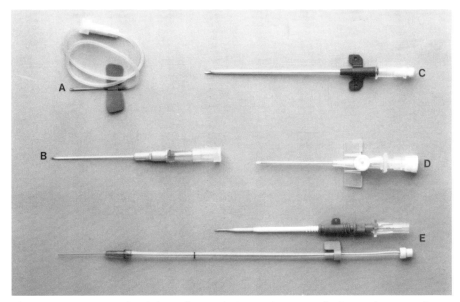

Fig. 6.5 *Intravenous cannulae. A, butterfly cannula; B, cannula over needle; C, cannula over needle with wings; D, cannula with injection port; E, Seldinger needle*

The Seldinger technique is not currently recommended for pre-hospital use, although it is common in the accident and emergency department.

TECHNIQUE

The superficial veins are situated immediately under the skin in the superficial fascia along with a variable amount of subcutaneous fat. The veins are relatively mobile within this layer and are also capable of considerable variation in their diameter. These details are of particular importance when it comes to inserting an intravenous cannula. The size of cannula used will depend upon its purpose: large ones are required for rapid fluid administration, smaller ones for drug administration.

In principle the largest cannula possible should be inserted. There is no point, however, in attempting to insert a large cannula into a very small vein. If the only visible or accessible vein is small, insert a *small* cannula; subsequent infusion of fluid with or without a tourniquet will enable a larger vein to fill and be cannulated.

> As with any procedure where there is a risk of contact with body fluids, gloves should be worn by the operator

Cannula over Needle

1. Choose a vein capable of accommodating the size of cannula needed, preferably one that is both visible and palpable (Figure 6.6). The junction of two veins is often a

good site as the 'target' is larger. If possible avoid veins over joints or those distal to fractures.

2. Encourage the vein to dilate as this increases the success rate of cannulation. In the limb veins this is usually achieved by using a tourniquet which stops venous return from the limb, but permits arterial flow into the limb. Further dilatation can be encouraged by gently tapping the skin over the vein. In the patient who is cold and vaso-constricted, topical application of heat from a towel soaked in warm water can also be useful, if time and facilities permit. If it is safe to do so, the patient can be tipped slightly head-down to encourage the external jugular vein to dilate.

3. The skin over the vein should be cleaned. Ensure there is no risk of allergy if iodine-based agents are used. If

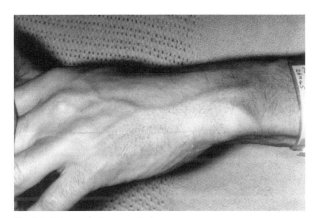

Fig. 6.6 *Vein ready for cannulation*

alcohol-based agents are used, they must be given time to work (2–3 minutes), ensuring that the skin is dry before proceeding further. This is not appropriate when rapid access is needed, such as during a cardiac arrest.

4. The vein should now be immobilized to prevent it being displaced by the advancing cannula. This is achieved by pulling the skin over the vein tight, with the operator's free hand (Figure 6.7).

5. Holding the cannula firmly, at an angle of 10–15 degrees to the skin, advance it through the skin and into the vein. Often a slight loss of resistance is felt as the vein is entered. This should be accompanied by the appearance of blood in the flashback chamber of the cannula (Figure 6.8). However, the appearance of blood indicates only that the tip of the needle is within the vein, not necessarily any of the plastic cannula.

6. While keeping the skin taut, the next step is to reduce the angle of the cannula slightly and advance it a further 2–3 mm into the vein. This is to ensure that the first part of the plastic cannula lies within the vein. Care must be taken at this point not to push the needle out of the back of the vein.

7. The needle is now withdrawn 5–10 mm into the cannula so that the point no longer protrudes from the end. As this is done, blood will often be seen to flow between the needle body and the cannula, confirming that the tip of the cannula is within the vein (Figure 6.9).

8. The cannula and needle are advanced along the vein together. The needle is retained within the cannula to provide support and prevent kinking at the point of skin puncture (Figure 6.10).

9. Once the cannula is inserted as far as the hub, the tourniquet should be released, and the needle completely removed and disposed of safely.

10. Confirmation that the cannula lies within the vein should be made by injection of a saline flush or by attaching an intravenous infusion where appropriate. The tissues

around the site must be observed for any signs of swelling that may indicate that the cannula is incorrectly positioned. Finally, the cannula should be secured using adhesive tape (e.g. Elastoplast) or a specific cannula dressing (e.g. Vecafix).

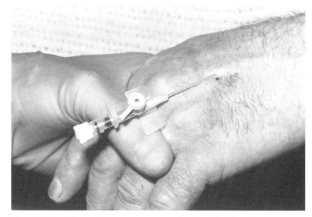

Fig. 6.8 *Inserting an intravenous cannula: the 'flashback'*

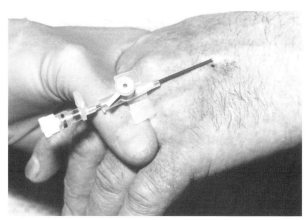

Fig. 6.9 *Inserting an intravenous cannula: withdrawing the needle*

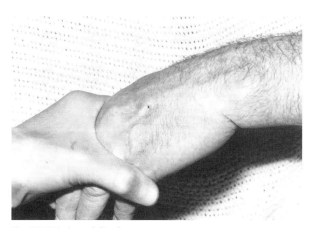

Fig. 6.7 *Vein immobilized*

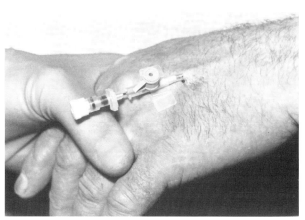

Fig. 6.10 *Inserting an intravenous cannula: the cannula inserted*

COMPLICATIONS

There are a large number of complications associated with venous cannulation. Most of them are minor; however, this must not be used as an excuse for carelessness and poor technique. The complications are conveniently divided into 'early' and 'late'.

Early Complications

Failure of cannulation
Failed cannulation is the most common complication. It usually occurs as a result of pushing the needle completely through the vein, and is due to inexperience. If possible, it is always best to start distally in a limb and work proximally. In this way, if further attempts are required, fluid or drugs will not leak from previous puncture sites.

Haematoma
Haematomas are usually secondary to failed cannulation when inadequate pressure has been applied to prevent blood leaking from the vein. They are made worse by forgetting to remove the tourniquet! Simply bending the arm is not adequate to prevent bleeding from a puncture site – direct local pressure is required.

Extravasation
Extravasation of fluid or drugs is commonly a result of failing to recognize that the cannula is not within the vein before beginning infusion. Placing a cannula over a joint or prolonged use to infuse fluids under pressure also predispose to leakage. Once the problem is identified, the cannula must no longer be used. Damage to the overlying tissues will depend primarily upon the nature of the extravasated fluid.

Damage to local structures
Damage to other local structures is secondary to poor technique and lack of knowledge of the local anatomy. This is seen most often in attempts to cannulate the external jugular vein.

Air embolus
Air embolus occurs when the pressure in the veins is lower than in the right side of the heart and air is entrained. It is usually prevented from occurring via the peripheral veins as they collapse when empty, but a cannula will splint the vein open. It is most likely to happen in the external jugular vein, particularly if the patient is in a head-up position. If unrecognized it can be fatal.

Breakage of the cannula
The plastic cannula can be sheared, allowing fragments to enter the circulation. This is usually a result of trying to reintroduce the needle into the cannula after it has been withdrawn. The safest action is to withdraw the whole cannula and attempt cannulation at another site with a new cannula.

Needle breakage
The needle may fracture as a result of careless, excessive manipulation with the finer cannulae. This complication requires surgical intervention to remove the fragment, but is fortunately very rare.

Late Complications

Inflammation of the vein, thrombophlebitis, is related to the length of time the vein is in use and irritation caused by the substances flowing through it. Drugs in high concentration and fluids with extremes of pH or high osmolality are the main causes. Once a vein shows signs of thrombophlebitis (tenderness, redness and deteriorating flow), the cannula must be removed to prevent subsequent infection or thrombosis which may spread proximally.

Infection, either local or systemic, is not a major problem when time is taken to clean the skin before cannulation.

INTRAOSSEOUS ACCESS

Percutaneous venous cannulation is often technically more difficult in children, particularly when they are critically ill. The intraosseous route has been demonstrated to provide rapid and effective access to the circulation in children. It allows the administration of fluids and drugs, with circulating levels of drugs being comparable to those achieved when given via a central vein. Furthermore, aspirated marrow can be used to cross-match blood in the absence of a blood sample. It is a technique most suited to children less than 6 years old, as beyond this age the vascular red marrow is gradually replaced by fatty yellow marrow.

Anatomy

The proximal tibia in the lower limb is the most commonly used site for intraosseous access, alternatives being the distal tibia and distal femur. Occasionally none of these sites is possible, and the upper limb can be used.

The lower limb
Three sites can be used for intraosseous access (Figure 6.11).

- The antero-medial surface of the tibia, 2–3 cm below the tibial tuberosity
- The distal tibia, just proximal to the medial malleolus
- The anterior surface of the femur, 3 cm above the lateral condyle

These sites are relatively free of other local important structures. The most relevant feature to be borne in mind is the

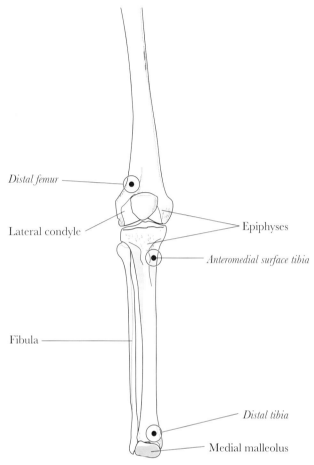

Fig. 6.11 Sites for intraosseous access in the lower limb

Labels: *Distal femur*, Lateral condyle, Epiphyses, *Anteromedial surface tibia*, Fibula, *Distal tibia*, Medial malleolus

proximity of the epiphyses (growth plates). Damage to these could interfere with subsequent bone growth and development.

The upper limb

The upper limb site is the distal humerus, just proximal to the lateral epicondyle.

Equipment

Although bone marrow biopsy needles can be used, needles specifically produced for intraosseous access are now available. As they have to pierce the bone cortex they are made entirely of metal. They come in a variety of designs, but they all have certain features in common. The needles have a short shaft, with a central solid trocar, which has a large handle attached. The trocar must be unscrewed before it can be removed from the needle. The external end of the needle has a standard Luer fitting. Some needles have a screw thread to improve their security in the bone (Figure 6.12).

Intraosseous needles come in a range of sizes

- 16–20 G for children younger than 18 months
- 12–16 G for children older than 18 months

Technique

1. An appropriate site is chosen, taking care to avoid placing the needle in a fractured bone or distal to fractures in the same limb. If the proximal tibia is used, it may help to place a firm support behind the knee.
2. If time permits, the skin over the site should be thoroughly cleaned. If the patient is conscious, local anaesthetic solution should be infiltrated into the skin and underlying periosteum.
3. The needle is then introduced at 90 degrees through the skin to make contact with the bone and then advanced using a twisting action, at the same time applying firm pressure.
4. A loss of resistance is felt as the cortex is penetrated and the marrow cavity entered. The needle should feel to be 'gripped' by the bone and hold its position once released (Figure 6.13).
5. The trocar is unscrewed and removed, and correct placement confirmed by the ability to aspirate bone marrow. Further confirmation is provided by being able to flush 5 ml of saline through the needle without resistance or signs of extravasation.

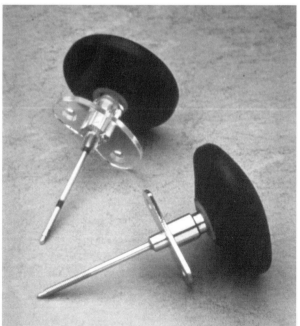

Fig. 6.12 Intraosseous needles

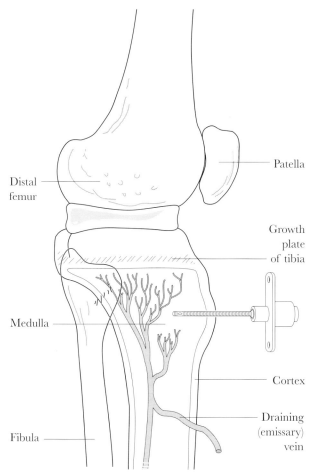

Fig. 6.13 An intraosseous needle in place in the proximal tibia

Labels: Distal femur, Medulla, Fibula, Patella, Growth plate of tibia, Cortex, Draining (emissary) vein

Complications

Complications are fortunately very rare and are mainly theoretical.

- Failure to enter the bone marrow cavity is the most common problem. This may occur more often when the distal femur is used, owing to the difficulty in identifying the correct landmarks

- If the needle is incorrectly placed, fluid may extravasate and prolonged infusion could cause a compartment syndrome. A second attempt at placement in the same bone will result, if successful, in leakage from the hole left by the previous attempt
- Infection in the skin, abscess formation and ultimately osteomyelitis may occur, but these complications appear to be related to prolonged use of a needle
- Fat and marrow emboli can occur, particularly if excessive pressure is used to infuse drugs or fluid
- Damage to the growth plate of the bone could happen as a result of careless placement, and in very young children a fracture could occur if excessive force is used

Intraosseous access to the circulation is a life-saving procedure and not a definitive route for resuscitation of a sick child. Once alternative routes of venous access have been achieved, the intraosseous needle should be removed.

FLUID FLOW THROUGH CANNULAE AND CATHETERS

There are four factors that affect the rate at which fluid will flow through a cannula or catheter (Table 6.1):

- *The diameter*: this is the most important factor, with flow theoretically being proportional to the fourth power of the radius. This means that doubling the diameter should result in flow increasing sixteen-fold (2^4). This is rarely achieved in practice, but an increase of four-fold to five-fold can be expected
- *The length*: flow is inversely proportional to the length of the cannula, therefore doubling the length will halve the flow
- *The viscosity of the fluid*: flow is inversely proportional to the viscosity, therefore increasing viscosity reduces flow. Hence colloids and blood flow much more slowly than a crystalloid, particularly when they are cold
- *The pressure applied*: increasing the pressure across the cannula will increase the flow. This is usually achieved by increasing the pressure of the fluid being administered,

Table 6.1 Rate of water flow through different sizes of Venflon cannulae

Colour	Diameter (mm)	Gauge	Length (mm)	Flow (ml/min)
Pink	1.0	20	32	54
Green	1.2	18	45	80
Grey	1.7	16	45	180
Brown	2.0	14	45	270

either by raising the height of the drip above the patient or by using external pressure

All these factors are related by *Poiseuille's law.*

Flow Through Intraosseous Needles

Using gravity alone, with a 1 metre head of pressure, the flow through intraosseous needles is similar to that achieved through a cannula of the same diameter. Using a 16 G needle, a flow approaching 200 ml/min is possible. With small-diameter needles, fluid (and drugs) can be infused more rapidly by using a syringe and three-way tap.

FURTHER READING

Driscoll PA, Gwinnutt CL, Mackway-Jones K & Wieteska S, eds (1997) *Advanced Cardiac Life Support – The Practical Approach*, 2nd edn. London: Chapman & Hall (in press).

Evans RJ, McCabe M & Thomas R (1994) Intraosseous infusion. *British Journal of Hospital Medicine* 51: 161–164.

Handley AJ & Swain A, eds (1994) *Advanced Life Support Manual*. London: Resuscitation Council (UK).

Tonks A (1992) How to put up a drip. *Student British Medical Journal* 1: 57–59.

3

MEDICINE

chapter seven

TAKING A MEDICAL HISTORY

Obtaining a medical history is a core skill for any health-care professional. It takes practice, discipline and empathy for the patient, and it requires a structure. This structure serves two purposes. Firstly, it acts as an *aide-mémoire* so that the practitioner does not omit any vital questions or observations, and secondly, it facilitates the recording of the information in a way that will be accessible to other practitioners. Obtaining the medical history must not interfere with initial management priorities of airway, breathing and circulation. Assessment and immediate appropriate action for any compromise of airway, breathing or circulation must take place immediately. Some elements of the history can be obtained during this action but the priorities of opening an airway, establishing adequate ventilation and establishing adequate circulation to allow organ perfusion take precedence at all times.

This chapter describes a structure which is widely used in medicine and the allied professions. Obtaining a complete medical history in difficult circumstances in a time-efficient way takes practice. The skills of observation and retaining information until it can be written down must be practised over and over again until they become second nature.

In medical illness the history affords 70% of the information on which most diagnoses are made. If at the end of history-taking you do not have a list of differential diagnoses, then you probably never will have. It is much more important than physical examination in establishing a diagnosis.

Purpose of history-taking

- Establish what has happened (the history)
- Establish what the patient feels to be wrong (the symptoms)
- Establish the background to the current events (the past medical history)
- Help establish a list of possible diagnoses (the differential diagnosis)
- Help establish priorities for treatment

- Obtain information that will not be available later (e.g. from the scene)
- Establish a baseline from which subsequent monitoring can start (e.g. of the conscious level)

STRUCTURE OF THE HISTORY

While at the scene a detailed history is not usually appropriate. A brief outline history is ample – and 'AMPLE' is a useful mnemonic to remember what constitutes an adequate history from the scene.

A > Allergies: in all emergencies other than cardiac arrest it is important to try to establish any known allergies before drugs are administered

M > Medicines: the presence of medications in the blood stream may influence the response to injury or illness or to any other drugs which may be given. A knowledge of what medication the patient has been taking gives an indication as to the severity and duration of any pre-existing illness

P > Past medical history: this has a major bearing on responses to treatment and possible outcomes from illness or injury. It also offers vital clues as to what may be the current problem. Make particular note of any known cardiac disease, respiratory disease or diabetes

L > Last food and drink: a full stomach is a major risk factor for regurgitation

E > Events leading up to the current problem: this is the core of the history. The other elements are important but this is the key to understanding what is happening to the patient now

You do not need to go through the questions in the order in which they appear above. The events leading up to the current problem and the past medical history are usually the first two to be addressed. Not all of the information needs to be acquired at the scene. Some of it can be acquired *en route*.

SOURCES OF INFORMATION

The Scene

Gleaning information from the scene of an illness requires the practitioner to be a trained observer. If you do not specifically look for something then you are unlikely to see it. Two pairs of eyes are better than one. If you have a colleague with you then his or her observations should be collated with your own before they are recorded. There may be vital clues at the scene and only you have the chance of interpreting them and carrying the information to those who will be subsequently caring for the patient. The following is an example of a scenario and the information that may be gleaned from it.

You are called to a patient lying ill in bed:
  are the patient and the surroundings clean and tidy?
  are there carers present?
  is it an environment to which a patient could return?
  are there bottles of medication which could be taken to the hospital?
  are there empty pill bottles indicating the nature of a possible overdose?
  is there evidence of alcohol or drug abuse?
  if the patient is unconscious are there any clues at the scene that might help establish the duration or cause of the unconsciousness?

The Patient

Whenever dealing with a conscious patient, direct your opening questions to the patient, even if he or she appears confused or aggressive. The response to initial questioning may or may not be meaningful but will give information as to the degree of cooperation you can expect with subsequent questions. If you establish no meaningful response then turn to bystanders or witnesses for further information.

The Witnesses

Even if the patient is conscious and cooperative, witnesses may help with information about the mechanism of injury not necessarily known to the patient. If the patient is unconscious then ask witnesses for the duration of the unconsciousness and specifically ask if the patient is getting worse, getting better or staying the same.

Some witnesses or bystanders may know the patient and be able to give background information.

Medical Information Devices

Only a few patients in this country wear Medic-Alert bracelets or necklaces but they are always worth looking for. Horse riders often carry medical information in a recess inside their crash-helmet.

Many patients have lists of medication on their person.

THE ART OF QUESTIONING

Obtaining information from frightened, ill or injured patients is made easier by a positive, confident and friendly approach. Try to make sure that the patient can see you before you speak. Patients who are confused or deaf may be reassured more by a smile than by the words that are spoken.

Introduce yourself early in your approach. Tell the patient your name and who you are, and that you are there to help.

Establish the patient's name and age and then use the name during your conversation. Whenever possible position yourself at the same level as the patient; for example, kneel beside a patient who is lying on the floor. Make sure you are in a position so that you can maintain eye contact. These manoeuvres take seconds but help establish empathy with the patient and make it likely that your subsequent questions will be answered helpfully.

The questions which you ask will be dictated by the circumstances. Assessment and correction of any problems in airway, breathing and circulation will take priority. The circumstances and the urgency which you perceive around the situation will dictate how many questions you need to ask at the scene, how many can be asked *en route* and how many will need to be left to the hospital staff.

In general terms you should start your questioning with broad, open questions, e.g.

  '*Tell me what's the matter*'. Questions such as this allow patients to express what they perceive to be wrong. You can follow up an open question with a more focused question. For instance, if the answer to the question above is, 'I've got a pain in my chest', then the next question might be along the lines of, 'Tell me about the pain'. If, after the patient has volunteered more information, you still need more detail then questions can become more focused, as follows:

  '*What's the pain like?*'
  '*How long have you had it?*'
  '*Have you ever had a pain like this before?*'

The transition from open questions to more focused questions is dictated by the knowledge of what information you need to glean to help with your decision-making in any given clinical situation. Knowing the right questions to ask requires a thorough knowledge of the conditions in your differential diagnosis. It requires discipline to remember all the answers so that you can formulate them into a chronological statement of what the patient has told you. Be careful not to change the history as you write it down. Whenever possible use the patient's own expressions in inverted commas to describe the symptoms.

PASSING ON THE INFORMATION

The key points of the history should be recorded with brevity and clarity. In many situations a printed form assists recording of the history and findings at the scene. Such documentation makes it easier for subsequent carers to refer back to information that might be lost if it is not recorded and kept with the patient.

Another way to transmit information is by telling the receiving doctor, or other professional, what you have found. This can be done succinctly and quickly, but summarizing all that you have found takes practice and discipline. The summary should include the patient's name (if known), the patient's age (if known), the events surrounding the involvement of the emer-gency medical services and any past history you have been able to glean. Most people cannot receive more information than that at the early part of the hand-over. Many receiving rooms have a chalkboard or flipchart on which pre-hospital personnel can record information that may be useful later. The receiving doctor or other professionals usually have more time to receive information after they have completed the primary survey, which may only take a very few minutes. It can be helpful if pre-hospital personnel are actively involved in the hand-over and do not leave until they have handed on all the information that they think is relevant to the case. A copy of the pre-hospital record must accompany the inpatient notes to allow a holistic picture of the injury or illness to be recorded.

FURTHER READING

Munro (1996) *Macleod's Clinical Examination*. Edinburgh: Churchill Livingstone.

chapter eight:

INTRODUCTION TO PHARMACOLOGY

This chapter provides an overview of pharmacology for the pre-hospital provider. The first section addresses general issues and definitions relating to pharmacology, the second is a list of drugs commonly used in pre-hospital care. Every effort has been made to avoid the complex mathematical models that all too often alienate the reader and taint their view of pharmacology.

WHAT IS A DRUG?

Put simply, drugs are chemicals that have a variety of effects on the function of the body. Pharmacology is the study of drugs and their effects; it is subdivided into *pharmacokinetics* – the study of how a drug passes into, around and out of the body – and *pharmacodynamics* – the study of the biochemical and physiological effects the drug produces.

WHERE DO DRUGS COME FROM?

There are many sources of drugs. Some drugs are derived from plants (e.g. atropine from deadly nightshade), others exist as natural minerals (e.g. sodium bicarbonate). Many drugs, however, have been specifically designed and chemically engineered, a process that may take some 20 years at a cost of many millions of pounds to the drug company.

WHICH ORGANIZATION REGULATES DRUGS?

The body responsible for the licensing of drugs in the UK is the Department of Health. Before a drug is allowed on the commercial market it must undergo a period of intense research. The safety profile of a drug is established using both animal and human studies. Eventually a drug may be granted a Product Licence, allowing the drug to be legally sold. Such licences are granted country by country, so a drug that may be used on a day-to-day basis in Great Britain may not be legally allowed in the USA.

Depending on the drug's safety record and potency, it may be given one of several legal categories. Although there are many categories, they can essentially be divided into those medicines that do not require a prescription (e.g. aspirin or paracetamol) and those that have to be prescribed by a doctor (e.g. adrenaline or atropine). The latter drugs are called Prescription Only Medicines (POM).

HOW CAN PRE-HOSPITAL PROVIDERS PRESCRIBE POM?

The use of POMs in the UK is controlled under the Medicines Act of 1968. Under this Act exemption is given to suitably trained ambulance personnel to use specified drugs without consultation with a doctor or dentist. The list was compiled by the Joint Colleges and Ambulance Service Liaison Committee (JCALC), a group of doctors who advise the government on the medical aspects of ambulance service provision.

WHY SO MANY NAMES?

Each drug has several 'names'. The first of these, the *chemical name*, describes the drug's chemical structure. It is often too long and unwieldy to use on a day-to-day basis, and hence each drug is given a simplified version known as its *generic name*. As different drug companies will sell the same drug in a competitive market, each company will give the drug a third or *trade name* that identifies it to their company. Hence for metoclopramide, a drug commonly used with morphine to prevent nausea, the following names exist:

> chemical name – 4-amino-5-chloro-*N*-[2-(diethylamino)ethyl]
> 1-2-methoxybenzamide
> generic name – metoclopramide
> trade names – Maxolon, Primperan

PHARMACOKINETICS

Pharmacokinetics is the study of how drugs pass into, around and out of the body. For a drug to have a desired effect it should:

- Reach its target organ in a timely manner
- Reach its target organ in an appropriate dose
- Reach its target organ in active form
- Stay at the target organ for an appropriate period of time

These elements of the pharmacokinetic process are described in more detail below.

Modes of Administration

The route by which a drug is delivered should be considered carefully for several reasons. Firstly, the speed with which a drug has its effect can be drastically altered. For example, drugs given by the oral route in cardiac arrest would be patently useless as the process of absorption from the gastrointestinal tract is far too slow. Secondly, the metabolism of a drug may be different with different routes. For example, lignocaine when given orally is absorbed through the gut and passes to the liver before entering the central circulation. In the liver it is metabolized to a functionless state and rendered useless. To have an effect it must therefore be given intravenously when it can pass directly to its site of action at the heart.

The routes of drug administration are either *enteral* (i.e. via the alimentary tract – oral, rectal or sublingual) or *parenteral* (not via the alimentary tract – intravenous, intramuscular, subcutaneous).

Enteral routes

Oral The oral route is the most common and convenient method of administration. It is often the cheapest and simplest, with little risk of infection. Effects are seen some 30–45 minutes after administration.

Rectal Drugs may be given rectally in the form of suppositories or tubes. This method is ideally suited to patients who are nauseated, unconscious or unable to swallow. Effects are seen 5–15 minutes after administration.

Sublingual Tablets may dissolve or an aerosol may be sprayed under the tongue. The effect is rapid, in 2–3 minutes. This route is ideal where rapid and routine prescription is required, where patients are unable to swallow or where they are nauseated.

Parenteral routes

Dermal patches Patches impregnated with drug are placed on the skin and the drug absorbed through the layers of the skin. Ideal for drugs that can be given slowly and that are rapidly inactivated (metabolized) when they enter the body.

Intradermal The intradermal route involves injection directly into the layers of the skin. Absorption is slow. This method is most commonly used for allergy testing.

Subcutaneous Injection of drug into the fatty tissue beneath the skin leads to slower absorption than that of intravenous or intramuscular injection. It is an ideal method for drugs that can have drastic consequences if given too quickly, such as in anaphylactic shock or severe asthma where adrenaline is needed but rapid administration may cause a fatal arrhythmia.

Intramuscular The intramuscular (IM) route involves injection into muscle tissue where the blood supply absorbs the drug. This is a simple technique requiring less training than the administration of an intravenous injection. Absorption is slower than intravenous administration but faster than subcutaneous. The advantages are similar to subcutaneous injection.

Intravenous Either as a slow intravenous (IV) injection or as an infusion where a drug is diluted in a bag of fluid. This method has the fastest rate of absorption, and consequently also the highest risk of infection and side-effects.

Endotracheal The endotracheal route permits rapid absorption; it is useful when rapid administration is required and IV access is difficult or unobtainable. Drugs are injected via an endotracheal tube at double the usual dose.

Inhaled or nebulized Administration of drugs as fine droplets in oxygen or air gives rapid effects, occurring in minutes.

Sublingual injection Sublingual injection is a rapid absorption method that can be utilized when neither an IV injection nor an endotracheal tube can be placed.

Intracardiac (ventricular) The intracardiac route has the advantage of rapid absorption, but is plagued by many complications including damage to the heart and its blood vessels. It is of potential use during cardiac arrest when intubation and IV placement have failed.

Distribution

Once in the body a drug may pass to many tissues. This is termed its *distribution*. In a perfect world a drug would go to the one organ where its effect is desired. In reality, however, a drug may be widely distributed throughout the body with the ever-existing threat of side-effects. An example of this is seen with lignocaine, where an excess dose affects the brain and may result in seizures.

Bioavailability

After a drug has been administered the body may change the drug's chemical structure. This may have the effect of switching the drug off or turning it on. How much drug is finally available to do its 'work' is termed its *bioavailability*. The example has already been given of how an oral dose of lignocaine is rendered ineffective by the liver. In contrast, diazepam is an example of a drug that is chemically changed to become more active once it is within the body.

Clearance or Elimination

Eventually each drug is removed or eliminated from the body, via the kidneys into urine, via the liver into bile, via the lungs into the air or via the intestine into faeces. Failure of any of these organs can allow drug concentrations to rise to toxic levels.

PHARMACODYNAMICS

In order for a drug to produce an effect, be it desired (therapeutic effect) or undesired (side-effect), it must interact with the body on a cellular or biochemical level. From this reaction there may be a biochemical or physiological change. For example, the binding of an adrenaline molecule to its specific cellular receptor and the consequent change in heart rate or blood pressure is an expression of the pharmacodynamic process.

Drugs may act through a variety of other mechanisms: they may prevent chemicals moving across cell walls, they may alter enzyme function or they may simply change the chemical characteristics of other body chemicals.

DRUG PROFILES

The following list of drugs does not include all the drugs used in pre-hospital care but does include many that are named in the Medicines Act 1968 and its subsequent revisions. Where possible each drug is addressed in a broad context, allowing for a more complete understanding of its action. However, it should be remembered that local protocols should be strictly adhered to.

Adrenaline

- *Class*
  sympathomimetic

- *Action*
  increases heart rate
  increases blood pressure
  increases myocardial contraction force
  bronchodilation

- *Kinetics*
  if given orally, rapidly metabolized to inactive form by gut and liver
  inactive form then excreted in urine

- *Indications*
  cardiac arrest

- *Other uses*
  anaphylaxis
  hypotension
  severe asthma

- *Side-effects* (dose-related)
  tachycardia
  hypertension
  anxiety
  pallor

- *Route of administration*
  IV, IM, endotracheal

- *Dosage*
  give 1 mg during cardiac arrest; repeat according to advanced life support (ALS) protocol
  double dose if given by endotracheal route

Aspirin

Aspirin is contraindicated in children as it is associated with the development of Reye's syndrome.

- *Class*
  painkiller
  antithrombotic (prevents or limits formation of a blood clot)

- *Action*
  antiplatelet activity limits formation of clots
  decreased perception of pain
  antipyretic (lowers temperature)

- *Kinetics*
  well absorbed orally
  metabolized in blood and liver
  excreted by kidney

- *Indications*
  possible myocardial infarction

- *Contraindications*
  known hypersensitivity
  children < 12 years (see above)
  patients on anticoagulants
  patients with known clotting disorders
  pregnancy

- *Other uses*
  pain relief
  prevention of strokes

- *Side-effects*
  gastric irritation
  bronchospasm

- *Route of administration*
  oral

- *Dosage*
  75–600 mg

Atropine

- *Class*
  anticholinergic

- *Action*
  increases heart rate

- *Kinetics*
  rapidly metabolized by the liver if given orally, therefore given parenterally

- *Indications*
  bradycardia with associated hypotension

- *Side-effects*
  dilation of pupils and blurred vision
  dry mouth
  urine retention
  confusion

- *Route of administration*
  IV, endotracheal (requires double dose)

- *Dosage*
  bradycardia – 500 μg repeated if required
  cardiac arrest – 3 mg according to ALS protocol

Diazepam

- *Class*
  benzodiazepine sedative

- *Action*
  anticonvulsant
  skeletal muscle relaxant
  sedation

- *Kinetics*
  can be given orally
  chemically modified to a more active form and eventually degraded by the liver
  poorly absorbed if given IM, therefore if given parenterally better given IV

- *Indications*
  seizure

- *Contraindications*
  known hypersensitivity

- *Other uses*
  muscle relaxation
  sedation

- *Side-effects*
  local irritation if given at injection site
  decreased level of consciousness
  hypotension
  decreased respiratory rate

- *Route of administration*
  IV, per rectum, oral
  Note: intravenous diazepam should be given as diazepam emulsion (Diazemuls) a non-irritant white suspension, and in aliquots of no more than 5 mg

- *Dosage*
  adult   5–10 mg slow IV injection, repeated if necessary
            10 mg per rectum, repeated if necessary
  child (under 3 years old): 5 mg per rectum

Ergometrine

- *Class*
  oxytocic (uterus-stimulating) agent

- *Action*
  uterine contraction
  lactation

- *Kinetics*
  naturally occurring body hormone
  if given orally digested by gut enzymes, therefore given parenterally
  once in the body metabolized in blood, kidney and liver to inactive form

- *Indications*
  postpartum bleeding

- *Side-effects*
  anaphylaxis
  cardiac arrhythmias
  abdominal pain
  nausea and vomiting

- *Route of administration*
  IV, IM, subcutaneous, nasal

- *Dosage*
  250 μg IV

Glucagon

Glucagon is the drug of choice in the pre-hospital treatment of hypoglycaemia.

- *Class*
  antihypoglycaemic agent

- *Action*
  breaks down glycogen (a reserve form of glucose found in the liver and other tissues), raising blood glucose levels
  increases heart rate
  increases myocardial contractility

- *Kinetics*
  naturally occurring body hormone
  digested by gut hormones if given orally
  metabolized in blood, kidney and liver

- *Indications*
  suspected hypoglycaemia

- *Contraindications*
  known hypersensitivity

- *Other uses*
  treatment of beta-blocker overdose

- *Side-effects*
  few in emergency situation

- *Route of administration*
  IV, intradermal

- *Dosage*
  adult: 1.0 mg IM
  child: 0.5 mg IM

Glyceryl trinitrate

Glyceryl trinitrate (GTN, occasionally called 'TNT' by patients!) may be given as tablets or as an aerosol spray. The spray has a much longer shelf-life and is therefore more suitable for occasional use.

- *Class*
  vasodilator

- *Action*
  dilates coronary arteries
  reduces cardiac workload by dilating veins and arteries

- *Kinetics*
  metabolized by the liver if given orally
  given sublingually or intravenously if rapid effect desired

- *Indications*
  angina

- *Contraindications*
  severe hypotension

- *Other uses*
  heart failure

- *Side-effects*
  hypotension
  headache

- *Route of administration*
  IV, sublingual, transdermal, oral

- *Dosage*
  400 µg sublingual, repeated as necessary

Heparin solution

- *Class*
  anticoagulant

- *Action*
  prevents formation of blood clot

- *Kinetics*
  because of its chemical structure heparin is not absorbed by the gut, therefore it requires SC or IV administration
  eventually metabolized by the liver and excreted in the urine

- *Indications*
  priming of intravenous cannulae when fluids are not being used

- *Contraindications*
  known hypersensivity

- *Other uses*
  prevention of clot formation in cases of venous thrombosis, or artificial valves

- *Side-effects*
  haemorrhage

- *Route of administration*
  IV, SC

- *Dosage*
  10 units in 1 ml IV, repeated if necessary as flush

Lignocaine

- *Class*
  antiarrhythmic

- *Action*
  suppresses ventricular ectopy
  reduces fibrillation threshold
  slows conduction of impulses through the Purkinje system

- *Kinetics*
  if given orally, metabolized to inactive form by the liver
  inactive metabolites then excreted in urine

- *Pre-hospital indications*
  ventricular fibrillation
  ventricular tachycardia

- *Contraindications*
  patients in heart block
  premature ventricular contraction with bradycardia

- *Other uses*
  local anaesthetic

- *Side effects* (dose-related)
  central nervous system toxicity producing nausea,
    vomiting, drowsiness, seizures
  bradycardia
  hypotension

- *Route of administration*
  IV, IM, endotracheal

- *Dosage*
  100 mg IV bolus, repeated if necessary
  double dose if given by endotracheal route

Nalbuphine

Nalbuphine may reduce the effectiveness of subsequent opiate or opioid analgesics; medical staff must therefore be clearly informed that it has been given.

- *Class*
  synthetic analgesic

- *Action*
  central nervous system depressant
  pain relief

- *Indications*
  moderate to severe pain

- *Contraindications*
  opiate dependency
  pregnancy
  decreased level of consciousness
  impaired respiration

- *Side-effects*
  decreased level of consciousness
  nausea and vomiting

- *Route of administration*
  IV, IM

- *Dosage*
  10 mg slow IV injection
  repeated if necessary

Naloxone

- *Class*
  opiate antagonist

- *Action*
  in the context of opiate excess will increase respiratory
    rate and level of consciousness

- *Kinetics*
  rapidly metabolized by liver if given orally
  requires prescription if given parenterally

- *Indications*
  opiate excess

- *Contraindications*
  known hypersensitivity

- *Precautions*
  may precipitate a withdrawal syndrome in those
    dependent on opiates
  duration of action short (minutes); repeated doses may
    therefore be necessary

- *Route of administration*
  IV, IM

- *Dosage*
  400 µg IV, repeated if necessary

Nitrous oxide

Nitrous oxide (N_2O) is normally used in the form of Entonox, an equal mixture of nitrous oxide and oxygen. It is an effective analgesic if given in adequate doses; asking the patient to take a few breaths before a manipulation will not be effective. Nitrous oxide is extremely soluble and will diffuse rapidly into any gas-filled cavity; it may thus increase the size of a pneumothorax. Nitrous oxide is therefore contraindicated if there is any possibility of a pneumothorax. At temperatures below −6°C Entonox may separate into nitrous oxide and oxygen. Bottles should therefore be shaken thoroughly and used in a horizontal position. Under these conditions frosting may occur on the bottle, which should be kept away from the patient's skin.

Entonox should not be used in any patient (for example a victim of major trauma) who requires 100% oxygen, as its use reduces the inspired oxygen concentration to 50%. An alternative form of analgesia should be used, together with 100% oxygen by high-flow mask.

- *Class*
  anaesthetic gas

- *Action*
  central nervous system depression
  decreased sensitivity to pain

- *Kinetics*
  eliminated unchanged through lungs

- *Indications*
  moderate to severe pain

- *Contraindications*
  any possibility of pneumothorax
  gastrointestinal obstruction
  decompression sickness ('bends')

- *Side-effects*
  decreased level of consciousness
  nausea, vomiting

- *Route of administration*
  inhalation

- *Dosage*
  self-administered

Oxygen

Under normal conditions the stimulus to breathe is paradoxically the amount of carbon dioxide in the blood, and not a deficit of oxygen. In patients with chronic obstructive pulmonary disease (COPD), however, the stimulus to breathing is a deficit of oxygen as the poor function of their lungs has produced high levels of CO_2 in the blood for a long period of time. If these patients are given high quantities of oxygen they will stop breathing, CO_2 levels will rise and the blood will turn acidic rendering the patient unconscious and at risk of cardiac arrhythmias. (Under normal conditions the kidneys of COPD patients can remove or compensate for excess CO_2, but this process takes days.)

- *Class*
  odourless, tasteless gas

- *Action*
  essential component of the chemical reaction that occurs in all cells and supports life
  combines with glucose to liberate energy and carbon dioxide

- *Indications*
  hypoxia

- *Contraindications*
  patients with COPD (see above)

- *Side-effect*
  respiratory arrest in COPD patients

- *Route of administration*
  inhaled

- *Dosage*
  trauma patients: 100% via non-rebreathing reservoir masks
  asthma patients: 100% via non-rebreathing reservoir masks
  COPD patients: 28% via appropriate mask (except in life-threatening trauma when 100% should be given)

Salbutamol

- Class
  selective sympathomimetic

- *Action*
  reverses bronchospasm

- *Indications*
  asthma
  COPD

- *Side-effects*
  tremor
  palpitations
  tachycardia

- *Route of administration*
  inhaled as nebulized solution, IV, oral

- *Dosage*
  adult: 5 mg as nebulized solution, repeated as necessary
  child (under 5 years old): 2.5 mg as nebulized solution, repeated as necessary

chapter nine:

RESPIRATORY EMERGENCIES

Respiratory emergencies arise commonly, and all paramedics should be able to deal with them quickly and effectively. Delays in diagnosis and treatment can lead to the patient's death.

Common life-threatening respiratory problems

- Asthma
- Pulmonary oedema
- Airway obstruction
- Anaphylaxis
- Chronic obstructive pulmonary disease

ANATOMY OF THE RESPIRATORY TRACT

Trachea

The anatomy of the upper airway has already been described in Chapter 4. Below the level of the cricoid cartilage, the airway continues as the trachea. This is a flexible tube which is strengthened by incomplete hoops of cartilage and is lined with mucous membrane. In the chest the trachea divides into two main bronchi, one going to either lung (Figure 9.1). The right one lies more vertically and so receives most of the foreign objects that manage to overcome all the defences in the upper airway. The bronchi subsequently divide, much like a tree, into smaller and smaller branches. Ultimately small branches known as respiratory bronchioles are produced.

The respiratory bronchioles, and the alveoli and ducts they give rise to, are known as the respiratory portion of the lung. They are so named because they are the only places in the lungs where oxygen is taken up from the inspired air and carbon dioxide released from the blood. As this gas exchange occurs by diffusion, the walls of the airway and blood vessels have to be extremely thin, closely applied to one another and have a large surface area.

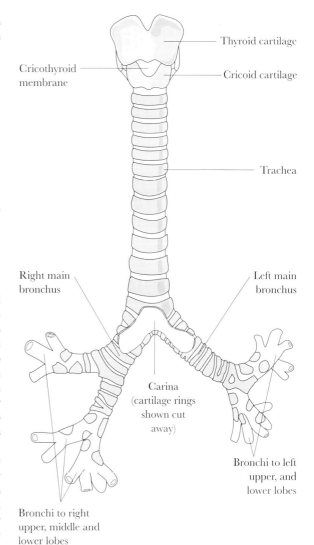

Thyroid cartilage

Cricothyroid membrane

Cricoid cartilage

Trachea

Right main bronchus

Left main bronchus

Carina (cartilage rings shown cut away)

Bronchi to left upper, and lower lobes

Bronchi to right upper, middle and lower lobes

Fig. 9.1 *The lower airways*

Chest Wall

The lungs lie in the thorax (chest cavity) on either side of the heart, trachea, oesophagus and great vessels. The lungs and chest wall are both lined by a tough tissue layer (the pleura) with a potential cavity between the layers known as the intrapleural space.

It is important to realize that both the lung and chest wall comprise elastic tissue which is pulling in opposite directions, i.e. the chest wall is trying to open out and the lungs are trying to collapse. The interface between these two opposing forces results in a vacuum (negative pressure) in most of the intrapleural space. This stretches the lungs so that their outer surfaces are closely applied to the chest wall.

During inspiration the muscles lying between each rib (intercostal muscles) contract and move the ribs upwards and outwards. At the same time the muscular floor of the thorax (the diaphragm) contracts and moves downwards. These actions cause the volume inside the chest to increase and the intrapleural pressure to fall. As a result the lungs are stretched even further and air is drawn in. The opposite process occurs in expiration.

Mediastinum

The trachea, oesophagus, heart and major blood vessels lie in close proximity to one another in the centre of the chest. They are collectively named the *mediastinum*.

RESPIRATORY PATHOPHYSIOLOGY

The main functions of the lungs are oxygen uptake and carbon dioxide elimination. To achieve this, air (or more accurately, oxygen) has to flow to the alveoli (ventilation), blood has to flow to the pulmonary capillaries (perfusion) and oxygen (O_2) and carbon dioxide (CO_2) have to move between the alveoli and blood in the pulmonary capillaries (diffusion). Finally, the balance between ventilation and perfusion has to be correct. Impairment of any of these processes can lead to a low level of oxygen in the blood (hypoxaemia) and a high level of carbon dioxide in the blood (hypercarbia).

Ventilation

The amount of air breathed in (or out) with each breath is called the tidal volume. It is normally equal to 7–8 ml/kg body weight (approximately 500 ml in a 70 kg patient). The volume of air inspired (or expired) each minute is the minute volume and can be calculated by multiplying the tidal volume by the respiratory rate. For a 70 kg patient this gives a value around 5 litres per minute at rest.

Not all of the air breathed in reaches the point where oxygen and carbon dioxide exchange takes place (i.e. the respiratory portion of the lung). Approximately 150 ml of each breath remains in the conducting airways and this area is known as the *anatomical dead space*. In some circumstances (e.g. following blood loss), the volume of this space is increased by the addition of areas of lung which are ventilated but not perfused with blood.

Diffusion

Blood with low levels of oxygen is pumped by the right ventricle through the pulmonary circulation. Gas exchange between the alveoli and blood takes place across the pulmonary membrane and occurs by passive diffusion. The lung is ideally suited for diffusion as the pulmonary membrane has a large surface area and is very thin. It is not surprising therefore that a reduction in surface area (e.g. from a pneumothorax) or an increase in thickness (e.g. from fluid in the alveoli) will reduce gas exchange. The rate of diffusion will also fall if the concentration of oxygen (or more accurately the partial pressure) in the alveoli falls, either as a result of decreased ventilation or a lowering of the inspired oxygen concentration.

ASTHMA

Asthma is a common condition from which approximately 10% of the population, in all age groups, suffer. The prevalence appears to be rising, and approximately 1000 people die in the UK each year from this condition. The young and the elderly are particularly vulnerable. Effective and rapid treatment is therefore vital.

There are three factors that lead to the generalized airway obstruction characteristic of asthma:

- Mucosal inflammation in the airway passages, leading to oedema and swelling of the tissues
- Increased production of thick mucus leading to plugging of bronchioles
- Generalized bronchial smooth muscle constriction leading to bronchospasm

In the early stages of an attack the obstruction is reversible. However, as the attack progresses it becomes increasingly difficult to reverse the process.

Precipitating causes include exercise, infection, allergy to drugs or other substances, and emotional upset; however, in many cases there is no obvious cause. Individuals susceptible to other atopic disorders such as eczema are more prone to developing asthma. There also appears to be a familial element.

Mild attacks are normally dealt with by the patient's general practitioner and it is usually the severe attacks with which ambulance staff become involved. The early symptoms include exercise-induced and night-time cough. As an attack progresses the patient will become increasingly breathless and start to wheeze. The wheeze is usually expiratory, but may also be inspiratory. The patient may have visible indrawing in the intercostal spaces with recession subcostally. In severe cases patients may be seen to fix the chest by splaying their arms out firmly, thereby allowing the accessory muscles of respiration to be used. The accessory muscles are those not normally used in respiration, and are principally the sternomastoids. The patient is usually anxious, and cyanosis may be present in a severe attack. It should be remembered that *a minor attack may develop into a life-threatening situation in a very short time.*

Clinical examination will show the patient to have a tachycardia, hyperresonant chest on percussion and reduced air entry. A polyphonic (more than one musical note) expiratory wheeze will be heard on auscultation. The peak flow rate is characteristically reduced in asthma: this is a measure of the maximum expiratory rate. The rate is measured using a peak flowmeter (Figure 9.2); the patient makes three attempts to breathe into the meter and the best result is compared with a standard chart of predicted values for individuals of the same sex, height, age and race. Each attempt must be a sudden short, hard blow into the meter.

In extreme cases the patient may have a 'silent chest'. This is a most ominous sign as it means that there is not enough air entry to generate a wheeze. Oximetry will show a reduced S_pO_2. In rare cases asthmatic patients develop spontaneous pneumothorax as a result of a ruptured bulla (lung cyst). They may also develop subcutaneous emphysema in the neck and anterior chest wall.

The differential diagnosis of a severe asthma attack includes pulmonary oedema, anaphylaxis, pneumothorax (Chapter 23) and airway obstruction (Chapter 3).

Management

1. Do not panic. Maintain an air of calm no matter how worried you may be.
2. Obtain a rapid history including recent episodes and current treatment.
3. Look for signs of severe or life-threatening asthma (Tables 9.1 and 9.2).
4. Consider and exclude other possibilities.
5. Measure peak flow rate and calculate the predicted figure if not known to patient.
6. Begin immediate treatment of asthma.
7. *Transport the patient to hospital as quickly as possible.* There can be no exceptions to this rule.

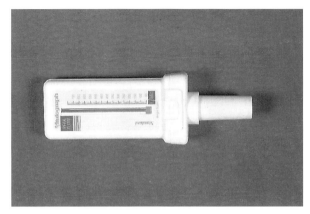

Fig. 9.2 Peak flowmeter

8. Advise the receiving hospital of impending arrival if there is no response to your treatment or the clinical situation is serious.
9. If a delay in transportation is anticipated it would be prudent to seek the assistance of the patient's general practitioner or a doctor from a local Immediate Care scheme, who may be able to provide additional treatment. However, *do not delay departure* to wait for this doctor.

Clinical Features

The clinical features of severe asthma are shown in Table 9.1, and the features of life-threatening asthma are shown in Table 9.2.

> Patients with severe or life-threatening asthma may not be distressed or have all of these features. Make the diagnosis if any feature is present

Pre-hospital Treatment of Severe and Life-threatening Asthma

All paramedics should be familiar with their own local treatment protocols and *should adhere to those protocols at all times.* The aim of emergency treatment is to reverse hypoxia with oxygen and reduce the bronchospasm using beta-2-adrenoceptor agonists. Oral or intravenous steroid therapy has no effect for at least 4 hours.

Table 9.1 Features of severe asthma

Adults	Children
Cannot complete sentences	Cannot talk or feed
Pulse > 110 per minute	Pulse > 140 per minute
Respiratory rate > 25 per minute	Respiratory rate > 50 per minute
Peak flow rate < 50% of predicted	

Table 9.2 Features of life-threatening asthma

Adults	Children
Exhaustion	Reduced conscious level
Cyanosis	Agitation
Bradycardia	Cyanosis
Hypotension	Silent chest
Silent chest	Coma
Peak flow < 33% of predicted	
Coma	

Adults

1. Give oxygen, high flow via reservoir mask (10–15 l/min).
2. Give salbutamol 5 mg or terbutaline 10 mg via an oxygen-driven nebulizer.
3. Establish intravenous access.
4. Give hydrocortisone 200 mg IV.
5. Monitor the ECG.
6. If asthma is life-threatening and local protocols allow, add ipratropium 0.5 mg to the nebulizer.

Children

1. Give oxygen, high flow via reservoir mask (10–15 l/min).
2. Give salbutamol 5 mg or terbutaline 10 mg via an oxygen-driven nebulizer (halve the dose in the very young).
3. Establish intravenous access.
4. Give hydrocortisone 200 mg IV.
5. Monitor the ECG.
6. If asthma is life-threatening and local protocols allow, add ipratropium 0.25 mg to the nebulizer (0.125 mg in the very young).

Transport to hospital

It is essential that time is not wasted in repeatedly attempting to perform clinical interventions that are not going according to plan. If problems are encountered you should immediately take the patient to hospital. All of the above procedures can be carried out in the back of a moving ambulance. Be prepared to intubate if respiratory arrest occurs; airway pressures are likely to be high and ventilation will therefore be difficult. Cardiac arrest may ensue and the standard protocols should be followed (Chapter 12).

Paramedics are well placed to deal with severe and life-threatening asthma, but they must act with speed and foresight to ensure a satisfactory outcome. Nebulized ipratroprium or intravenous hydrocortisone are not drugs in the standard armamentarium of a paramedic in the UK. However, local paramedic steering committees can recommend additional drugs if considered appropriate and beneficial.

PULMONARY OEDEMA

Pulmonary oedema is usually caused by acute left ventricular failure (LVF) and is a very common cause of death in the elderly.

Fluid collects in the interstitial tissues of the lung (the tissues between the alveoli), usually because of the heart's inability to pump properly. Ultimately, fluid leaks into the alveoli themselves, causing marked interference with oxygenation. Hypoxia rapidly develops and cardiac arrest follows soon afterwards. It is unlikely that ambulance staff will be expected to deal with patients with mild LVF as they usually present to their general practitioners. Paramedics will, however, have to deal with severe cases regularly.

The causes of 'pump failure' include acute myocardial infarction (AMI), dysrhythmias, overdose of antiarrhythmic drugs, inadequate heart rate (beta-blocking drugs or post-infarction), chronic valvular heart disease (usually aortic or mitral valve), cardiac tamponade and fluid overload. Cardiac tamponade occurs when fluid builds up around the heart within the pericardial sac, preventing the proper mechanical action of the heart.

The differential diagnosis of pulmonary oedema includes asthma and bronchopneumonia. All three conditions may coexist.

The early symptoms of pulmonary oedema are breathlessness on exertion, paroxysmal nocturnal dyspnoea (waking at night with severe shortness of breach, which often resolves after sitting or standing), and breathlessness on lying down (orthopnoea). Wheeze and cough are often reported. In severe cases acute respiratory distress is present and the patient often coughs up pink froth or blood. If AMI is the cause the patient may have chest pain, but beware that a 'silent infarct' may present as acute pulmonary oedema.

Clinical examination in severe cases will often reveal an anxious, pale, cold, and clammy patient, who will be cyanosed, tachypnoeic and have a tachycardia. The patient is likely to be hypotensive. Electrocardiographic monitoring *may* reveal the injury pattern of AMI (ST elevation), or a dysrhythmia. Fine crepitations ('crackles') may be heard on auscultation of the chest, and occasionally wheeze. When there is wheeze, there may be diagnostic confusion with asthma or chronic obstructive pulmonary disease (COPD); wheeze in a cold, clammy, sweaty patient is usually due to LVF – asthmatic and bronchitic patients are usually warm and well perfused. If pulmonary oedema is severe the patient may be unconscious and may progress to cardiac arrest.

Treatment

Treatment is aimed at improving oxygenation, reducing the volume of blood returned to the left ventricle and treating the underlying cause. Definitive treatment of acute pulmonary oedema is the responsibility of the doctor, and includes the use of diamorphine and diuretics. However, there is a great deal that the paramedic can do:

1. Keep calm and act swiftly.
2. Sit the patient up with feet or legs dependent.
3. Take a rapid history of events. Note the patient's current medication.
4. Give high-flow oxygen via a reservoir mask. *Note:* give oxygen if there is a history of severe underlying lung disease, *but monitor respiration very closely.*
5. Give two glyceryl trinitrate sprays under the patient's tongue. Warn of headache as a side-effect, and be vigilant for the development of hypotension. Do NOT shake before use (mixing the propellant with the drug reduces the metred dose). Ideally, check the blood pressure is at least 100 mmHg before giving this drug.
6. Establish intravenous access.
7. Give intravenous frusemide (a diuretic) according to local protocols.
8. Monitor the three-lead ECG. Be prepared to treat any dysrhythmia and cardiac arrest.
9. Transfer the patient to hospital as rapidly as possible.
10. Warn the hospital of your impending arrival.
11. If a delay in transportation is anticipated, it would be prudent to seek the assistance of the patient's general practitioner or a doctor from a local Immediate Care scheme, who may be able to provide additional treatment. *Do not delay departure* from the scene awaiting this doctor's arrival.

AIRWAY OBSTRUCTION

> **HYPOXIA KILLS**
> **An obstructed airway is a dire emergency:**
> **Evaluation of the airway is ALWAYS the first step**
> **in the primary survey of EVERY patient**

Airway obstruction and the resultant hypoxia is the most fundamental and preventable cause of death in trauma and medical collapse. It is a tragedy if simple airway obstruction, causing hypoxia, is the sole cause of death, as it is so readily treated. The maintenance of the airway is central to both basic life support (Chapter 4) and advanced life support (Chapter 5). The aggressive resuscitation of a bleeding multiple trauma victim with IV fluids may be futile if the airway is not secured and adequate oxygenation maintained.

There are many causes of airway obstruction, but perhaps the most common is the tongue falling back onto the posterior pharyngeal wall. Others include a foreign body (e.g. food, false teeth); severe facial injury (Chapter 22); acute anaphylaxis resulting in airway oedema; and burns with inhalation of hot gases, which can similarly lead to laryngeal oedema and airway

obstruction (Chapter 29). Medical conditions such as epiglottitis are a rare cause of acute obstruction. Carcinoma of the throat leads to chronic obstruction that can be suddenly exacerbated by haemorrhage or infection.

Treatment

The treatment of airway obstruction is aimed at removing the cause of obstruction, and maintaining a secure airway thereafter. The essential features of treatment of a simple obstructed airway and choking are covered fully in Chapter 3. Advanced airway techniques may be required if the patient does not recover consciousness (Chapter 5). Expeditious treatment and transportation are essential if casualties are to have the best chance of survival.

The use of simple airway techniques, augmented with 100% oxygen, is often all that is required as pre-hospital treatment, although advanced techniques such as intubation are within the scope of paramedical staff when the need arises. If difficulty with airway management is encountered medical help should be sought *quickly.* This means that crews should be ready to move immediately. Alternatively, if rapid evacuation is not possible because of entrapment, they should call on the expertise of their local Immediate Care scheme or hospital mobile medical team. Paramedics should be able to anticipate problems and lay plans to prevent them, rather than simply responding to problems when they do occur.

Intrinsic causes of obstruction such as carcinoma may not be amenable to pre-hospital treatment, and indeed in many cases treatment may not be appropriate. If there is any doubt the patient's general practitioner should be contacted for guidance. If this doctor is not available the patient should be taken to hospital.

Epiglottitis

Epiglottitis warrants special mention as injudicious examination can precipitate complete airway obstruction. Epiglottitis is a bacterial infection of the epiglottis, seen most often in children. It leads to marked swelling of the epiglottis, with a typical 'cherry red' appearance. It is usually associated with fever and malaise. The patient will often be grey, distressed, drooling at the mouth and leaning forward. There is severe continuous stridor.

> **Examination of the mouth and pharynx must not be**
> **attempted in suspected epiglottitis**

Complete airway obstruction can develop within minutes. Any procedure that can cause crying or gagging, including simple examination of the throat, can precipitate laryngeal spasm and airway obstruction. *Although most children will need intubation, it should only be attempted by a senior anaesthetist in hospital.* If the condition is suspected the patient should be calmed, given high-concentration oxygen, sat forward and transported quickly to hospital. A paediatric team and senior anaesthetist should be requested to stand by. If airway obstruction occurs before arrival at hospital a surgical airway may be required (Chapter 5).

ANAPHYLAXIS

Anaphylaxis is an acute hypersensitivity (allergic) reaction to foreign protein. True anaphylaxis does not occur on the first exposure to a substance; it occurs only in patients who have been exposed, or 'sensitized', to that protein in the past. Repeated exposure leads to outpouring of histamine and histamine-like substances that mediate the acute reaction, with each subsequent attack often being worse than the last. *Anaphylactoid* reactions can occur with first exposure to certain severe stimuli, such as insect stings and snake bites (including the British adder). *Anaphylactic* reactions involve the release of the immunoglobin IgE, *anaphylactoid* reactions do not.

Common triggers for anaphylaxis are exposure to antibiotics (particularly the penicillins), insect stings, shellfish, strawberries and nuts (e.g. peanuts). Colloid intravenous fluids (Haemaccel, Gelofusine) have been identified as a rare cause. In essence, *any* substance can cause a reaction. Many patients will be aware of their own triggers and will avoid them wherever possible – but in many cases, and especially in first attacks, the cause is unknown. Some hypersensitive patients carry their own adrenaline injection or nasal spray.

Allergic responses vary in severity, from a simple urticarial rash ('nettle rash') to a full-blown acute anaphylactic reaction with cardiorespiratory arrest. The symptoms are very variable and include itchy skin, running eyes and nose, and urticarial rash in the early stages. As the process develops, there is swelling of the face, eyes and lips, and occasionally the tongue and fauces also become swollen. Laryngeal oedema leads to airway obstruction. Bronchospasm and wheeze may be noted. In severe attacks tachycardia, tachypnoea and hypotension can be expected – indeed all the signs of profound shock (Chapter 20). The speed of onset is variable, and patients with marked sensitivity can progress to a severe reaction in a matter of minutes.

Management

1. Maintain a calm atmosphere.
2. Establish the history and the precipitating cause.
3. Check what treatment has been taken (antihistamines, adrenaline).
4. Initiate the treatment of anaphylaxis (see below).
5. Transport the patient to hospital as soon as possible.
6. Advise the hospital of your impending arrival.

If a delay in transportation is anticipated it would be prudent to seek the assistance of the patient's general practitioner or a doctor from a local Immediate Care scheme who may be able to provide additional ongoing treatment. *Do not delay departure from the scene awaiting the arrival of this doctor.*

Table 9.3 Paediatric doses of adrenaline solutions (1:1000 contains 1 mg/ml, 1:10,000 contains 1 mg/10 ml)

Age (years)	Adrenaline 1:1000 (ml)	Adrenaline 1:10,000 (ml)
< 1	0.05	0.5
1	0.1	1
2	0.2	2
3	0.3	3
5	0.4	4
6–12	0.5	5

Treatment of acute anaphylaxis

1. Open, clear and secure the airway. If the airway is obstructed, intubate immediately.
2. If intubation fails, move on. A surgical airway is required: *either* call for immediate medical support *or* move the patient rapidly to hospital.
3. Give 100% oxygen (15 litres per minute via reservoir mask).
4. Give 0.5–1.0 ml of adrenaline 1:1000 IM or 5–10 ml of adrenaline 1:10,000 IM, at once. Be prepared to repeat with either IM or slow IV doses. For children the dose should be 0.01 ml/kg IM or IV, or see Table 9.3. The adult dose of adrenaline is 0.5–1.0 mg. Use the 1:1000 solution when available as there is 1 mg in 1 ml – as compared with 1 mg in 10 ml of 1:10,000 solution.
5. Establish IV access. Give crystalloid rapidly according to the patient's requirements and local protocols.
6. If bronchospasm is present, treat as asthma (see above).
7. Give hydrocortisone 100–200 mg IV* (children 100 mg)*, and if local protocols permit give chlorpheniramine 10 mg IV. Neither hydrocortisone nor chlorpheniramine (Piriton) is effective immediately in the treatment of anaphylaxis but if given early both will subsequently be useful in reducing the anaphylactic response. Chlorpheniramine must be given slowly.

* Not generally approved for paramedic use.

CHRONIC AIRFLOW LIMITATION

Chronic airflow limitation is caused by chronic bronchitis and emphysema, or 'chronic obstructive pulmonary disease' (COPD); some asthmatics may also suffer chronic airflow limitation. Chronic bronchitis is clinically defined as the production of sputum for at least 3 months each year in 2 consecutive years. It causes obstruction by plugging the airways (bronchioles) with mucus, and by inflammation and thickening of the airway mucosa. Emphysema is the dilation of alveolar air spaces by the destruction of their walls. The elastic recoil that holds the airways open in expiration is lost and obstruction to air flow occurs. Both conditions usually coexist to some degree.

The main cause of COPD is smoking, although some cases are attributable to a rare inherited enzyme deficiency (alpha-1 antitrypsin).

The patient with chronic bronchitis will usually present with an acute exacerbation of breathlessness, often precipitated by infection. The complexion will be bluish, hence the description 'blue bloater'. The patient will have a moist, productive cough, severe dyspnoea and wheeze. Auscultation may reveal reduced air entry, scattered wheezes and coarse crepitations throughout the lung fields. Arterial blood gases are abnormal with a raised carbon dioxide concentration (hypercarbia) and a decreased oxygen concentration (hypoxaemia). The patient may have associated heart disease and right heart failure (*cor pulmonale*).

A patient with emphysema tends to have fewer symptoms and is able to maintain reasonably normal blood gas levels. The chest is often barrel-shaped. The patient will be breathless and will often purse the lips on expiration; the term 'pink puffer' is often used.

The pure bronchitic and the pure emphysematous patient represent opposite ends of a clinical spectrum. The majority of patients demonstrate features of both.

Patients with COPD rely on hypoxia as their drive to breathe because their respiratory centre, normally driven by a high carbon dioxide concentration, becomes relatively insensitive to carbon dioxide. People without this disease use an elevation of their blood carbon dioxide level (hypercarbia) as a respiratory stimulus.

Pre-hospital Management of COPD

Patients with acute exacerbations of COPD are hypoxic.

Emergency treatment is aimed at general supportive measures and relief of hypoxia. Rapid transport to hospital is mandatory.

> **Hypoxia kills**

The pre-emptive siting of an IV cannula may be helpful in case of cardiorespiratory arrest.

Patients with acute respiratory decompensation need supplemental oxygen. However, it is potentially dangerous to give supplemental oxygen to these patients *unless* they are carefully observed and the paramedic is prepared to assist ventilation if required. It is possible that administering oxygen will raise the oxygen concentration in the blood (PO_2) to a level whereby the hypoxic drive is switched off, resulting in hypoventilation or apnoea. Patients can be verbally instructed to take additional breaths, and can be assisted with a bag and mask with oxygen reservoir if necessary.

> **Never withold oxygen from a patient who needs it**

Patients who die, do so from *hypoxia*, either because oxygen therapy is withheld or because paramedical staff fail in their duty to support ventilation when the hypoxic drive is lost.

> **HYPOXIA KILLS QUICKLY**
> **HYPERCARBIA KILLS SLOWLY**
> **So give oxygen, and support ventilation should the 'hypoxic drive' be lost**

chapter ten:

THE HEART: ANATOMY, PHYSIOLOGY AND THE ECG

In 70 years of life the human heart beats well over 3 billion times and propels well in excess of 300 million litres of blood. *How does the heart achieve this?* A thorough knowledge of the anatomy (structure and design) and physiology (function) of the human heart and circulatory system enables the paramedic to understand and manage cardiovascular emergencies, shock, arrhythmias and cardiac arrest.

ANATOMY

Location and Size

The heart is a muscular, hollow organ located in the thoracic cavity (Figure 10.1). It is enclosed in the pericardial sac (or pericardium) in a space called the mediastinum. The mediastinum

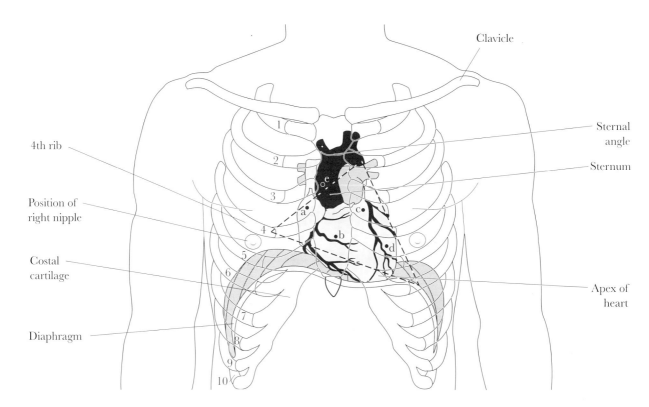

Fig. 10.1 *The anatomical location of the heart: a, right atrium b, right ventricle; c, left atrium; d, left ventricle; e, aortic arch*

is sandwiched between the lungs laterally, the sternum and its connecting costal cartilages anteriorly, and the ribs and the thoracic spinal column posteriorly. The cone-shaped heart rests on the diaphragm and points with its apex towards the left nipple. The heart thus lies obliquely in the mediastinum with two-thirds of the muscle to the left of the midline of the sternum. The heart size is about the same as the person's clenched fist.

Pericardium and Myocardial Wall

The pericardial sac (Figure 10.2) consists of tough fibrous tissue which is inelastic and limits any sudden cardiac distension. Within the fibrous pericardium there is a delicate double-layered membrane, the serous pericardium, which surrounds the heart and extends to the great blood vessels – the aorta and pulmonary trunk.

Between the outer and inner layer of the serous pericardium is the pericardial cavity which contains a slippery secretion, the pericardial fluid. This fluid reduces the friction between the membranes when the heart expands. The wall of the heart is formed by three layers: the outer layer of the serous pericardium (outermost layer, also called the epicardium), the myocardium (middle layer) and the endocardium (innermost layer).

The myocardium is the cardiac muscle tissue itself. It makes up most of the wall thickness of the heart and is responsible for its pumping function. Cardiac muscle consists of a network of muscle fibres, which branch and connect with each other. If one muscle fibre contracts, this contraction spreads throughout

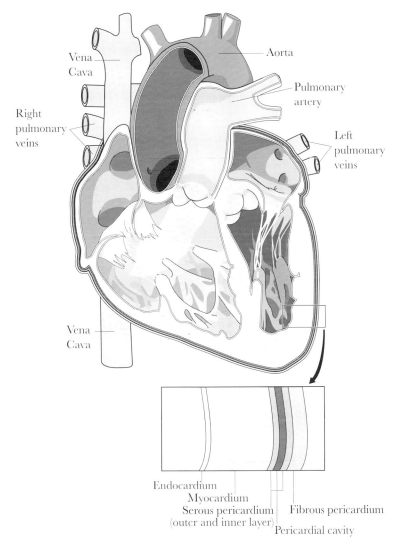

Fig. 10.2 Pericardium and myocardium

the entire network of cardiac muscle cells. Blood vessels and lymphatic vessels, nerves and specialized cardiac conduction fibres lie within the myocardial muscle bulk.

The endocardium provides a smooth lining inside the heart, and covers the heart valves. It is continuous with the innermost layer of the great blood vessels and the rest of the cardiovascular system.

The Chambers and Valves of the Heart

The heart consists of four chambers: right atrium and left atrium (plural 'atria') separated by connective tissue from the right and left ventricles (Figure 10.3). The interatrial and interventricular septum divides the right side of the heart from the left side.

Heart valves direct blood flow and prevent backflow. The right atrium opens into the right ventricle through an atrioventricular (AV) valve called the *tricuspid* valve. Similarly, the left atrium opens into the left ventricle through an AV valve called the

bicuspid or *mitral* valve. The pulmonary artery arises from the right ventricle and has a *pulmonary* valve. The aorta arises from the left ventricle and has an *aortic* valve. The pulmonary and aortic valves are also called *semilunar* (SL) valves because of the three half-moon shaped cusps.

Pacemaker Cells and the Conduction System of the Heart

Specialized cardiac muscle cells in the right atrium near the junction of the superior vena cava have the ability to continuously and rhythmically generate spontaneous impulses (*action potentials*) which cause the heart muscle to contract.

In order for the heart to pump effectively, all cardiac chambers must contract in a coordinated manner. This is achieved by the conduction system (Figure 10.4) which consists of five specialized components:

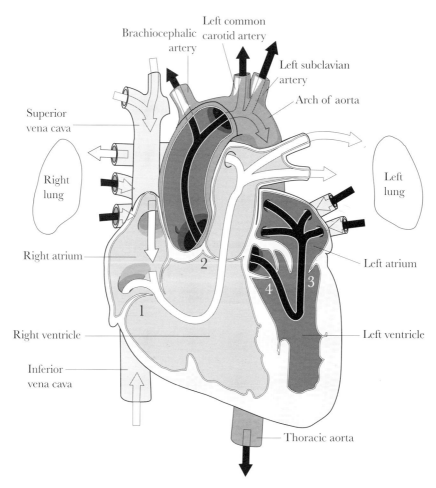

Fig. 10.3 *Chambers and valves of the heart: 1, tricuspid valve; 2, pulmonary valve; 3, bicuspid valve; 4, aortic valve*

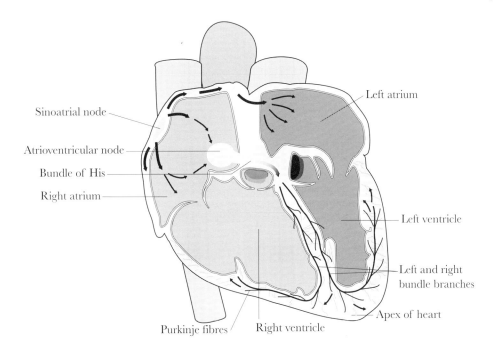

Fig. 10.4 *The conducting system of the heart*

- The sinoatrial (SA) or sinus node
- The atrioventricular node
- The atrioventricular bundle (bundle of His)
- The right and left bundle branches
- The Purkinje fibres

It is the SA node which normally acts as the primary pace-maker and is responsible for the heart rate in sinus rhythm. The SA node generates a repeated impulse which travels in all directions through every muscle fibre of both atria, causing them to contract.

The impulse then reaches the AV node located in the septum between the two atria, and travels down the AV bundle (bundle of His). The AV bundle is important because it is the only normal electrical pathway between the atria and ventricles (additional pathways exist in some conditions, e.g. Wolff–Parkinson–White syndrome). The cardiac impulse continues to spread through the right and left bundle branches within the interventricular septum towards the apex of the heart. Purkinje fibres (muscle fibres specialized for conduction) rapidly excite the muscle bulk of the left and right ventricle.

Any part of the conduction system or any myocardial cell can potentially act as a pacemaker, and is then called a secondary or *ectopic* pacemaker.

Myocardial Blood Supply

In order to perform the enormous amount of work the heart muscle does, it needs its own blood supply. It could not obtain nearly enough nutrients from the blood by simple diffusion through the endocardium and myocardium. Two coronary arteries, the right and left coronary artery, arise from the ascending aorta at the point where the aorta leaves the left ventricle (Figure 10.5).

The *left main coronary artery* divides into the *left anterior descending artery* and the *circumflex artery*. Together these supply the left atrium and most of the left ventricle muscle bulk as well as a small part of the right ventricle. The *right coronary artery* transports oxygen-enriched blood to the right atrium and right ventricle. It also gives off an important small branch to supply the SA node.

Anatomically, the myocardial blood supply does vary between individuals. There is a rich network of connections between the right and left coronary arteries, but these vessels are very small. Furthermore, they cannot enlarge in the event of a sudden blockage in an adjacent branch.

Most venous blood is drained via the cardiac veins into the *coronary sinus*. The coronary sinus opens directly into the right atrium. Some of the smaller veins empty directly into the heart chambers.

Circulatory System

A complex system of branching arteries arises from the left ventricle. The arterial system carries blood away from the heart through arterioles into the capillary network of body tissues. The

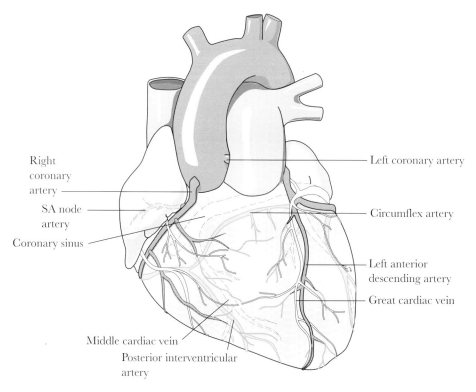

Right coronary artery

SA node artery

Coronary sinus

Left coronary artery

Circumflex artery

Left anterior descending artery

Great cardiac vein

Middle cardiac vein

Posterior interventricular artery

Fig. 10.5 *Myocardial blood supply*

capillary network is responsible for the exchange of nutrients and waste products at tissue level and is often referred to as the *micro-circulation*. From there the circulating blood returns through venules and the venous system to the right side of the heart.

Arteries

The aorta arises from the left ventricle and gives off important main branches: the *brachiocephalic artery, left common carotid artery* and *left subclavian artery* in the chest, before it ultimately divides into two common iliac arteries in the abdomen (Figure 10.6A). These large vessels are elastic conducting arteries. They actively propel blood to the various organs and tissues of the body and adjust blood flow according to the demand of the individual organ. Their vessel walls are thick owing to a large smooth muscle layer, which allows vasoconstriction (narrowing of the vessel lumen) and vasodilation (widening of the vessel lumen).

Arterioles are the smallest arteries and deliver blood to the capillaries. They are also capable of vasoconstriction and vasodilation.

Capillaries

Capillaries are very small, thin-walled vessels which connect arterioles to venules (Figure 10.6B). They often form extensive branching networks, particularly in body tissues with high metabolic activity, for example the liver, kidney or central nervous system. The capillary walls are a single layer of cells with a basement membrane to anchor these cells. Their structure allows a rapid exchange of nutrients and waste products with surrounding tissue cells. This process is further enhanced by the large total surface area of the capillary network.

Veins

Several capillaries unite to form *venules*, or small veins. Venules drain the blood collected from the capillaries into the veins. Veins are blood vessels that carry blood from the tissues to the heart. They become progressively larger in diameter and ultimately drain into the right atrium via the superior and inferior vena cavae (Figure 10.6C). In order to aid blood flow towards the heart, veins contain valves, particularly in dependent tissues, which prevent the backflow of blood.

Content of the Circulatory System

The normal circulating volume is variable, but in a 70 kg adult it is about 5 litres (equivalent to about 70 ml/kg body weight). The adult blood volume is fairly constant in good health (Table 10.1).

Blood consists of a fluid phase (plasma) and three types of cells: red blood cells (erythrocytes), white blood cells (leucocytes), and platelets (thrombocytes).

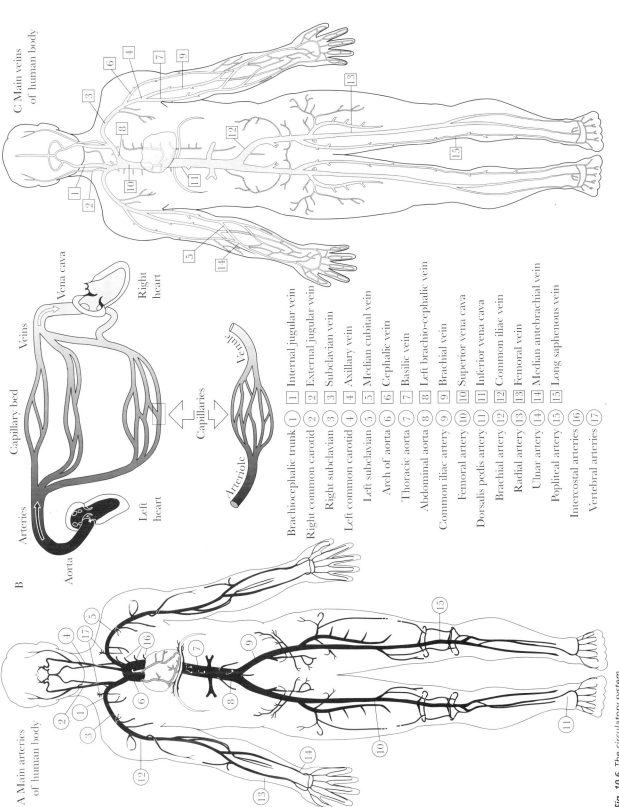

A Main arteries of human body

B

Capillary bed

Veins

Vena cava

Right heart

Arteries

Aorta

Left heart

Capillaries

Arteriole

Venule

C Main veins of human body

Brachiocephalic trunk ①
Right common carotid ②
Right subclavian ③
Left common carotid ④
Left subclavian ⑤
Arch of aorta ⑥
Thoracic aorta ⑦
Abdominal aorta ⑧
Common iliac artery ⑨
Femoral artery ⑩
Dorsalis pedis artery ⑪
Brachial artery ⑫
Radial artery ⑬
Ulnar artery ⑭
Popliteal artery ⑮
Intercostal arteries ⑯
Vertebral arteries ⑰

① Internal jugular vein
② External jugular vein
③ Subclavian vein
④ Axillary vein
⑤ Median cubital vein
⑥ Cephalic vein
⑦ Basilic vein
⑧ Left brachio-cephalic vein
⑨ Brachial vein
⑩ Superior vena cava
⑪ Inferior vena cava
⑫ Common iliac vein
⑬ Femoral vein
⑭ Median antebrachial vein
⑮ Long saphenous vein

Fig. **10.6** *The circulatory system*

Table 10.1 Circulating blood volume in relation to age

Age group	Blood volume (ml/kg body weight)
Adult	70
Child	80
Neonate	90

Red blood cells are responsible for the transport of oxygen and carbon dioxide. White blood cells are involved in defending the body against bacteria, viruses, fungi and parasites. Platelets primarily stop bleeding by plugging any holes in the vessels, in conjunction with other blood clotting mechanisms.

Proteins in the plasma include albumin, alpha- and beta-globulins, and fibrinogen. Plasma proteins play an important role in maintaining *homeostasis* within the body – a constant, stable internal environment, which is essential for optimal tissue function. Fibrinogen helps to form a web of protein fibres when blood clotting mechanisms are activated. Albumin and alpha- and beta-globulins assist in transporting other proteins and lipids. Gamma-globulins provide immunity and defence against infection.

Nerve Supply to the Heart

The heart can beat even if it is removed completely from the body owing to the inherent pacemaker function of the SA node. However, the heart receives nerve impulses from the cardiovascular regulatory centres in the midbrain and medulla oblongata (Figure 10.7). These are transmitted via sympathetic and parasympathetic nerve fibres. Both of these can increase or decrease the heart rate, and the strength of the pumping action of the heart.

PHYSIOLOGY

Cardiac Pump

The heart is a double pump which serves two circulations: the pulmonary and the systemic circulation (Figure 10.8). The right atrium and right ventricle pump blood at low pressure into the pulmonary vasculature via the pulmonary trunk, while the left atrium and left ventricle pump blood at high pressure into the systemic vasculature via the aorta.

The right atrium receives deoxygenated blood (blood that has lost oxygen to the cells and taken on carbon dioxide) from the systemic circulation via the superior and inferior vena cavae. Blood from the heart itself also drains into the right atrium from the coronary sinus. Deoxygenated blood flows through the tricuspid valve into the right ventricle which pumps it through the pulmonary valve into the pulmonary trunk and consequently into the left and right lungs. From there the blood

enters the pulmonary capillary bed, where it is re-oxygenated and carbon dioxide is lost to be exhaled. The oxygenated blood then flows through four pulmonary veins back into the left atrium. The mitral valve opens and blood reaches the left ventricle to be propelled through the aortic valve into the aorta. Blood is then distributed throughout the body via the systemic arterial circulation.

Cardiac Cycle

The adult human heart beats about 70 times per minute at rest. One heart-beat within a single cardiac cycle therefore lasts about 0.8 seconds or 800 milliseconds (ms). During a cardiac cycle the atria and ventricles alternately contract and relax (Figure 10.9). The phase of contraction is called *systole*, the phase of relaxation is called *diastole*. Blood movement through the heart is caused by pressure changes within the heart chambers. During atrial diastole, which lasts approximately 700 ms, both atria fill with blood from the superior and inferior vena cavae on the right, and the pulmonary veins on the left.

The two atria contract for about 100 ms during atrial systole while the two ventricles are still relaxed. Thus the right and left atria actively support filling of the ventricles by squeezing approximately 20–30% of the blood into the ventricular chambers; 70–80% of the blood contained in the atrial reservoirs flows passively down a pressure gradient through the opened atrioventricular valves into the ventricles.

As the ventricles begin to contract during ventricular systole, the pressure in the ventricles rises above the pressure in the atria and the AV valves shut. Ventricular pressure continues to rise until it exceeds pressure in the pulmonary trunk of the right side of the heart and in the aorta on the left side. The pulmonary and aortic valves are forced open and blood is ejected from the ventricles into the pulmonary and systemic circulation respectively. As the ventricular volumes decrease owing to outflow of blood after 300 ms, ventricular diastole or relaxation begins. Ventricular pressure now falls below pressure in the pulmonary trunk or aorta and the pulmonary and aortic valves close. Once ventricular pressure is lower than atrial pressure, the tricuspid and mitral valves open and blood flows from both atria into the ventricles.

Heart sounds are due to closure of the heart valves at different phases of the cardiac cycle. The first heart sound is caused by the closure of the mitral and tricuspid valve and is soft in character ('lub'). The second is a higher-pitched sound ('dup') and is due to the closure of the aortic and pulmonary valve. Hence: *lub-dup – lub-dup – lub-dup.*

Coronary blood flow to the cardiac muscle takes place almost exclusively during diastole or relaxation of ventricular muscle. During systole coronary blood flow is very limited owing to compression of the coronary arteries. As the heart rate rises, the duration of diastole is shortened and there is less time for nourishment of the cardiac muscle despite increased requirements.

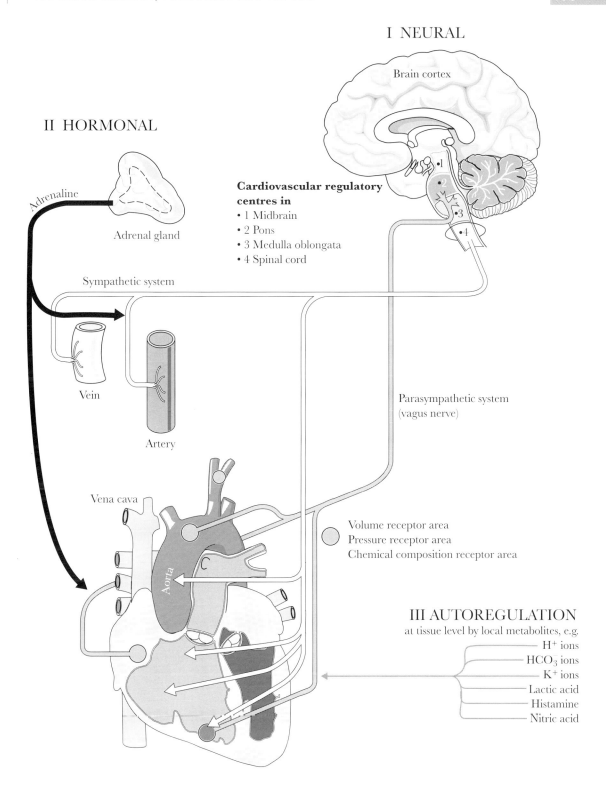

I NEURAL

Brain cortex

II HORMONAL

Adrenaline

Adrenal gland

Cardiovascular regulatory centres in
- 1 Midbrain
- 2 Pons
- 3 Medulla oblongata
- 4 Spinal cord

Sympathetic system

Vein

Artery

Parasympathetic system
(vagus nerve)

Vena cava

Aorta

Volume receptor area
Pressure receptor area
Chemical composition receptor area

III AUTOREGULATION
at tissue level by local metabolites, e.g.

H^+ ions
HCO_3 ions
K^+ ions
Lactic acid
Histamine
Nitric acid

Fig. 10.7 Regulatory control of the cardiovascular system

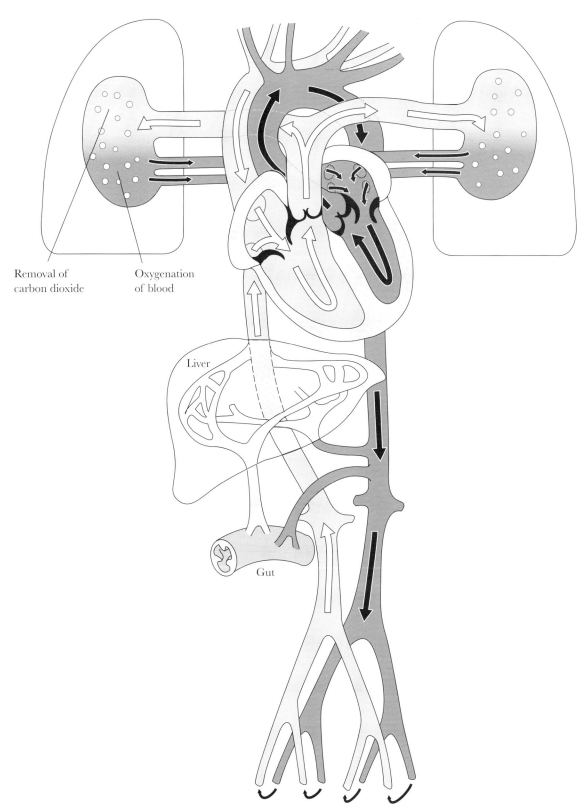

Removal of
carbon dioxide

Oxygenation
of blood

Liver

Gut

Fig. 10.8 *The pulmonary and systemic circulations*

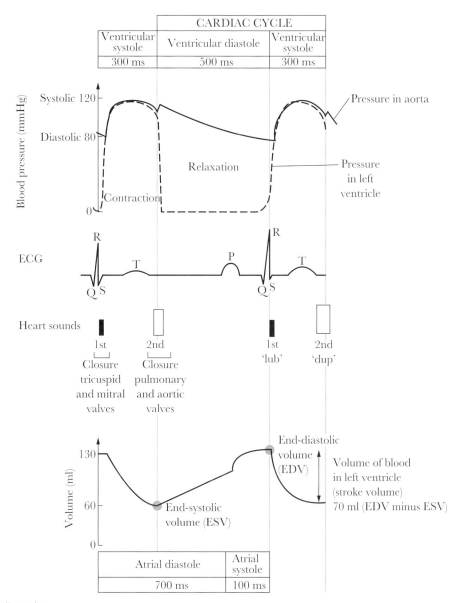

Fig. 10.9 The cardiac cycle

Cardiac Output

Cardiac output is defined as the volume of blood ejected by each ventricle per minute. At rest the cardiac output amounts to 5000 ml (5 litres) per minute. During severe exercise the cardiac output can be increased up to six-fold to reach 30 litres per minute. Cardiac output is calculated by multiplying the heart rate by the *stroke volume* (volume ejected per heart-beat).

Cardiac output = stroke volume × heart rate

Stroke volume

The stroke volume is the amount of blood ejected from each ventricle during a single contraction during the cardiac cycle. It amounts to 70–80 ml at rest, but can be doubled with exercise. The heart rate, on the other hand, can treble with exercise. Thus cardiac output can be varied by changing the heart rate, the stroke volume, or both. Three factors determine stroke volume :

- Pre-load – the filling of the heart during diastole
- After-load – the resistance in the arterial circulation against which the heart has to pump
- Contractility – the intrinsic performance of the heart muscle at a given pre-load and after-load

Pre-load The degree of filling of the heart determines pre-load. Ventricular performance depends on the pre-load. Frank and later Starling stated that within certain limits the higher the degree of venous filling of the heart, the higher its stroke volume and therefore cardiac output (Figure 10.10). In other words, Starling's law of the heart states that the more myocardial fibres are stretched the more forcefully they contract.

However, if the load increases beyond physiological limits, the heart begins to fail owing to overstretching of myocardial fibres. The degree of venous filling depends on the venous return or the amount of circulating blood volume entering the right side of the heart.

After-load After-load is the resistance against which the heart has to pump during ejection. This opposing force to ejection depends on the pressure in the systemic arterial circulation. After-load is increased in a patient with hypertension (high blood pressure) due to arteriosclerosis. Stroke volume and therefore cardiac output decrease. If after-load is reduced, the left ventricle is able to contract more quickly and forcefully, and therefore the stroke volume and cardiac output increase.

Myocardial contractility Myocardial contractility is defined as the strength of contraction of myocardial fibres at any given stretch or pre-load. Naturally produced hormones and drugs such as adrenaline and noradrenaline increase myocardial contractility and are called *positive inotropes*. They increase the stroke volume and cardiac output. Hypoxia and acidosis have a negative inotropic effect on the myocardium.

Regulation of heart rate

Cardiac output depends on the heart rate as well as the stroke volume. Regulation of the heart rate is extremely important in cases of decreased stroke volume. Stroke volume falls after damage to the myocardium, for example in an acute myocardial infarction, or if the circulating blood volume decreases, for example owing to extensive haemorrhage. In order to maintain a constant cardiac output the heart rate must increase. This is achieved by nervous system control of the cardiovascular system, and chemical regulation of the heart rate by hormones and ions.

Autonomic nervous system control of heart rate Both sympathetic and parasympathetic fibres of the autonomic nervous system innervate the heart (Figure 10.11). There is a balance between these two systems. At rest the parasympathetic effects slow the SA node down to a resting heart rate of 70 beats per minute. Parasympathetic fibres reach the heart via the right and left vagus nerve, which supply the SA node, AV node and both atria, and can slow the heart down to 20–30 beats per minute or even result in vagal sinus arrest.

Sympathetic fibres extend from the medulla oblongata in the brain into the spinal cord and reach the SA node, AV node, atria and ventricles. They increase the heart rate to a maximum of 250 beats per minute. The highest cardiac output is achieved at heart rates of 160–200 beats per minute. Sympathetic and parasympathetic parts of the autonomic nervous system receive input from higher brain centres such as the cerebral cortex.

Regulation of heart rate by hormones and ions The stress hormones adrenaline and noradrenaline are released from the adrenal glands in the 'fight or flight' response. They both increase heart rate (chronotropism) and contractility (inotropism).

Myocardial cells are surrounded by extracellular fluid which is composed of water containing small electrically charged particles called ions, for example sodium (Na^+), potassium (K^+), and calcium (Ca^{++}). For optimal cell function (Table 10.2) a balance is essential between intracellular (inside the cell) and extracellular (outside the cell) fluid composition. Any electrolyte or ion imbalance will compromise cardiac function. Elevated levels of K^+ or Na^+ will decrease the heart rate and contractility. Increased Ca^{++} in the extracellular fluid speeds up the heart and strengthens its pumping action.

Haemodynamics of the Circulation

The systemic circulation is responsible for supplying all organs

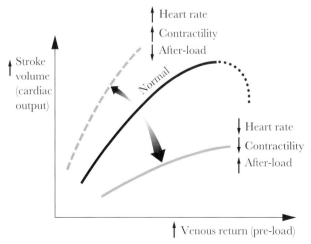

Fig. 10.10 Starling's law

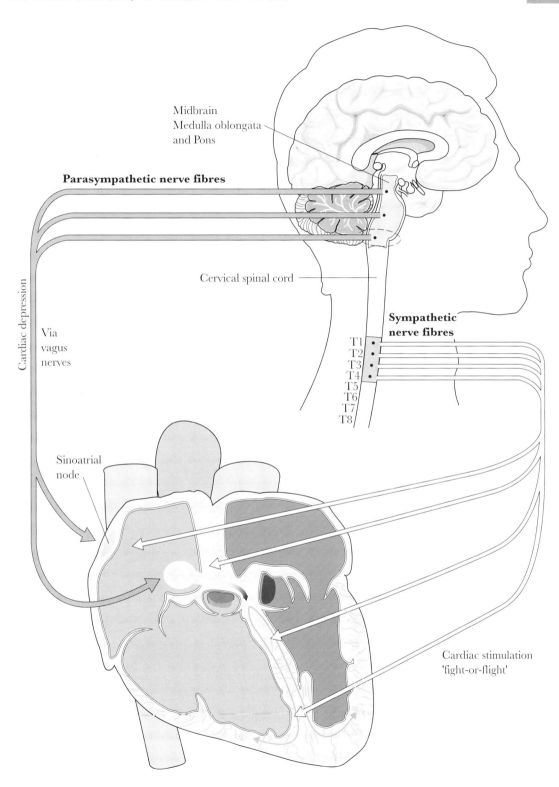

Fig. 10.11 *Autonomic control of the heart*

Table 10.2 Role of electrolytes in cardiac function

Electrolyte	Symbol	Role
Sodium	Na^+	Initiates depolarization of myocardial cell
Potassium	K^+	Initiates repolarization of myocardial cell
Calcium	Ca^{++}	1. Initiates depolarization of pacemaker cells
		2. Sustains cardiac action potential
		3. Increases myocardial contractility

and tissues according to their needs with oxygen and nutrients. The flow rate of the blood or cardiac output is influenced not only by the stroke volume and the heart rate, but also by two other factors:

- blood pressure
- total peripheral resistance in the systemic circulation

Blood pressure

Blood pressure (BP) is the pressure that the blood exerts upon a vessel wall. In the systemic circulation the term refers to the pressure generated by contraction of the left ventricle in the aorta. During systole the BP rises to about 120 mmHg (equivalent to 16 kilopascals) and falls to about 80 mmHg (11 kPa) during diastole in the aorta and larger systemic arteries (Table 10.3). Blood pressure progressively decreases as blood flows from the aorta to reach the capillary beds and returns via the great veins to the right atrium.

Total peripheral resistance

Total peripheral resistance refers to the sum of all vascular resistances of the systemic blood vessels. Arterioles, capillaries and venules (Figure 10.12) are mainly responsible for resistance. They oppose blood flow. Arterioles in particular are able to control blood pressure by changing their vessel diameter. The smaller the radius of a blood vessel, the greater the resistance it offers to blood flow. The longer the blood vessel, the greater the resistance as blood flows through it. The velocity of blood flow is lowest in the capillary beds where resistance is highest. This principle is important as it enables capillary exchange of oxygen and carbon dioxide, nutrients and waste products to take place.

Circulation time

It takes about 1 minute in a resting adult for an intravenous

drug in the blood stream to travel from the right atrium through the pulmonary circulation, to the left ventricle and onward into the systemic circulation, and back to the right atrium.

Electrical Activity of Cardiac Cells

Cardiac cells, like all other cells in the body, are electrically charged. In its resting state the interior of a myocardial cell is negatively charged in comparison to the outer surface of the cell membrane. This resting cell membrane potential is caused by the uneven distribution of ions in the extracellular and intracellular fluid. Ions are small particles that are either negatively or positively charged. Potassium (K^+) is the main intracellular ion and tries to escape to the outside of the cell membrane down a concentration gradient. Sodium (Na^+) is the main extracellular ion and tries to intrude into the cells. At rest, energy-consuming ion pumps keep potassium ions inside the cell and sodium ions outside. Once a cardiac cell is stimulated or activated by a spontaneous rhythmical impulse arising from the SA node, the electrical charges inside and outside the cell change. The inside becomes positively charged due to a large influx of sodium ions through special cell membrane channels. Potassium ions flow out of the cell. Positively charged calcium ions (Ca^{++}) also travel into the cells. The resting membrane potential, which amounts to minus 90 millivolts, thus becomes positive (plus 20 mV): a cardiac action potential has been generated (Figure 10.13). A *depolarization* has taken place, lasting for about 200 milliseconds. After this time the resting membrane potential is restored by the opening of special potassium channels, and potassium ions diffuse out of myocardial cells along their concentration gradient. Simultaneously Na^+ and Ca^{++} channels start closing, and fewer and fewer sodium and calcium ions enter the cells. Recovery of the resting membrane potential is called *repolarization*. It is important to realize that events described above do not just apply to a single myocardial cell. Electrical depolarization is 'contagious' (Figure 10.14) . Owing to close contact of all myocardial cells with each other an electrical wave sweeps rapidly across all heart chambers. Electrical excitation must always occur before mechanical contraction of myocardial cells can take place, although the two processes are closely coupled with each other.

Cardiac muscle cells in the depolarization phase are refractory to a subsequent electrical stimulation for a period of 250 ms,

Table 10.3 Normal blood pressure in healthy, young adults

	Normal blood pressure (mmHg)	(kPa)	Range
Systolic	120	16	+/– 10%
Diastolic	80	11	+/– 10%

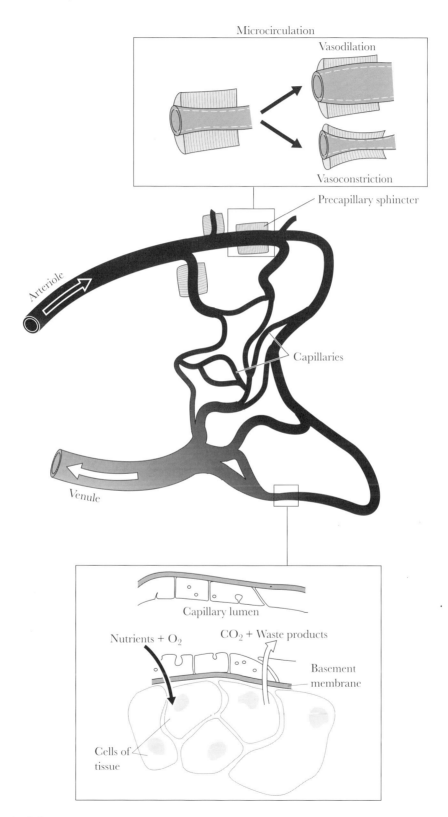

Fig. 10.12 *The microcirculation*

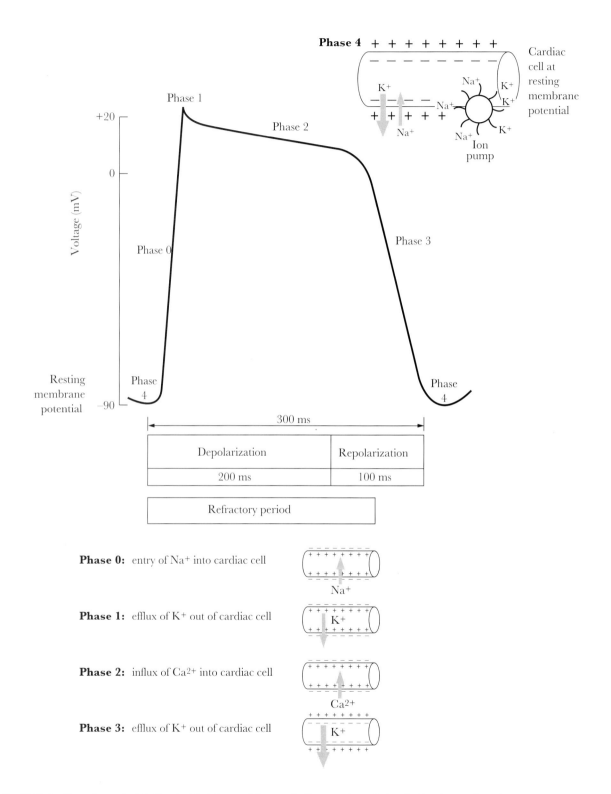

Fig. 10.13 *Cardiac action potential. The electrical charge of the muscle fibre membrane is denoted by plus or minus signs*

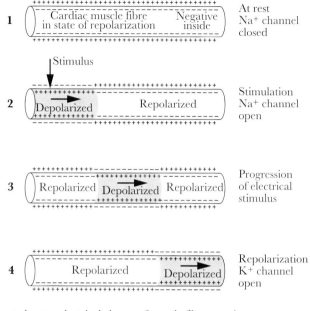

Positive outside

1 Cardiac muscle fibre in state of repolarization — Negative inside — At rest Na+ channel closed

Stimulus

2 Depolarized — Repolarized — Stimulation Na+ channel open

3 Repolarized — Depolarized — Repolarized — Progression of electrical stimulus

4 Repolarized — Depolarized — Repolarization K+ channel open

± denotes electrical charge of muscle fibre membrane

Fig. 10.14 *Progression of the cardiac action potential along cardiac muscle fibre. Plus or minus signs denote the electrical charge of the muscle fibre membrane*

which lasts slightly longer than the mechanical contraction itself. The refractory period allows the heart to alternate between contraction and ejection of blood and relaxation with refilling.

The spontaneous action potentials which are normally fired off in the pacemaker cells of the SA node are created by similar ionic movements of Na$^+$ and Ca^{++} as in ordinary myocardial cells.

The pathway of cardiac conduction is shown in Figure 10.4. If secondary pacemakers are responsible for excitation of the heart, the rate of intrinsic automaticity decreases: the AV node fires at 40–60 beats per minute, and the bundle of His and Purkinje fibres at 20–40 beats per minute.

Mechanical Activity of Cardiac Muscle Fibres

Cardiac excitation is closely coupled to mechanical activity. Excitation-contraction coupling needs optimum concentrations of Na$^+$, K$^+$ and Ca^{++} ions. Calcium is essential for cardiac contraction, and the force and velocity of contraction are directly related to the intracellular concentration of calcium ions. The calcium ions activate the sliding mechanism with myocardial fibres which results in contraction. Once the contraction has taken place calcium ions are rapidly pumped out of the cells, in order for the excitation-contraction to start again with the next heart-beat.

Overall Regulatory Control of the Cardiovascular System

The entire body must be supplied with enough blood containing oxygen and nutrients to meet tissue demands either at rest or under stress. All organs need a minimum blood flow. Active tissues, for example muscles in severe exercise, require more blood, which is therefore redistributed at the expense of other resting organs, for example the gastrointestinal tract.

The cardiovascular centre for overall regulatory control of the cardiovascular system is situated in the medulla oblongata and pons in the brain (Figure 10.7). Peripheral receptors in the heart chambers, aortic arch and carotid arteries send signals to these specialized brain regions. Baroreceptors provide a constant feedback of blood pressure and stretch, and chemoreceptors are sensitive to the chemical composition of the blood. The cardiovascular centre integrates this information and sends nerve impulses back to the heart and blood vessels via the vagus nerves and nerve fibres of the sympathetic nervous system. These nerve impulses regulate heart rate, cardiac contractility and the vasomotor tone of blood vessels, which is reflected in their degree of vasodilation or vasoconstriction. Apart from the nervous system control of the cardiovascular system, blood pressure and blood flow are affected by several hormones circulating in the blood, for example adrenaline, noradrenaline and antidiuretic hormone. A third factor which adjusts blood flow in organs is local control or *autoregulation*. Autoregulation is particularly important in the brain, kidney and heart. Local metabolites (hydrogen ions, carbon dioxide and potassium ions), lactic acid, lack of oxygen, and vasoactive substances such as histamine and nitric oxide produce a local vasodilation of arterioles. This results in an increased flow of blood into the tissue which restores tissue oxygen supply.

ELECTROCARDIOGRAPHY

The electrocardiogram (ECG) represents the electrical activity of the heart generated by depolarization and repolarization of both atria and ventricles. It can be represented graphically on the screen of a cardiac monitor, or printed on a paper rhythm strip (Figure 10.15).

Understanding the ECG

The normal heart beats (and therefore pumps) regularly, owing to orderly transmissions of electrical impulses along the cardiac conducting system. These electrical impulses stimulate the muscle cells of the myocardium to contract at a physiologically appropriate rate. Contraction of cardiac muscle cells is accompanied by the flow of sodium ions across the cell membrane producing a brief charge in cell wall polarity (relative electrical charge). All cardiac muscle cells have their own in-built rhythm and rate of contraction and it is the role of the conducting

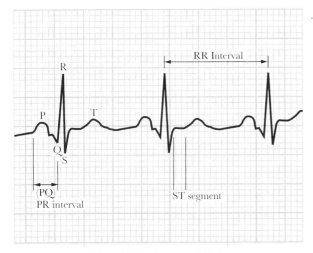

Sinus rhythm: heart rate 80/min

Fig. 10.15 *An ECG trace (rhythm strip)*

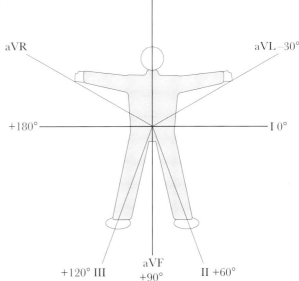

Fig. 10.16 *The standard leads*

system to coordinate the action of these cells to produce an efficient pumping mechanism. The electrocardiograph assesses the state of the conducting system and hence of the heart itself. Before considering ECG analysis, a number of conventions must be accepted.

Electrocardiograms are conventionally recorded from 12 leads: the standard leads named I, II, III, aVR, aVL and aVF, and the chest leads V_1, V_2, V_3, V_4, V_5 and V_6 (Figures 10.16 and 10.17). Each lead 'looks' at the heart from a different position:

- aVR may be remembered as the *right* (a**V**R) arm lead
- aVL may be remembered as the *left* (a**V**L) arm lead
- aVF may be remembered as the *foot* (a**V**F) lead

The position of these leads is described in degrees clockwise from lead I (0 degrees), thus lead aVF is 90 degrees, lead III is 120 degrees and lead aVR is 210 degrees. It is apparent therefore that leads II, III and aVF look at the heart from 'underneath' – these are the *inferior* leads; whereas lead aVL looks at the heart from 'above' (i.e. from the left shoulder).

The chest leads (Figure 10.17) form an incomplete arc around the chest.

The ECG does not enable any conclusions to be made about mechanical events taking place in the heart, the force of contraction or the blood pressure. The ECG serves as a tool to diagnose cardiac abnormalities such as abnormal heart rate, abnormal rhythm and abnormal conduction pathway. Furthermore, it serves to locate ischaemic areas of cardiac muscle, or an acute myocardial infarction. It may also provide indirect clues to electrolyte abnormalities, hypothermia and drug intoxication. It is essential in good paramedical practice to

evaluate ECG findings in conjunction with a thorough clinical history and assessment of the patient.

In the pre-hospital setting it is standard to monitor a single lead (lead II) to recognize abnormalities of the heart rhythm.

Lead II is the standard pre-hospital monitoring lead. Three electrodes are required: right arm electrode (negative) to lower left abdomen (positive) with third electrode (neutral) on left shoulder.

In hospital, however, a 12-lead ECG is usually recorded to evaluate electrical activity of the heart in three dimensions by utilizing six limb leads and six chest leads.

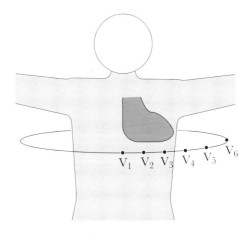

Fig. 10.17 *The chest leads*

A bipolar ECG lead is defined as a record of cardiac electrical activity sensed by two electrodes of opposite polarity (one positive and one negative). Lead II is most frequently used in pre-hospital rhythm monitoring. The negative electrode is attached to the upper right anterior chest wall (or the right arm) and the positive electrode to the lower left anterior chest wall, midclavicular line, below the left nipple (or the left leg). A third, electrically neutral electrode or *ground electrode* is most commonly attached to the upper left chest. This electrode serves to eliminate or reduce electrical interference.

Lead II 'looks at' the heart from below

ECG recording paper

In order to allow ECG analysis and comparison of ECGs recorded at different times for the same patient, the paper used is standardized. The ECG machine, or the printer of a defibrillator or ECG monitor, runs with a paper speed of 25 mm per second (Figure 10.18).

The graph paper is divided into small squares of side 1 mm. A large square consists of 25 small squares and measures 5 mm × 5 mm. At the standard paper speed each small square (1 mm) represents 0.04 seconds and each large square (5 mm) represents 0.20 seconds. The graph paper moves under the heated stylus of the ECG machine at this fixed rate. Time is represented along the horizontal axis of the paper strip. Amplitude of the electrical impulse is indicated along the vertical axis. A 10 mm deflection (two large squares) represents a 1 mV electrical signal provided that the ECG machine is properly calibrated.

The horizontal axis of the ECG trace is time

Components of the ECG

The ECG machine is 'wired' so that it records a positive deflection when electrical charge is flowing towards it (Figure 10.19) or a negative deflection when electrical charge flows away (Figure 10.20). When current is flowing at 90 degrees to the electrode (Figure 10.21) either no deflection, or more commonly one with equal negative and positive deflection (Figure 10.22), is produced.

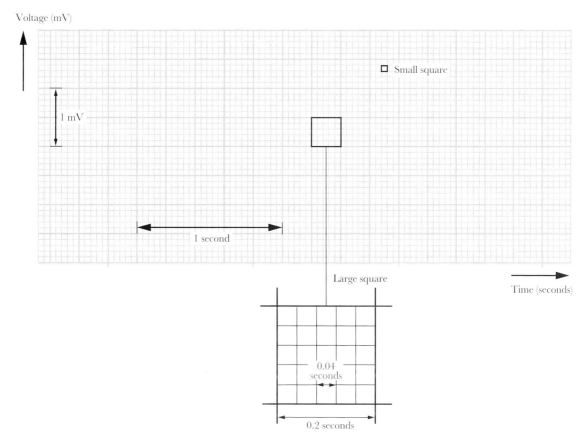

Fig. 10.18 *ECG recording paper*

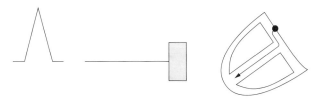

Fig. 10.19 *Trace recorded when electrical charge flows towards ECG machine*

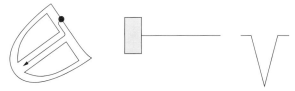

Fig. 10.20 *Trace recorded when electrical charge flows away from ECG machine*

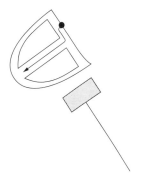

Fig. 10.21 *Current flowing at 90 degrees to the electrode*

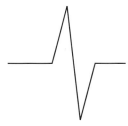

Fig. 10.22 *Trace recorded when current flows at 90 degrees to electrode*

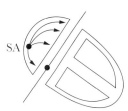

Fig. 10.23 *Atrial depolarization; SA, sinoatrial node*

It is important to understand that although in reality the heart has four chambers, as far as the ECG is concerned it only has two: atrium and ventricle.

Depolarization of the heart begins at the sinus node in the right atrium. The sinus node has its own rate of spontaneous depolarization, but it is also affected by nerve impulses and hormones. The rate of spontaneous depolarization of the sinus node is higher than that of other areas in the heart, hence in the normal heart it can override the spontaneous depolarization of other cells which would occur at a slower rate. From the sinus or sinoatrial (SA) node depolarization spreads through the atria (Figure 10.23); this produces the P wave due to depolarization of atrial cells (Figure 10.24).

From the atria the depolarization passes to the atrioventricular node, then down the normal conducting pathway to the ventricles.

Depolarization first passes down the bundle of His, then simultaneously up the left bundle (to the left ventricle) and the right bundle (to the right ventricle). The pathway is made of special cells which transmit depolarization very rapidly through the large muscle mass of the ventricles (Purkinje fibres) (Figure 10.25).

Depolarization of the ventricles produces the QRS complex on the ECG. Remember that any depolarization of the ventricle that does not follow the normal depolarization pathway will take much longer to occur as it passes from individual cell to individual cell. This will produce a wide, abnormal QRS complex on the ECG.

The time from the beginning of atrial depolarization to the beginning of ventricular depolarization is the PR interval (Figure 10.26). It is normally 0.12–0.20 seconds, i.e. three to five small squares on the ECG paper.

Following depolarization (and contraction) of the ventricles, they repolarize and return to their resting electrical state to await the next depolarization. This is represented on the ECG as the T waves.

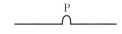

Fig. 10.24 *The P wave*

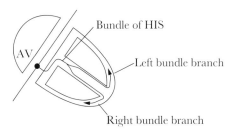

Fig. 10.25 *The conducting pathway in the ventricles; AV, atrioventricular node*

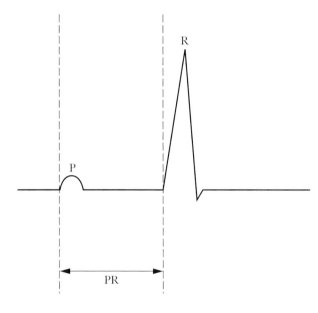

Fig. 10.26 *The P wave, and QRS complexes and the PR interval*

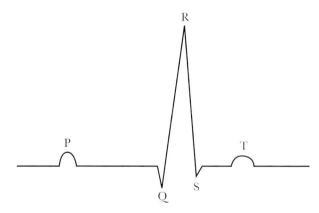

Fig. 10.27 *The normal ECG complex*

Thus the normal ECG trace consists of a series of waves: the P wave, the QRS complex and the T wave (Figure 10.27). Other components of importance include the PR interval and the ST segment (Table 10.4).

> Remember 0.04 second equals one small square
> 0.20 second equals one large square

Summary

P wave The P wave represents depolarization of the atria and in lead II is a small positive (upward) deflection. It lasts normally less than 0.10 seconds, is less than 2.5 mm in height, and precedes each QRS complex.

QRS complex The QRS complex represents depolarization of the ventricles. It consists of one or more waves: a negative deflection before the R wave is always called a Q wave (a Q wave may not always be present). The first positive deflection after the P wave is the R wave. A negative deflection following the R wave is called an S wave. A QRS complex that consists of a single, large negative deflection is called a QS wave. The duration of a normal QRS complex is less than 0.12 seconds (less than three small squares) in adults. The height or amplitude is variable from 2 mm to 15 mm. The QRS complex in lead II usually shows a large positive (upward) R wave.

T wave The T wave represents repolarization of the ventricles and is positive (upright) in lead II. Its duration is variable (0.10–0.25 second) and its amplitude is less than 5 mm. Note that there is no recognizable wave equivalent for atrial repolarization which occurs physiologically during ventricular depolarization. Thus the atrial T wave is hidden in the QRS complex.

PR interval The PR interval represents the time it takes for an electrical impulse generated in the SA node to reach the ventricles via the AV node and bundle branches. The PR interval begins with the onset of the P wave and terminates at the onset

Table 10.4 Cardiac events related to ECG components

Cardiac event	ECG component	Normal value (s)
Electrical activation of atria	P wave	0.10
Electrical activation of ventricles	QRS complex	0.12
Repolarization of ventricles and return to resting membrane potential	T wave	0.15–0.25
Spread of excitation from SA node through AV node to ventricular muscle	PR interval	0.12–0.20
Early part of repolarization of ventricles	ST segment	0.20
Time between two successive ventricular depolarizations	RR interval	

of the QRS complex (this is normally the point of the beginning of a Q wave, but may be at the start of the R wave, if a Q wave is not present); strictly speaking the PR interval should be called a PQ interval. The duration of the PR interval is normally 0.12–0.20 second (three to five small squares). A normal PR interval indicates that no conduction delay has occurred between the SA node through the AV node and bundle of His.

ST segment The ST segment represents the early part of repolarization of the ventricles. It stretches from the end of the S wave or QRS complex to the beginning of the T wave. It lasts for 0.20 second (five small squares) or less, although its length is dependent on the heart rate – the ST segment shortens with faster heart rates. Normally the ST segment is flat or identical with the isoelectric line.

Systematic Analysis of the ECG in Seven Steps

The main purpose of a systematic approach to analysing a patient's ECG is to be able to recognize a heart rhythm disorder or *arrhythmia*. Furthermore, it may be possible for the paramedic to suspect myocardial ischaemia, acute myocardial infarction or an electrolyte imbalance. However, the patient's overall condition – not just isolated ECG findings – will determine diagnosis and further management.

The seven steps in analysis of an ECG

1 Determine the heart rate
2 Determine the heart rhythm
3 Analyse the P waves
4 Analyse the QRS complexes
5 Measure the PR interval
6 Analyse the T waves
7 Analyse the ST segments

Step 1: Determine the heart rate

The heart rate is most easily calculated by dividing 300 by the number of large squares between two consecutive R waves of QRS complexes, the RR interval (Table 10.5).

This method is accurate if the heart rhythm is regular. The normal heart rate is between 60 and 100 beats per minute. A *bradycardia* is defined as a heart rate below 60 beats per minute. If the heart rate is above 100 beats per minute it is called a *tachycardia*. If the rhythm is irregular, the rate can be calculated by measuring the number of large squares between 5 or 10 'R' waves, dividing by 5 or 10, and then dividing into 300.

Step 2: Determine the heart rhythm

The heart rhythm is determined by comparing the length of several RR intervals on a sufficiently long strip of the ECG trace from left to right. The heart rhythm is regular if the distances between R waves counted in large or small squares are equal. If RR intervals vary and the difference between the shortest and longest is greater than 0.16 second (equivalent to four small squares) the rhythm is irregular. Irregular rhythms can be either 'regularly irregular' or 'irregularly irregular'. The latter describes a rhythm where there is no relationship between the RR intervals whatsoever.

Step 3: Analyse the P waves

In sinus rhythm there is a P wave before each QRS complex. In atrial fibrillation P waves are absent. In atrial flutter the P wave rate is at 300 per minute, and appears as a 'saw-tooth' pattern. If there are more P waves than QRS complexes, an atrioventricular block may be present. Before analysing the QRS complex, determine the length of the PR interval. If it measures less than 0.12 second (three small squares) it is shortened. If it lasts longer than 0.20 second (five small squares) it is prolonged.

Step 4: Analyse the QRS complex

The QRS complexes are normal if they are narrow and last less than three small squares or 0.12 second. The QRS complexes appear widened or bizarre if there is extra time taken for depolarization of the ventricles. If the QRS duration is greater than 0.12 second (three small squares) conduction through the ventricle is abnormally slow.

Step 5: Measure the PR interval

If the PR interval is less than 0.12 second (three small squares) or greater than 0.20 second (five small squares) the electrical impulse has not progressed from the atria to the ventricles via the normal conduction pathway. A prolonged PR interval occurs in atrioventricular block.

Step 6: Analyse the T wave

A normal T wave is upright and oriented in the same direction as the R wave of the QRS complex in that lead. Inversion of

Table 10.5 Calculation of heart rate

Number of large squares between two adjacent R waves		Heart rate (beats/min)
1	300/1	300
2	300/2	150
3	300/3	100
4	300/4	75
5	300/5	60
6	300/6	50
7	300/7	43
8	300/8	37
9	300/9	33
10	300/10	30

Remember: 1 large square = 0.2 second; 1 large square consists of 5 × 5 small squares

the T wave may indicate that an acute myocardial infarction has occurred in the past, and this pattern is often permanent. The T wave may also be inverted or flattened if the patient's serum potassium level is low, an electrolyte imbalance called *hypokalaemia*. The T wave appears tall and symmetrically peaked if the patient has a high serum potassium level, an electrolyte imbalance called *hyperkalaemia*.

Step 7: Analyse the ST segment

Elevation of the ST segment can signify an acute myocardial infarction if it is greater than two small squares above the isoelectric line. An ST segment depression can occur in acute cardiac ischaemia, but should only confidently be diagnosed on a 12-lead ECG (Figure 10.28).

Analysis of Rhythm

Heart rhythms can be divided into three groups:

- normal sinus rhythm
- slow rhythms (bradyarrhythmias)
- fast rhythms (tachyarrhythmias)

Slow and fast rhythms may or may not be associated with cardiac arrest (Figure 10.29).
Fast rhythms (VF and pulseless VT) and slow rhythms (asystole) that do cause cardiac arrest are discussed in Chapter 12.

Sinus rhythm

Sinus rhythm (Figure 10.30) is defined as a heart rate between 60 and 100 beats per minute; greater than 100 beats/min constitutes tachycardia, less than 60 beats/min is bradycardia.

Fast rhythms

Any rhythm with a rate exceeding 100 beats/min is a tachycardia; if the rhythm originates in the sinoatrial node, it is a

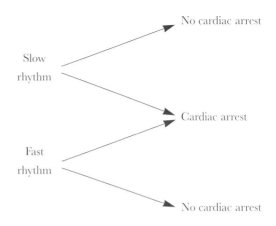

Fig. 10.29 Slow and fast rhythms

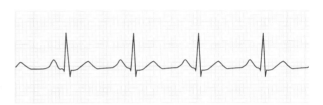

Fig. 10.30 Sinus rhythm

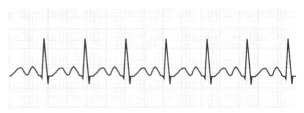

Fig. 10.31 Sinus tachycardia

sinus tachycardia (Figure 10.31). Sinus tachycardia is unlikely with a heart rate of greater than 150 beats/min.

Remember: electrocardiographically the heart only has two chambers

The atria are separated from the ventricles by a fibrous septum which is normally penetrated only at the AV node. The normal heart rhythm is usually initiated by the SA node, but because of the inbuilt rhythmicity of all cardiac cells a rhythm may be generated by other parts of the heart. If a discharging focus occurs in the muscle of the atria (Figure 10.32), depolarization passes through the atria following an abnormal pathway; the P wave is therefore broad and abnormally shaped. Once the depolarization reaches the AV node, the normal pathway is followed. The

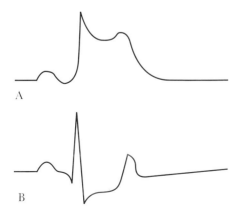

Fig. 10.28 ST segment elevation (A) and depression (B)

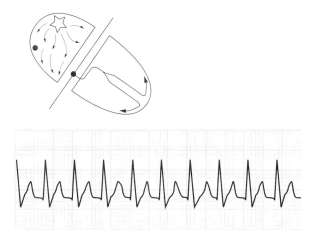

Fig. 10.32 Atrial tachycardia

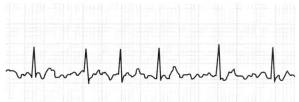

Fig. 10.34 *Atrial fibrillation*

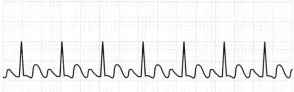

Fig. 10.35 *Atrial flutter*

QRS therefore looks normal. This is an *atrial tachycardia*. This rhythm is often so fast that the abnormal P waves cannot be seen. An isolated complex arising from an abnormal atrial focus is called an *atrial premature beat* or *atrial ectopic* (Figure 10.33).

Atrial tachycardia: abnormal P wave, normal QRS

In some people, particularly the elderly, there is no coordinated atrial activity, but a continual chaotic contraction of individual muscles. This is *atrial fibrillation*; because only single muscles are involved, atrial contraction is not seen on the ECG. Eventually, however, depolarization reaches the AV node and ventricular contraction (following the normal pathway) produces a normal QRS. Because the atrial cells are depolarizing chaotically, depolarization reaches the AV node randomly and the ventricular rate is irregular (Figure 10.34).

Atrial fibrillation: no P wave, normal QRS

Atrial flutter occurs when an atrial focus depolarizes at a regular rate (usually 300 per minute) with a proportion (100% or less) of atrial depolarizations being transmitted to the ventricles (Figure 10.35).

Atrial contraction produces a regular 'saw-tooth' pattern on the ECG. Once again, ventricular depolarization and the QRS complexes are normal.

Atrial flutter: abnormal (saw-tooth) P wave, normal QRS

The most common form of atrial flutter has only 50% of atrial depolarizations transmitted to the ventricles: *this is known as 2:1 block*. Consequently a ventricular rate of 150 per minute occurs.

Any ECG showing a ventricular rate of *exactly* 150/min is atrial flutter with 2:1 block until proved otherwise

An abnormal rhythm may also arise at the AV junction (Figure 10.36). When this happens, retrograde depolarization occurs at the same time as normal depolarization of the ventricles (Figure 10.37). Because of this, no normal P waves are seen on the ECG (late and inverted P waves may be seen). However, because it arises from the AV node, the resulting rhythm is regular and the ventricular depolarization and QRS normal: this is *junctional tachycardia* (Figure 10.38). This rhythm is sometimes incorrectly known as supraventricular tachycardia. In fact *all* tachycardias arising from the AV node or above are 'supraventricular'.

Junctional tachycardia: no P wave, normal QRS

It should now be clear that all supraventricular tachycardias (except sinus) have an absent or abnormal P wave and a *normal* QRS.

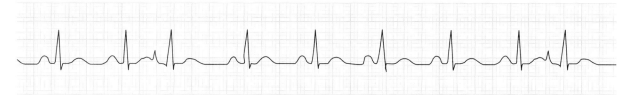

Fig. 10.33 *Atrial ectopics*

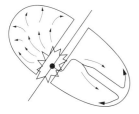

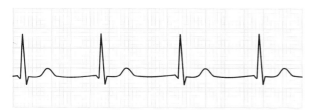

Fig. 10.36 *Junctional rhythm*

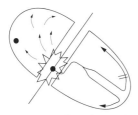

Fig. 10.37 *Simultaneous retrograde and normal depolarization of the ventricles*

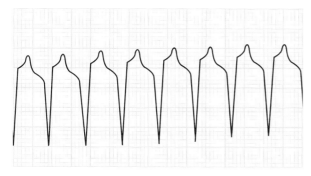

Fig. 10.38 *Junctional tachycardia*

Ventricular tachycardia An abnormal rhythm may arise from a focus in the ventricles (Figure 10.39). Depolarization therefore must follow an abnormal path through the ventricular muscle, producing a slower contraction and a wide, abnormal QRS complex. The effect is similar in origin to the abnormal QRS of bundle branch block. The contraction produced by a ventricular focus is less coordinated than normal: it is therefore less mechanically efficient, and may precipitate heart failure. The patient may be hypotensive, and can progress to cardiac arrest. Ventricular tachycardia may be the primary arrhythmia in sudden cardiac arrest (Figure 10.40).

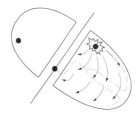

Fig. 10.39 *An abnormal rhythm arising from a focus in the ventricles*

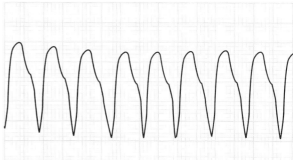

Fig. 10.40 *Ventricular tachycardia*

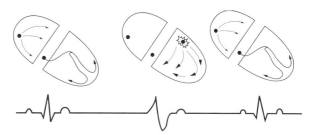

Fig. 10.41 *Ventricular ectopic beat between normal beats*

When a single complex arises from a ventricular focus, it is known as a ventricular premature beat or ventricular ectopic (Figures 10.41 and 10.42).

Summary of tachycardias All myocardial cells have 'inherent' rhythmicity, and contraction is initiated by the area with the fastest spontaneous rate of depolarization: this is the SA node, and its rapid depolarization rate overrides other areas producing a coordinated contraction using the normal conduction pathway.

Tachycardias (which can be divided into *supraventricular* or *ventricular*) occur when a pathological process or stimulant causes some other area of the heart to override the SA node as pacemaker at a higher rate. The characteristic ECG findings are summarized in Table 10.6.

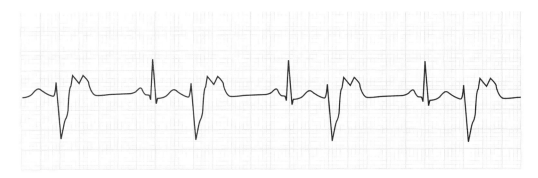

Fig. 10.42 *Ventricular ectopic beats*

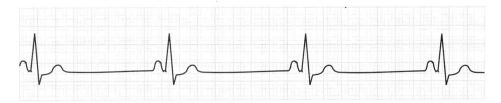

Fig. 10.43 *Sinus bradycardia*

Bradycardia and heart block

Sinus bradycardia occurs when the pulse is less than 60 beats/min, but the ECG is otherwise normal (Figure 10.43). Treatment is rarely required.

The PR interval (0.12–0.20 second, three to five small squares) indicates the time taken for depolarization to pass from the SA node through the atria to the ventricles. When this depolarization takes longer than 0.2 s it is termed *first degree heart block* (Figure 10.44). First degree heart block can only be diagnosed on ECG.

> **In first degree heart block atrial depolarization is always transmitted to the ventricles**

If some waves of atrial depolarization fail to be transmitted to the ventricles, *second degree heart block* has occurred. Because atrial depolarization has occurred normally, the P wave is normal whether or not it is followed by a QRS complex (Figure 10.45). *Second degree (Mobitz) type I heart block* (also known as the Wenckebach phenomenon) occurs when successive depolarization takes longer to transmit to the ventricles until one fails to be transmitted at all, causing progressive lengthening of the PR interval (Figure 10.46). Once again the P wave is normal as normal atrial depolarization has occurred. The abnormality is the increasing time taken for transmission of atrial depolarization to the ventricles.

Alternatively the PR interval may remain constant with occasional depolarizations failing to transmit to the ventricles. The missed (or dropped) beat may be regular (e.g. every third or

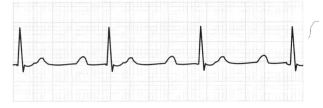

Fig. 10.44 *First degree heart block*

fourth beat) or irregular (random) (Figure 10.47). This is *(Mobitz) type II second degree heart block*. Causes of slow or absent conduction to the ventricles include ischaemia and connective tissue disorders.

Table 10.6 Summary of tachycardias: these are known as 'narrow complex' arrhythmias, except for ventricular tachycardia which is a 'broad complex' arrhythmic

Supraventricular	P	QRS
Sinus tachycardia	Normal	Normal
Atrial tachycardia	Abnormal	Normal
Atrial fibrillation	Absent	Normal
Atrial flutter	Abnormal (saw-tooth)	Normal
Junctional tachycardia	Absent	Normal
Ventricular		
Ventricular tachycardia	Absent	Abnormal

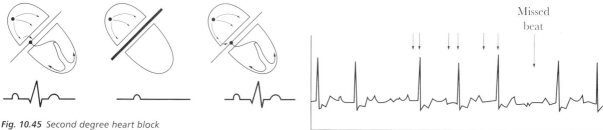

Fig. 10.45 *Second degree heart block*

Fig. 10.46 *Wenckebach phenomenon*

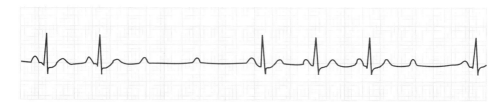

Fig. 10.47 *Mobitz type II second degree heart block*

In second degree heart block some atrial depolarizations are not transmitted to the ventricles

Sometimes no atrial depolarizations at all are transmitted to the ventricles (Figure 10.48). This produces isolated regular P waves on the ECG, and unless an *escape* mechanism occurs (ventricles contracting regularly from a ventricular ectopic focus) it will be rapidly fatal. This is *third degree heart block*.

As previously stated, all myocardial cells spontaneously and regularly contract. Normally ventricular cells do this at a slow rate and are overridden by impulses from the SA node via the AV node and conducting system. When the ventricles become electrically isolated from the atria in third degree heart block, spontaneous ventricular depolarization may therefore begin (Figure 10.49). This produces a wide QRS complex which is not related in any way to the normal P waves (Figure 10.50). This rhythm will prevent the patient suffering sudden cardiac death. Because there is no relationship between the electrical activity of the atria and the ventricles, this is often known as atrioventricular dissociation.

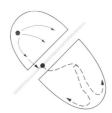

Fig. 10.48 *Third degree heart block*

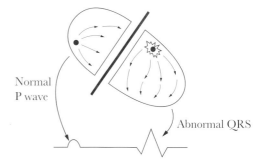

Fig. 10.49 *Spontaneous ventricular depolarization in third degree heart block*

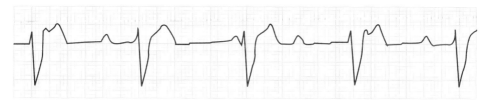

Fig. 10.50 *Complete (third degree) heart block*

> In third degree heart block there is no transmission of depolarization from atria to ventricles

The treatment of arrhythmias is discussed in Chapter 13.

CONCLUSION

Coronary heart disease is the most common cause of death in the UK. The paramedic will frequently encounter cardiac arrest and cardiac emergencies (see Chapters 12 and 13). Knowledge of the anatomy and physiology of the cardio-vascular system and of the ECG will enable the paramedic to strengthen the *chain of survival*, by recognizing the mechanism of cardiovascular dysfunction and commencing definitive and life-saving treatment at the scene and *en route* to hospital.

FURTHER READING

Anderson JE (1983) *Grant's Atlas of Anatomy*, 8th edn. Baltimore: Williams and Wilkins.

Epstein O, Perkin CD, de Bono DP & Cookson J (1992) *Clinical Examination*. London: Gower Medical Publishing.

Hampton JR (1992) *The ECG Made Easy*, 4th edn. Edinburgh: Churchill Livingstone.

Lamb JF, Ingram CG, Johnston IA & Pitman RM (1991) *Essentials of Physiology*, 3rd edn. Oxford: Blackwell.

Lumley JSP (1990) *Surface Anatomy: The Anatomical Basis of Clinical Examination*. Edinburgh: Churchill Livingstone.

chapter eleven:

MONITORING AND DEFIBRILLATION

The paramedic will monitor a number of physiological parameters in patients who become acutely unwell. Documentation of the baseline cardiac rhythm, blood pressure and oxygen saturation will allow the patient's progress to be monitored and may play a vital role in subsequent management. In some situations the results will indicate the need for immediate treatment.

Recent developments, particularly in electronics, have made it possible to equip ambulances with portable cardiac monitors and pulse oximeters, thereby allowing sophisticated monitoring of patients outside hospital. The availability of such equipment does not mean, however, that traditional clinical measurements are any less valid. On the contrary, clinical assessment of the patient's pulse, blood pressure, cardiorespiratory status, and cerebral function (assessed either by using the Glasgow Coma Scale, or by 'AVPU and pupils' – see Chapter 21) remains as important as ever.

In this chapter the monitoring techniques available to the paramedic are considered, and their application is discussed. Defibrillators are also considered here because most cardiac monitors used by the ambulance service also serve this function; furthermore, the use of defibrillators is dependent on the results of cardiac monitoring. The actual technique of defibrillation is discussed in Chapter 12.

CLINICAL ASSESSMENT

Much can be learnt about the cardiac and respiratory status of a patient by careful examination of the patient's colour, pulse rate, blood pressure and respiratory rate.

Colour

The presence of pallor may signify anaemia. This may be long-standing or have arisen suddenly because of blood loss; it may also be present in a patient who has developed shock from other causes. The presence of anaemia is assessed by examination of the mucous membranes, particularly the conjunctiva or oral mucosa. This may be difficult outside hospital because of poor light, the influence of ambient temperature, or the presence of dirt, grease or other contaminants. Examination of the nail beds is especially difficult and unreliable under these circumstances.

The term *cyanosis* refers to the bluish-grey discolouration of the skin or mucous membranes that results from reduced haemoglobin oxygen saturation. Two types are recognized: central and peripheral cyanosis. In *central cyanosis* inadequate oxygenation of the blood occurs because of imperfect oxygenation of blood in the lungs, or rarely a mixing of oxygenated and deoxygenated blood in the heart (deoxygenated blood may bypass the lungs with septum defects in the heart). It is, for example, frequently seen in patients with chronic bronchitis. The condition is assessed by examination of the oral mucosa which shows the characteristic bluish-grey colouration.

Peripheral cyanosis occurs when increased extraction of oxygen occurs in the periphery; it is most readily recognized in the fingers, particularly in the nail beds. The important differentiating feature from central cyanosis is that in peripheral cyanosis blood is oxygenated normally so that the warm oral mucosa is a normal colour. Peripheral cyanosis may be recognized in the hands when the peripheral circulation is slowed; this may be caused by cold, and its presence does not necessarily indicate disease.

Pulse

In a collapsed patient a central pulse in a prominent artery should be palpated. In most cases the carotid artery will be used; the femoral pulse is also suitable, although less accessible. The role of pulse assessment during the management of cardiac arrest is covered in Chapter 12. Valuable information may be obtained from the rate, strength and character of a central (carotid or femoral) pulse. Assessment of a peripheral pulse (radial, brachial or foot pulse) is less reliable, although the brachial pulse is recommended for palpation in cardiac arrest in infants (see Chapter 35). The cardiac rate may be assessed by counting the pulse, and the radial pulse in the wrist is most commonly used for this purpose. It is unreliable in conditions of reduced cardiac output – in this situation a central pulse should always be employed. In many cases the ECG or the pulse oximeter will be used to document the pulse rate.

Respiratory Rate

The respiratory rate should be assessed in all cases where cardiac or respiratory function is compromised or where central control of respiration may be reduced – for example after head injury or drug overdose. The respiratory rate is usually expressed in breaths per minute. The normal rate is highest in neonates and babies, and falls progressively with age until the adult range of 12–18 breaths per minute is reached.

Blood Pressure

The accurate measurement of blood pressure is an important part of the assessment of the patient. Successive readings may be compared and allow the patient's progress and response to treatment to be monitored. The familiar mercury sphygmomanometer widely used to measure blood pressure in hospital is not robust enough for field use – loss of mercury may occur if the machine is dropped, broken or stored incorrectly. It is also difficult to read in adverse lighting conditions. For these reasons aneroid sphygmomanometers (Figure 11.1) or electronic methods are usually employed when a portable machine is used. Care is necessary to ensure that the zero level does not change with time and these machines should be regularly standardized against a known reference pressure to ensure consistent accuracy.

Manual methods

The sphygmomanometer cuff should be the correct size for the patient's arm if accurate readings are to be obtained. Smaller cuffs are appropriate for children while larger cuffs should be employed for obese adults. The ideal size of cuff may not always be available with the restricted equipment carried on an

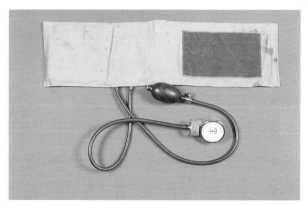

Fig. 11.1 An aneroid sphygmomanometer

ambulance, but where an inappropriate cuff size has been used the cuff size should be recorded.

The blood pressure cuff is applied to the upper arm. Most modern cuffs have a method of indicating the correct position of the cuff over the brachial artery. Velcro fastenings are more convenient than the traditional wrap-around type of cuff as they are more secure and easier to apply. The cuff is inflated above the systolic blood pressure; this point may be determined by palpating the radial pulse while inflating the cuff. An estimate of systolic blood pressure may be obtained by determining the point at which the radial pulse returns when the cuff is subsequently deflated. This may be the only measurement possible if the Korotkoff sounds (those sounds heard with a stethoscope over the artery distal to the cuff) are difficult to hear when the blood pressure is low, or because of adverse circumstances in pre-hospital care. The blood pressure is best determined by slowly deflating the cuff while listening for the return of Korotkoff sounds through a stethoscope diaphragm placed over the brachial artery in the antecubital fossa. The systolic blood pressure is taken at the point when the sounds return (i.e. when systolic blood pressure exceeds the pressure in the cuff). The diastolic pressure is measured at the point of disappearance of the sounds.

Electronic blood pressure monitoring

Electronic devices that measure blood pressure non-invasively are available; sometimes this facility is incorporated into other monitoring equipment, for example a pulse oximeter. In most cases a blood pressure cuff is applied to the upper arm in the conventional manner and connected to the monitoring unit through tubing that permits inflation and deflation of the cuff. The circuit incorporates a sensor (microphone or oscillotonometer) that monitors brachial artery pulsation, thereby allowing the systolic and diastolic pressure to be determined. The blood pressure reading obtained is displayed digitally on a screen. Most modern units also display the pulse rate. (Microphone sensor units are cheap and unreliable. They may be readily available in high street retailers, and paramedics should be dissuaded from buying these for their own use.) The frequency with which the blood pressure is measured can be pre-set according to the patient's requirements and allows progress to be monitored. Although these units offer convenience (particularly where limited help is available or access to the patient is difficult), it is essential that the manufacturer's instructions are followed precisely if consistently accurate readings are to be obtained. The units require regular checking and standardization to ensure accuracy.

Intra-arterial blood pressure monitoring

Intra-arterial measurement is performed when continuous monitoring of arterial pressure is required, most often in the operating theatre or intensive therapy unit. A catheter is inserted directly into an artery and the pressure wave is monitored by a transducer connected to the catheter. Such intra-arterial monitoring lines may be *in situ* when a patient is transferred between hospitals; paramedics should be aware of their presence and clarify any precautions necessary during the journey with the appropriate staff.

PULSE OXIMETRY

In recent years pulse oximetry has become established as the most convenient non-invasive method of monitoring arterial oxygen saturation (Figure 11.2). It is widely used outside hospital and is particularly useful where there is delay in moving a patient (for example in cases of entrapment), or for monitoring the patient during transport.

Hypoxia is an important cause of neurological damage and the early detection (and adequate treatment) of hypoxia plays a vital role in its prevention. Pulse oximetry offers many advantages over clinical methods of assessing oxygenation; the detection of cyanosis is subject to considerable observer bias and is often difficult outside hospital because of bad light or other adverse conditions. There are further problems with polycythaemic patients who may appear cyanosed despite an adequate oxygen tension.

Pulse oximeters measure the saturation of the blood with oxygen in terms of the percentage saturation of haemoglobin (the blood's oxygen carrier), by measuring the differential absorption of light by total haemoglobin and the oxyhaemoglobin (i.e. saturated) constituent of this. A probe containing a light source is attached to a finger: light traverses the finger and nail bed and is monitored on the opposite side of the finger from the light source. A pulsatile flow of blood (usually in the bed of the fingernail) is required for measurements to be made, so problems may arise when the peripheral circulation is impaired. Rapid fluctuations in ambient light levels may produce false pulsatile signals, and movement during patient transport may also cause inaccurate readings. Carboxyhaemoglobin present in cases of carbon monoxide poisoning may cause a pulse oximeter to over-

estimate the true oxygen saturation: in carbon monoxide poisoning pulse oximetry will measure the total percentage saturation of haemoglobin with oxygen (oxyhaemoglobin) and carbon monoxide (carboxyhaemoglobin). Dirt, grease and nail varnish (dark and metallic colours only) also lead to inaccurate measurements. Skin colour has no effect on oxygen saturation recording.

Incorrect pulse oximeter readings may be caused by

- Poor circulation
- Fluctuating light levels
- Carbon monoxide poisoning
- Skin, dirt and grease
- Nail varnish (dark and metallic colours only)

The relationship between arterial oxygen tension (Pao_2) and arterial oxygen saturation is described by the oxyhaemoglobin dissociation curve (Figure 11.3). The relationship between arterial oxygen tension (content) and the oxygen saturation forms an S-shaped curve, which implies that there may be a marked drop in arterial oxygen content before this is reflected in a fall in oxygen saturation. Normal values are shown in Table 11.1. The most serious pitfall of pulse oximetry arises when alveolar hypoventilation causes respiratory failure; this may arise from lung disease, muscular weakness or central respiratory depression. A rise in arterial and alveolar carbon dioxide tension (Pco_2) occurs, and alveolar Po_2 falls with resultant arterial hypoxaemia. If a patient is breathing air the oxygen saturation

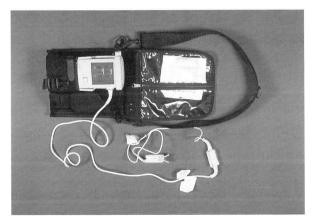

Fig. 11.2 *A pulse oximeter*

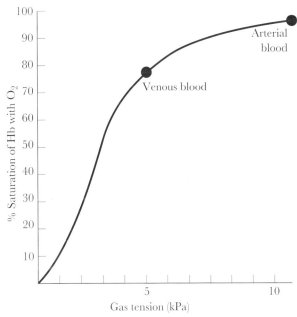

Fig. 11.3 *The oxygen dissociation curve for haemoglobin (Hb)*

Table 11.1 Arterial oxygen saturation values

Normal range	97–100%
Mild hypoxia	90–97%
Moderate hypoxia	85–90%
Severe hypoxia	< 85%

will fall quickly and provide a reasonably early warning of hypoventilation. If, however, the patient is receiving supplementary oxygen the alveolar Po_2 will be much higher, and the alveolar Pco_2 will have to rise much further before hypoxaemia sufficient to produce measurable desaturation occurs. *It must be stressed that a normal oxygen saturation in the presence of an increased inspired oxygen concentration gives no information about the adequacy of ventilation.*

Pulse oximetry does not measure carbon dioxide

Pulse oximetry has been used to assess the vascular supply to a limb when arterial trauma is thought to be present, but has proved to be unreliable and even misleading when used for this purpose. A trend of falling oxygen saturation readings is likely to be more valuable than an isolated reading and several readings should therefore be recorded if used for this purpose. Alternatively the saturation values in an injured and an uninjured limb can be compared.

Despite these limitations, the pulse oximeter is a valuable development in the monitoring of arterial oxygen saturation to detect the presence of serious hypoxaemia easily and non-invasively. A sustained trend of falling oxygen saturation is always a clinically important observation, despite doubts about the precision of individual readings.

ELECTROCARDIOGRAPHIC MONITORING

Electrocardiographic (ECG) monitoring is undertaken to define the cardiac rhythm. Documentation of an abnormal cardiac rhythm may play a vital part in the patient's subsequent management. In some circumstances treatment of an abnormal cardiac rhythm will be instituted by the paramedic before arrival at hospital; accurate rhythm monitoring and interpretation are particularly important in the management of cardiac arrest (described in Chapter 12). In other circumstances cardiac monitoring may allow measures to be taken to correct an arrhythmia before cardiac arrest takes place. This applies particularly in cases of chest pain, collapse, syncope, palpitation or shock.

Cardiac Monitors

Many types of cardiac monitoring system are available, but in the ambulance service the cardiac monitor is usually an integral part of the defibrillator. Manual defibrillators and cardiac monitors feature a screen for displaying the cardiac rhythm and usually incorporate an arrangement for obtaining a printout of the ECG. Automated external defibrillators (AEDs) often store the ECG electronically and a hard copy is obtained from the appropriate playback device.

Many cardiac monitors incorporate a heart rate meter which is triggered by the QRS complex of the ECG. An alarm will sound automatically should the heart rate fall outside pre-set limits; lights and audible signals may also provide additional indications of the heart rate. Traditional (analogue) monitors display the ECG on a cathode-ray oscilloscope screen. Many modern cardiac monitors convert the electronic signals into a digital form; the rhythm may then be displayed on a liquid crystal screen and computer-aided rhythm analysis of the ECG becomes possible. Digital signals are also easier to store electronically for subsequent playback and analysis.

Monitoring Electrodes

In most circumstances paramedics will instigate ECG monitoring by attaching adhesive electrodes to the patient's chest. The positions illustrated in Figure 11.4 will allow records that approximate to leads I, II or III of the conventional ECG. The configuration that displays the most prominent P wave (if organized atrial activity is present) with sufficient QRS amplitude to trigger the rate meter should be adopted; this will usually be lead II (see Chapter 10). Electrical interference may be minimized by applying the electrodes over bone rather than muscle; the precordium must be left unobstructed so that chest compression and defibrillation may be carried out if necessary. Hair should be removed from the areas where the electrodes are to be attached and the skin should where possible be cleaned with alcohol to remove skin oil. Some adhesive electrodes incorporate a wrapping on the electrode which is used to abrade the skin and improve electrical contact. Movement artefact will be minimized in conscious, cooperative patients by keeping them warm.

Monitoring after Cardiac Arrest

It is important to obtain a read-out of the cardiac rhythm as soon as possible after cardiac arrest. Modern monitor-defibrillators enable the cardiac rhythm to be monitored through the defibrillator electrodes (semiautomatic) or paddles (manual) applied to the chest wall. If ventricular fibrillation is present defibrillation can be carried out immediately, while if the original rhythm appears to be asystole different paddle positions may be employed to exclude fine ventricular fibrillation.

Defibrillator paddles do not make ideal monitoring electrodes: they need to be kept in position by hand and are really only suitable for a quick look at the rhythm, otherwise chest compression will be interrupted for an unacceptable time. Electrode

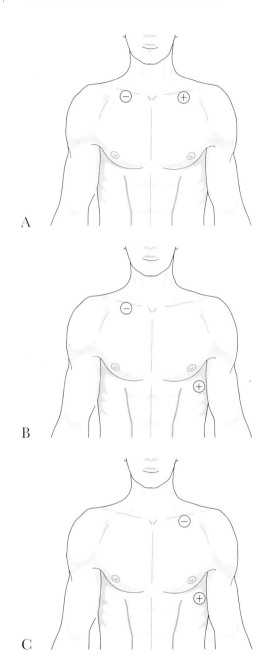

Fig. 11.4 ECG electrode positions. A (positive left shoulder, negative right shoulder) equivalent to lead I; B (Positive left lower chest, negative right clavicle) equivalent to lead II; C (positive left lower chest, negative left clavicle) equivalent to lead III

gel, necessary to obtain good electrical contact, tends to become dispersed over the chest during subsequent chest compression with a danger of arcing when defibrillation is carried out – special defibrillator gel pads offer a considerable advantage in this regard and are strongly recommended.

A better ECG signal is obtained from adhesive electrodes; these should be applied as soon as convenient, so that continuous monitoring and recording of the rhythm may take place.

> Ensure that your defibrillator is changed to read from leads when the electrodes have been attached

Diagnosis from Cardiac Monitors

The displays and printouts from cardiac monitors are suitable only for rhythm recognition and not for analysis of ST segment changes or more sophisticated ECG morphology interpretation. The printout of the ECG should be inspected carefully to diagnose the cardiac rhythm and retained for transfer to the patient's records on arrival at hospital. The time that the trace is recorded is essential information and should be added manually at the start of the record if this is not done automatically by the monitor.

DEFIBRILLATORS

All front line ambulances in the UK are now equipped with defibrillators. Defibrillators are of two types: manual and automated. With manual defibrillators (Figure 11.5) the operator interprets the cardiac rhythm, decides whether a defibrillatory countershock is required, charges the machine and administers the shock. Skill in ECG interpretation is required, and training takes much longer than with an automated defibrillator. It was the introduction of the automated external defibrillator (AED), which may be used by paramedics and less highly trained staff, that enabled the rapid introduction of defibrillators throughout the ambulance service. Automated external defibrillators may be semi-automatic (SAD) or fully automatic. Paramedics in a number of ambulance services will use a manual defibrillator. With the SAD (Figure 11.6) the process of rhythm recognition and preparation for defibrillation are automated. All that is required of the operator is to recognize that cardiac arrest may have occurred and attach two electrodes to the patient's chest. These serve the dual purpose of cardiac rhythm monitoring and delivery of the direct current (DC) countershock. The SAD converts the ECG signal into digital format and applies an electronic algorithm to enable ECG interpretation. The machine will recognize ventricular fibrillation and certain other arrhythmias likely to require DC countershock. During the analysis period (which in most models is less than 10 seconds) no contact must be made with the patient to avoid the chance of movement artefact interfering with rhythm analysis. If a rhythm requiring DC shock is detected the machine will charge itself to a predetermined level and indicate to the operator that

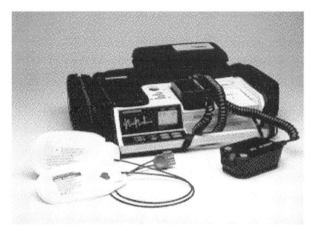

Fig. 11.5 A manual defibrillator

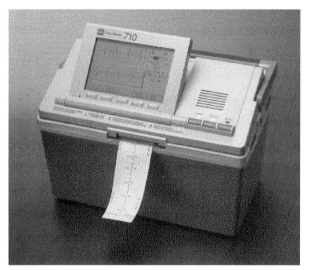

Fig. 11.6 A semiautomated external defibrillator (SAD)

a shock is indicated. Many models incorporate written on-screen instructions and some models also feature synthesized voice instructions to guide the operator.

Where monitoring is instituted with an SAD in patients at risk of cardiac arrest it is more economical to employ standard ECG electrodes as these are considerably cheaper than the electrodes used to perform defibrillation. In such patients defibrillation electrodes must be available immediately should cardiac arrest occur.

The AED is accurate in the interpretation of shockable rhythms and only rarely is a DC shock advised inappropriately. Clinical trials have shown that defibrillation may be accomplished more quickly with these models than with manual defibrillators, and the ease and rapidity of training in their use has enabled the rapid introduction of defibrillation into the

ambulance service throughout the UK. This has brought defibrillation within the scope of a much wider range of personnel than was possible with manual models. Ambulance technicians as well as paramedics may use the automated machine; first-aid and other workers have also employed them successfully.

A recent development of the SAD is the first responder defibrillator (fully automated external defibrillator). Essentially this is a basic SAD designed to be stored for prolonged periods without use. The devices available offer the usual instructions and prompts during use but do not display the cardiac rhythm; the ECG storage and playback capacity is also limited. A limited number of DC shocks is possible, before servicing and battery replacement are required. First responder AEDs are considerably cheaper than the standard model, and ambulance personnel may encounter these devices in use by first-aid personnel.

Fully automated defibrillators administer a DC shock on recognition of a shockable rhythm without involvement of *the operator*. An override key can be used to convert an automated external defibrillator into a manual one.

Defibrillator Battery Care

Two types of battery are in widespread use: the lead-acid battery and the nickel-cadmium cell. The lead-acid battery works on the same principle as the accumulator used in the motor car; however, the acid is present as a gel and these units are less susceptible to the effects of movement and position. Lead-acid batteries hold their charge for prolonged periods, losing approximately 1% per month. They can be recharged rapidly after use and may be left on charge when already fully charged without the problems caused by similar treatment of nickel-cadmium cells.

Nickel-cadmium cells have been widely used in defibrillators. They are designed for regular use and ideally should be fully discharged before recharging. Regular charging when fully charged or when the cells are not greatly depleted reduces the efficiency of the battery and must be avoided. Regular reconditioning cycles (where the battery is fully discharged before being recharged) are required to maintain optimal battery condition and should be performed in accordance with the maker's recommendations. Nickel-cadmium cells lose approximately 1% of their charge per day and are less suitable than lead-acid cells for equipment that is used infrequently.

Dry batteries have a prolonged shelf-life and are used in certain type of first responder defibrillator. They are replaced when the machine is used, or if their shelf-life is exceeded before use.

Defibrillator Safety

Defibrillators are potentially dangerous pieces of equipment. A high-energy shock of several thousand volts is administered to the patient. It is essential that no part of the operator or any assistant is in electrical contact with the patient when the shock is administered. The operator must shout, 'Stand clear!' and visually check that no person is touching the patient. There are hazards for the unwary, particularly where the patient is lying on a metal table or when the surroundings are wet. Care must be taken with defibrillator gel to ensure that electrical arcing across the chest or from the electrodes to the operator's hands is not possible. This can be avoided by the use of gel pads which are now commonplace and have almost completely replaced the gel. Intravenous fluid giving sets may act as a potential conductor and helpers should not be holding these while a shock is administered. Defibrillation in the rain is normally safe unless the rain is torrential, providing the chest is wiped dry first. Patients lying in a pool of water should be moved before defibrillation and the carers must ensure they are not connected to the patient by standing in water.

Defibrillation in Patients with Pacemakers

Increasing numbers of patients are now fitted with permanent pacemakers. A generator is implanted in the chest wall usually under one clavicle and an electrode leads from the generator to the heart. In dual-chamber systems (that pace both atria and ventricles) two electrodes are employed.

Occasionally the pacing electrodes may be screwed into the heart from the epicardial surface; these are connected to a generator often implanted into the upper abdominal wall.

Modern pacemaker generators incorporate protection circuits that prevent the discharge from a defibrillator damaging the pacemaker. An electric current may, however, travel through the pacing electrode and cause an electrical burn at the point of contact with the myocardium. This may cause a subsequent rise in pacemaker threshold with loss of pacing. When defibrillation is successful this rise in threshold may not be apparent until some weeks later, and to minimize the chances of this occurring, defibrillator electrodes should be placed as far away from the generator as possible – at least 12 cm whenever possible. With temporary pacing, an external generator is connected to a temporary pacing electrode (usually inserted through the subclavian or jugular vein). Paramedics may encounter these during the transfer of patients between hospitals. Should defibrillation be necessary, the same precautions that apply to permanent pacemakers should be followed, placing the defibrillator electrodes as far away as possible from the point where the temporary pacing wire enters the skin. Care with electrode gel is also necessary to prevent electrical arcing to the pacing electrode or its attached wires.

> Glyceryl trinitrate patches must be removed prior to defibrillation to avoid the risk of explosion

FURTHER READING

Beevers D (1988) *The ABC of Hypertension*. London: BMJ Publications.

Bossart L & Koster R (1992) Defibrillation: methods and strategies. *Resuscitation* **24**: 211–225.

Colquhoun MC, Handley AJ & Evans TR (1995) *ABC of Resuscitation*, 3rd edn. London: BMJ Publications.

Crockett PJ, Doppert BM & Higgins SE (1991) *Defibrillation: What You Should Know*, 3rd edn. Physio Control Corporation.

Handley AJ & Swain AH, eds (1994) *Advanced Life Support Manual*. Resuscitation Council (UK).

Hutton P & Clutton-Brook T (1994) The benefits and pitfalls of pulse oximetry. *British Medical Journal* **307**: 457–458.

chapter twelve:

CARDIAC ARREST IN ADULTS: ADVANCED LIFE SUPPORT

Cardiac arrest is the most serious emergency confronted by paramedics. It is the final common pathway for death in the pre-hospital environment (whether from acute illness, injury or environmental causes such as drowning). The prevention of cardiac arrest in a deteriorating patient also represents one of the greatest challenges to the paramedic.

The term *primary cardiac arrest* is used in this chapter to denote an arrest that is primarily of cardiac origin. It may be associated with acute obstruction of a coronary artery and infarction of cardiac muscle, but more frequently results from critical coronary ischaemia which disturbs electrical activity within the heart and produces a potentially lethal arrhythmia. Arrhythmias may also result from severe physiological or metabolic stresses, notably hypoxia. In the UK 150–200 cardiac arrests occur every day.

The management of cardiac arrest occupies a significant proportion of the time devoted to paramedical training. Optimal management of cardiac arrests requires:

- Knowledge of the theoretical aspects of cardiac arrest and the more effective and scientifically justified forms of treatment recommended by the European and UK Resuscitation Councils
- Training in the practical techniques required to achieve the best chance of successful resuscitation
- Regular retraining and review of theoretical and practical aspects

With all emergency work, one is working against the clock. Practical skills must be applied promptly and in a coordinated manner, ensuring that not a second is wasted. The balance between speed and efficiency is delicate and can only be achieved by regular training.

DEFINITION AND CAUSES OF CARDIAC ARREST

Cardiac arrest may be defined as the absence of a major arterial pulse in an unresponsive patient. It must be understood that this is a clinical diagnosis; there may in fact be a very weak and undetectable pulse, but the course of action is the same. An electrocardiogram is not required to establish the initial diagnosis, but may be helpful when death is to be pronounced.

The majority of sudden deaths occur from arrhythmias associated with ischaemic heart disease, or from clot formation (thrombosis) when a plaque of fatty material (atheroma) breaks through the internal lining of a coronary artery and its exposure to the circulating blood activates the clotting mechanism (see Chapter 13). Cardiac arrest may also occur as a secondary result of respiratory arrest, or from other physiological causes such as hypothermia, electrolyte imbalance, poisoning, electrocution or anaphylaxis (allergy). Whatever the root cause, the arrest can manifest in one of three ways determined from the electrocardiogram (ECG) in a pulseless patient (Figure 12.1).

- Ventricular fibrillation/pulseless ventricular tachycardia
- Asystole
- Electromechanical dissociation

THE PLACE OF ADVANCED LIFE SUPPORT

Advanced life support may be defined as cardiopulmonary resuscitation performed with the assistance of monitor-defibrillators, advanced airway techniques (usually tracheal intubation) and first-line cardiac drugs (administered intravenously).

Advanced life support (ALS) must be considered in the context of the whole resuscitation attempt, that is the chain of survival.

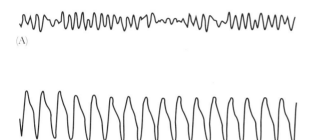

(A)

(B)

(C)

(D)

Fig. 12.1 *Traces of rhythms causing cardiac arrest: A, ventricular fibrillation; B, pulseless ventricular tachycardia; C, asystole; D, electro-mechanical dissociation*

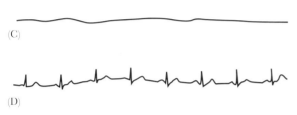

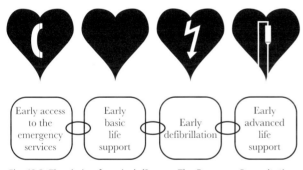

| Early access to the emergency services | Early basic life support | Early defibrillation | Early advanced life support |

Fig. 12.2 *The chain of survival. (Source: The European Resuscitation Council)*

(Figure 12.2). This emphasizes the importance of immediate contact with the ambulance service, correctly performed bystander basic life support (BLS) or cardiopulmonary resuscitation while the ambulance is *en route* to the scene, rapid defibrillation in the presence of ventricular fibrillation or pulseless ventricular tachycardia, proceeding to the application of other ALS skills.

Advanced Life Support Approach

The first principle of advanced life support is to avoid compounding the situation: the ambulance crew must not be exposed to any avoidable hazard whether physical or infectious. The next stage is to assess the patient following the standard basic life support principles of:

- Safe approach
- Establish unresponsiveness
- Open the airway
- Assess breathing
- Assess the circulation

In this way, cardiac arrest is confirmed. However, in ALS the emphasis moves from ventilation and chest compressions to attempting definitive treatment for the underlying rhythm which is assessed either by monitoring the heart through the paddles of the defibrillator or by connecting monitoring electrodes to the front of the patient's torso – one over the outer end of each clavicle and a third close to the upper part of the left iliac crest (hip). Placing the electrodes over bone reduces muscle artefact and ensures that the chest is clear for defibrillation. Speed is essential and the application of gel pads below the right clavicle and in the vicinity of the V_5 chest electrode position allows almost instantaneous monitoring of the ECG trace through the defibrillator. This can be charged immediately allowing a 200 J shock to be administered to a pulseless patient within a few seconds. However, the detailed sequence of treatment depends on the underlying rhythm as described below.

VENTRICULAR FIBRILLATION OR PULSELESS VENTRICULAR TACHYCARDIA

Ventricular tachycardia without cardiac output usually rapidly degenerates into ventricular fibrillation as electrical activity in the ventricles becomes more disorganized. The treatment is therefore the same for both conditions (Figure 12.3). Ventricular fibrillation is the most common arrhythmia causing cardiac arrest, but it may deteriorate from coarse to fine ventricular fibrillation and then asystole before the paramedic arrives. Effective basic life support is vital between the moment of collapse and the arrival of an ambulance crew and defibrillator, but BLS at best represents a holding manoeuvre which is incapable of converting ventricular fibrillation to sinus rhythm in its own right. Abnormal electrical activity needs to be treated with electrical therapy, in the form of defibrillation. Despite its limitations, it is nevertheless very important that hospital staff know whether, how competently, and for how long BLS was administered before the arrival of ALS skills.

Not infrequently, ventricular fibrillation or pulseless ventricular tachycardia develop in the presence of the ambulance crew during transportation to hospital. It is essential that good, supportive treatment is given to patients at risk of cardiac arrest: the administration of oxygen, glyceryl trinitrate and analgesics may help to prevent the ailing heart from stopping. However, if cardiac arrest is witnessed despite these interventions, the first

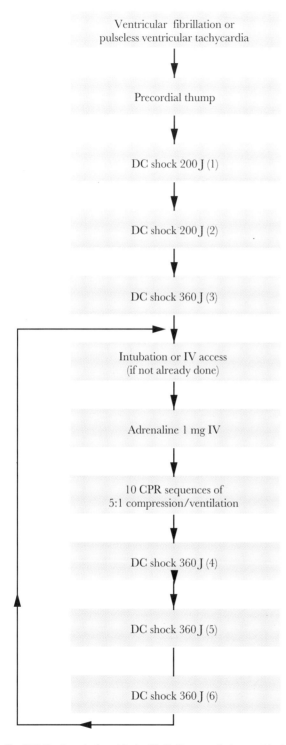

Ventricular fibrillation or
pulseless ventricular tachycardia

↓

Precordial thump

↓

DC shock 200 J (1)

↓

DC shock 200 J (2)

↓

DC shock 360 J (3)

↓

Intubation or IV access
(if not already done)

↓

Adrenaline 1 mg IV

↓

10 CPR sequences of
5:1 compression/ventilation

↓

DC shock 360 J (4)

↓

DC shock 360 J (5)

↓

DC shock 360 J (6)

Fig. 12.3 Treatment of ventricular fibrillation or pulseless ventricular tachycardia. The interval between shocks 3 and 4 should not be more than 2 minutes. Adrenaline should be given during loops every 2–3 minutes. Continue as long as defibrillation is indicated, but after three loops consider giving bicarbonate or antiarrhythmic agents

approach in the monitored patient is to administer a precordial thump in the normal position for chest compression (two fingers' breadth above the xiphisternum). The thump should be given from a height of approximately 15 cm above the chest to avoid unnecessary trauma. However, the success rate of this manoeuvre is only 2% in cases of ventricular fibrillation, increasing to over 10% in ventricular tachycardia. Although not a particularly effective technique, it can be recommended as it only takes a second or two to perform and can be administered easily while preparations for defibrillation are being made. After the precordial thump, a further pulse check must be made immediately and if the patient remains pulseless, the paramedic must progress rapidly to defibrillation. In cardiac arrest following trauma, the precordial thump is not recommended.

As BLS is a holding manoeuvre intended to prevent further deterioration in the biochemical state of the heart, its administration must not hold up definitive treatment of ventricular fibrillation or pulseless ventricular tachycardia. In a witnessed arrest, a reasonable degree of oxygenation should have been maintained until the moment of collapse and the main priority is to restore cerebral circulation within approximately 3 minutes. A colleague can administer BLS while the defibrillator is rapidly prepared, but nothing should interfere with defibrillation, as the time taken to administer the first shock is crucial. Up to three direct current shocks should be administered in rapid sequence. The reason for this is that the impedance (resistance to current flow) through the chest wall is reduced by each shock given in close succession, and the current flow is correspondingly increased. As only approximately 5% of the current passing between the paddles actually goes through the heart, the prospect of successful defibrillation is increased when shocks are given in close succession. The rapid sequence also serves to maximize the number of attempts at defibrillation during the most receptive phase of early resuscitation. Other factors such as expiration also reduce impedance.

The effectiveness of defibrillators is related to the current flow (measured in amperes) rather than the energy (measured in joules).

With modern defibrillators, three shocks can be administered within 45 seconds (and often in under 30 seconds); BLS is only necessary during this period if the shocks are delayed by technical or practical difficulties. With automated external defibrillators, BLS is not performed between shocks anyway because it interferes with rhythm analysis. An initial energy level of 200 J provides as good a chance of successful defibrillation as higher settings, and less risk of myocardial damage. Any tissue through which an electric current is passed will sustain some degree of injury and it is not in the interest of the patient to use the maximum energy level (360 J) from the beginning. After each shock, the pulse must be checked immediately for 5 seconds. If ventricular fibrillation persists after the first, a second shock of 200 J is given. As each shock reduces transthoracic impedance, the second will in fact transmit about 8% more current than the first, even though the energy level is unchanged. If the second shock is unsuccessful, the third shock is given at 360 J which is considered the maximum energy that the myocardium will satisfactorily tolerate. There is evidence that shocks of higher energy tend to generate rather than reverse arrhythmias.

When the first shock sequence proves unsuccessful, attention must be directed to basic life support. The priority at this stage has shifted from direct attempts to restore cardiac output, to establishing a degree of cerebral perfusion and oxygenation by means of cardiopulmonary resuscitation (albeit at 30% of the normal cardiac output). Cardiopulmonary resuscitation (CPR) is commenced with ten cycles of 5 chest compressions to 1 ventilation (five cycles of 15 compressions to 2 ventilations if a single operator). Immediately, the paramedic has to make preparations for a longer resuscitation. Tracheal intubation is undertaken to protect the airway and optimize oxygenation. The establishment of venous access allows drugs to exert their effects more reliably than in the bronchial tree, where administration causes transient hypoxia and absorption is erratic, especially if pulmonary oedema is present. Thirty seconds are allowed for tracheal intubation (the NHS Training Directorate recommendation of 15 seconds is recognized, but Resuscitation Council guidelines are more generous), which means that during the first ten cycles of CPR, an ambulance crew of two will not normally have time to intubate, establish venous access *and* administer drug therapy. The second period of CPR allows these tasks to be completed and every remaining cycle provides an opportunity for further attempts at interventions. Venous access is normally obtained in a peripheral upper limb vein. If permitted, the external jugular vein can be recommended as it is superficial, often distended in cardiac arrest and closer to the heart than the forearm veins.

Good oxygenation and basic life support during this stage is accompanied by the administration of 1 mg of adrenaline as soon as intravenous access is established. Adrenaline is *the* first-line drug in cardiac arrest, irrespective of the underlying arrhythmia. It acts by constricting peripheral vessels and diverting blood to the brain and coronary arteries. If for whatever reason (e.g. failure to establish intravenous access) adrenaline cannot be given at this stage, further attempts at defibrillation must not be held up.

After ten cycles of CPR, a rapid sequence of three shocks is given as before, but this time the maximum energy (360 J) is used on each occasion. The monitor and pulse must be checked carefully after each shock to see whether cardiac output has been restored or the arrhythmia has changed. With a manual defibrillator, three shocks are most rapidly administered if the paddles remain on the chest and an assistant checks the pulse after each shock.

A dose of 1 mg of intravenous adrenaline should be repeated between each sequence of shocks (i.e. at the start of every ten cycles of CPR). Adrenaline may be administered down the tracheal tube at a dose of 2 mg which should be blown in with vigorous ventilations, but the drug will produce pulmonary vasoconstriction and thereby inhibit its own absorption. If the

rhythm changes, necessitating use of a different treatment algorithm, and then reverts to ventricular fibrillation, treatment should start again at the top of the first algorithm, but omitting the precordial thump which should only be given once.

After four triplets of shocks, drugs other than adrenaline may be considered. The most frequently used antiarrhythmic agent is lignocaine at a dose of 100 mg intravenously (200 mg down the tracheal tube). However, the prospects of success are waning at this stage and although a change of paddle position (to anterior/posterior) or the use of a different defibrillator has been recommended, the prognosis becomes increasingly bleak. Furthermore, the effectiveness of lignocaine is disputed.

The outcome of defibrillation depends on many factors. The chance of successful defibrillation is at its greatest for approximately 1½ minutes after the onset of cardiac arrest. It is therefore the first and second sequence of shocks that are most important. Success is influenced not only by transthoracic impedance and the factors that affect it, but also by the wave form and the direction of the fibrillating current at the precise moment the shock is given.

A greater amount of time can justifiably be spent at the scene when the patient is in ventricular fibrillation, since the only treatment for this condition is defibrillation which cannot be administered in a moving ambulance. At least five sequences of three shocks are recommended before transfer to hospital is considered, thereby allowing lignocaine to be given before the fifth group of shocks. Resuscitation must not be abandoned by ambulance crews in the presence of ventricular fibrillation.

ASYSTOLE

Although asystole carries with it an adverse prognosis in adults (overall survival rate approximately 5%), this is partly because it tends to be the terminal stage of primary cardiac arrest. However, when asystole is secondary to other causes such as respiratory arrest or drug intoxication, the prognosis may be more favourable. Treatment of asystole is summarized in Figure 12.4.

The diagnosis of asystole is confirmed by the presence of an almost flat ECG trace in a pulseless patient. Asystole rarely produces a completely flat (isoelectric) line. In all cases of presumed asystole, a rapid check must be made to confirm that the leads are connected correctly, that the chest electrodes remain attached, and that the amplitude setting (gain) on the monitor has not been set too low. All monitor-defibrillators have design idiosyncrasies, and confusion often arises with manual machines that automatically monitor through the paddles when first switched on. If you are monitoring from the paddles, make sure the defibrillator is set to 'paddles'. If leads are connected to the patient, make sure they are connected to the monitor which is set to 'leads' (usually lead II).

Semi-automated external defibrillators may mistake fine

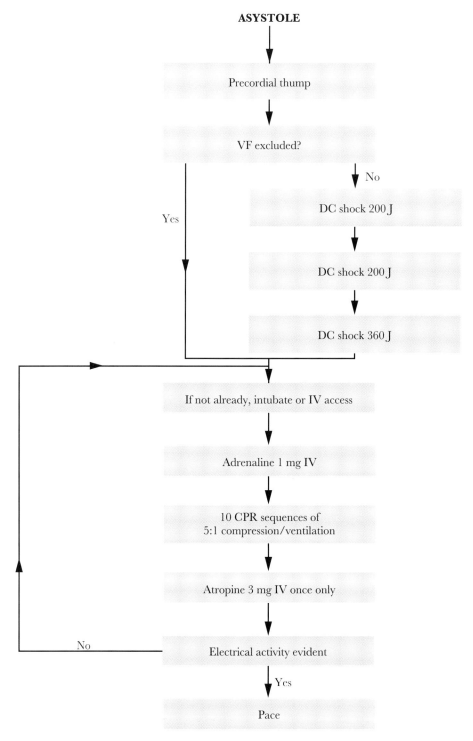

ASYSTOLE

Precordial thump

VF excluded?

No

Yes

DC shock 200 J

DC shock 200 J

DC shock 360 J

If not already, intubate or IV access

Adrenaline 1 mg IV

10 CPR sequences of
5:1 compression/ventilation

Atropine 3 mg IV once only

No

Electrical activity evident

Yes

Pace

Note: if no response after 3 loops, consider high dose adrenaline 5 mg IV

Fig. 12.4 Treatment of asystole

ventricular fibrillation (VF) for asystole and fail to 'allow' defibrillation. In the absence of an override key this situation can only be avoided by use of a manual defibrillator.

Asystole may be more evident in the presence of occasional P waves (ventricular standstill) or an occasional, aberrant QRS complex. When no such features are demonstrated and there is some irregularity of the baseline, it may not be possible for the paramedic to exclude fine ventricular fibrillation. In this situation, it is worthwhile monitoring through another lead configuration as more obvious evidence of ventricular fibrillation may be seen in one of the other standard leads. If this cannot be achieved, the message is simple: in the early stages of an arrest, VF is the most common rhythm, is more responsive to treatment and carries a better prognosis, so any patient who may be in fine ventricular fibrillation should receive a standard sequence of three shocks. This may successfully defibrillate the patient or alter the pattern of VF, rendering it more apparent on the monitor. In the absence of any response, a provisional diagnosis of asystole can be reached more comfortably.

If there is any doubt at all treat as VF

While preparing to defibrillate or administer drug therapy for asystole, it is worthwhile administering a single precordial thump as this can on occasions stimulate bursts of QRS complexes and associated cardiac contractions. If a precordial thump does generate QRS complexes, it may be repeated as necessary ('fist pacing').

Most patients in asystole are very hypoxic or have been in cardiac arrest for some time. It is therefore essential that they are preoxygenated before intubation and ventilation and that intravenous access is obtained immediately afterwards. Throughout this period, CPR must be maintained by an assistant. Effective oxygenation may in its own right help to restore a perfusing rhythm, but the other most effective intervention is adrenaline (1 mg intravenously or 2 mg endobronchially). The adrenaline serves to stimulate electrical (and hopefully myocardial) activity as well as to dilate the coronary arteries and transfer blood from the peripheries. Atropine, which accelerates the spontaneously beating heart by depressing parasympathetic tone, has not been proved to have any benefit in cardiac arrest but some patients are tipped into asystole by parasympathetic stimulation (for example, suction of the pharynx or intubation). It is therefore considered sensible to block the effect of parasympathetic activity, and a single dose of 3 mg atropine intravenously (or 6 mg endobronchially in concentrated solution, e.g. 10 ml of 600 µg/ml) will block parasympathetic activity for the duration of the cardiac arrest. A dose of 60 ml of atropine 1 mg in 10 ml is not appropriate for endobronchial use.

After adrenaline and atropine have been administered, they need to be circulated by means of effective CPR employing ten cycles of 1 ventilation to 5 chest compressions (two rescuers). Progress through these cycles is facilitated if the person responsible for ventilation counts each insufflation and indicates when the tenth cycle is approaching, so that a further dose of adrenaline can be prepared and administered.

There is little more that can be done for the asystolic patient. One exception is the patient with ventricular standstill whose ECG trace demonstrates P waves or an occasional ventricular complex. Such a patient may respond to electrical pacing which is usually administered in the accident and emergency department by means of temporary external electrodes (the same electrodes as the defibrillating electrodes in some models). At present, external pacing is only occasionally available in the pre-hospital situation and the presence of P waves should normally encourage the ambulance crew to transfer the patient as rapidly as they can while maintaining CPR to the best of their ability. In the absence of P waves, there needs to be a cut-off point. Asystole that is going to respond to the approaches described above will normally do so within a few cycles of CPR, so that once ventilation and adrenaline are being reliably administered, the patient should be transported directly to hospital.

ELECTROMECHANICAL DISSOCIATION

Electromechanical dissociation (EMD) may be defined as the presence of an ECG trace compatible with but not producing any detectable cardiac output. It is diagnosed on the basis of clinical signs of cardiac arrest (unconsciousness and an absent major pulse) in the presence of QRS complexes on the monitor. In adults, several causes of EMD are potentially treatable, especially those exerting a mechanical effect that impairs cardiac output to a level that produces no detectable pulse. Conditions potentially responsive to treatment include hypovolaemia, tension pneumothorax, cardiac tamponade and pulmonary embolism. Other causes of EMD that exert their effects biochemically and may not respond so readily to medical intervention include drug intoxication, hypothermia and electrolyte imbalance. However, prolonged resuscitation is indicated in the latter conditions (particularly hypothermia and drug intoxication), so all the following conditions merit consideration as soon as EMD is diagnosed.

Causes of electromechanical dissociation

- Hypovolaemia
- Tension pneumothorax
- Cardiac tamponade
- Pulmonary embolism
- Drug overdose or intoxication
- Hypothermia
- Electrolyte imbalance

Certain other causes of EMD such as rupture of the ventricle

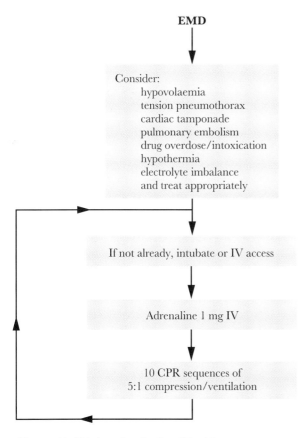

EMD

↓

Consider:
hypovolaemia
tension pneumothorax
cardiac tamponade
pulmonary embolism
drug overdose/intoxication
hypothermia
electrolyte imbalance
and treat appropriately

↓

If not already, intubate or IV access

↓

Adrenaline 1 mg IV

↓

10 CPR sequences of
5:1 compression/ventilation

*Note: consider high dose adrenaline 5 mg IV, calcium,
pressor agent and alkalising agents after 3 loops*

Fig. 12.5 *Algorithm for the management of electromechanical dissociation (EMD)*

or cords attached to a heart valve (*chordae tendineae*) invariably prove fatal.

In practical terms, treatment is initiated in the normal manner with BLS, followed by ventilation with oxygen and early intubation (Figure 12.5). Defibrillation has no place in the treatment of EMD. Attention must then focus on the list of potentially treatable conditions, each of which poses questions for the paramedic:

- Hypovolaemia – is there a history or clinical evidence of trauma, internal bleeding or external bleeding?
- Tension pneumothorax – are high inflation pressures required to ventilate the patient? Is the trachea deviated? With the tracheal tube properly placed, are inflation sounds reduced on one side of the chest?
- Cardiac tamponade – has the patient been subjected to recent cardiac surgery or trauma to the front of the chest (particularly penetrating injury)?

- Pulmonary embolism – is there a history of venous thrombosis in the lower limbs or any previous passage of clots from the legs into the lungs?
- Drug intoxication – are there any empty tablet bottles, drugs or signs of overdose at the scene?
- Hypothermia – do the patient's chest and abdomen feel cold?
- Electrolyte imbalance – does the patient suffer with renal failure or any medical condition known to be associated with electrolyte disturbance?

At present, paramedics can only intervene to a limited degree in the treatment of these conditions. Hypovolaemia should be treated by rapid administration of crystalloid or colloid (preferably warmed) through at least two large cannulae (14 G if possible). Some authorities allow paramedics to pass a cannula through the second intercostal space in the midclavicular line on the front of the chest to decompress a tension pneumothorax (see Chapter 23). Cardiac tamponade and pulmonary embolism are difficult to diagnose, even in hospital, and the emergency treatment of these conditions requires particular skills. However, in pulmonary embolism, vigorous chest compressions may help to dislodge the clot. The remaining, physiological causes of EMD are not readily addressed in the pre-hospital environment.

With practice, the list of possible causes of EMD can be rapidly considered, and in the majority of cases no underlying cause for the condition will be diagnosed. The majority of cases of EMD seen by paramedics are of primary cardiac origin, and for these patients the prognosis is similar to that of asystole. The treatment too is not dissimilar. Tracheal intubation and intravenous access are established and intravenous or endobronchial adrenaline is given in the standard dose after every ten cycles of 5 chest compressions to 1 ventilation. There is little more the paramedic can do, and once cycles of CPR are under way, the patient should be transported with haste to the nearest accident and emergency department.

High-dose Adrenaline

In the asystole or EMD algorithms, the use of an intravenous bolus of 5 mg adrenaline may be considered after ten cycles of CPR have been performed three times. Such a regimen has been effective in children and an initial impact has also been observed in adults. However, survival has not been improved and therefore no firm recommendation can be made. Paramedics may not have sufficient adrenaline in their possession to be able to administer such a dose.

Bicarbonate

The use of bicarbonate in early resuscitation has fallen out of favour. When blood is rendered more alkaline, oxygen dissociates less readily from haemoglobin and is therefore less available to hypoxic tissues than it is in more acid blood. Furthermore, bicarbonate releases carbon dioxide as it neutralizes acid, and if the carbon dioxide is not conveyed adequately to the lungs and removed by means of effective ventilation, it will diffuse across cell membranes and also the blood-brain barrier to increase acidity within cells as well as the brain.

Sodium bicarbonate is an irritant which can produce tissue necrosis if it leaks from the site of intravenous infusion. Although this must never preclude its use in an emergency situation, it is best administered in hospital where blood gas analysis allows the acidity of the blood to be accurately assessed and the amount of bicarbonate required to be calculated.

> The best way to reduce acidosis is to achieve good oxygenation

Calcium

Calcium is rarely of benefit in the treatment of cardiac arrest. It is a vasoconstrictor and is involved in cell death. However, it may be helpful if the patient is known to have a low blood level of calcium or a high potassium level, or to be taking drugs of the calcium antagonist type (Table 12.1). These drugs are used in the treatment of angina and hypertension. In pre-hospital care the value of calcium is therefore very limited.

DIFFICULT DECISIONS IN THE APPLICATION OF ALS

Certain guidelines may help the paramedic take decisions which will always be influenced by the prevailing circumstances.

1. Was the arrest primarily or secondarily cardiac in nature? Cardiac arrests that are a secondary to other conditions generally have a better prognosis because the myocardium did not fail primarily. Examples of such conditions include near-drowning, hypothermia, electrocution, respiratory disease, poisoning and anaphylaxis. These patients are often younger, and treatment should be continued even if basic life support was delayed. Every attempt must be made to restore cardiac output and the decision to terminate resuscitation can only be made in hospital.

Table 12.1 Calcium antagonists

Commonly encountered agents	Less common agents
Nifedipine	Amlodipine
Nicardipine	Felodipine
Verapamil	Isradipine
Diltiazem	Lacidipine
	Nimodipine

2. It is well established that for basic life support to be effective, it must be administered within 4 minutes of collapse and advanced life support must be initiated within 8 minutes. Careful consideration must therefore be given to timings and delays in the administration of basic or advanced life support. The 80-year-old patient who is reached by ambulance 15 or more minutes after collapse, has an obstructed airway and has had no basic life support will not survive. However, local policies may address this situation.

3. More time can justifiably be spent at the scene when the patient is in ventricular fibrillation, since the only treatment is defibrillation which cannot be safely or properly performed in a moving ambulance. At least four sequences of three shocks are recommended before transfer to hospital is considered. No such delay is necessary in cases of asystole or EMD, and the patient can be moved once cycles of CPR and adrenaline administration are under way.

4. Paramedics often feel compromised by instructions or information given to them by doctors at the scene. It takes confidence, tact and experience to reason with doctors, some of whom will have less up-to-date training in resuscitation than the paramedics. It is often necessary for paramedics to apprise doctors of local resuscitation protocols. This should be done tactfully but firmly, as the protocols are the rules by which paramedics are expected to operate.

5. It must be remembered that the patient is the responsibility of the paramedic once *en route* to hospital, and if the paramedic chooses at that stage to administer what he or she considers to be justifiable treatment, this should be done in accordance with local protocols.

6. Resuscitation may be deemed clinically inappropriate, but there may be pressure from relatives or bystanders to initiate it. Ideally, the decision to resuscitate or not should be taken at the start, but if pressure from others makes this difficult, the appropriate decision can be made in the paramedic's own domain, namely the ambulance. Some ambulance services are assessing an arrangement whereby paramedics may discontinue resuscitation in the presence of persistent asystole.

7. It is rarely necessary for a paramedic to request medical assistance at the scene of a cardiac arrest. However, the volume of equipment used nowadays is such that the assistance of a second crew is invariably welcome. If another crew cannot be obtained, an Immediate Care doctor can be extremely helpful. Control of the scene, removal to hospital and the care of relatives can all be achieved more effectively if additional support is recruited.

CONTINUITY OF CARE – THE HAND-OVER

While driving to hospital, consideration should be given to the essential information required by hospital staff. This includes:

- Approximate time from collapse to arrival at scene
- Administration and efficiency of any bystander CPR
- Any available medical history
- Primary diagnosis
- Response to resuscitative efforts

The enthusiasm to convey this information may distract the ambulance crew from their main responsibilities, which are to transfer the patient rapidly on to the resuscitation trolley or coronary care bed and allow hospital staff to gain control of the airway, breathing and circulation as priorities.

PREVENTION

The importance of effective management of patients at risk of cardiorespiratory arrest cannot be overstated. Prevention is always better than cure and patients with chest pain, respiratory difficulties or arrhythmias must receive the best support available within paramedic protocols (see Chapters 9 and 13). Compromising arrhythmias such as bradycardia, supraventricular tachycardia or ventricular tachycardia may predispose to cardiac arrest. Oxygen, reassurance, intravenous access, pain relief and appropriate treatment of arrhythmias (e.g. severe bradycardia) are essential.

ETHICAL MATTERS AND BEREAVEMENT

Although the problems of ethics and bereavement mainly involve medical and nursing staff in the community or at hospital, consideration must be given to the paramedic's obligations in these areas (see Chapters 54 and 60). As with all health-care workers, emotional stress can be underestimated and paramedics should always have an opportunity to receive feedback and debrief following a stressful incident.

CONCLUSION

It must be emphasized that the paramedic represents the arm of acute medical care reaching out to those who collapse with sudden illness. As such, paramedics are better placed than any other health-care provider to administer promptly the most effective life-saving skills. General practitioners are not so well equipped, and hospital staff cannot be present at the critical moment when therapeutic interventions have the greatest chance of success. The role of the paramedic in the timely provision of advanced life support in the community is therefore paramount, and the application and retention of up-to-date knowledge and skills are constant challenges.

It must be appreciated that cardiac arrest is not a homogeneous entity: its cause, presentation and prognosis differ from one individual to another. To afford the patient the best chance, the paramedic must understand the scientific principles underlying the European Advanced Life Support protocols, be fully familiar with them and regularly review the theoretical and practical aspects of resuscitation. Difficult decisions often have to be faced, and efforts do not terminate on arrival at hospital when, after an efficient hand-over, feedback and support may be needed from other members of the emergency team.

FURTHER READING

ALS Working Party of the European Resuscitation Council (1992) Guidelines for Advanced Life Support. *Resuscitation* **24**: 111–121.

chapter thirteen:

CARDIOVASCULAR EMERGENCIES

Diseases of the cardiovascular system account for the majority of medical emergencies encountered by paramedics. In the UK the picture is dominated by ischaemic heart disease, and in particular acute myocardial infarction ('heart attack'). Cardiopulmonary arrest due to lethal cardiac arrhythmias is the most dramatic medical emergency, and in recent years many studies in both the USA and Europe have reported successful treatment of the condition by ambulance personnel. Policies on the training of ambulance paramedics and the provision of equipment (particularly defibrillators) have consequently been profoundly influenced.

Ischaemic heart disease is considered in detail in this chapter because it remains the most common cause of all cardiac emergencies and in particular of cardiopulmonary arrest. The optimal treatment of patients with myocardial infarction may prevent more serious complications. Arrhythmias causing cardiopulmonary arrest are the subject of Chapter 12, but it is important to realize that the appropriate treatment of other arrhythmias may prevent subsequent cardiac arrest. The principles of their treatment are discussed in this section, which should be read in conjunction with the section on electrocardiography in Chapter 10.

ISCHAEMIC HEART DISEASE

Ischaemic or *coronary heart disease* (IHD, CHD) accounts for more deaths in the UK than any other condition. Approximately one in three men and one in four women die from the disease: this represents around 170,000 people per year. Approximately 2 million patients suffer from angina and there are in excess of 300,000 episodes of myocardial infarction per year.

The economic consequences of IHD are staggering, with an estimated 5 million working days lost every year in the UK, costing industry £3 billion in lost production. There are enormous financial implications for the taxpayer – £463 million spent annually on invalidity benefit payments and a cost to the National Health Service of approaching £1 billion spent on treatment.

Risk factors for IHD

- Cigarette smoking
- High blood cholesterol levels
- Hypertension
- Diabetes
- Family history

Several important factors have been identified that contribute to ischaemic heart disease: cigarette smoking is a leading cause and theoretically one of the most easily modified. A high blood cholesterol level, particularly when a feature of familial hypercholesterolaemia, is also a significant risk factor for development of the disease, as are hypertension and diabetes mellitus. The association of two or more risk factors greatly increases the chance of developing ischaemic heart disease. Certain racial groups seem at particular risk; in the UK immigrants from the Indian subcontinent have a high prevalence. A strong family history of ischaemic heart disease is often found in patients suffering from the condition.

It is important to realize, however, that in an individual patient no identifiable risk factors may be present. It follows, therefore, that the absence of risk factors in an individual patient does *not* help exclude the diagnosis of ischaemic heart disease.

Pathology

The term *ischaemic heart disease* implies that the supply of oxygenated blood to the myocardium is reduced. The usual cause is coronary atheroma – the accumulation of lipid-rich atheromatous deposits in the wall of the coronary arteries. These cause narrowing of the lumen with restriction of blood supply to the myocardium. This is most apparent during conditions of increased myocardial oxygen requirement, typically during exertion. Angina pectoris is the clinical syndrome that results from this.

Changes in a plaque of atheroma situated in the wall of the artery may result in the rupture of the plaque through the inner wall of the artery (the intima) covering the plaque. Platelet aggregation and thrombus formation occur on the surface of the ruptured plaque leading to occlusion of the artery. Loss of blood supply to the area of myocardium supplied by the vessel results (in the absence of an alternative blood supply through collateral vessels), leading to myocardial infarction with death of myocardium.

Ischaemic Cardiac Pain

Angina pectoris

The discomfort of angina is caused by reversible myocardial ischaemia, and usually occurs during conditions of increased oxygen demand, most typically during exertion. When the patient ceases the activity and rests the discomfort passes off rapidly (within 2–3 minutes) as myocardial oxygen requirements fall. Patients with angina often describe a feeling of tightness in the chest ('like a tight band') or liken the discomfort to a weight on the chest; sometimes it is described as a squeezing sensation. The pain is felt retrosternally (behind the sternum) and may radiate across the chest, spreading into the arms. In some patients the pain may also radiate into the throat or jaw and occasionally through to the back. The characteristic relationship to exertion is the cardinal feature in the diagnosis of angina. Patients may volunteer that the discomfort is provoked more easily after heavy meals, when walking up hill or into the wind, and in the early morning.

Where there is doubt about the origin of a patient's pain, because possible ischaemic pain is atypical in site or nature, it is the characteristic relationship to exertion that may provide the clue to its nature. Approximately 20,000 patients develop angina for the first time every year and there is a high incidence of infarction in the first few months after its appearance.

Unstable angina

The term *unstable angina* is used to describe a rapidly progressive, deteriorating pattern of angina often occurring in patients whose angina has been previously stable. The patient's exercise tolerance is reduced and ischaemic pain occurs more frequently. The consumption of glyceryl trinitrate is often increased. Ischaemic pain occurring at rest or on only minor exertion is a particularly worrying feature. Unstable angina is a medical emergency and most patients are admitted to hospital for investigation and treatment, as there is a high instance of subsequent myocardial infarction.

Myocardial infarction

The pain of myocardial infarction is similar in nature, site and distribution to that of angina. It is usually felt retrosternally and may spread across the chest into the arms, or into the throat and jaw. Pain may also be felt in the epigastrium (upper abdomen) and may initially be thought to arise from the gastrointestinal tract. Occasionally the pain may radiate through to the back, between the shoulder blades. Patients with pre-existing angina often describe the pain of infarction as being similar, although much more severe; it is not usually relieved by glyceryl trinitrate. Many patients will not have a previous history of angina.

To complicate matters further, pain (particularly in elderly people) may be a minor feature or absent altogether: the diagnosis will then only be made if a high index of suspicion is maintained.

MYOCARDIAL INFARCTION

Loss of functioning myocardium occurs in the area deprived of its blood supply. The mechanical effects depend on the extent and location of the muscle loss, although the consequences will also depend on the pre-existing state of the myocardium. The loss of a small volume of muscle may be tolerated badly in a patient whose ventricle has been damaged by previous episodes of infarction. When the ability of the ventricular myocardium to act as a pump is impaired, ventricular failure results. Fluid collection in the pulmonary circulation causes pulmonary oedema. With severe impairment of cardiac output cardiogenic shock results as the blood pressure falls. Other mechanical effects may arise: where the area of infarction involves the papillary muscles of the mitral valve, its function may be impaired with resultant mitral regurgitation. Rupture of infarcted myocardium may also occur with loss of blood into the pericardium, usually with disastrous haemodynamic consequences. Occasionally the interventricular septum may rupture with the creation of a ventricular septal defect; shunting of blood occurs from left to right ventricle, and severe heart failure is the usual result.

Clinical Features

A patient with acute myocardial infarction is usually middle-aged or elderly and may have a history of preceding angina or previous infarction. Risk factors for the development of ischaemic heart disease (for example cigarette smoking, hypertension, diabetes or hypercholesterolaemia) may be present, but the absence of these features should not prevent the diagnosis.

Symptoms of myocardial infarction

- Chest pain
- Fear and anxiety
- Nausea
- Vomiting
- Sweating

- Shortness of breath
- Palpitation

The dominant symptom of myocardial infarction is chest pain, the characteristics of which are discussed above. The patient is usually apprehensive, in pain, and appears distressed. Nausea, vomiting and sweating are commonly associated features, and when pulmonary oedema is present the patient will be short of breath. The blood pressure should be recorded in all cases: it may be high in patients with pre-existing hypertension, or in the presence of severe pain. A low blood pressure with reduced cardiac output occurs in cardiogenic shock and is an ominous sign.

A presumptive diagnosis of myocardial infarction can be made from the history and associated clinical features. Other conditions, for example dissecting aortic aneurysm or pulmonary thromboembolism (PE), may produce a similar clinical picture and be very difficult to distinguish from myocardial infarction (without further investigation in hospital). This should not concern ambulance personnel unduly as the principles of treatment before hospital admission are broadly similar.

Treatment

The British Heart Foundation recommends that the optimal treatment for cases of early infarction is by a combined response from the patient's general practitioner and the ambulance service. This recommendation recognizes the frequency with which cardiac arrest occurs in the early phases of myocardial infarction and the importance of admitting patients to hospital as rapidly as possible for confirmation of the diagnosis and the institution of thrombolytic ('clot busting') treatment. Ideally the general practitioner would be familiar with the patient's medical history and be able to provide diagnostic skills, while the ambulance service can respond very rapidly, making a defibrillator available with the minimum of delay. The treatment of an individual patient will depend very much on whether the general practitioner is present at the scene. In some cases a doctor will be able to confirm the diagnosis of infarction by performing an electrocardiogram in the patient's home, and will liaise with ambulance personnel to provide optimal treatment. The patient will usually be most comfortable sitting upright and *high concentration oxygen* should be given. Venous access should be secured at an early stage, usually with an intravenous cannula placed in a forearm vein. Intravenous access is required for the administration of opiate analgesia, antiemetic drugs, and other drugs if required. If a cardiac arrest should occur it is a great advantage if an intravenous cannula is already *in situ*. A heparinized saline flush may be used to prevent clotting in the cannula.

Analgesia

The relief of pain is a major priority in the treatment of patients with infarction. Diamorphine or morphine are the agents of choice, but both are controlled drugs and not widely available in the ambulance service. General practitioners attending the patient will usually administer one of these drugs. Many ambulance services now have protocols for paramedics to administer nalbuphine for treating the severe pain of myocardial infarction; tramadol has also been used successfully. Whichever analgesic agent is used, it should be given by slow intravenous injection, with careful observation of its effect. Opiate analgesics not only relieve the pain of myocardial infarction, but also have beneficial effects on ventricular filling pressures, acting to reduce myocardial workload and oxygen requirements.

In the absence of any other analgesic, nitrous oxide inhalation (Entonox) is effective against the pain of myocardial infarction.

Aspirin

A daily dose of soluble aspirin (150 mg) has been shown to reduce the mortality from myocardial infarction and should be started as soon as possible after the diagnosis has been established. Under certain circumstances and according to established local protocols, it may be appropriate to give the first dose pre-hospital. Active peptic ulceration and bleeding disorders are contraindications. The first dose is recommended as 300 mg, and should be chewed.

Antiemetic drugs

Opiates and related analgesics will worsen the nausea that frequently accompanies myocardial infarction, and produce vomiting. An antiemetic drug should therefore be administered intravenously; metoclopramide (Maxolon) is licensed for use in this fashion. Prochlorperazine (Stemetil) is not licensed for intravenous use because of its potential to produce severe hypotension. Drugs with vasoconstrictor properties, for example cyclizine, may increase myocardial workload and are not recommended for use in patients with myocardial infarction.

Glyceryl trinitrate

By reducing ventricular pre-load, cardiac workload and oxygen consumption are reduced. The beneficial action of the drug in angina is largely due to this action, and patients with infarction may have already taken the drug. The same actions are also beneficial during evolving myocardial infarction, and where the drug has been approved for use by the local paramedical steering committee, the protocol should be followed. The sublingual administration of 400–800 µg either by tablet or spray should therefore be considered at this point.

Atropine

Vagal overactivity is relatively common in the early stages of myocardial infarction and may cause sinus bradycardia with hypotension and reduced cardiac output. The pain of infarction contributes to this vagal overactivity and effective analgesia may help considerably. Where bradycardia with hypotension or other evidence of reduced cardiac output persists, atropine should be given intravenously with continuous ECG monitoring. Comparatively small doses (0.2–0.4 mg) may be adequate to increase the heart rate with significant improvement in cardiac output and blood pressure. Local protocols should be followed in all cases.

Diuretic drugs

Intravenous diuretic agents are employed when heart failure is present, particularly in the presence of pulmonary oedema. Treatment will usually be administered by a doctor who is in attendance. Frusemide (40–120 mg) given intravenously is the agent employed most frequently.

Antiarrhythmic drugs

In the past much importance has been attached to the occurrence of ventricular ectopic activity. Certain patterns of ectopic activity were thought to predict a high risk for the development of ventricular fibrillation. Antiarrhythmic drugs, particularly lignocaine, have been widely employed to suppress such ectopic activity, and these agents may reduce the incidence of ventricular fibrillation. The routine use of such drugs prophylactically, however, has not been shown to reduce mortality and in some surveys has been disadvantageous. The drugs employed are usually administered by injection followed by slow intravenous infusion; this is difficult to do accurately in an ambulance during transport. There is also a risk of serious adverse effects with inadvertent overdosage. In the absence of more conclusive evidence of benefit, few paramedical steering committees have approved protocols for the use of prophylactic antiarrhythmic agents in patients with acute infarction.

Thrombolytic therapy

Myocardial infarction is usually caused by the formation of thrombus (clot) in a major coronary vessel. Thrombolytic agents activate the natural mechanism for producing clot breakdown (lysis); dissolution of the obstructing thrombus occurs with reperfusion of ischaemic myocardium. Several large trials have clearly demonstrated reduced mortality in cases of myocardial infarction treated with intravenous thrombolytic agents. Treatment has been shown to be most effective when given as soon as possible after the onset of symptoms, and when used in combination with oral aspirin.

Many strategies have been adopted to minimize delay in the administration of thrombolytic drugs; in the USA and several European countries treatment has been instituted in the patient's home or during ambulance transport to hospital. However, these schemes have usually employed ambulances carrying doctors, nurses or specially trained ambulance staff and have often relied on telephonic transmission of the ECG, which is interpreted in the base hospital. In the UK, general practitioners have provided thrombolytic treatment safely with a valuable saving of time compared with later administration in hospital. This practice may increase in the future and be more frequently encountered by ambulance staff. Other procedures to reduce the 'door-to-needle' time include the direct admission of patients to the coronary care unit for rapid diagnosis and institution of therapy, and the 'fast-tracking' of patients with possible infarction through rapid assessment and treatment in the accident and emergency department. Locally agreed arrangements will dictate the policy adopted by the ambulance service in a given area.

Primary treatment of myocardial infarction

- Oxygen
- Analgesia
- Antiemetic
- Glyceryl trinitrate
- Thrombolysis
- Aspirin

Treatment of complications

- Treatment of arrhythmias
- Treatment of heart failure

Sudden Cardiac Death

Sudden, apparently unheralded cardiac death remains a distressingly common occurrence. It has been recognized for many years that the majority of patients who die from coronary heart disease do so outside hospital, very often before medical help arrives. Ventricular fibrillation complicating the early stages of acute myocardial infarction is responsible for many cases, while a lethal arrhythmia complicating severe coronary disease, without actual evidence of infarction at post-mortem, accounts for many more. Non-coronary disease may also cause sudden cardiac death: valvular heart disease (especially aortic stenosis), arrhythmias complicating cardiomyopathy, metabolic, iatrogenic or inherited conditions explain some cases.

The Development of Out-of-Hospital Coronary Care

With the realization that the majority of deaths from myocardial infarction occur in the early stages (around half of all patients who die do so in the first hour after the first onset of symptoms), special units where prompt resuscitation is available became part of the routine hospital management of patients at high risk of developing cardiac arrest. Once the effectiveness of resuscitation in hospital became established, attempts were made to provide coronary care and, in particular, defibrillation in the community. The credit for this goes to Pantridge in Belfast who pioneered the first mobile coronary care unit staffed by a doctor and a nurse. Early experience confirmed the high incidence of lethal arrhythmias at the onset of myocardial infarction, and many patients attended by mobile units were successfully resuscitated from cardiac arrest before hospital admission. The successful experience in Belfast led to a reappraisal of the role of the ambulance service and laid the foundation for the development of the paramedic. Pantridge and his co-workers also drew attention to the value of cardiopulmonary resuscitation (CPR) initiated by a bystander when cardiac arrest occurred before the arrival of medical help.

In the early 1970s Leonard Cobb, a cardiologist in Seattle, was inspired by these results and equipped paramedics with defibrillators and also trained firefighters to perform basic life support. The fire service in Seattle is highly coordinated and a standard fire appliance can reach any part of the city within 4 minutes, enabling CPR to be started before the arrival of the more highly trained ambulance crew. The most crucial determinant of survival from cardiac arrest was found to be the speed with which defibrillation was performed. To accelerate this further the firefighters were equipped with defibrillators, a process facilitated by the development of the semiautomatic advisory model that requires less training to use. (AED)

Vicary, the chief of the fire service in Seattle, made the crucial suggestion that citizen CPR might be the first stage in the provision of coronary care outside hospital. With Cobb, he inaugurated training in resuscitation techniques for the public to increase the practice of CPR. Research in Seattle and the surrounding area of King County confirmed the importance of rapid access to the emergency medical services, the rapid institution of basic life support together with early defibrillation, and the early application of advanced life support techniques including advanced airway management and the use of drugs in determining survival from cardiac arrest occurring outside hospital. These stages should be seen as an interrelated sequence of events, each one constituting a link in the *chain of survival* (Figure 13.1). Intensive efforts to reduce delays to the minimum have resulted in survival rates from cardiac arrest of 40% being reported from that part of the USA.

Scotland became the first country in the world to equip every front-line ambulance with a defibrillator. England and Wales followed shortly afterwards. It is planned that in the near future every ambulance will also carry at least one trained paramedic. Cobbe and his co-workers in Glasgow have demonstrated the value of community resuscitation programmes; survival rates were approximately 15% when cardiac arrest took place before the arrival of the ambulance, whereas survival rates of 50% have been reported following cardiac arrest witnessed by an ambulance crew.

DISSECTING AORTIC ANEURYSM

A dissecting aortic aneurysm is one of the most serious cardiovascular emergencies. The condition is more common in men, and hypertension is an important predisposing factor. However, the patient may not have been known to be hypertensive. The condition starts with a tear in the intima of the aorta, usually in the ascending part of the arch of the aorta. Blood dissects a pathway between the layers of the aortic wall extending proximally to the aortic valve, and runnning distally for a variable distance. On occasions 're-entry' may occur, when the distal part of the dissection re-establishes continuity with the lumen forming a 'double-barrelled' aorta. The dissection may involve one or more major branches of the aorta, including the coronary arteries. The proximal dissection around the root of the aorta may distort the aortic valve and cause aortic regurgitation. Rupture of the aorta into the pericardium or pleura may occur and is usually rapidly fatal (Figure 13.2).

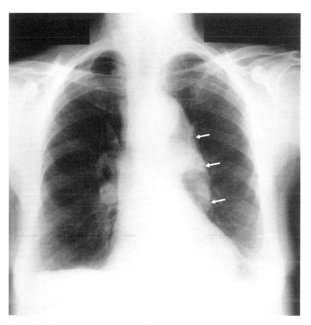

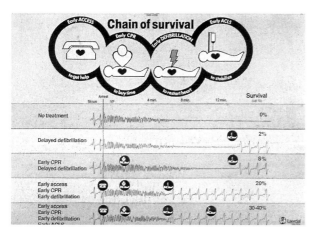

Fig. 13.1 The 'chain of survival'

Fig. 13.2 Dissecting aneurysm of the aorta

The clinical manifestations of dissecting aortic aneurysm include severe chest pain, aortic regurgitation, restriction of blood flow through branches of the aorta, and the consequences of aortic rupture. The pain of dissecting aneurysm is similar to that of myocardial infarction. It is sometimes described as having a 'tearing' quality and often radiates into the back between the scapulae. It may also be felt in other parts of the chest, or in the lumbar area, and on occasions in the abdomen; the site of the pain may change as the aneurysm extends. The most frequent clue that a dissecting aneurysm is the cause of the patient's pain (as opposed to myocardial infarction or other causes of severe chest pain) is evidence of obstruction to blood flow in the major branches of the aorta caused by the dissection. This is sometimes manifested as a discrepancy in the pulses in the arms, or a marked difference in blood pressure on the two sides. The same may occur with the carotid or femoral vessels: disturbance of consciousness occurs with interruption of cerebral blood supply. Myocardial infarction (from obstruction of the coronary arteries) or paraplegia (from obstruction to spinal blood flow) may be seen, while gastrointestinal symptoms and haematuria may also occur when the mesenteric or renal vessels are involved.

The occurrence of severe chest pain, often reaching a rapid peak of intensity, followed within minutes or hours by signs of arterial occlusion as outlined above, should suggest the diagnosis. In practice the diagnosis is rarely made before hospital admission. The presence of sustained hypertension may occur with dissection, but also occurs in patients with myocardial infarction; profound hypotension may also occur in both conditions.

Management

In many cases the patient will be suspected to be suffering from myocardial infarction. Electrocardiographic monitoring, oxygen therapy and analgesia are equally appropriate in both conditions, while sublingual nitrates will do no harm in dissection. Venous access will be established at an early stage and used to provide effective analgesia. In summary, if a paramedic mistakes aortic dissection for acute infarction little harm is likely to result. Where consciousness is disturbed owing to involvement of the cerebral blood vessels in the dissection, the diagnosis will usually be clear, and appropriate treatment for an unconscious patient (with careful attention to airway maintenance and adequate ventilation) becomes an important priority.

PULMONARY EMBOLISM

Pulmonary embolism is a frequent finding at post-mortem, the inference being that it frequently contributes to the death of patients. The diagnosis, however, is only infrequently made before death – perhaps in only 25% of cases. Pulmonary embolism occurs when a thrombus that has formed in a large vein in the leg or pelvis becomes dislodged and is carried through the venous system and right ventricle into the pulmonary circulation. Three main factors have been identified in the cause of such thrombi: abnormalities in the blood vessel, blood that clots more easily, and obstruction to venous flow resulting in stasis. Conditions associated with a high risk of thromboembolism include pregnancy, the postoperative period, chronic heart failure or pulmonary disease, fractures and other injuries of the legs, chronic venous insufficiency affecting the lower leg, prolonged bed rest and the presence of carcinoma.

The immediate result of pulmonary thromboembolism is obstruction of part of the pulmonary arterial bed, and the consequences will depend on the size of the area of vascular bed obstructed. The increased resistance to pulmonary blood flow that results from obstruction, when severe, will lead to pulmonary hypertension with acute right ventricular failure, tachycardia and a decline in cardiac output. It is the extent to which the embolism obstructs the pulmonary circulation that determines outcome. The status of the patient before the embolism is also important: a relatively small embolism may have limited impact on an otherwise healthy individual yet have serious consequences in a patient with pre-existing cardiac or pulmonary disease.

Clinical features of pulmonary embolism

- Chest pain
- Central cyanosis
- Tachycardia
- Dyspnoea
- Remember to check for deep vein thrombosis

Diagnosis

In milder cases examination findings may be entirely normal. With more severe emboli, pleuritic chest pain (pain made worse by breathing), central cyanosis, tachycardia and dyspnoea occur. The presence of deep vein thrombosis (DVT), usually in the legs, provides an excellent clue to diagnosis but is often absent. On clinical grounds it is difficult to make a firm diagnosis of pulmonary embolism and many of the diagnostic features are beyond the scope of the paramedical examination. Detailed hospital investigation is often necessary, the results of which determine the most appropriate treatment.

Treatment

Outside hospital, treatment will centre on the administration of oxygen, instituting cardiac monitoring and securing intravenous access. Where a strong analgesic is required, the same agents recommended for the treatment of myocardial infarction may be employed, although it is unusual for a pulmonary embolism to cause the same severe pain.

Treatment of pulmonary embolism

- Oxygen
- Cardiac monitoring
- Intravenous access
- Opiate analgesia

CARDIAC TAMPONADE

Cardiac tamponade occurs when fluid collects in the pericardial cavity in quantities sufficient to obstruct venous return. If the condition develops rapidly (as may occur with the collection of blood following trauma), 250 ml may be sufficient to produce severe consequences. Where fluid accumulates more slowly and the pericardium has time to stretch and adapt to the accumulation of fluid, up to 1000 ml may be present. Tamponade occurs most commonly from bleeding into the pericardial space as a result of trauma, surgical procedures, or cardiac rupture following myocardial infarction. Tumours invading the pericardium (most commonly from the bronchus or breast) may also cause the accumulation of fluid. Bacterial infection occasionally causes purulent fluid to accumulate in the pericardium, particularly in immunocompromised patients. A pericardial effusion may follow acute pericarditis from viral or other causes and produce similar mechanical effects.

Causes of cardiac tamponade

- Trauma
- Following myocardial infarction
- Following surgery
- Malignancy
- Infection

Diagnosis

The cardinal diagnostic feature of cardiac tamponade is a reduction in cardiac output associated with systemic venous congestion. With rapidly developing effusions, as may occur with cardiac trauma, quiet heart sounds occur, but the recognition of this sign is difficult outside hospital. The absence of this feature does not exclude the diagnosis. When tamponade develops slowly, the clinical features may resemble heart failure: dyspnoea, tachycardia, congestion of the neck veins, hepatic engorgement and peripheral oedema. Immediate treatment may be life-saving and in most cases will be undertaken in hospital after confirmation of the diagnosis by echocardiography. Only very rarely is pericardial aspiration by medical staff required before hospital admission. Treatment by the paramedic will be the provision of oxygen, establishment of intravenous access and cardiac monitoring. Where trauma is responsible, the treatment of associated injuries may dominate the picture.

CARDIAC ARRHYTHMIAS

The treatment of asystole, pulseless ventricular tachycardia and ventricular fibrillation is considered in Chapter 12: these arrhythmias are not considered further in this chapter.

> All arrhythmia patients require oxygen

In pre-hospital care, treatment of arrhythmias is relatively simple. The golden rule is to treat the patient and not the arrhythmia.

> Treat the patient, not the arrhythmia

Treatment of Tachycardia

All treatments for tachycardia have their own risks and are therefore most safely undertaken in hospital. Pre-hospital treatment should therefore only be undertaken if the arrhythmia presents a significant threat to the patient's cardiovascular status or life.

Sinus tachycardia

Treatment should be directed towards the cause of the tachycardia (for example, hypovolaemia due to haemorrhage).

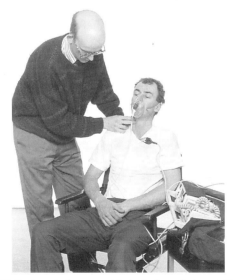

Fig. 13.3 *Treatment of supraventricular tachycardia by carotid sinus massage*

Atrial tachycardia and atrial flutter

Drug treatment may be considered after rapid transfer to hospital. Carotid sinus massage (Figure 13.3) or the Valsalva manoeuvre ('Take a huge breath in and strain as if you were on the toilet') may increase the degree of atrioventricular block, but only rarely terminates the arrhythmia. Both of these are 'vagal manoeuvres', and are *more effective in the younger patient and when lying flat*. Do not perform carotid sinus massage (massage over the carotid artery level with the upper border of the larynx) for more than 5–10 seconds. Vagal stimulation with a Valsalva occurs on *release* of the manoeuvre. The patient with acute paroxysmal cardiovascular compromise is best treated by synchronized cardioversion which should be performed by a doctor in hospital.

Atrial fibrillation

Atrial fibrillation with a moderate ventricular response (pulse rate < 120/minute) usually responds to a course of oral digoxin. In the patient with pronounced tachycardia, intravenous digoxin or cardioversion (if there is haemodynamic compromise) are effective; treatment should be undertaken in hospital.

Junctional tachycardia

Junctional tachycardia may respond to vagal manoeuvres – carotid sinus massage, the Valsalva manoeuvre, plunging the face into cold water – and these should be tried first. If vagal manoeuvres fail the patient should be transferred rapidly to hospital where medical treatment is with adenosine 3 mg by rapid IV injection, followed if unsuccessful after 1–2 minutes by 6 mg, and followed again if unsuccessful by 12 mg. Cardiac monitoring must be maintained during the treatment. Adenosine is not currently licensed for paramedical use. Verapamil 5 mg IV (and repeated once if necessary) is also effective in the treatment of junctional tachycardia, but is *absolutely contraindicated* if the patient is taking oral beta-blockers. Direct current (DC) cardioversion is effective in terminating

junctional tachycardia, but should be undertaken after transfer to hospital.

> **Remember to print a rhythm strip**

Ventricular tachycardia

If ventricular tachycardia (Figure 13.4) is pulseless the resuscitation algorithm for ventricular fibrillation should be followed. If a pulse is present, oxygen should be given, followed by immediate rapid transfer to hospital. Medical administration of intravenous lignocaine is indicated, followed if necessary by DC cardioversion.

Isolated ventricular complexes – ventricular premature beats – do not require treatment unless they occur in runs in which case 100 mg of lignocaine should be given IV.

Treatment of Bradycardia

First and second degree heart block rarely require treatment. Very occasionally, enough complexes fail to be transmitted in second degree heart block to cause bradycardia with cardiovascular compromise. Atropine 500 µg (repeated if necessary) should then be given.

If third degree heart block ('complete heart block') is accompanied by an adequate cardiovascular status, it may be appropriate to delay treatment until arrival in hospital. Otherwise treatment is with intravenous atropine (500 µg, repeated if needed). If this is unsuccessful, external pacing (if available) should be attempted. It is important to remember, however, that this is uncomfortable in the conscious patient.

In summary, bradycardia or heart block requires the following treatment:

- First degree block – none
- Second degree block – none or atropine
- Third degree block – none, external pacing or atropine
- Sinus bradycardia (Figure 13.5) – none or atropine

FURTHER READING

Colquhoun MC, Handley AJ & Evans TR eds (1995) *ABC of Resuscitation*, 3rd edn. London: BMJ Publications.

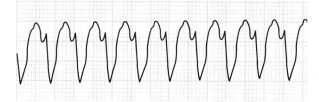

Fig. 13.4 *Ventricular*

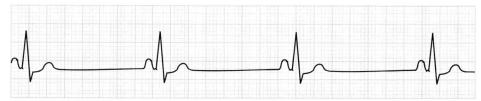

Fig. 13.5 *Sinus bradycardia*

chapter fourteen:

THE UNCONSCIOUS PATIENT

The unconscious patient is a person in danger. Many of the normal protective reflexes are lost, and unconscious individuals cannot actively protect themselves from the environment. Paramedical staff who attend an unconscious casualty have several roles: they must assess and treat any potentially or immediately life-threatening conditions; they should ensure that the patient comes to no further harm; and finally they should safely transfer the patient to the nearest definitive care facility and communicate their findings to the receiving medical personnel.

DEFINITIONS

Consciousness is best thought of as a scale. At the highest level, a patient is fully aware of the environment and can be described as 'alert'. Patients who have lost all awareness of their surroundings can be described as 'unconscious'. As the conscious level falls the eyes close, speech may become confused or cease and motor responses change. An individual who is not rousable from unconsciousness is said to be in coma. At the deepest levels of coma the patient will be totally unresponsive to any stimulus.

MANAGEMENT OF THE UNCONSCIOUS PATIENT

The initial assessment of the unconscious patient should follow the standard system of the 'ABC' system.

Approach

Always make sure that you are safe when you approach the unconscious patient. The victim of an assault may still be surrounded by assailants who present a danger to the paramedic. There may be other potential risks such as noxious fumes or smoke, and invisible dangers such as carbon monoxide. Only approach the patient when you are sure that you will be at no risk. Use the SAFE approach:

S > SHOUT for help (when necessary)
A > APPROACH with care
F > FREE from danger
E > EVALUATE the ABCs

Awake

The next stage is to see if the patient is conscious. Speak to the patient with sentences such as, 'Can you hear me?', and gently rock the shoulders while stabilizing the forehead to see if the patient is rousable (be wary of rocking if the patient is a victim of trauma). If the patient responds by speaking to you then there is no immediate airway problem. If there is no verbal response, proceed to check the airway.

Airway

The unconscious patient is at risk from airway obstruction from the tongue falling back into the oropharynx. A patient with a partially obstructed airway will make grunting or snoring noises in an effort to overcome the obstruction. The patient may also have lost normal protective reflexes and may aspirate food or vomit into the lungs, so make sure that there is no debris in the upper airway. Look into the mouth and remove any obvious foreign body. If there is vomit present, aspirate it, using a portable suction device. Open the airway using the head tilt or chin lift manoeuvres as described in Chapter 3, but avoid head tilt in patients who are known to be victims of trauma. If the airway cannot be maintained with simple manoeuvres it may be necessary to introduce a correctly sized oropharyngeal (Guedel) airway (Chapter 5). Be careful if inserting an oral airway into a patient who is only lightly unconscious: it may promote gagging and vomiting. Once the airway has been opened, cleared and secured, move on to assess the patient's breathing. If there is any suspicion that the patient may have been a victim of trauma, immobilize the neck in a rigid cervical collar while the airway is being assessed.

Breathing

Look, listen and feel for signs of breathing. The respiratory rate may be very slow if the patient has taken an overdose of an opiate. Breath sounds may be absent on one side if the patient has a pneumothorax. Abnormal breathing patterns are seen in some patients with head injuries. If the patient is breathing, supplemental oxygen should be administered via a face mask as soon as possible. After assessment of breathing proceed to assess the circulation.

Always give high concentration oxygen

Circulation

Check that the patient has a pulse. If both spontaneous breathing and the pulse are absent, proceed with cardiopulmonary resuscitation. If the patient is not breathing but has a pulse, ventilate the patient using a bag and mask. If the patient has a pulse, measure the blood pressure, then site an intravenous cannula. If the patient is a victim of trauma use a wide-bore cannula (16–14 G) and start immediate fluid resuscitation. *Do not delay transfer of the patient to hospital if you are having difficulty placing the cannula.*

Diabetes and Disability

If there is any evidence that the patient may be a diabetic suffering from hypoglycaemia, intravenous glucose should be given. Look for a diabetic warning bracelet or insulin syringes in the patient's pocket. Test a finger-prick blood sample (or use blood from the cannula) for glucose with a reagent strip (e.g. BM stix®). A result of 2.5 mmol/l or below supports the diagnosis of hypoglycaemia, but treat the patient even if the result is normal and you suspect the diagnosis – the tests can be inaccurate at very low and very high values.

Next perform the rapid neurological checks – 'AVPU' (see below) and assessment of pupillary responses. If both pupils are constricted (like pinpoints) consider the diagnosis of opiate overdose. Other signs of opiate overdose are needle marks from previous injections, and slow, shallow respiration. If your ambulance service allows the use of naloxone (Narcan), then 0.8–2 mg should be given intravenously and the patient observed for a response. Otherwise, simply protect the patient's airway, support respiration as necessary with a bag and mask, and transport the patient as quickly as possible to hospital.

Further Information

When the patient's condition has been stabilized, try to obtain more information about the collapse. The unconscious patient will be unable to offer any history, so any details obtained from relatives and witnesses may be crucial. Important questions to ask can be remembered using the mnemonic 'AMPLE':

A > Allergies
M > Medication
P > Past illnesses
L > Last ate
E > Event

The patient may have suffered an allergic reaction and collapsed with anaphylactic shock: a relative may be aware of an allergic history, or the patient may be wearing a warning bracelet or carrying a treatment pack of injectable adrenaline. Knowledge of the patient's medication may indicate a likely cause of collapse. Ask also about the use of recreational drugs and alcohol. Medicines may be found by the patient or may be carried in a pocket.

Ask relatives if the patient has had any previous episodes of collapse or serious illness.

It is important to know when the patient last ate. Someone who has recently had a meal presents a much higher risk of aspiration of food into the airway.

Ask about the sequence of events with questions such as, 'Please describe exactly what happened', 'Did the patient collapse suddenly?' and, 'Was he assaulted?'

The collection of this information should not delay the transport of the patient to hospital. The definitive diagnosis of the cause of collapse will in many cases not be made until the patient has had extensive further investigation in hospital. The unconscious patient who is breathing, has a pulse and is not a victim of trauma should be transferred to hospital in the recovery position in order to protect the airway (Figure 14.1). The unconscious trauma victim patient should be immobilized on a long spinal board with a rigid collar. Suction must be immediately available in case of vomiting.

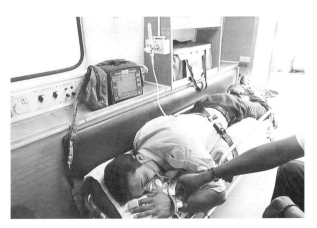

Fig. 14.1 *Transport of a patient in the recovery position*

During transport the patient's condition should be re-evaluated. Routine observations and neurological checks should be regularly repeated. If you have time, perform further neurological checks (Glasgow Coma Scale and lateralizing neurological signs) and check the patient's temperature. A limited secondary survey may help to determine the cause of the collapse. Signs to look for include:

- Battle's sign and 'racoon eyes' (base of skull fracture)
- A bitten tongue and urinary incontinence (epileptic fit)
- Temperature and rash (meningococcal septicaemia)

If any of the patient's routine observations change, then reassess airway, breathing and circulation and treat as necessary. Deterioration in the neurological status (decreasing AVPU score, decreasing Glasgow Coma Scale score or development of lateralizing signs) is ominous: ensure that the patient reaches the definitive care centre as soon as possible.

The management of the unconscious patient is summarized in Figure 14.2.

ASSESSMENT OF NEUROLOGICAL STATUS IN THE UNCONSCIOUS PATIENT

The assessment of the airway, breathing and circulation should always take priority. After 'A', 'B' and 'C' proceed to 'D' (disability), the preliminary examination of the patient's neurological status. This is an important part of clinical assessment and allows you to determine the conscious level of the patient. The more deeply unconscious the patient, the more he or she is at risk from the environment. The assessment may indicate possible causes of the unconscious state and it serves as a baseline so that progress of the patient's condition can be monitored.

There are two neurological checks that you should perform when assessing disability: an assessment of conscious level, and a check of the pupillary reactions. These checks should be repeated regularly to look for any changes in the patient's neurological state.

Basic neurological checks

- Conscious level
- Pupillary responses

Conscious Level

Conscious patients are alert and aware of their surroundings. As conscious level falls, individuals may respond to vocal

stimuli, and then only to painful stimuli. Finally they may be totally unresponsive. The first letter of each of these responses spells the mnemonic 'AVPU', used to describe a simple tool to assess conscious level.

A	>	Alert
V	>	Vocal stimuli
P	>	Painful stimuli
U	>	Unresponsive

Using the AVPU scale

On initial assessment the patient who is awake, knows his or her name and is aware of the surroundings, scores 'A'. This is usually noted down in this format:

$$\underline{A} \quad V \quad P \quad U$$

The next step is to talk to a patient who does not speak spontaneously. A response by speech or movement scores 'V'. If there is no response, you should try a painful stimulus. The best stimulus to use is pressure over the supraorbital ridge, above one of the eyes (see Figure 14.3). A response to this stimulus scores 'P', no response scores 'U'.

Remember to repeat the assessment regularly. A change in conscious level is the most important single sign in the assessment of the unconscious patient with a head injury.

Pupillary Responses

The state of the pupils can provide important information that may help to determine the cause of collapse. Causes of pupillary changes are noted in Table 14.1. Bilateral pinpoint pupils are a particularly valuable sign, as they virtually always indicate opiate overdosage (although a brain stem stroke can produce the same sign). Bilateral dilated pupils are less helpful because there are a multitude of potential causes. It must be remembered that patients with fixed dilated pupils are not necessarily dead, and this sign is not an indication to terminate cardiopulmonary resuscitation. Pupils of different sizes may be highly significant. A person with a head injury, for example a subdural or extradural haematoma (see Chapter 21), may initially have normal pupils. As the haematoma expands pressure increases inside the head and presses on one of the third cranial nerves. This will cause the pupil *on that side* to dilate. As intracranial pressure increases further the third nerve on the opposite side will be affected and the other pupil will dilate.

To assess the pupils, first gently open the eyelid. Signs of local trauma such as haemorrhage under the conjunctiva may be present. Look at the pupils: note the pupillary size and shape (an irregular pupil may indicate local trauma or previous surgery to the eye). Compare the two pupils to see if they appear the same, and shine a light in each eye in turn to see if the pupils show the normal reflex constriction.

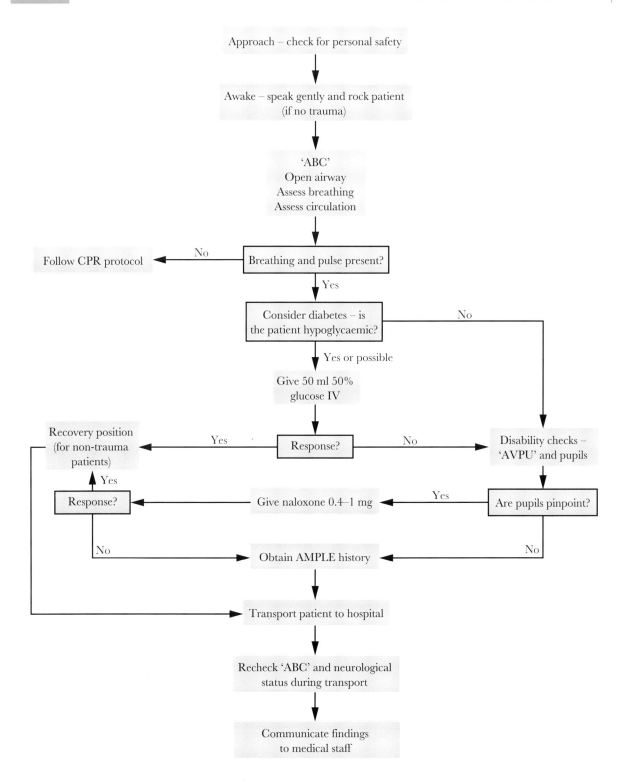

Fig. 14.2 *Algorithm for management of the unconscious patient*

Table 14.1 Pupillary changes and possible diagnosis

Pupillary signs	Possible diagnosis
Bilaterally fixed and dilated	Death; hypovolaemic shock; drugs such as atropine, adrenaline and Ecstasy
Unilaterally fixed and dilated	Head injury; stroke
Bilateral pinpoint constriction	Opiate overdose
Bilateral constriction	Brain stem stroke
Irregular pupil	Trauma; previous eye operation

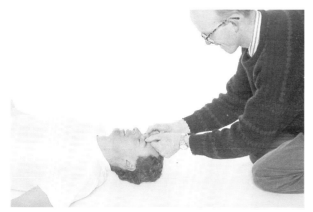

Fig. 14.3 *Supraorbital pressure*

Pupillary assessment

- Size
- Shape
- Comparison with other pupil
- Reaction to light

Remember that the most important sign of deterioration in neurological status is a change in the clinical signs. This can only be determined if the conscious level and the pupillary signs are repeatedly checked.

Regularly repeat AVPU and pupillary assessment

FURTHER NEUROLOGICAL EXAMINATION

An important priority with the unconscious patient is early transfer to hospital for further assessment and management. A more extensive neurological evaluation of the patient can usually be deferred until the patient has arrived at the receiving medical facility. However, if time arises *during transport* two other useful neurological checks can be performed: a more detailed assessment of the conscious level of the patient using the Glasgow Coma Scale, and a brief neurological examination to determine if the patient has any areas of localized weakness or paralysis (focal neurological deficit).

Further neurological checks

- Glasgow Coma Scale
- Focal neurological deficit

The Glasgow Coma Scale

The Glasgow Coma Scale uses three areas of patient response to determine a score that indicates coma level: these are *eye opening*, *speech* and *best motor response*. Eye opening is scored from 1 to 4, speech from 1 to 5, and best motor response from 1 to 6. The highest score (the alert patient) is therefore 15, and the lowest (in deep coma or dead) is 3. The scoring system is shown in Table 14.2. 'Coma' is officially recognized as a score of 8 or less.

The components of the system can be incorporated into the ambulance service initial assessment sheet (report form) as an aid to remembering the individual scores. A patient in 'coma' will give no verbal responses (scores 1), the eyes will remain closed (scores 1) and the patient will at best localize to pain (scores 5) – that is, a maximum score of 7. The best response is recorded if it differs between the two sides.

Focal Neurological Deficit

A full neurological assessment is inappropriate in the pre-hospital care of the unconscious patient. However, useful information can be obtained by close observation. On close examination of the face, note should be made of a drooping of the smile on one side indicating a facial paralysis (Figure 14.4), common in patients who have had a cerebrovascular accident (stroke).

After a painful stimulus, movement of the patient's limbs should be observed, which may reveal paralysis in one or more of the limbs. Weakness and paralysis are signs of 'focal neurological deficit', and should be recorded and communicated to the receiving doctor at the medical facility.

Table 14.2 The Glasgow Coma Scale

Component	Response	Score
Best motor response	Obeys commands	6
	Localizes to pain[a]	5
	Withdraws from pain[b]	4
	Flexor response to pain[c]	3
	Extensor response to pain[d]	2
	No motor response to pain	1
Best verbal response	Oriented	5
	Confused conversation[e]	4
	Inappropriate speech[f]	3
	Incomprehensible speech[g]	2
	No speech	1
Eye opening	Spontaneous	4
	In response to speech	3
	In response to pain	2
	No eye opening	1

[a] Moves hand towards pain; [b]moves away from pain; [c]bends arm at elbow and wrist in response to a painful stimulus; [d]straightens at elbow and knee in response to a painful stimulus; [e]disorientated in time and place; [f]inappropriate response to question; [g]moans and groans.

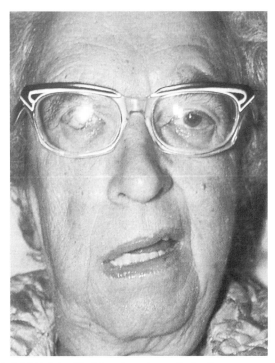

Fig. 14.4 *Unilateral facial weakness in a patient with a cerebrovascular accident. From Forbes CD & Jackson WF (1993)* A Colour Atlas and Text of Clinical Medicine. *London: Wolfe Publishing*

COMMON CAUSES OF COMA

The causes of collapse can be remembered with the mnemonic 'CID, CID' (*think of who investigates – the CID*). The two Cs stand for *Cerebral causes* (such as cerebrovascular accident, subarachnoid haemorrhage and epilepsy) and *Cardiac causes* (including the simple faint, myocardial infarction and cardiac arrhythmias). The Is stand for *Injury* to the head and major trauma elsewhere and for *Infection* (for example meningitis). The Ds refer to *Diabetes* and other metabolic emergencies, and to *Drugs*, poisons and alcohol. A final rare cause of unconsciousness that can be added to this mnemonic is *Failure* – both of organs (such as respiratory, cardiac or renal failure) and failure to maintain normal body temperature. (*If CID will not give the answer, think of failure*).

C	>	CEREBRAL
I	>	INJURY TO THE HEAD
D	>	DIABETES AND METABOLIC
C	>	CARDIAC
I	>	INFECTION
D	>	DRUGS, POISONS AND ALCOHOL
F	>	FAILURE OF ORGANS

Cerebral Causes of Unconsciousness

The most common cerebral causes of unconsciousness are epilepsy, cerebrovascular accident (stroke) and subarachnoid haemorrhage. Head injury and meningitis are considered later in the chapter.

Cerebrovascular accident

Cerebrovascular accidents (CVAs) or strokes have two basic causes. They may result from haemorrhage from a cerebral blood vessel – a *haemorrhagic stroke* – or from blockage of the blood supply to part of the brain – a *cerebral infarct*. A blood vessel can either become blocked by atheroma (fat deposits that build up on the vessel wall with increasing age) or by an embolus (a clot of blood or other material that has come from another part of the body, often the heart or neck, and lodged in the brain).

The two types of stroke cannot be distinguished clinically and present with the same features. The patient's conscious level may be decreased and there will be localizing neurological signs, such as paralysis on one side, facial asymmetry and dysarthria (difficulty articulating speech). If the features are transient and resolve completely over the space of several hours then the episode is known as a *transient ischaemic attack* (TIA). TIAs are often precursors of full-blown strokes.

Little treatment is available at present for people who have cerebrovascular accidents. Close attention should be paid to the ABCs to ensure that the airway is protected and the patient is well oxygenated. A cannula should be sited so that emergency drugs can be given. The patient should then be transferred to hospital so that a definitive diagnosis can be made and treatment started.

Remember that the term 'right-sided stroke' implies right-sided weakness; a 'right-sided CVA', however, implies involvement of the right side of the brain and hence *left-sided* weakness.

Subarachnoid haemorrhage

Subarachnoid haemorrhage is a bleed into the fluid that surrounds the brain. It is usually caused by the sudden bursting of a small swelling (an aneurysm) of a cerebral vessel. The results of the haemorrhage can be rapidly fatal. The condition affects all ages and may be precipitated by a sudden rise in blood pressure.

The characteristic history is a patient who develops a sudden headache (often described as 'like being hit on the back of the head with a hammer') and who then collapses. The patient may develop focal neurological signs and convulse. The airway should be secured, ventilation assisted as necessary, a cannula sited and rapid transfer arranged to the nearest hospital with emergency facilities.

Epilepsy

Epilepsy is a condition of abnormal brain activity which presents with convulsions or 'fits'. Any associated decrease in conscious level is transitory – although full recovery may take several hours or even longer. The most common type of epilepsy is 'grand mal' epilepsy. The patient may present in one of three phases. A paramedic should be able to recognize these phases, and be able to treat the patient appropriately.

Initially the patient collapses and the whole body contracts – the *tonic phase*; this usually lasts for a period of up to 30 seconds. There then follows a period of generalized contractions and relaxations, the *tonic-clonic phase* (the 'fit'), the duration of which can be very variable. If the tonic-clonic phase continues for more than 15 minutes the patient is said to be in *status epilepticus*. Finally, the convulsion stops and consciousness slowly returns: this is the *post-ictal phase*. The patient may at first be confused before gradually returning to full awareness.

If the patient is still convulsing when you arrive at the scene, ensure that he or she comes to no further harm. If possible, a bite guard should be inserted into the mouth to prevent damage to the lips and tongue – do not, however, open the mouth forcibly to insert a guard. An oxygen mask should be placed on or near the face of the patient. If the convulsion shows no sign of ceasing, the patient should be transported rapidly to the nearest available hospital with resuscitation facilities. Care should be taken to ensure that the individual is protected from self-injury during the ambulance journey. Remember to check the patient's blood glucose level with a reagent strip to exclude hypoglycaemia as the underlying cause.

Most diagnostic difficulty is encountered when a patient is found in the post-ictal state. Look for an epilepsy warning bracelet and antiepileptic medication in the patient's pocket. Ask any witnesses for a description of the event. Examine the recovering patient for signs of a bitten tongue or urinary incontinence. The patient who is immediately alert after an episode of collapse is unlikely to have had a grand mal fit .

Neurological abnormalities (for example unequal pupils or focal weakness) may not be of significance after a fit and can only be properly assessed once the patient has fully recovered, when many such abnormalities will have resolved.

Other forms of epilepsy may occasionally be seen. The patient with temporal lobe epilepsy often experiences a warning 'aura' prior to the fit. This may take the form of an unusual smell or taste. Focal fits occur when only one area of the body is involved. Some forms of epilepsy can be triggered by flashing lights or repetitive patterns. 'Petit mal' fits are otherwise known as 'absence' attacks, because the patients appear not to be listening, and are unaware of their surroundings for a short time. There is no tonic or tonic-clonic phase. These types of epilepsy are commoner in the younger patient and may disappear with age.

It is extremely unlikely that paramedical assistance will be requested for a patient having a petit mal seizure.

Injury

Head injury

The diagnosis of head injury should not be overlooked, particularly with the drunk or intoxicated patient. Signs of trauma such as a head wound or palpable depressed fracture may be present. Other, more subtle signs that indicate a base of skull fracture are bruising around both eyes ('raccoon eyes'), bruising over the mastoid process (Battle's sign – usually takes a number of hours to develop) and blood or cerebrospinal fluid leaking from an ear. However, the patient with a head injury may have no external signs at all.

Patients with more severe head injuries may have areas of haemorrhage inside the skull. An extradural haemorrhage occurs when blood leaks out of a ruptured artery outside the covering of the brain (the *dura mater*). Characteristically this occurs with trauma to the temporoparietal region and damage to the middle meningeal artery. Initially, the patient may fall unconscious but then recover for a short time. As the bleed enlarges the patient falls unconscious again and may then develop localizing neurological signs. Unless the blood is evacuated urgently the patient is likely to suffer permanent handicap or die.

A bleed inside the dura mater but surrounding the brain is known as a subdural haemorrhage. This usually results from bleeding from ruptured small veins and can develop suddenly or gradually. A subdural haemorrhage is associated with more extensive injury to the brain (and a worse prognosis) than an

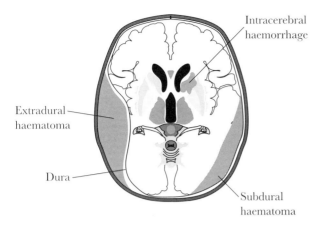

Fig. 14.5 *The anatomy of intracranial bleeding*

extradural haemorrhage. Subdural haemorrhages are common in alcoholic patients who have impaired blood clotting and who suffer frequent head injuries (Figure 14.5).

Trauma can also occur to the brain tissue itself. If blood leaks into the brain tissue it is known as an intracerebral haemorrhage. If it extends into the fluid surrounding the brain it can be described as a traumatic subarachnoid haemorrhage. Sometimes the brain swells without any bleeding, with resultant damage to the brain cells.

None of these diagnoses can be made before hospital admission. Attention should be aimed at ensuring the ABCs are fully assessed and treated. Of particular importance is the patient's breathing: the underventilated patient retains carbon dioxide, which dilates the cerebral blood vessels and results in a rise in the intracranial pressure.

When adequate ventilation has been achieved and the patient's condition has been stabilized, the patient should be transported to the nearest unit capable of offering definitive neurological care. This should be a hospital that offers diagnostic CT scanning and access to neurosurgical facilities.

Injury elsewhere

Cellular hypoxia of the brain will result in unconsciousness. Hypoxia can be caused by obstruction of the airway, breathing difficulty (for example a tension pneumothorax) and mechanical obstruction from cardiac tamponade or from fluid loss (the human body requires 50% of its normal circulating blood volume to be able to maintain consciousness). The treatment of hypoxia and hypovolaemia during the initial assessment using the ABC method is therefore vital in the management of the unconscious trauma victim. *Do not assume that coma is due to a head injury* and so neglect management of the airway, breathing and circulation.

Assess and treat any immediately life-threatening injury, stabilize the patient's cervical spine and then transport the patient to the nearest available centre capable of treating major trauma.

Diabetes and Other Metabolic Emergencies

Hypoglycaemia

A low blood glucose level is one of the most common causes of coma found in the community. It is seen most commonly in diabetic patients who have taken too much insulin in relation to their food intake and activity level. However, it can also occur in non-diabetic patients. People who are chronic alcoholics have very low sugar stores and may develop acute hypoglycaemia after a bout of drinking – a patient debilitated by malignancy or chronic liver disease may be similarly affected.

The features of hypoglycaemia develop rapidly, usually over a period of a few minutes. The first symptoms may be of dizziness and light-headedness. Profuse sweating often occurs. As the condition worsens changes of behaviour are seen. The patient may become confused and aggressive, and appear as if drunk. Weakness and incoordination develop. With further progression the patient's level of response will reduce, and the patient is likely to be cold and clammy. Unless treatment is given rapidly convulsions will ensue, with potential secondary brain damage.

Hyperglycaemia

A very high blood glucose level can also result in loss of consciousness. This can occur in patients who are developing diabetes, or in those in whom the established condition is out of control, for instance if they have a coincidental infection. This is known as diabetic ketoacidosis. The patient may have complained of thirst, weight loss and passing large amounts of urine prior to their collapse. On examination the patient will look dehydrated, with dry skin and sunken eyes. You may be able to detect a sweet smell of ketones on their breath (not all people can smell ketones). These patients also have a characteristic respiratory pattern with deep, sighing breaths, known as Kussmaul's respiration.

If you suspect the diagnosis of diabetic ketoacidosis you should quickly assess the ABCs and transfer the patient to hospital. A glucose testing strip (e.g. BM stix®) will read high. If you have a diabetic patient who has collapsed and you cannot decide if the cause is hypo- or hyperglycaemia then *assume hypoglycaemia* and give the patient glucose. Untreated hypoglycaemia can kill, while hyperglycaemia will not significantly worsen with a single injection of intravenous glucose.

> **If you are unsure why a diabetic patient has collapsed, assume hypoglycaemia and give glucose**

Other metabolic emergencies

Other metabolic emergencies are rare and difficult to diagnose out of hospital. Addison's disease is a failure of the patient's adrenal gland, responsible for secreting the body's natural steroids. This results in an electrolyte imbalance, a low blood pressure and collapse. Patients who have been on high doses of steroids that are suddenly stopped can develop a similar condition. Treat any hypotension with a normal saline fluid infusion and transfer the patient to the nearest emergency hospital.

Cardiac Causes of Unconsciousness

Cardiac arrhythmias

Major cardiac arrhythmias such as ventricular fibrillation result in collapse and should be treated using the cardiac arrest protocols (see Chapter 12). Non-arrest arrhythmias may only cause transitory upset in cardiac output and result in a brief loss of consciousness. The most common of these episodes are known as Stokes–Adams attacks, in which a patient (usually elderly) has a short run of a haemodynamically compromising arrhythmia. Patients have no warning symptoms of the collapse and recover quickly. They may report previous similar episodes. On examination, note the presence of any irregularity of the cardiac rhythm or slowness of the rate. A cannula should be inserted and the patient transported to hospital (with ECG monitoring) for cardiological investigation.

Simple faint

The simple faint or syncope is characterized by a sudden transient loss of consciousness. It is caused by a temporary decrease of blood flow to the brain. This may be precipitated by a number of factors: emotional triggers include fright, desire and the sight of blood; physical triggers such as pain, drugs (e.g. glyceryl trinitrate), standing up too quickly and anaemia may also be responsible.

The patient should be laid flat with the feet raised or in a head-down position. If the patient does not recover rapidly an alternative diagnosis should be suspected. When the patient awakes, ask about any possible precipitating causes of the faint. If there is any suspicion that there may be underlying disease, if the patient does not recover fully, or if there is concern about their safety alone at home, transport the patient to hospital for further investigation.

Infection

Infection is a rare but serious cause of collapse. It is most commonly encountered in the young child who develops meningococcal septicaemia. The child rapidly becomes unwell with a high fever. There may be the symptoms of meningitis with a stiff neck and photophobia (light hurting the eyes) before the collapse, but the septicaemia can occur without meningitis. On examination look for the characteristic rash which resembles widespread bruising (Figure 14.6). These children should be transported to hospital as rapidly as possible. Any delay in giving them intravenous antibiotics can be fatal (from onset of symptoms to death is often less than a day, and sometimes only a matter of hours). If transfer to hospital is likely to be delayed or will take a long time it may be appropriate to call the general practitioner to give the first dose of antibiotics at home prior to departure.

Other infections of the brain such as encephalitis (infection of

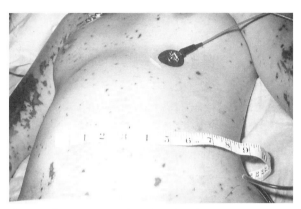

Fig. 14.6 *The meningococcal septicaemic rash*

the tissues of the brain) and cerebral abscess can also cause collapse. These patients are likely to exhibit abnormal neurological signs.

Overwhelming septicaemia, whatever the organism, may cause unconsciousness. Consider the diagnosis in an unconscious patient who is tachycardic with a low blood pressure and has no signs of blood loss. Start intravenous fluids and transport the patient to hospital as soon as possible.

Drugs, Alcohol and Poisons

Alcohol

Alcohol is the great deceiver when assessing the unconscious patient. A drunk patient is not necessarily unconscious because of the alcohol; the cause may be a head injury, hypoglycaemia or an overdose. Furthermore, the drunkard has the same risk of respiratory obstruction and of aspiration of fluid and food into the lungs as any other unconscious patient.

When attending a collapsed drunkard remember to check the blood glucose level with a reagent strip. Hypoglycaemia may be present and should be treated with intravenous glucose. The patient should be transported to hospital for further assessment to exclude other pathological conditions and in order to monitor recovery. *Be wary of leaving an apparently drunk patient in police custody* when other possible causes of decreased consciousness have not been excluded.

Opiate poisoning

Injecting drug abuse with opiate drugs such as morphine, diamorphine (heroin) and pethidine is an increasing problem. Opiates are also contained in tablets such as co-proxamol (Distalgesic) and may be taken in overdose. The features of opiate overdose are pinpoint pupils, respiratory depression and coma. The diagnosis should be suspected in any collapsed patient who has pinpoint pupils. Management should follow the ABC routine. If opiate overdose is suspected, the opiate antagonist naloxone (Narcan) should be given. This drug reverses all the side-effects of the drug, in particular the respiratory depression and the coma. However, it is short-acting, with a half-life of about 40 minutes. All patients with overdose must therefore be transported to hospital for further assessment and observation. Naloxone is given intravenously in a dose of 0.8–2.0 mg. Response to the drug is rapid, with wakening within a minute. If intravenous access is not possible, naloxone can be given intramuscularly. If your ambulance service does not have a protocol for the use of naloxone, transport the patient to hospital as quickly as possible while assisting respiration as necessary.

Other drugs that can cause coma

The next most common group of drugs causing coma is the antidepressants, particularly tricyclic antidepressants such as amitriptyline and mianserin. Signs that may indicate tricyclic overdose include dilated pupils, convulsions and respiratory depression. These overdoses can also cause severe cardiac arrhythmias. Monitor the patient's cardiac rhythm during transport to hospital.

The benzodiazepines are a group of drugs that are used to relieve anxiety. They include such drugs as diazepam, temazepam and nitrazepam. When taken in overdose they can cause drowsiness, but only very rarely result in coma.

The list of drugs that can cause coma is long. Drugs are often taken in combination with alcohol. The effects of the drugs may then be additive. However, the principles of management remain the same: protect the airway, ensure good ventilation, stabilize the circulation and transport the patient to hospital.

A final agent that should be considered when thinking of poisoning as a cause of coma is the gas carbon monoxide. Poisoning can result from faulty gas central heating and major fires, as well as attempted suicides from car exhaust fumes. The toxic effects are due to hypoxia. Remove the patient from the source of carbon monoxide and give high-concentration oxygen via a face mask. Remember that carbon monoxide is odourless and invisible and may endanger your own safety.

> **Consider the diagnosis of carbon monoxide poisoning for all unconscious patients found in an enclosed space**

Failure

Organ failure

The failure of major body organs can result in coma. Organ failure can be acute, for example the respiratory failure that occurs with a severe asthma attack, or chronic as in chronic obstructive pulmonary disease. Chronic organ failure is usually accompanied by other signs of disease that indicate the responsible organ. The patient who is suffering hepatic failure and is in coma is likely to be jaundiced, the patient in respiratory failure may be cyanosed, and the patient with cardiac failure will have a weak, thready pulse. Renal failure can be more difficult to diagnose clinically. Patients with severe renal disease usually have a sallow complexion and in the end stages of the disease may develop a crystalline 'frost' on their brows. Treatment of these conditions out of hospital is difficult. Stabilize the ABC as far as possible and transport the patient to the nearest hospital.

Failure to maintain body temperature

Hypothermia, a core body temperature of less than 35 °C, can be a cause of or a result of coma. As body temperature falls, the conscious level deteriorates. At first, patients are listless and drowsy. Suspect the diagnosis in the collapsed elderly patient, or in anyone who has been unconscious for a long period or has been exposed to the environment (such as the entrapped trauma victim). The diagnosis is best confirmed with a low-reading rectal thermometer, but this should not be performed in the pre-hospital environment. *Do not* atttempt to intubate these patients unless absolutely necessary as fatal cardiac arrhythmias can be provoked. Remove any wet clothes, wrap the patient in warm woollen blankets, and then transport the patient to the nearest hospital (see Chapter 38).

chapter fifteen:

THE ACUTE ABDOMEN

Abdominal emergencies usually present with acute abdominal pain in association with other symptoms and signs. The causes range from life-threatening conditions that require immediate resuscitation and laparotomy to those that require more conservative management.

Even in a hospital with ample facilities it can be difficult to assess and diagnose an abdominal emergency. It is therefore particularly difficult to carry out this task in the pre-hospital environment. Consequently the paramedic should concentrate instead on assessing the severity of the patient's condition and on managing it appropriately. In particular it is important to detect patients who require immediate resuscitation and urgent transfer. This chapter discusses the essential parts of the medical history and examination which will enable the paramedic to assess the severity of the patient's condition. For correct assessment it is important that the clinically relevant aspects of abdominal anatomy are understood.

APPLIED ANATOMY

Boundaries

The abdomen is a bony and muscular cavity supported by the lumbar and sacral elements of the spine and the pelvis. The back wall is a semirigid structure being made from the spine and paraspinal muscles. In contrast, the flanks and anterior abdominal wall are formed by deformable layers of muscles and sheet-like fibres; these musculotendinous layers are hung from the costal margins of the thoracic cage above, and are attached to the bones and ligaments of the upper aspect of the pelvic girdle below (Figure 15.1).

The abdomen's internal boundaries are defined by two other sheets of muscle. The diaphragm divides the upper abdomen from the thoracic cavity. As this major muscle of respiration moves down with inspiration, it alters the relationship of the thoracic and abdominal contents. The lower boundary is formed by the pelvic floor muscles. These separate the abdomen from the buttocks, the perineum and the genital areas of the external pelvis. However, this lower boundary does allow access of the femoral vessels and nerves anteriorly into the bulk of the thigh muscles. The former represent the main blood supply and drainage of the lower limbs.

Peritoneum

The internal aspect of the abdominal cavity is lined by a thick, double-layered sheet of peritoneum (Figure 15.2), which divides the abdominal organs into those that are intraperitoneal and those that are extraperitoneal (retroperitoneal). The outermost layer is supplied by nerves which also supply the skin overlying that area of peritoneum, making it possible to localize accurately areas of injury and inflammation. In contrast, the internal layers have a different nerve supply which does not allow precise localization of pathological problems. The peritoneal cavity is a potential space between the layers which normally contains small amounts of fluid and cells.

The layers of peritoneum covering the intraperitoneal structures provide not only structural support, but also vascular and nervous access to and from the abdominal organs. The majority of the small bowel is intraperitoneal and is mobile. Consequently the blood supply of the small bowel may be interrupted if its mobile vessels are sheared from the immobile aorta as well as from the caval and portal venous systems.

The liver, spleen and stomach are intraperitoneal but their mobility is dependent upon their diaphragmatic attachments. This results in these organs being pushed below the partial protection of the lower ribs and costal margins when the diaphragm descends during deep inspiration. The liver and spleen are vascular organs and are vulnerable to blunt traumatic forces causing shearing of their solid tissue. This can lead to fractures or lacerations of these organs with consequent life-threatening blood loss. In addition, shearing forces can result in vascular disruption especially where mobile vessels join ones that are more fixed. Thus a laceration may extend from the surface of an organ into its core, where the major vessels are usually found.

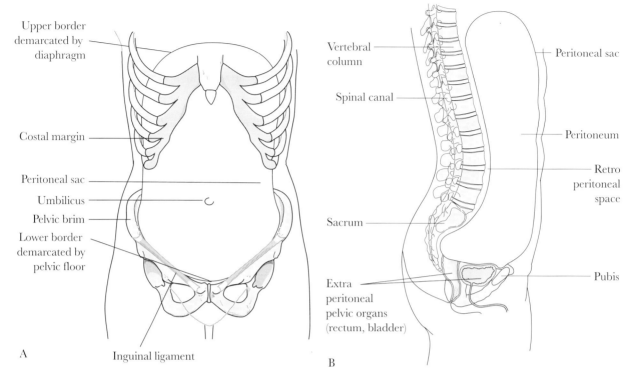

Fig. 15.1 *The abdomen: A, front view; B, side view*

Retroperitoneum

Some structures lie behind the peritoneum (retroperitoneally) on the semirigid posterior abdominal wall and in the pelvis (see below). The pelvis forms a firm support for the major vessels and branches of the abdominal aorta and inferior vena cava (IVC) which are adherent to it. Distally the aorta and IVC supply both the pelvic contents and lower limbs via the internal and external iliac vessels respectively.

Retroperitoneal structures

- Aorta
- Inferior vena cava
- Large bowel (ascending and descending parts)
- Duodenum
- Pancreas
- Kidneys and ureters

As the retroperitoneal structures have limited mobility they cannot move out of the way following penetrating injury. Consequently viscera such as the ascending and descending parts of the large bowel are more likely to be damaged following this mechanism of injury than the small bowel and transverse colon.

The duodenum lies coiled around the pancreas gland high up in the retroperitoneal space. These organs can therefore be damaged together following significant blunt trauma or penetrating injury. In either case the leakage of pancreatic and duodenal contents presents late because of the deep location of these structures within the abdomen.

The mobility of the kidneys and ureters is closely related to diaphragmatic movement during respiration. In general these organs are well protected by the lower ribs and lumbar musculature, but are prone to direct blunt trauma and shearing forces acting through its vascular connection with the aorta.

Hernias

The abdominal muscle layers allow certain organs and structures to pass into and out of the abdominal cavity. In doing so they leave potential weaknesses in the muscular layers which may lead to a hernia. Protrusions of abdominal contents into these hernias can cause a range of problems varying from general discomfort to bowel obstruction and perforation.

> HERNIA: a protrusion of an organ or tissue out of the body cavity in which it normally lies

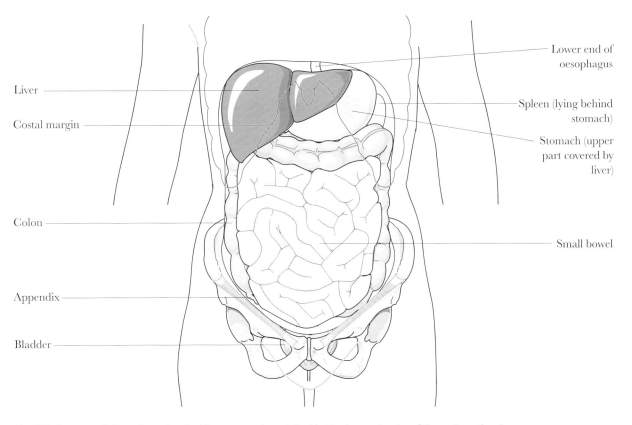

Liver

Costal margin

Colon

Appendix

Bladder

Lower end of oesophagus

Spleen (lying behind stomach)

Stomach (upper part covered by liver)

Small bowel

Fig. 15.2 *Anatomy of the peritoneal cavity. The upper surface of the bladder forms a border of the peritoneal cavity*

Types of hernia

- Inguinal
- Femoral
- Hiatus
- Epigastric
- Lumbar
- Incisional

ASSESSMENT

When this knowledge of applied anatomy is combined with the important aspects of the medical history and examination (Table 15.1) a reliable assessment of the severity of the patient's condition can be made.

Pain

Pain is the major symptom of abdominal emergencies. It also has characteristics that can provide a clue to the underlying problem. It is important to ask the following questions:

Where is the pain?
What type of pain is it (i.e. inflammatory, colicky or ischaemic)?
Does the pain move?
What makes the pain better?
What makes the pain worse?
How long has the pain been present?
Have you had this pain before – if so what happened?

As mentioned previously, the nerve fibres of the outer peritoneal layer also supply the skin overlying that area of peritoneum. This enables any pathological condition to be precisely located by the site of the pain the patient is experiencing or by eliciting tenderness and guarding by pressing on the inflamed area. If the pressing hand is suddenly withdrawn, the patient will

Table 15.1 Important aspects of the medical history and examination

History	Examination
Pain	Shock
Vomiting	Distension
Bleeding	
Altered bowel habit	

experience an increase in pain as the stretched, inflamed peritoneum springs back into place. This is known as *rebound tenderness*. This local area of peritonitis gives rise to inflammatory pain which is usually throbbing and persistent, but may also increase in intensity as the disease develops.

Signs of peritonitis

- Patient can localize the area of tenderness precisely (early)
- Coughing precipitates abdominal pain in the area of tenderness (early)
- There is rebound tenderness in the painful area (intermediate)
- No abdominal movement with expansion of the chest on inspiration (late)
- Generalized rigidity of the abdominal wall (very late)

This type of pain can be eased by intravenous opiate analgesia. Before it is given, however, the patient will tend to lie still and be unwilling to move since movement aggravates the pain. Occasionally this can lead to splinting of the diaphragm and elimination of abdominal breathing. Toxins are released into the general circulation from the inflamed area and this leads to the patient becoming pyrexial. In extreme cases general peritonitis develops and there is involuntary spasm of the abdominal muscle with 'board-like' rigidity of the abdominal wall.

The inner layer of peritoneum and its contents have nerve fibres that cannot localize injuries or inflammation precisely. Nevertheless, these deep nerves are particularly sensitive to stretching or spasm of tissue. This gives rise to colicky pain whereby the intensity of the discomfort increases and decreases repeatedly. During these attacks of pain the patient is usually very restless in an attempt to find a position of comfort. This type of pain is also usually eased with intravenous opiate analgesics.

In contrast, ischaemic pain can be a mixture of both inflammatory and colicky pain and usually requires larger amounts of intravenous opiate analgesia. The important factor in this type of pain is the time from onset to restoration of normal blood flow, because this affects the degree of necrosis with consequent life-threatening or organ-dependent damage. Therefore if a condition giving rise to this pain is suspected (see below), urgent transfer to the accident and emergency department is required and the staff must be warned of the patient's imminent arrival. Some areas of the abdomen have a nerve supply that also supplies distant areas of skin. For example, the nerve supplying the diaphragm comes from an area of the spinal cord that also gives rise to the innervation of the skin overlying the ipsilateral shoulder. This conjoint nerve supply can lead to pain occurring at a site distant from its cause. This phenomenon is known as *referred pain*, and there are several examples specific to the abdomen (Table 15.2 and Figure 15.3).

Awareness of this phenomenon can help reduce the chances of making an incorrect diagnosis. In particular, retrosternal chest pain should not be automatically assumed to be due to a myocardial infarct or angina. Instead the paramedic must look for further clues in the patient's history or examination to support or disprove this conclusion (see Chapter 13).

If the intraperitoneal disorder develops it may eventually impinge on the outer peritoneal surface. To the patient, it seems that the pain has moved. A good example of this is seen when a patient develops appendicitis. Initially the intraperitoneal nerves are involved and pain is referred to the periumbilical area. Eventually, however, the inflamed appendix begins to irritate the overlying outer peritoneal surface. Consequently, as far as the patient is concerned, the pain has 'moved' to the right iliac fossa.

Vomiting

Vomiting may accompany severe pain or be directly caused by the abdominal disease. It is a common presentation in most acute abdominal conditions.

Intestinal obstruction is one of the causes of vomiting but its onset is dependent upon the site of the obstruction. Vomiting will present early with proximal obstructions such as those

Table 15.2 Sites of referred pain from abdominal pathological conditions

Site of referred pain	Site of abdominal disease
Shoulder tip	Diaphragm
Retrosternal	Oesophagus and upper stomach
Epigastrium	Distal stomach to the second part of the duodenum
Periumbilical	Second part of the duodenum to the mid-transverse colon
Hypogastrium	Mid-transverse colon to the rectum
Right loin and back	Abdominal aortic aneurysm
Flank and genital pain	Ureter
Back	Pancreas
Back	Duodenum
Hip and knee	Pelvic organs

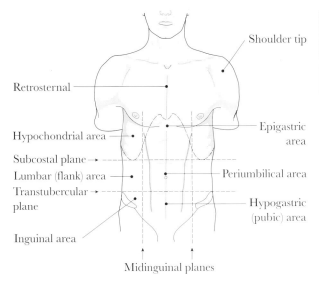

Fig. 15.3 *Areas of referred pain*

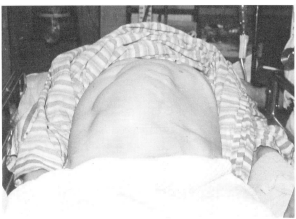

Fig. 15.4 *Intestinal obstruction secondary to intestinal adhesion from previous surgery. Loops of distended bowel and previous abdominal scars are seen*

sited in the oesophagus, stomach, duodenum and jejunum. Obstruction in these areas can cause the patient to lose significant amounts of water and electrolytes.

Vomiting blood indicates disease of the upper gastrointestinal tract. Unaltered, bright red blood suggests an oesophageal lesion, whereas altered blood, resembling 'coffee grounds', indicates a gastric or duodenal site.

Upper gastrointestinal bleeding can also give rise to *melaena*, altered blood being lost as sticky, black, 'tarry' stools with a characteristic smell. In contrast, bleeding from the lower gastrointestinal tract is seen as altered blood if the lesion is in the proximal part of the large bowel (e.g. caecal or small bowel carcinoma) or as bright-red blood if it lies more distally (e.g. haemorrhoids or rectal carcinoma).

Shock

Hypovolaemic shock associated with an abdominal emergency is indicative of severe or prolonged disease.

Abdominal causes of hypovolaemic shock

- Severe gastrointestinal bleeding
- Ruptured abdominal aortic aneurysm
- Trauma leading to abdominal vessels or organs being torn or ruptured
- Intestinal obstruction
- Mesenteric infarction
- Continuous vomiting or diarrhoea without fluid replacement
- Ectopic pregnancy (ruptured)

Shock can also result from an uncontrolled release of digestive juices into the peritoneal cavity following pancreatitis, or perforation of the stomach or duodenum. In addition, shock may be secondary to sepsis in fulminant peritonitis when it has reached a premorbid stage.

Altered Bowel Habit

Diarrhoea and constipation are two very common presentations with abdominal emergencies but are not very specific for any abdominal disorder. Altered bowel habit is a characteristic sign of intestinal obstruction, and the chances of it being an early sign are higher if the site of the obstruction is in the large bowel. These distal obstructions also allow greater retention of gas and fluid and are therefore associated with intestinal distension.

Abdominal Distension

Abdominal distension is a common presentation which again is non-specific. However, when it is associated with severe, colicky abdominal pain, vomiting and absolute constipation (i.e. failure to pass faeces, fluid or flatus) it is pathognomonic of intestinal obstruction (Figure 15.4).

COMMON EXAMPLES OF ABDOMINAL EMERGENCIES

Stomach and Proximal Duodenum

Mild cases of gastritis and duodenitis lead to epigastric or retrosternal inflammatory pain and mild epigastric tenderness.

This is frequently associated with nausea and haematemesis. Gastroenteritis presents as mild to severe, colicky abdominal pain which is poorly localized. It is commonly associated with vomiting, especially initially, and this may be followed, or replaced by, diarrhoea. Depending upon the duration of the disease, and its causative agent, this can lead to dehydration. The patient usually has a raised temperature and diffuse, mild abdominal tenderness. Guarding and rebound tenderness are uncommon findings.

Severe tenderness with localized signs of peritonitis (guarding and rigidity) suggests that the bowel may have perforated. If this is left untreated, the area of tenderness and pain increases as more of the gastric contents leaks into the peritoneal cavity. Ultimately the patient will become shocked and critically ill, and may die.

Biliary Tree

Biliary tract obstruction presents initially as epigastric colicky pain and may be provoked by eating fatty meals. Nausea, vomiting and belching are also common associated features and occasionally the patient is jaundiced. Later, when the inflamed gallbladder touches the outer peritoneum, tenderness and inflammatory-type pain are localized to the right hypochondrium. This pain may radiate to or from the right shoulder-blade on the back. Occasionally, when the inferior surface of the diaphragm is also involved in this inflammatory process, right shoulder tip pain occurs.

Secondary infection is common in the stagnant bile trapped in the biliary tree proximal to the obstruction. This increases the local inflammation and can give rise to pyrexia, tachycardia, tachypnoea and, in severe cases, rigors.

Intestines

Colic from small and large bowel obstruction is usually localized to the periumbilical and hypogastric regions respectively. The pain is not commonly related to any specific trigger and the patient may be comfortable between bouts, while remaining apprehensive about a subsequent spasm. As described previously, the frequency of vomiting and dehydration as an early associated feature increases with the more proximal location of the intestinal obstruction. Conversely, obstruction of the large bowel is associated with an early presentation of an altered bowel habit and loss of blood *per rectum*.

Appendicitis

The initial presentation and the change in characteristics of the site of the pain in appendicitis have been described above. Appendicitis is usually associated with poor appetite, vomiting and a mild pyrexia. As with all inflammatory conditions, if it is left untreated the patient's condition will become more pyrexial and toxic as infection and necrosis develop.

Pancreas

Patients with pancreatitis have epigastric tenderness and severe inflammatory pain. The latter gradually increases in intensity and may radiate into the back. There are many causes, but it is frequently associated with a history of either gallstones or the recent excessive intake of alcohol. In order to gain some relief, the patients will either sit and lean forward, or lie curled up on their side. Nausea and vomiting are common. Severe cases are associated with dehydration and a major metabolic disturbance due to the release of pancreatic enzymes, resulting in the digestion of the pancreas itself. Bruising of the flanks and abdomen indicates a more fulminant presentation with internal haemorrhage.

Kidneys and Ureters

Obstruction in the kidneys or ureters presents as ipsilateral colicky pain localized to the posterior aspect of the flank (renal angle). This is typical of renal and proximal ureteric obstruction. With a more distal ureteric location, however, pain may radiate anteriorly and distally from the flank to the ipsilateral iliac fossa, and even into the testis or labia majora. Severe pain is commonly associated with vomiting. In addition, urinary symptoms of frequency and dysuria can accompany lower ureteric problems, especially when the obstruction lies near the junction with the bladder. Occasionally the ureteric obstruction is complete and permanent, enabling infection to develop proximally. In these serious cases pyrexia, rigors and other signs of sepsis can occur, and can progress to a fulminant form of septic shock if the obstruction is not relieved quickly.

Pathological lesions at any site in the urinary tract can give rise to dark urine owing to the presence of blood in the urine. However, provided there is no torrential bleeding source, a good rule of thumb is the more red the blood looks, the more distal the lesion is located. Renal or ureteric colic associated with visible blood or clots is a common presentation of a renal tumour.

Blood Vessels

Aortic aneurysm

Aortic aneurysms develop progressively with age, and enlargement may be relatively painless until catastrophic haemorrhage occurs following rupture or dissection. Commonly an aneurysm presents as collapse, sweating and abdominal ischaemic pain. However, because of its retroperitoneal position, this pain can be referred to the back or even the left flank, and consequently can be misinterpreted with disastrous consequences. An abdominal pulsatile mass may be palpable, but tenderness and the patient's respiratory and circulatory problems make this examination difficult. Occasionally there is vomiting, haematemesis, lower limb pain and neurological deficit. A brachiofemoral pulse delay or asymmetrical femoral pulses will indicate a dissection – and may herald ischaemic problems for the intestines, kidneys, lower limbs and spinal cord.

Patients with aortic aneurysms giving rise to abdominal pain require an urgent operation. It is therefore essential that they are rapidly transferred to hospital and that time is not wasted attempting to insert intravenous lines. A pneumatic antishock garment (PASG) may be helpful in maintaining the abdominal tamponade and should be applied if it is available and the transfer is likely to be prolonged.

Mesenteric artery embolus

Mesenteric artery embolism has a sudden onset. Initially there is colicky abdominal pain, which after about an hour becomes unrelenting and poorly localized. With the exception of nausea and vomiting there may be very few signs and symptoms in the initial stages. The hallmark of this condition therefore is severe pain with very few signs on abdominal examination. Occasionally shock develops early on. With subsequent progression localized peritonitis and dehydration develop, the latter being due to impaired absorption, vomiting and fluid becoming trapped in the atonic bowel. Later, when the bowel wall becomes gangrenous and necrotic, generalized peritonitis and septic shock occurs.

Genital Tract

Pelvic inflammatory disease

Pelvic inflammatory disease is a blanket term used to cover inflammation of the female upper genital tract and the adjacent peritoneum and bowel. The patient invariably has bilateral inflammatory iliac fossa pain and tenderness. Usually there are also signs of infection such as pyrexia, tachycardia and occasionally rigors. In addition there is frequently a history of menstrual irregularities, abnormal vaginal discharge and dyspareunia (pain on sexual intercourse).

Ectopic pregnancy

Ectopic pregnancy occurs when a fertilized ovum becomes implanted outside the uterus. Usually the patient develops recurrent episodes of inflammatory lower abdominal pain, tenderness and guarding. This is associated with amenorrhoea, transient 'fainting' feelings and irregular vaginal bleeding.

Occasionally there is rupture of a fallopian tube and significant bleeding. This gives rise to severe inflammatory pain in the iliac fossa or hypogastrium, generalized tenderness and guarding, and syncope due to blood loss. Shoulder tip pain can occur when there is much free intraperitoneal blood and the patient has been lying with her head down. In these circumstances the free blood irritates the inferior surface of the diaphragm and gives rise to the referred shoulder pain described previously. These patients require vigorous resuscitation and urgent transfer to hospital so that haemostasis can be achieved surgically.

Ovarian cyst torsion

Ovarian cyst torsion presents as sudden onset of recurrent colicky pain in the ipsilateral iliac fossa. Nausea and vomiting are common associated features. In addition the abdominal wall overlying the torsion is tender and may be rigid during the attacks.

Testicular torsion

Twisting of the testis on its cord causes intense ischaemic pain localized in the testis. Usually there is localized tenderness and vomiting (which may be the sole presenting feature) but no significant swelling. These patients require urgent surgery to salvage the testis and must be transferred immediately to hospital.

SUMMARY

Paramedics managing a patient with an abdominal emergency must concentrate on assessing the severity of the condition, carrying out appropriate treatment and transporting the patient safely to hospital. All immediately life-threatening conditions must be corrected first. If this is not possible, for example in cases of major haematemesis, then the patient must be rapidly transferred to hospital, and the accident and emergency department forewarned. Any further resuscitation can be provided in transit, but must not delay the patient's transfer.

If the immediately life-threatening conditions can be corrected, relevant aspects of the patient's history should be obtained and adequate intravenous analgesia provided. The abdomen can then be examined if the severity of the condition is still unclear. With these two elements completed the paramedic can transport the patient to hospital with the appropriate degree of urgency.

chapter sixteen:

POISONING

Poisoning takes a variety of forms. Harmful substances may be ingested, inhaled or absorbed through the skin. The exposure to the poison may be accidental (as with most childhood poisonings), or deliberate as part of an attempted suicide or following 'recreational' activities. The role of paramedical workers is crucial in the management of poisonings in the community: without their detailed assessment of the situation and immediate management, the task of the emergency physician is difficult and occasionally futile.

GENERAL CONSIDERATIONS

The assessment of a patient with suspected poisoning is often difficult. The patient found unconscious with a suicide note and an empty bottle of pills poses no problem to diagnosis, but the information at the scene may not be that clear-cut. The patient may be just behaving oddly, or have cardiovascular or respiratory problems. If there are no witnesses and the patient is unable to give a history, the diagnosis of poisoning becomes increasingly difficult. Fortunately, however, the majority of poisoned patients will require little in the early stages other than standard emergency care – i.e. protection of the airway, and support of breathing and circulation.

Approach

The patient with suspected poisoning is managed with the 'SAFE' approach used for all medical emergencies (see Chapter 3).

The paramedic must remember that the patient may have been poisoned by exposure to dangerous substances which may still be in the immediate environment. It is of benefit to no-one if the paramedical crew become secondary casualties – therefore exercise caution in approaching the patient, remaining alert to clues in the environment that may suggest inhalational or dermal exposure to a toxic substance.

If you can approach safely, the next task is to ensure that no further harm comes to the patient. If the patient is in a dangerous position, for example lying unconscious in the middle of the road, then he or she should be moved immediately. Similarly, a patient who has been exposed to an inhalational poison and is still in the poisoned atmosphere, for example a smoky room in a house fire or a garage full of carbon monoxide, again needs to be moved immediately.

Once the patient is in a place of safety, an assessment of the patient's clinical state needs to be made, and a history taken. If the situation permits, these tasks should be undertaken simultaneously. If this is not possible then it is for the paramedic to decide which of these tasks takes priority. If the patient is extremely ill or unconscious, the first priority is to secure and maintain the airway and support the circulation. If the patient is stable, then the history should be taken, both from the patient if possible and from any witnesses.

History

When taking the history, three crucial questions must be asked:

- What was taken?
- How much was taken?
- When was it taken?

Without a knowledge of the nature of the substance, the quantity taken and the time elapsed between ingestion and presentation, it is extremely difficult to assess the severity of the poisoning, or to make any predictions as to the patient's subsequent course.

If possible, the paramedic should take any medicine containers found at the scene to the hospital along with the patient. Note also the presence of any additional substances such as alcohol, which may contribute to the patient's condition. In up to 30% of cases of deliberate ingestion of a poison, two or more substances have been taken.

Examination

The immediate examination of the patient should be to establish the stability of the vital signs. Many poisons depress the level of consciousness, and adults who deliberately ingest poisons have often also taken alcohol. In many of these cases the actual poison will not cause serious harm to the patient other than by endangering the airway as a result of the altered mental state. Simple attention to the airway may be all that is needed to treat this patient's poisoning, but if omitted a relatively 'harmless' poisoning may be fatal.

As a general rule, most cases of poisoning require no treatment other than maintenance of the vital signs. If this is achieved, the majority of patients will have a favourable outcome.

Once the ABC has been assessed a more general examination should follow, both to give an indication of the patient's general state and also hopefully to obtain information relating to the nature of the poisoning (Table 16.1).

A rapid pulse rate may indicate ingestion of substances such as tricyclic antidepressants, antihistamines, amphetamines or other arrhythmogenic agents. Similarly, a low blood pressure will result from ingestion of anticholinergic medications or vasodilators such as alcohol. An increased respiratory rate is associated with substances that cause shock, but it also occurs in the early stages of salicylate overdose. A decreased respiratory rate occurs with opiate ingestion. The pupils may be dilated (tricyclic antidepressant and amphetamine ingestion), or constricted (opiate ingestion). The presence of nasal bleeding or perioral sores suggests solvent abuse.

It should be emphasized that the gathering of this information should in no way delay the stabilization and transport of the patient to the nearest hospital. As noted earlier, most cases of poisoning require little other than maintenance of the airway and circulation. However, this may require skills and techniques only available in the hospital setting.

Similarly, in cases where further absorption of the poison can be prevented, or where there is a specific antidote to the poison, any delay in hospitalization will decrease the chances of a successful outcome.

Poisoning in Children

Poisoning in children is common, but not commonly serious. A typical case of poisoning in childhood is the accidental ingestion of a mildly toxic substance by a child aged 1–3 years. Most incidents are minor.

In the UK, the majority of children ingest therapeutic agents – paracetamol, iron, benzodiazepines, tricyclic antidepressants and the contraceptive pill are the most common. The remainder are usually poisoned by a variety of household products (see later). The accidental ingestion is usually noticed early by the parents, and therefore the children often present very soon after ingestion (unlike the situation in many adult poisonings).

Some parents keep syrup of ipecacuanha in the house for use as an emetic in case of accidental poisoning. The use of this substance is controversial, as it can result in aspiration pneumonitis and gastrointestinal haemorrhage. In addition, it is only effective in removing the poison if given within 5 minutes of ingestion. As a general rule, however, it should not be used in the pre-hospital setting. If ipecacuanha has been given, the paramedic needs to be aware that up to 15% of children will develop prolonged vomiting, diarrhoea and drowsiness. Because its effects are delayed, the child may become drowsy as a result of the poisoning before the ipecacuanha induces vomiting, increasing the risk of aspiration.

The vast majority of poisoned children can be expected to recover if vital functions are preserved. Aspiration pneumonitis is far more dangerous to the patient than most poisons.

SPECIFIC POISONS

Medications

Almost any medication can be harmful if taken in excess. Unfortunately, members of the public often perceive a difference in the toxicity of prescription medications compared with over the counter medications, believing the former to be more dangerous than the latter. This leads to the tragic consequence of a patient 'crying for help' by taking an overdose of paracetamol, believing it to be of limited toxicity, with a fatal outcome. Conversely, the patient who takes a relatively innocuous overdose of benzodiazepines may genuinely believe that the drug may be toxic enough to be fatal, as it is only available on prescription.

Table 16.1 Diagnostic clues following drug overdose

Clinical sign	Drug
Tachycardia	Tricyclic antidepressants, antihistamines, amphetamines
Increased respiratory rate (tachypnoea)	Salicylates (aspirin), substances causing shock
Decreased respiratory rate	Opiates
Hypotension	Anticholinergic drugs, vasodilators, alcohol
Pupillary dilation	Tricyclic antidepressants, amphetamines
Pupillary constriction	Opiates
Nasal bleeding or perioral sores	Solvent abuse ('glue sniffing')

The prescription medications most commonly taken in overdose in the UK are the benzodiazepines. These usually just cause drowsiness or unconsciousness, although if taken with alcohol they may cause respiratory depression. The management of these patients consists of clearing and maintaining the airway, and supporting the breathing with bag–mask ventilation if required. Although there is a specific antidote to benzodiazepines (flumazenil), there are dangers with its use in the pre-hospital setting. The patient may develop seizures as a result of benzodiazepine withdrawal, or because other medications (e.g. tricyclic antidepressants) may also have been ingested. Should this happen, the seizures are extremely difficult to treat as the usual anticonvulsant in this situation – diazepam – will not work in the presence of the flumazenil. A further problem arises with the patient who revives following the administration of flumazenil, refuses further treatment and leaves the scene; because the effects of the flumazenil are short-lived, unlike the effects of the benzodiazepines, the patient may succumb again to the overdose, possibly when no witnesses are present to call for help.

The most common over-the-counter medication taken in overdose is paracetamol. As noted previously, the great danger of this drug is that it is perceived as harmless. Because there are often no immediately felt ill-effects after taking this drug, there may be a prolonged delay in seeking treatment. The tragedy is that such a delay may be fatal. Paracetamol is an extremely toxic drug when taken in overdose, and although there is a specific antidote, it is most effective if given within 15 hours of ingestion. A delay in presentation, therefore, may render the antidote ineffective and lead to a preventable death. For the paramedic, the management of such cases is usually just transporting the patient to hospital for specific treatment. However, it should be remembered that the patient may perceive the overdose to be harmless, and may decide to refuse treatment or transport to hospital. The paramedics must use all their powers of communication and persuasion in these cases, as the patient may die if not treated.

So, for the two most common adult poisonings, the treatment is support of the vital signs and rapid transportation to hospital. However, there are other medications commonly taken in overdose, for which there are specific treatments that are available to the paramedic, as follows.

Tricyclic antidepressants

Tricyclic antidepressants are commonly prescribed to the patients who are most at risk of attempted self-harm. It is unfortunate that this group of drugs are amongst the most toxic medications taken in overdose.

Poisoning by these drugs affects the central nervous system, causing depressed consciousness followed by seizures. They also affect the cardiovascular system, producing cardiac arrhythmias ranging from sinus tachycardia in the early stages of poisoning, to ventricular tachycardia in the later stages of severe poisoning. The patient usually has a degree of vasodilatation,

which causes hypotension. Together with the impaired function of the heart, this leads to poor perfusion of organs and a metabolic acidosis. With the depressed conscious level impairing ventilation, respiratory acidosis is also a common finding in these patients.

The management of these patients can be very challenging; however, the ABC approach will be sufficient pre-hospital care for most of them. The airway should be cleared and protected, and oxygen given via a face mask. Ventilation may be needed, and this should initially be via a bag–valve–mask system. Hyperventilating the patient will help correct both metabolic and respiratory acidosis. Hypotension should be treated with intravenous fluid challenge, and an ECG monitor should be applied to determine and monitor the cardiac rhythm.

Should seizures occur, these can be treated in the normal manner with intravenous or rectal diazepam, remembering that this may well depress respiration further. Cardiac arrhythmias such as sinus tachycardia need no specific treatment. If the patient develops a ventricular arrhythmia with a pulse, specific urgent in-hospital investigations and treatment will be required. The specific in-hospital treatment will include repeated boluses of sodium bicarbonate until the rhythm normalizes, or the pH reaches 7.55.

The decision to intubate these patients is fraught with difficulties. Although intubation will protect the airway from vomit and facilitate ventilation, the procedure can cause marked cardiac stimulation and may precipitate a life-threatening arrhythmia. It is usually safer to use a bag–valve–mask system for ventilation, with the patient in the recovery position and slightly head-down. Should the patient need intubation, this can more safely be accomplished in the hospital setting with the aid of sedating and paralysing agents.

Tricyclic antidepressant overdose

- **Clinical features**
  Tachyarrhythmias
  Hypotension
  Tachypnoea
  Depressed conscious level
  Fits

- **Management**
  Airway and oxygen
  Breathing – support ventilation
  Circulation – maintain circulation, rapid transfer, *monitor ECG* (bicarbonate in hospital only)
  Control seizures with diazepam

Beta-blockers

Beta-blockers are widely prescribed to the elderly. This section of the population is at risk of poisoning for two reasons: poor vision and impaired memory predispose to accidental overdose of prescription medications; and intentional overdose, although less common in this age group, is usually undertaken with more determination.

The results of beta-blocker overdose reflect the *function* of the drug, namely to produce bradycardia and hypotension (unlike tricyclic antidepressants where overdose reflects the *side-effects* of the drug). The patient may also have a depressed conscious level as a result of cerebral underperfusion. The treatment follows ABC principles: the airway is secured and breathing is assessed. Hypotension is treated with intravenous fluid, and bradycardia is treated with 0.5 mg atropine intravenously. A further dose may be given if there is no effect, or if the patient deteriorates after transient improvement. Glucagon 0.5–1.0 mg given intramuscularly or intravenously (and repeated) has been shown to be of benefit in severe beta-blocker poisoning. In severe cases the patient may require insertion of an intravenous pacemaker, therefore there should be no delay in taking the patient to the nearest hospital.

Insulin

It is uncommon for insulin to be taken as a deliberate overdose, but accidental overdoses occur frequently. The patient may be comatose, in which case the diagnosis and management are paradoxically easy: protection of the airway, breathing and circulation, a simple thumb-prick blood glucose assay to confirm the diagnosis, and the administration of intravenous dextrose or intramuscular glucagon (depending on local policy) will result in a gratifying return to consciousness and normality. More difficult is the assessment and management of the combative, apparently drunk patient in the early stages of hypoglycaemia. It should be emphasized that every minute's delay in the treatment of hypoglycaemia will have a cumulative effect. It is important, therefore, to make the diagnosis and institute appropriate therapy as rapidly as possible.

After receiving treatment from the paramedic, with associated clinical improvement, a diabetic patient who has frequent hypoglycaemic episodes may be reluctant to travel to hospital once 'cured'. In such cases the paramedic will need to be persuasive, for the patient requires careful assessment in hospital to determine the reason for the hypoglycaemic event. The patient's diabetic regimen may need altering, there may be another cause for the hypoglycaemia, and – most importantly – if the overdose was of a long-acting insulin, the patient may need a period of observation to ensure that the episode does not recur.

Opiates

Opiates may be taken in overdose accidentally (in the case of the patient with chronic pain); intentionally, with a view to self-harm; or recreationally, by injecting drug abusers. The effects of opiate poisoning are a depressed level of consciousness, depressed respiration (breathing tends to be slow and deep) and hypotension. The greatest dangers are of aspiration of stomach contents while comatose, hypoxia and respiratory acidosis.

The diagnosis of opiate poisoning may be obvious: witnesses may be aware of the patient's medication or lifestyle, there may be labelled medication nearby, or the patient's physical characteristics may suggest opiate abuse (e.g. needle tracks). On examination, the patient is usually comatose, with pinpoint pupils and sighing respiration. Hypotension may be present. The treatment, fortunately, is simple. After securing the airway, supplying oxygen, assisting breathing and establishing intravenous access, naloxone should be administered intravenously in boluses of 0.8–2 mg, allowing a few minutes for effect, and repeated until the patient begins to recover.

The danger of using naloxone in these cases, which the paramedic must constantly bear in mind, is that the half-life – and therefore the effect – of naloxone is shorter than the effect of most commonly used opiates. The result of this is that the improvement in the patient's condition may be short-lived and coma may return. Unfortunately, the patient may take advantage of being 'cured' to refuse transport to hospital or further treatment. A patient who is allowed to leave the scene may well lapse into another coma, possibly with no witnesses to summon help. There are practical and medicolegal problems associated with taking such patients to hospital against their will. One method that may be used in such cases is to administer intramuscular naloxone to the poisoned patient before giving the intravenous dose. In this way, if the patient leaves the scene following recovery, naloxone will be slowly released into the circulation from the IM dose, and may prevent a relapse.

The specific teatments for overdosage are summarized in Table 16.2.

Household Substances

Almost any product designed for household use can be (and has been!) ingested, whether accidentally or intentionally. This chapter cannot hope to deal with all of them, but considers some of the more common substances ingested and looks at the general principles of management.

Most household products in current use are of low systemic toxicity if accidentally ingested. Commonly ingested substances include bleaches, turpentine substitute, paraffin and household cleaning products. The treatment of ingestion of these substances is to administer oral fluids (milk) and rapidly transfer the patient to hospital. There may be local irritation of the mouth or oesophagus, but systemic toxicity is unusual. The patient should *not* be encouraged to vomit, as this may lead to a potentially fatal pneumonitis.

Plants and Fungi

It is unusual for adults to eat poisonous plants, though mistakes occur occasionally. More commonly it is children who ingest berries, seeds or other parts of plants in the wild, the garden or around the home. Fortunately the quantities involved are usually small.

Table 16.2 Treatment for overdosage of specific drugs

Drug	Effects	Treatment
Tricyclic antidepressants	Heart rate increased Blood pressure lowered Drowsiness Convulsions	ABC IV fluids Diazepam (for fits) Bicarbonate (in hospital)
Beta-blockers	Heart rate increased Blood pressure lowered Possible drowsiness	ABC IV fluids Atropine Glucagon May need external pacer
Opiates	Drowsiness Respiration reduced Pinpoint pupils Blood presure lowered	ABC Naloxone
Insulin	Agitated Conscious level lowered Pale, clammy appearance Low blood glucose level	ABC Dextrose Glucagon

The most common plant poisoning in Britain is the ingestion of laburnum seeds. If more than ten seeds have been ingested, the effects listed below may occur. However, fatalities are extremely rare.

Effects of laburnum ingestion

- Burning mouth and throat
- Nausea
- Abdominal pain
- Vomiting
- Diarrhoea
- Drowsiness
- Incoordination
- Delirium
- Twitching
- Coma

The treatment of laburnum poisoning is the same as that for all plant ingestions: evaluate and support the airway, breathing and circulation, and transport the patient to hospital. It is of vital importance that a sample of the ingested plant is also taken to hospital for identification.

Many poisonous fungi can be eaten by mistake, but serious poisoning is rare in Britain. Usually, patients who have ingested fungi have a violent but self-limiting attack of abdominal pain, diarrhoea, nausea and vomiting about 2 hours later. Rarely, there may be signs of excessive cholinergic stimulation (bronchospasm, bradycardia, constricted pupils and collapse). This can be treated with boluses of intravenous atropine, but it should be remembered that this may exacerbate any agitation or hallucinations. As with plant ingestion, the patient and the fungi should be taken to the nearest hospital as soon as possible.

> **Wherever possible take a sample of the ingested plant to hospital**

Other Substances

Inhalational agents

Several substances are harmful if inhaled. The two main groups of inhalational 'poisons' are the recreational drugs (opiates, cocaine and solvents – see Chapter 51), and substances inhaled accidentally or for deliberate self-harm (carbon monoxide and other gases). The treatment of the first group is rapid assessment of the airway, breathing and circulation, supportive care, administration of naloxone in the case of opiate poisoning, and rapid transport to hospital. The second group is important because in these cases there is a danger to the paramedic. Care should be taken that the paramedic does not become a secondary casualty by inhaling the toxic fumes. If it is possible to approach safely, remove the patient from the environment and give high-concentration oxygen. The patient should then be taken to the nearest hospital.

Recreational drugs

There are unfortunately many harmful substances that are inhaled, ingested or injected for 'recreational' purposes. Some of these have already been discussed. The general effect of these drugs is to affect the central nervous system, producing depression (opiates and benzodiazepines) or stimulation (Ecstasy, amphetamines and cocaine). The treatment of poisoning by these substances is the assessment and support of airway, breathing and circulation, the administration of naloxone in opiate poisoning, and rapid transport to hospital (see Chapter 51).

SUMMARY

Poisoning is common, and likely to become more common, with the increase in medications being dispensed and the growth of substance abuse. The paramedic has a crucial role in the care of poisoned victims, being in the best position to gather vital information at the scene and provide immediate life-saving treatment.

Immediate evaluation and support of airway, breathing and circulation, the administration of specific antidotes, and rapid transport to hospital will ensure that the patient is given the best chance of survival. Most patients will survive with no further treatment, other than a continuation of support of ABC.

chapter seventeen

RISK OF INFECTION

Paramedical workers will encounter many patients who are suffering from infectious diseases. Only a small minority of these patients present any risk of infection to paramedical, medical and nursing staff. Furthermore, the chances of becoming infected from contact with one of these patients while at work is very small indeed. A basic knowledge of the common causes of infectious diseases and of methods of avoiding their spread is necessary to ensure that risk of infection is minimized.

TERMINOLOGY

The two most common causes of infection are bacteria and viruses. Bacteria are small, unicellular organisms that have evolved to live in very specialized environments. Bacterial infections usually respond to antibiotics. Viruses are much smaller organisms that cannot be seen with a normal light microscope. They do not respond to antibiotics and there are few drugs available to treat the illnesses that they cause. Other organisms such as protozoa and fungi can also cause infection. They do not usually represent an infection risk to paramedical staff.

A person is *infected* if he or she has an illness caused by a micro-organism. The disease is *infectious* if it can be transmitted from person to person. Some people may have harmful organisms in their body and yet not exhibit signs of the infection. These individuals are known as *carriers* and may transmit infection to others The area in which the micro-organism grows is known as the *source*, while the vehicle of transport of infection (e.g. the finger in a faecal–oral transmitted infection) is known as the *reservoir*. The *incubation period* of a disease is the time during which the micro-organism is multiplying in body tissue before signs and symptoms of illness have developed. The *infectious period* is the time during which the infection may be transmitted to other people.

ROUTES OF INFECTION

Infection can be spread by a number of different routes.

Droplet spread is the common route of infection for respiratory disease. Coughing or sneezing propels showers of small fluid droplets through the air. These contain bacteria and viruses which others may inspire, resulting in transmission of the infection.

Many wound infections are caused by direct contact, for instance when an unwashed hand touches a surgical wound. Direct contact may also be a route of transmission of disease during mouth-to-mouth contact in artificial ventilation. If the direct contact actually punctures the skin, for example with a bite or a needle-stick injury, the risk of infection is much higher. The risk is highest when foreign material such as blood is injected, for example from a hollow needle.

Dirty hands can also act as the reservoir for spreading infection from the lower gastrointestinal tract. This occurs when unwashed hands are placed near the mouth. This is known as faecal–oral spread and is the route of infection of many gastrointestinal infections and diseases such as hepatitis A.

Finally, infections can be spread by indirect contact when clothing, dressings or medical equipment contaminated with bacteria or viruses from an infected patient are used for another casualty. For this reason all medical equipment should be kept scrupulously clean.

IMPORTANT INFECTIOUS DISEASES IN THE UK

Bacterial Infections

Tuberculosis

Tuberculosis is a disease that mainly affects the respiratory system, causing shortness of breath and cough. It can also affect the lymph nodes of the neck and may cause discharging sinuses to the skin. It is caused by the bacterium *Mycobacterium tuberculosis* and other related mycobacteria. The incidence of the disease has recently risen in the UK, possibly owing to the increasing number of immigrants, decrease in the uptake of vaccination and poor living standards in inner cities. The disease is spread by the droplet route and occasionally by direct contact with infected debris from a tuberculous lymph node.

The typical patient is an emaciated homeless person, who presents coughing up small amounts of blood. The incubation period of the disease is 4–8 weeks and patients continue to be infectious until their illness has been treated. All paramedical staff should ensure that they are fully immunized against tuberculosis and have a Heaf test (intradermal tuberculin) every 3 years to check immunity. Those who do not show a good response to the Heaf test should have a chest radiograph to ensure that they do not have the disease.

If a patient with active tuberculosis has been transported you should thoroughly air the ambulance, launder the linen and ensure that all contaminated respiratory equipment such as face masks and tubing is destroyed. If you are worried that you might contact the disease you should attend the occupational health department who will arrange further investigation.

Meningitis

Meningitis is an infection of the membranes that surround the brain. It can be caused by bacteria or viruses. The presenting symptoms are headache, photophobia (light hurting the eyes) and neck stiffness. The common bacteria that cause meningitis are *Haemophilus influenzae*, *Neisseria meningitidis* and *Streptococcus pneumoniae*. Meningitis secondary to *Neisseria* infection (meningococcal meningitis) represents an infection risk to close contacts of the patient. It has an incubation period of 2–3 days and presents in young people. Alternatively, *Neisseria meningitidis* infection may cause a widespread bruising rash (purpura) which represents meningococcal septicaemia (Figure 14.6). The child with meningococcal disease may deteriorate very rapidly and must be transported to hospital as soon as possible to receive intravenous antibiotics.

If you transport such a patient, wear a face mask and ensure that you, the ambulance and all equipment are thoroughly cleaned afterwards. If the final diagnosis is proved to be meningococcal meningitis you should attend your occupational health department. They will consider giving a course of antibiotics to reduce any possible risk of your acquiring the infection – but prophylactic antibiotics are *not* usually given to paramedical or medical staff unless they have been 'kissing' contacts (mouth-to-mouth ventilation).

Whooping cough

Whooping cough is a bacterial respiratory infection caused by the bacterium *Bordetella pertussis*. It mainly affects children and is most severe in those under 6 months of age. Characteristically after an incubation period of 7–10 days the child develops what appears to be a mild cough. This gradually worsens and the child develops a whooping noise when coughing (an inspiratory whoop between bouts of coughing). The disease often lasts several months and may be complicated by vomiting, weight loss and pneumonia.

The incidence of the disease has fallen with increased use of the pertussis vaccine. Whooping cough does not represent a great risk to paramedical staff, but an ambulance should be thoroughly cleaned and aired if a child with the illness has been transported.

Viral Infections

Hepatitis

Hepatitis is the name given to infective conditions affecting the liver. There are several different viruses that can cause hepatitis, which present different risks to paramedical staff. *Infectious hepatitis* is caused by the *hepatitis A virus* and is spread by the faecal–oral route. It is common in conditions of poor sanitation and tends to occur in outbreaks, for instance in prisons or mental health institutions. The incubation period of the disease is 2–6 weeks and the patient presents with general malaise, jaundice, nausea and vomiting. The disease tends to run a benign course and usually resolves over a period of 1–2 months. Infection with *hepatitis B virus* results in a much more serious illness, sometimes known as *serum hepatitis*. This condition is spread by the intravenous route or by sexual contact and causes a much more severe hepatitis which can result in death or the patient being left as a chronic carrier of the disease. It is most common in Britain in injecting drug abusers who share needles. It is much easier to contract hepatitis B than the more widely feared human immunodeficiency virus (HIV) from needle contact with an infected person. An effective vaccine is available to immunize against hepatitis B. All ambulance staff should ensure that they are vaccinated and have their antibody levels checked every 3 years. Another virus causing hepatitis has recently been discovered. It is called *hepatitis C virus* and causes a very similar condition to hepatitis B. It is also spread by the intravenous or sexual routes. There is no effective vaccine against hepatitis C to date. The paramedic can prevent spread of these diseases by being extremely careful whenever using sharp instruments or needles.

HIV infection and AIDS

There have been few diseases that have generated such widespread public interest and dread as the acquired immunodeficiency syndrome (AIDS). It can be caused by either of two viruses, HIV-1 or HIV-2, which are spread by sexual contact or by the intravenous route. The disease causes fear because as yet there is no vaccine, no cure and all patients eventually die of their illness. However, the virus is very fragile when outside the human body and is easy to destroy. The risk of becoming infected from a needle-stick injury is ten times lower for HIV than for hepatitis B virus, taking equivalent inoculating doses of the virus. The chances of acquiring HIV while at work are very small, but disease transmission has occurred in medical and nursing staff through needle-stick injury and there are occasional instances of contamination through non-intact skin.

The duty of care to a patient with AIDS remains the same as for any patient. The nature of the illness should not affect the standard of care that is given. If universal precautions are used the infection risk can be minimized. The ambulance should be thoroughly cleaned and disinfected after use and all disposable items placed in labelled double bags and sent for incineration.

Herpes virus infections

The herpes viruses cause a variety of different blistering eruptions. Herpes simplex type 1 causes cold sores on the mouth and on the fingers ('whitlow'). Herpes simplex type 2 causes similar lesions on the genitalia. Type 1 infections are common on the fingers of nursing staff who deal with patients with exposed cold sores. Spread of the infection can be prevented by wearing gloves when dealing with such patients, and regularly washing the hands.

The chickenpox virus is another herpes virus. Chickenpox is a widespread blistering eruption that is common in children and is highly infectious. The incubation period of the disease is 14–21 days and the vesicles first appear on the face and scalp before spreading to the trunk and finally the limbs. It remains infectious until the vesicles are dry. Chickenpox can affect adults more seriously, so try to avoid carrying an infected patient if you have not had the illness as a child.

The virus remains dormant in nerve endings and may reactivate at a later date resulting in 'shingles' or herpes zoster. This is characterized by vesicles erupting in small areas corresponding to the spinal nerves that supply the skin (dermatomes). It commonly occurs in the elderly, precipitated by stress or underlying disease, and can be very painful. Chickenpox and shingles are usually self-limiting diseases. However, both can become severe if the patient is immunosuppressed, for example with AIDS, or if pregnant. After carrying such a patient, clean the ambulance thoroughly to avoid the possibility of spreading the infection to other casualties.

Other childhood infectious diseases

There are a number of other childhood infectious diseases caused by viruses, of which the paramedic should be aware. The incidence of these illnesses is on the decrease because of the widespread uptake of the vaccination programme.

Measles Measles is a viral illness transmitted by droplet spread. After an incubation period of 10 days the child develops fever, cough and conjunctivitis. A rash appears 2–4 days later. The disease is infectious from the beginning of symptoms until 4 days after the appearance of the rash. The incidence of measles has decreased markedly because of the use of the measles, mumps and rubella (MMR) vaccine. The illness is not always benign and can result in deafness and brain damage. Patients with measles do not present any particular risk to paramedical staff, but the ambulance and equipment should be thoroughly cleaned after use to prevent transmission of infection to others.

German Measles (Rubella) Rubella is similar to measles but is a less severe disease, with a transient rash and lymphadenopathy (swelling of the lymph nodes). The incubation period is 14–21 days and the disease is infective from 1 week before until 4 days after the onset of the rash. The most important aspect of rubella infection is the potential fetal damage which can result when mothers are exposed to the virus in the early months of their pregnancy. For this reason all British girls are immunized against rubella prior to leaving school. The national immunization programme has now been extended to cover all teenagers, to lower the incidence of the illness in the community. All female ambulance staff should ensure that they are immunized against the disease, and if pregnant should not transport patients who are suspected of having the disease.

Mumps Mumps is a viral illness which results in swelling of one or both parotid glands (the salivary glands situated near the angle of the jaw). The incubation period of the illness is 14–21 days and the patient is infectious for several days before the parotid gland swells and for the subsequent 5 days. The child with mumps looks exceptionally miserable, with general malaise and parotid swelling. Mumps in adult life can result in inflammation of the testes (orchitis) with subsequent sterility. Adult males who have not had mumps should therefore avoid transporting children who are suspected of having the illness. Inflammation of the ovaries (oophoritis), thyroid (thyroiditis) and pancreas (pancreatitis) can all result from mumps infection. The common and serious infectious diseases encountered in the UK are summarized in Table 17.1.

MINIMIZING THE SPREAD OF INFECTIOUS DISEASES

The risk of catching an infectious disease is small. This risk can be minimized by the observation of some simple precautions.

Measures to avoid the spread of infectious disease

- Ensure you are fully immunized
- Observe good general hygiene
- Use disposable equipment when possible
- Have a regular cleaning schedule for equipment and the ambulance
- Use 'universal precautions' (see below)
- Take extreme care when using sharps

Immunization

Paramedical staff should ensure that their immunization schedules are up to date. In addition to routine childhood immunization, the following immunizations are essential:

- Tetanus – a booster should be given every 10 years
- Tuberculosis – a Heaf test is necessary every 3 years to check on immunity
- Hepatitis B – a full course of three injections should be given and then antibody levels checked. If levels are low a further booster dose may be necessary. Antibody levels should be checked every 3 years
- Rubella – antibody titres should be checked and immunization offered to female personnel who are not immune

Check these immunizations: Tetanus; Tuberculosis; Hepatitis B; Rubella

General Hygiene

All health-care professionals should observe general standards of personal hygiene. Hands should be thoroughly washed in a surgical scrub solution after each patient. Nails must be kept clean and regularly trimmed otherwise they may act as a reservoir for bacteria. Hair should be kept short or tied back so that

Table 17.1 Common and serious infectious diseases in the UK

Disease	Mode of transmission	Incubation period	Infectious period	Symptoms and signs
AIDS	Sexual contact, dirty needles	Months to years	Unknown	Unusually susceptible to infections
Chickenpox	Droplet spread, direct and indirect contact	14–21 days	For 2 days before rash until vesicles dry	Fever, blistering rash that comes in crops
German measles	Droplet spread	14–21 days	From 7 days before until 4 days after rash	Fever, rash and sore throat
Glandular fever	Mouth-to-mouth contact	2–6 weeks	Unknown	Generally unwell, swollen lymph glands
Hepatitis A	Faecal–oral	15–40 days		Lethargy, jaundice
Hepatitis B, C	Sexual contact, dirty needles	40–160 days	Variable, beware of chronic carriers	Lethargy, jaundice
Herpes virus infections	Sexual contact/ direct contact	2–10 days	For 2 days before rash until vesicles dry	Blistering eruption
Measles	Droplet spread	10 days	From beginning of symptoms to 4 days after appearance of rash	Fever, cough, conjunctivitis, rash
Meningococcal disease	Droplet spread and contact	2–3 days	Until treated	Fever, stiff neck, haemorrhagic rash
Mumps	Droplet spread	14–21 days	For 2 days before parotid swelling to 5 days after	Malaise, swollen parotid glands, orchitis
Tuberculosis	Droplet spread	4–8 weeks	Until patient treated	Cough, haemoptysis, weight loss
Whooping cough	Droplet spread	6–10 days	From 7 days after exposure to 21 days after first symptoms	Fever, characteristic cough

it cannot contaminate a wound. A paramedic with any large wound or open weeping areas should not work until the injury has healed. Small lacerations should be cleaned and dressed with a waterproof dressing to decrease the risk of infection.

Equipment

Medical equipment, particularly items such as airway tubing, can act as a reservoir of infection. Whenever possible, use disposable equipment and replace as it is used. Disposable sharps should be kept in puncture-resistant containers. Other disposables should be placed in plastic bags and clearly marked before being sent to be destroyed.

> Have a regular equipment cleaning schedule

The ambulance is another potential reservoir of infection. It should be aired regularly and the interior cleaned thoroughly at least once a day. All non-disposable equipment should be scrubbed with an antiseptic solution after each patient. Linen should be changed and sent for cleaning to the laundry. All uniforms should be clean and ideally impermeable to blood and other bodily secretions. If a uniform does become contaminated during use, the paramedic should shower and change to remove any skin contamination that may have occurred through the garment.

Universal Precautions

A small number of people in the general community may represent an infection risk. Unfortunately, there is no easy way of identifying this group. Therefore all patients should be assumed to represent a potential risk and *universal precautions* to prevent contact with blood or other bodily fluids should be taken, as follows.

1. Ensure that protective equipment is always available. If it is not immediately to hand it will not be used. Make sure your ambulance is well stocked with gloves, masks and aprons and develop the routine of using them.
2. Gloves. Latex gloves should be worn whenever contact with bodily fluids is anticipated, e.g. in venepuncture or in dressing a wound. Hands should be washed thoroughly after the gloves have been removed. Thicker protective gloves should be worn to protect the extremities when there is a likelihood of sustaining an injury, e.g. when removing an entrapped patient surrounded by broken glass in a road traffic accident.
3. Face protection and gowns. If there is a possibility of blood or bodily fluids being splashed over the body additional protective measures should be taken. A mask and glasses may help to protect the face and eyes. Alternatively a face shield can be worn. A plastic apron may help to prevent seepage of blood through to the skin. Sensible measures such as the use of pressure on bleeding areas should be taken to minimize the spread of body fluids.
4. Wash if you become contaminated. If blood or other body fluid reaches your skin, wash immediately to reduce any possible chance of infection.

Universal precautions

- Ensure that protective equipment is always available in the ambulance
- Observe blood and body fluid precautions with ALL casualties
- Wear gloves whenever exposed to blood or other body fluids
- Protect eyes, face and trunk if blood is likely to be splashed
- Wash immediately if blood or body fluid is splashed onto skin

Sharps

Extreme care should be taken when using needles, blades and other sharps. They should be disposed of immediately in a puncture-resistant container, such as the Sharpsafe®. Needles should never be resheathed or broken because of the risk of needle-stick injury. Also beware of sharp items such as broken glass or edges of metal which can present a danger when attending accident victims.

Sharps

- Use extreme care whenever handling sharps
- Never break needles
- Never resheathe needles
- Dispose of sharps in a puncture-resistant container

HIGH-RISK SITUATIONS

There are several situations in which ambulance staff may be subjected to a higher risk of exposure to an infectious disease. In these situations further precautionary measures may be necessary.

Cardiopulmonary Resuscitation

There have been no case reports of HIV or hepatitis B infection caused by transmission of the virus during mouth-to-mouth ventilation. However, both viruses are present in saliva so a small risk may be present. In addition there have been isolated cases of transmission of herpes virus (responsible for cold sores), tuberculosis and meningitis. For these reasons mouth-to-mouth ventilation should be avoided if at all possible. Instead, ventilation should be performed using a Laerdal pocket mask® with a one-way valve or a self-inflating bag with mask.

Transport of High-Risk Patients

On some occasions an ambulance may be called upon to transport a patient with a known infectious disease. In this case some anticipatory measures can be taken. A crew with known immunity to the disease should be selected where possible. For example, a patient with mumps should be transmitted by a paramedic who has proven immunity or who has previously had the disease. Disposable linen should be used in the ambulance, and gowns and masks should be worn by the crew whenever they examine the patient. After the transfer of the patient all disposables should be placed in plastic bags and sent for incineration.

Action to Take in Case of Exposure to Infectious Disease

If you have been exposed to an infectious disease and are worried that you may have contracted the infection, you should contact your occupational health department. They will want to know the nature of the illness, the time of exposure and the way in which you were exposed to the disease. Try to obtain as much information about the infected patient as possible. Investigations and treatment will depend on the nature of the disease, for example antibiotics as prophylaxis against meningococcal meningitis (rarely required), and Heaf testing and chest X-ray for tuberculosis.

If you suffer a needle-stick injury immediately wash the affected area in running water (Figure 17.1). Ask the patient if he or she is known to have an infectious disease. If possible a blood sample should be taken from the patient to assess the hepatitis and HIV status (*the patient will need counselling before having these investigations*). Then attend the occupational medicine unit or local accident and emergency unit. Blood will be taken from you to check your hepatitis status and to ensure that you are immune. Any treatment will depend on your hepatitis status and that of the patient. The occupational health department may offer HIV counselling.

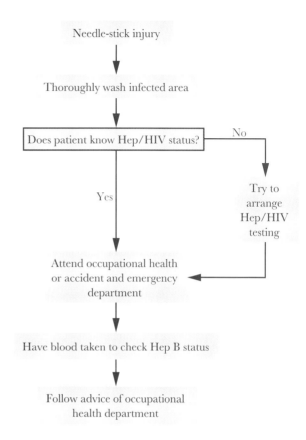

Fig. 17.1 Dealing with a needle-stick injury (Hep, hepatitis)

INFECTIONS TRANSMITTED FROM PARAMEDICAL STAFF TO PATIENT

It should be remembered that a patient can acquire an infection from a paramedic as easily as a paramedic can from a patient. All paramedical personnel therefore have a duty to ensure that they are healthy and are not harbouring any potentially infectious disease. Any concerns about illness should be discussed with the occupational medicine department or with a local general practitioner. Similarly, paramedical staff should not work if they have large open wounds and must ensure that any small cuts or abrasions are covered with waterproof dressings.

4

TRAUMA

chapter eighteen

OBTAINING A TRAUMA HISTORY

The trauma patient requires rapid assessment and management prior to removal to hospital for definitive care.

This early evaluation and resuscitation must be organized and methodical, and must identify time-critical cases where patients have life-threatening injuries. These patients will never be effectively managed with field resuscitation and need the urgent services of a major receiving hospital, trauma team and trauma surgeons. This forms a part of the '*golden hour*' concept, introduced by the Baltimore Shock-Trauma Unit surgeon, Dr R. Adams Cowley. The pre-hospital treatment phase of the *golden hour* should not exceed 10 minutes in critical patients, and taking a trauma history must be incorporated within this time-frame.

> The 'golden hour' is the time from injury to the time the patient must reach definitive treatment

The medical history of the patient and the mechanism of the accident are the two essential requirements of the trauma history, and must be obtained at a speed appropriate to the clinical state of the patient.

THE HISTORY OF THE PATIENT

After introducing yourself and offering reassurance, ask the patient about what has happened. A positive and appropriate response will also provide the information that the patient is conscious, has a patent airway, sufficient tidal volume to phonate, and sufficient cardiac output to provide adequate cerebral circulation.

The major complaints and location of pain must be sought next, followed by accompanying symptoms such as breathing difficulty and nausea. Any current or previous alteration of level of consciousness, and any events or symptoms prior to the accident, such as chest pain, must be checked for.

Finally, medication and past medical history, along with any history of alcohol or drug intake, must be obtained. Medication

allergies, and time of last food and fluid intake are also important history details.

The mnemonic 'AMPLE' is a helpful *aide-mémoire* for a history of key events.

A	>	ALLERGIES
M	>	MEDICATION
P	>	PAST MEDICAL HISTORY
L	>	LAST FOOD OR DRINK
E	>	EVENTS PRECEDING THE INJURY

Any interventions by bystanders prior to your arrival should be noted, and any relevant observations by them must be noted for passing on to the accident and emergency department staff.

The professional way a history is obtained while initially assessing and treating the patient does much to establish one's credibility with both the patient and the bystanders.

History-taking must not delay assessment and correction of vital functions in the primary survey, where both assessment and interventions must be performed simultaneously.

THE MECHANISM OF INJURY

Knowing the answer to two basic questions can significantly affect the outcome for patients with major trauma. These two questions are, 'What happened to the patient during the accident?', and 'What mechanisms caused the injury?'

Ambulance staff are the 'eyes and ears' of the accident and emergency department, and they are privileged to know far more about the mechanism of injury of the patient than anyone in the receiving department. They are under an obligation to pass on this information, and the department staff would be wise to listen with care. Failure on either side will harm only one person – the patient.

Road Traffic Accidents

Knowing the mechanism of an accident can alert the

paramedic, and subsequently the doctor, to the possibility of serious injury. Knowing, for instance, that a patient was ejected from a vehicle in a road traffic accident immediately increases the likelihood that the patient has sustained spinal cord and other serious injuries (Figure 18.1).

The so-called 'T-bone' type, side-impact vehicle accident with intrusion into the passenger compartment increases the likelihood of pelvic, chest, shoulder and intra-abdominal injury on the same side. These injuries tend to be caused by the massive lateral forces involved, and by intrusion into the passenger compartment of the vehicle B-post (the post between the side doors) and door structures. Injury to the cervical spine is also possible in this type of incident (Figure 18.2).

When examining wreckage, especially when assessing intrusion, always bear in mind that the elastic nature of metallic structures may allow some rebound of the intruded metal after the impact. This may lead to an initial underestimation of the actual degree of intrusion on impact.

> Entrapment for over 15 minutes is associated with an increased magnitude of injury severity.

Roll-over incidents tend to be associated with an increase in cervical spine injuries. This fits well with the forceful lateral bending and flexion-extension forces involved, and the increased likelihood of axial loading in this type of injury mechanism.

In head-on collisions, the unrestrained driver will travel forwards at the same velocity as the vehicle until collision with the steering column, windscreen and dashboard. The steering column tends to be forced upwards towards the windscreen on impact, so the chest, neck and face are commonly injured. Windscreen impact injuries tend to cause hyperextension to the neck, as well as axial loading to the cervical spine, and dashboard injuries commonly injure the knees, femurs and hips.

The restrained driver will normally be spared the majority of the above injuries, but facial injuries from the steering wheel are very common, as are 'seat-belt injuries' to the clavicles, sternum and ribs. Even with seat-belt restraint, intrusion of wreckage, especially the dashboard and floorpan around the feet, can still cause major lower limb injuries (Figure 18.3).

The introduction of driver and passenger airbags has undoubtedly enhanced the protection of vehicle front-seat occupants. Used with seat-belts, airbags will prevent many of the facial and neck injuries mentioned above. Their presence in the rescue situation when undeployed is still giving rise to concern for rescuer safety.

Rear-end collisions increase the likelihood of cervical spine injury through the 'whiplash' mechanism. Although in impacts at lower speed this is likely to take the form of ligamentous sprain and injury, the possible increased risk of fractures due to forced hyperflexion and extension must be remembered.

It is important to inform the hospital staff about a fatality in the same vehicle, as the types of forces sufficient to kill a patient in

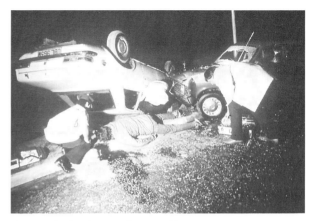

Fig. 18.1 *Ejection from a roll-over accident*

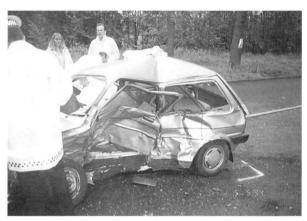

Fig. 18.2 *'T-bone' impact*

the vehicle have possibly been applied to all the vehicle occupants, and occult serious injury in the survivors is then possible.

Pedestrians hit at speed are vulnerable to major injuries, and information about this injury mechanism must be passed on to receiving clinicians.

> Consider taking Polaroid photographs of the scene

Falls from a Height

Falls from a height inevitably involve sudden deceleration on impact. The distance of the fall, type of surface contacted, and anatomical points of impact will determine the injury pattern in the patient.

Most adult falls involve lower limb fractures, often including the talus, femur and, by transmitted force, the pelvis. The spine, in particular the lumbar and thoracic areas, is frequently affected, with often multiple crush fractures of the vertebral bodies. In

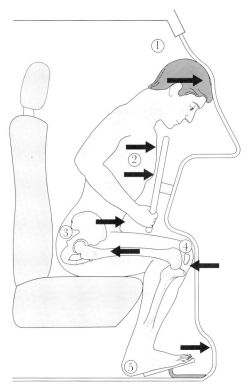

Fig. 18.3 Frontal impact injuries. 1, head and neck injuries; 2, chest injuries; 3, posterior hip dislocation; 4, knee injuries; 5, foot and ankle injuries with entrapment

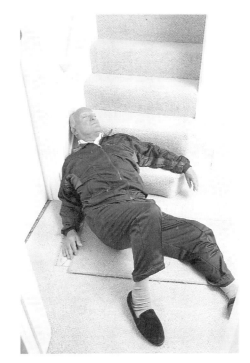

Fig. 18.4 The elderly are at risk of significant injury from simple household accidents

addition, the narrowness of the spinal canal in the thoracic area makes cord injury at this level more common.

Fractures of the forearms are common, along with internal injury due to rapid deceleration forces. In children, head injuries are common as they tend to fall head first, as a result of their proportionately larger head.

Remember, also, that even trivial falls may cause serious injury in the elderly. The elderly man who falls down two or three stairs and strikes his forehead on the ground, may hyperextend his relatively rigid cervical spine enough to produce a fracture (Figure 18.4).

Penetrating Trauma

Penetrating injuries from knife and bullet wounds are becoming more common in UK pre-hospital care practice.

Knife wounds cause direct injury in the direction of blade penetration. The damage depends on the length of the blade and the degree of penetration. Knife wounds to the neck and chest may be particularly dangerous owing to the presence of important blood vessels and organs. Abdominal wounds are less damaging, unless a major vessel or solid organ is injured.

Of particular concern are wounds to the upper abdomen and the lower thorax, as the diaphragm may be penetrated and intrathoracic or intra-abdominal structures injured, remote from the entry wound. A wound in the epigastrium may possibly penetrate the diaphragm, causing ventricular puncture and pericardial tamponade.

Civilian bullet wounds in the main tend to be from either a handgun or a shotgun. Lethal damage from these injuries depends largely on the anatomical area of injury and the type of projectile – for example, hollow point projectiles break up during the first 10 cm of penetration and cause increased tissue injury. The velocity of the projectile-tissue collision also determines the likely degree of injury, along with the degree of fragmentation.

Tissue response and damage are variable, depending on the tissue type, specifically its density and elasticity (a missile passing through dense tissue will result in greater energy transfer).

That a high-velocity projectile induces a more severe wound than a low-velocity projectile is a myth, and this fallacy has been revised in the light of more current research. It is now acknowledged that even a low-velocity handgun may cause extensive tissue damage (high-energy transfer), depending on the behaviour of the bullet when entering tissues, and the nature of the bullet design.

With high-energy transfer, injury may occur some distance away from the bullet's entry wound (a result of 'temporary cavitation'). Virtually all bullet wounds will require surgical exploration.

Blast Injuries

Four patterns of injury are commonly associated with explosions (Figure 18.5):

- Primary blast injury: the shock wave
- Secondary blast injury: injuries from flying debris
- Tertiary blast injury: injuries due to impact on the surroundings
- Flash burns

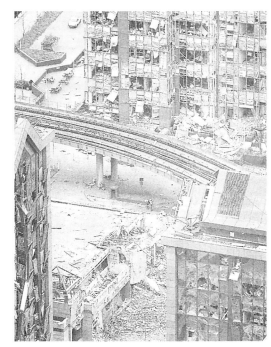

Fig. 18.5 A London bomb incident

Primary blast injuries are those caused by the blast wave arising directly from the explosion. Secondary injuries arise from the flying debris. Tertiary injuries arise from the blast wind, where the whole body may be projected, or exposed parts traumatically amputated. Flash burns arise from the intense, short-lived heat of the explosion.

Primary injury commonly causes damage to the ears, lungs and gastrointestinal tract. The injuries to the lung range from pinpoint haemorrhages to massive intrapulmonary haemorrhage ('blast lung'), which is often fatal at the scene. Secondary blast injuries are directly related to the types of flying debris and the sites of penetration. Tertiary injuries depend on many factors including the position of the casualty in relation to the blast. Flash burns tend to affect those nearest to the site of the explosion.

Blast injury can therefore produce a variety of injuries, which are considered in greater detail in Chapter 28. The incident history and the patient's 'AMPLE' history are vital information: the patient history is an essential part of the initial assessment, and the mechanism of injury may provide vital clues to underlying injuries not initially apparent on clinical examination.

chapter nineteen

THE PRIMARY AND SECONDARY SURVEY

ASSESSMENT OF THE SCENE

Prior to any assessment of the patient at the accident scene (Figure 19.1), the basic rules of personal safety, scene safety and incident resourcing must be addressed (see Chapter 1).

- Are additional ambulances required?
- Is the scene safe from hazards, are emergency vehicles parked safely, and is your equipment accessible?
- Have you brought the correct resuscitation equipment?
- Are the fire and rescue services or medical support required?

Assess the scene to evaluate casualty numbers, and note the mechanisms involved in the accident, while assessing the casualties for priority of intervention and evacuation.

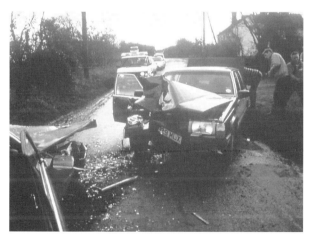

Fig. 19.1 *A typical road traffic accident*

ASSESSMENT OF THE PATIENT

The initial assessment requires basic clinical competence, and most important, a methodology to apply consistently and in priority order. Without this fundamental skill, all the resuscitation procedures applied may be either inappropriate or inadequate for the needs of the patient.

> Initial patient assessment is the most important clinical skill possessed by an ambulance paramedic or technician

The format of a primary assessment of vital functions and a more comprehensive and detailed secondary patient assessment where appropriate, is provided by the *primary and secondary survey* procedures. These procedures have their origins in trauma assessment, but the logic of the primary survey in particular should apply to the assessment of any seriously injured or ill patient.

The term 'survey' wrongly implies assessment only. The primary survey is both an assessment *and* an immediate treatment procedure, assessing for threats to life associated with compromise to the airway, breathing, circulation and impaired conscious level.

> Primary Survey = Assessment + Management

PRIMARY SURVEY

The primary survey should be completed in 1–2 minutes. Any critical deficit found on the primary survey must be immediately rectified before moving on to the next part of the assessment. The order in the primary survey of airway prior to breathing, which in turn precedes circulation, is purely related to the relative speed of the threat to life of each. Airway obstruction will cause death in a few minutes, breathing disruption will usually take a few additional minutes to cause death, and circulatory compromise will take longer again to threaten life. On that basis, immediate assessment and correction of the airway ('A'), while protecting the cervical spine, is followed by assessment and correction of any breathing ('B') compromise. Any circulatory deficit ('C') found on circulatory assessment is then rectified.

Next, the level of consciousness and pupil signs are assessed ('D, disability'), before proceeding to 'E' (expose and evaluate), once again looking for major injuries.

Primary survey

- Airway, with cervical spine immobilization
- Breathing, with oxygen
- Circulation, with control of external haemorrhage
- Disability – preliminary neurological examination
- Expose and evaluate

Trauma patients found to have a major problem in the primary survey require immediate removal to an appropriate hospital facility.

This immediate evacuation must incorporate highly organized on-site care. The aim is to prepare the patient for departure from the scene in *10 minutes* from the ambulance's arrival. This imposes enormous demands on both the paramedic and technician, and to achieve this takes teamwork and practice.

'Scoop and Run'

The modern 'scoop and run' method incorporates:

- Airway and cervical spine protection
- Breathing assessment and support
- Arrest of major haemorrhage
- Immobilization on a long spinal board
- Rapid evacuation to an appropriate hospital
- Infusion *en route*

This rapid evacuation of critical patients is not to be confused with what previously may have been implied by 'scoop and run'. To succeed, it requires impeccable airway care and ventilatory support. Arrest of major haemorrhage and basic splintage of major long bone fractures have also to be achieved. The patient is then secured, with cervical collar, head restraints and straps, to a long spinal board, and removed to the ambulance. Infusion and any further resuscitation measures may be performed *en route* to hospital, *but must not delay evacuation of the patient.* Trauma team reception, and precise radio communication with

the receiving hospital, are vital to the success of this high-speed method of critical trauma patient management.

It is something of an emotional conflict for experienced and well-trained paramedics to see a patient who has multiple injuries and demands the full array of skills they possess, rapidly loaded into the back of an ambulance and moved to hospital with minimal interventions performed. Despite these misgivings, there is an overwhelming logic in this approach.

Pre-hospital care is hampered in critical trauma situations by a shortage of skilled personnel at the accident scene. There is a limit to the speed with which invasive interventions can be performed by a single paramedic and a technician. There is no option but to perform each resuscitation skill individually, and not to move on to the next one until the first is complete. Otherwise, inadequately secured IV lines and endotracheal tubes will come adrift, and require resiting. This is unlike the situation in cardiac arrest, where the technician is perfectly able to perform defibrillation while the paramedic secures the airway. In trauma, however, infusion, intubation and drug administration are all paramedical sskills, and have to be performed 'linearly' (that is, one after the other) by the paramedic, which increases resuscitation time and hence the time at the scene. There is now evidence that in critical trauma prolonged scene times are associated with an increase in mortality.

In contrast, in hospital the patient should be tended by a well-led and skilled trauma team: one team member will secure the airway, while another secures IV lines the airway and another examines the patient. This simultaneous and co-ordinated application of resuscitation by several team members dramatically reduces resuscitation time, justifying the rapid transport to hospital of these patients with minimal care at the scene.

Intravenous fluid therapy is rarely worth attempting in critical cases where the transport times to hospital are short. If a trauma team is assembled to receive the patient, it is possible to establish up to four IV lines within minutes of arrival in the accident and emergency department. More fluid may be given in those first few minutes than would ever be achieved at the scene. Where transport times are longer, in rural areas for example, IV access and therapy should be established *en route* to hospital in critical patients, and reasonable volumes of fluid given. When patients are trapped, intravenous infusions must be established early and fluid therapy commenced.

On-site medical support is essential in dealing with entrapped patients with significant injuries from an early stage, to supervise frequently difficult patient assessments and to institute fluid therapy

In non-critical patients, found on primary survey not to have any evidence of life-threatening injury, a secondary survey should be performed. This is the more traditional and systematic head-to-toe examination to assess for injury to the various body parts and systems.

Performing the Primary Survey

The primary survey and resuscitation permit identification of life-threatening conditions and their simultaneous treatment.

Airway and cervical spine

Assessment Any injury severe enough to compromise the airway may put the cervical spine at risk. Managing the airway must therefore be performed while protecting the cervical spine. Airway impairment may arise from a direct obstruction such as vomit, or secondary to impaired consciousness, for example from a head injury. It may occur at any level from the mouth and nose to the larynx and trachea. Impaired level of consciousness and 'noisy' breathing are characteristic signs.

Management Gloved manual removal and aspiration of vomit and blood, followed by either chin lift or jaw thrust, will open most airways. These manoeuvres must only be performed while maintaining in-line cervical spine immobilization. Oropharyngeal or nasopharyngeal airway placement may be needed if the above measures are inadequate. Orotracheal intubation, and in the case of failure to provide an airway with any of the above methods, needle cricothyrotomy with translaryngeal jet insufflation at 15 litres per minute may be necessary. Following cricothyrotomy, oxygen is directed via a Y-piece through the cannula (size 14 G) for 1 second, followed by a 4 second pause to allow some exhalation. Carbon dioxide retention limits this technique to some 20–30 minutes use (see Chapter 5).

Once the airway is secure, continue to immobilize the neck, applying a correctly sized semirigid cervical collar and head immobilization device. Before the collar is applied it is sensible to examine the neck for wounds, a deviated trachea, distended neck veins and laryngeal integrity. The patient must be fully immobilized on a long spinal board with at least four body straps. Restless patients should only be fitted with a semirigid collar, as full immobilization may only exacerbate movement in the cervical spine if the rest of the body is flailing. Then assess breathing.

Stepped airway care

1. Airway clearance – manual and aspiration
2. Manual airway opening manoeuvres
3. Chin lift or jaw thrust
4. Oropharyngeal airway
5. Nasopharyngeal airway
6. Orotracheal intubation
7. Cricothyroid transtracheal jet ventilation

Breathing

Assessment *Clearing the airway does not assure adequate ventilation.* Breathing must be assessed for rate, adequacy and equal bilateral ventilation of the lungs. The chest must be visualized to assess movement, instability, flail segment and any wounds. The chest wall must be felt to detect surgical emphysema, tenderness from rib fractures and paradoxical movement. Percussion bilaterally may reveal one-sided hyperresonance over a large pneumothorax. Finally, auscultation for the presence of breath sounds bilaterally must be performed.

Remember the aim of the primary survey is to identify life-threatening problems.

Life-threatening breathing problems

- Tension pneumothorax
- Massive haemothorax
- Open chest injury
- Flail chest
- Cardiac tamponade

Distress, confusion and abnormally rapid or slow respiratory rate are alarming signs, and may require assisted ventilation.

Management Management of spontaneous ventilation in any patient with significant trauma requires the provision of supplemental oxygen, with a non-rebreathing reservoir mask, and oxygen flow rate of 10–15 litres per minute.

Inadequate ventilation demands assisted ventilation. In adults, a respiration rate of less than 10/min or more than 30/min suggests significant ventilatory inadequacy. This is most easily performed using a bag–valve–mask and reservoir device, with oxygen supplied at a minimum of 10 litres per minute.

Explanation, where appropriate, to the patient is followed by supplementing the patient's respiratory rate and volume. The self-inflating bag may be emptied to a maximum of 700–1000 ml, preferably with a two-handed technique, and at a rate of 15 breaths per minute. This will achieve an acceptable minute volume of about 10–15 litres.

Formal intermittent positive pressure ventilation with bag and mask or tube may be necessary in case of respiratory arrest. A time-cycled, pressure-limited mechanical ventilator may also be useful, especially for longer transfers. Care must be taken to assess for any indication of airway obstruction or loss of patency in transit, as well as continued vigilance for adequacy of ventilation.

Displacement of an endotracheal tube in transit, or development of tension pneumothorax secondary to positive pressure ventilation, may occur at any time. The use of pulse oximetry and end-tidal CO_2 monitors can assist greatly in transit, but repeated auscultation is essential.

Tension pneumothorax may be present initially, or appear secondary to positive pressure ventilation, where a simple, undetected pneumothorax is expanded by the pressure of the ventilating gases. It is characteristically detected by the combination of rapidly increasing breathlessness, and unilaterally absent breath sounds. Hyperresonance on percussion of the affected hemithorax, raised and congested neck veins, and hypotension are frequently noted. Finally, cyanosis and tracheal shift from the affected side complete the picture of this extreme respiratory emergency.

Increasing resistance to ventilation and unilaterally reduced breath sounds in a ventilated patient should alert the paramedic to a possible tension pneumothorax, once a right mainstem bronchus intubation has been excluded.

Treatment involves the immediate insertion of a 14 G intravenous cannula into the chest. It is inserted with aspiration, using a 10 ml syringe, over the top of the third rib in the midclavicular line on the affected side, in the second intercostal space.

Once air is expelled into the syringe, withdraw the syringe and needle leaving the cannula *in situ*. Secure firmly with a cannula fixing tape. A formal chest drain will be needed as soon as possible.

Open chest wounds must be covered with an occlusive dressing sealed on three sides or, alternatively (if local protocols permit), completely sealed and an intercostal cannula inserted.

Circulation

Skin colour and temperature, pulse rate and volume, capillary refill time (normal less than 2 seconds) and the site of palpable pulses provide a rapid circulatory assessment.

Pale, cool skin, tachycardia, delayed capillary return and altered mental state indicate significant blood loss. Hypotension frequently is not apparent until at least 30% of the blood volume has been lost.

Management Arrest any external blood loss, and insert two wide-bore (14 or 16 G) intravenous lines each connected to 500 ml of warmed Hartmann's solution. Take blood for haemoglobin estimate and cross-matching if an entrapment is likely to be prolonged, and consider arranging for it to be sent ahead for processing.

Check the response to the first 1000 ml of fluid by assessing pulse rate and perfusion. If there is no improvement, or if perfusion and pulse rate deteriorate again after a short interval, give a further 1000 ml rapidly and reassess. If there is a sustained improvement in haemodynamic status after the first 1000 ml, slow the rate down and maintain observation. No improvement, or no sustained improvement, suggests persisting haemorrhage and the need for urgent operation. Sustained improvement in haemodynamic status after 1000 ml only of Hartmann's solution suggests that bleeding has stopped, and that the initial infusion has corrected the volume deficit.

Care must be taken in severe haemorrhage not to elevate the blood pressure above 90 mmHg systolic during fluid resuscitation. This is important in a number of conditions, especially dissecting aneurysms where elevation of blood pressure may induce rebleeding.

Scene times in patients with critical trauma should not exceed 10 minutes. In these cases, intravenous infusion must be commenced *en route* to hospital, or cannulation achieved within a halt of no longer than 30 seconds *en route*.

Disability

The accident scene rarely provides the opportunity for detailed assessment of neurological status. A quick neurological examination is used, comprised of an assessment of the level of response plus the pupil size and reaction. The 'AVPU' mnemonic should be used:

A > Is the patient Alert?
V > Is the patient responding to Verbal stimulus?
P > Is the patient responding to Painful stimulus?
U > Is the patient Unresponsive?

The responses obtained are noted and form the baseline for repeated observations as necessary.

Expose and evaluate

The chest and neck area are exposed as part of the primary survey and management. If critical problems are found during primary survey, and not immediately resolved, the patient needs rapid transport to a major receiving hospital unit. Radio contact must be made *en route* to the receiving accident and emergency department, and the trauma team alerted.

If, during the primary survey, the patient deteriorates, the paramedic must return to airway reassessment and once the airway is cleared proceed to breathing, then circulation reassessment. If the paramedic follows this procedure meticulously, no critical cause of sudden deterioration will be missed. In non-critical patients, a secondary survey involving more detailed assessment may be appropriate.

THE SECONDARY SURVEY

The secondary survey is the more detailed 'head to toe' survey performed rapidly on *non-critical* patients at the accident scene, or *en route* to hospital (Figure 19.2). It allows more precise anatomical location and immediate management of non-life-threatening injuries. There is an ordered approach to this survey, as in the primary survey, so it can be rapidly performed to minimize time at the scene.

Patients initially assessed as non-critical may deteriorate from occult injury, and a degree of urgency during the secondary survey must be maintained.

Performing the Secondary Survey

Assessment of the head

Look for:
1. Lacerations
2. Bruising

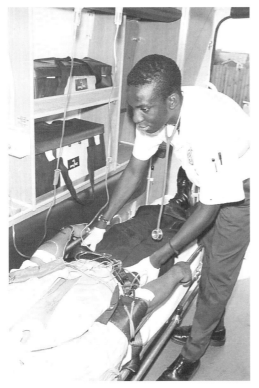

Fig. 19.2 *The secondary survey*

3. Blood and or cerebrospinal fluid from ears or nose (suggesting basal skull fracture)
4. Recheck pupil size and response
5. Battle's sign and 'raccoon' eyes (suggesting basal skull fracture)
6. Pallor and sweating
7. Cyanosis

Feel for:
1. Scalp haematomas
2. Depressed skull fractures
3. Facial tenderness and fractures

Listen for:
1. Airway 'noise' suggesting obstruction
2. Breathing adequacy and rate

Assessment of the neck
To assess the neck, the collar may need to be removed while maintaining in-line immobilization of the neck.

Look and feel for:
1. Lacerations and contusion
2. Surgical emphysema – skin 'crackling'
3. Spinal deformity, tenderness or haematoma
4. Recheck pulse rate and volume

5. Distension of neck veins
6. Laryngeal integrity
7. Tracheal deviation

Assessment of the chest
Look for:
1. Wounds and evidence of penetrating injury
2. Deformity and abnormal movements
3. Breathing distress and pain on inspiration

Feel for:
1. Tenderness
2. Instability and 'clunking' of flail segment
3. Surgical emphysema
4. Percussion revealing increased resonance over pneumothorax, or stony dullness over haemothorax

Listen for :
1. Presence of equal breath sounds
2. Unilateral absence or reduction of breath sounds suggestive of pneumothorax
3. Unilateral, usually basal reduction of breath sounds associated with haemothorax

Assessment of the abdomen
Look for:
1. Penetrating wounds and contusions
2. Seat-belt contusions and clothing imprints
3. Distension

Feel for:
1. Tenderness – either localized or generalized
2. Guarding – involuntary muscle spasm on gentle palpation

Assessment of the pelvis
Feel for:
1. Tenderness and instability from bilateral and antero-posterior compression

Assessment of lower and upper extremities
Look for:
1. Obvious wounds and contusions
2. Deformity and swelling associated with fractures
3. Voluntary movement

Feel for:
1. Tenderness and deformity
2. Distal pulses
3. Intact nerve supply – sensation to touch and pain, motor function
4. Normal movement in joints

On completion of the secondary survey, immediately stabilize any located injuries, for instance by the application of a traction splint to a femoral shaft fracture. The patient is then loaded into the ambulance.

The patient's condition is monitored frequently during this continued assessment to detect any deterioration, and if it becomes critical the survey is abandoned and the patient moved rapidly to an appropriate receiving hospital while undergoing resuscitation.

CONCLUSION

This process of primary and secondary surveys allows an organized, methodical and rapid assessment of a trauma patient. The patient's condition can be assessed by the findings of the primary survey into critical or non-critical, and a decision to go immediately to hospital reached in the first 2 minutes at the scene.

The secondary survey allows a methodical assessment of the more complete range of injuries, with interventions as needed. Any deterioration during the primary or secondary survey necessitates a rapid return to airway assessment, and rechecking of all the primary survey assessments and interventions in the ABCDE order.

> If the patient deteriorates at any point in the primary or secondary survey, check:
> Airway, breathing, circulation and disability
> Reassess these functions and your interventions

These procedures need practice every day, and are a good approach to any trauma and many medical emergencies. Unpractised, they will not come readily to hand when they are most needed, so use them all the time.

chapter twenty:

SHOCK

Shock is inadequate tissue perfusion resulting in hypoxia and ultimately in cell death.

Common causes of shock

- Hypovolaemic (blood loss, plasma loss or salt/water loss)
- Cardiogenic (myocardial ischaemia, infarction, contusion or conditions preventing normal cardiac function – tamponade, massive pulmonary embolism)
- Septic (bacterial, viral or fungal infection)
- Neurogenic (following head or spinal cord injury)
- Anaphylactic

By far the most common cause of shock in the pre-hospital environment is hypovolaemia (inadequate blood volume), usually related to blood or plasma loss from trauma, burns, ruptured aortic aneurysm, ectopic pregnancy or gastrointestinal haemorrhage. Less common causes of shock are discussed later in this chapter.

> **The most common treatable cause of shock is hypovolaemia**

HYPOVOLAEMIC SHOCK

The signs and symptoms of hypovolaemic shock are:

- Tachycardia (arrhythmias may develop)
- Change in blood pressure (initially reduced pulse pressure, later lowered systolic and diastolic pressures)
- Altered mental state
- Tachypnoea
- Cool, clammy skin
- Cyanosis
- Oliguria

Normal Compensatory Mechanisms and Pathological Responses in Hypovolaemia

There are many physiological responses that can compensate for blood loss in a healthy individual to maintain oxygen delivery and organ perfusion. These mechanisms involve a number of body systems, and the pathological processes that occur when the body can no longer compensate for further blood loss are described at organ and cellular level.

Cardiovascular system

The cardiac output is the volume of blood that is pumped around the body every minute. If the total circulating blood volume decreases (because of blood loss), tissue and organ perfusion can only be maintained by the heart working harder to increase the cardiac output. This may be achieved by two mechanisms. Firstly, the quantity of blood ejected by the heart with each cardiac cycle (the stroke volume) can increase. Secondly, the heart rate can increase in response to sympathetic stimulation, with systemic release of adrenaline and noradrenaline from the adrenal glands and sympathetic nerve endings throughout the vascular system.

> **Cardiac output = Stroke volume × Heart rate**

These compensatory mechanisms do have limits. At a critical level the heart muscle reaches the point where each fibre is stretched maximally, further compensation is impossible, and the heart begins to fail. Furthermore, the heart rate cannot rise indefinitely. The relaxation or diastolic phase of the cardiac cycle is essential to allow filling of the ventricles and hence 'prime' the cardiac pump. With extreme tachycardia the stroke volume is reduced and cardiac output drops. In addition, as the diastolic time decreases, the amount of oxygen reaching the myocardium via the coronary vessels falls, as diastole is the period during which blood enters the coronary circulation. As the heart continues to work in excess of its aerobic ability, anaerobic metabolism with the production of lactic acidosis develops. This results in a reduction of the strength of myocardial contraction and pump failure.

Finally, if blood loss continues, the decreased venous return to the heart results in distortion of the cardiac chambers and activation of cardiac C fibres. These cause vagal stimulation and slowing of the heart together with peripheral vasodilation, and a catastrophic (and usually terminal) fall in blood pressure ensues.

The state of the blood vessels into which the heart ejects its contents is also important. There is always a degree of resting tension in the walls of arteries. By increasing this tension under the control of the nervous system, the blood pressure can be maintained in hypovolaemia by effectively reducing the volume of the system. By selective activation of this system, blood can be redirected preferentially to vital organs by vasoconstriction in less important sites such as skin, gut and muscle. This mechanism acts to protect the heart, brain and kidneys, which can control their own blood supplies to a certain extent. The increase in arterial wall tension results from the action of receptors which detect falling blood volume, increasing blood acidity and rising arterial carbon dioxide levels ($Pa\text{CO}_2$).

Respiratory system

Shock results in tissue hypoxia. The response to shock therefore includes a compensatory increase in the frequency and depth of respiration. This tachypnoeic response is controlled by the respiratory centre in the brain which receives input from peripheral nerves and receptors, which in turn measure blood acidity and carbon dioxide levels.

To improve the uptake of oxygen and excretion of carbon dioxide in the lungs, preferential vasoconstriction diverts pulmonary blood flow to areas of high alveolar oxygen concentration, thus improving the ventilation/perfusion ratio. The oxygen-carrying capacity of the blood depends upon the haemoglobin concentration and its ability to bind with oxygen. The body has no immediate ability to increase haemoglobin concentration, so the mechanisms regulating oxygen-carrying capacity relate to changes in the affinity of the haemoglobin molecule for oxygen. Increases in acidity, $Pa\text{CO}_2$ or temperature allow a greater release of oxygen to the cells for a given oxygen saturation.

A number of factors contribute to eventual inadequate ventilation and oxygen uptake by the lungs. A drop in venous return with continued blood loss results in a fall in right heart filling pressures, leading to reduced pulmonary blood flow and oxygen uptake. Anaerobic metabolism producing lactic acid within the respiratory muscles causes muscle fatigue and eventually respiratory failure. Central respiratory depression caused by direct head injury, hypotension or the effects of drugs (such as opioids) will also result in hypoventilation.

Other physiological responses to hypovolaemic shock

Two hormones are released in increased amounts in response to hypovolaemia – aldosterone from the adrenal gland and antidiuretic hormone from the pituitary gland. These hormones act to maintain the circulating blood volume by reducing urine output.

The brain's blood supply is protected until late in the pathological process of worsening shock. Eventually, however, autoregulation and preferential supply cannot preserve cerebral perfusion pressure any longer. Once cerebral hypoxia occurs, a downward spiral of events ensues. Vasoconstriction of the reticular formation (that part of the brain concerned with level of consciousness) in some patients leads to marked agitation and apprehension, but as the process continues central stimulation of the respiratory centre is lost, resulting in hypoventilation and therefore worsening organ oxygenation. Vasomotor and cardiac centres are also depressed, causing slowing of the heart rate and peripheral vasodilation. Accumulation of lactic acid and other waste products of metabolism within cerebral neurones results in depression of the conscious level, and finally coma.

Like the brain, the kidneys are able to regulate their own blood supply during the initial stages of shock. As a consequence renal blood flow is maintained despite falling perfusion. However, as with other organs a critical period is reached when continued constriction of the renal vessels (increase in vessel wall tension) causes a reduction in renal perfusion and consequently a reduction in function evident by falling urine output.

Clinical Features of Hypovolaemic Shock

The common clinical features of hypovolaemic shock are listed above.

In an adult, the normal circulating blood volume is 7% of the *lean* body mass. In an average patient weighing 70–75 kg the total circulating blood volume will be about 5000–5500 ml. In children the blood volume is proportionately greater, 8–9% of body weight or 80–90 ml/kg (see Chapter 36). Knowledge of the clinical signs and symptoms of shock in a trauma patient is essential to enable resuscitative measures to begin at an appropriate time.

The clinical features of hypovolaemia depend upon the magnitude of circulating volume loss. However, these features can act only as general guides and have major limitations, especially in the pre-hospital setting where advanced monitoring and investigational facilities are unavailable.

Classification of haemorrhagic shock

To assist in the assessment of the severity of haemorrhagic shock the symptoms and signs can be subdivided into four grades depending on the extent of circulating volume lost (Table 20.1). This will vary depending on the patient's previous medical and drug history (see below). The extent and severity of soft tissue injury will also affect the degree of interstitial fluid formation and will decrease the accuracy of this classification, as a sizeable part of the soft tissue swelling is fluid that has leaked from the vascular compartment.

Table 20.1 Classification of hypovolaemic shock (adult)

Grade	Blood loss	Symptoms	Urine output
Grade I	Up to 750 ml < 15%	Minimal Blood pressure unchanged Occasionally tachycardia occurs	Normal
Grade II	750–1500 ml 15–30%	Pallor, tachycardia > 100/min, decreased pulse pressure Subtle changes in mood may be seen, e.g. anxiety, aggression or fright	Reduced to to 20–30 ml/ hour
Grade III	1500–2000 ml 30–40% This is the minimum volume loss that results in a decrease in blood pressure	Classic signs of inadequate perfusion are usually noticed: pallor, sweating, altered mental state (anxiety, confusion, aggression), tachycardia > 120/min, tachypnoea, hypotension	Reduced to to 10–20 ml/ hour
Grade IV	Over 2000 ml Life-threatening and catastrophic	Pulse is weak and thready Tachycardia may deteriorate to bradycardia Systolic blood pressure drops markedly with a very narrow pulse pressure or unobtainable diastolic pressure Drowsiness, lethargy or unconsciousness	Negligible

The classification in Table 20.1 must be used *only as a guide*; precise estimation of blood loss will never be possible. An easy way to remember the percentage losses is to compare them to the scores in tennis (love-fifteen, fifteen-thirty, thirty-forty, game over).

There are a number of pitfalls in the assessment of the patient with hypovolaemic shock. The following factors must be taken into consideration:

- Age (the elderly are less able to compensate for volume loss)
- Fitness (athletes and fit individuals may compensate and hence have few signs or symptoms even with major losses)
- Medications (drugs such as beta-blockers, antihypertensives and antianginals may mask normal responses such as tachycardia)
- Pre-existing disease (patients with underlying conditions such as ischaemic heart disease, cerebrovascular disease and pregnancy are less able to cope with the effects of shock)

The elderly are less able to compensate for blood loss and may consequently have the signs associated with a higher grade of shock with lower blood loss. Conversely, the very fit may compensate for blood loss, concealing significant haemorrhage until

the patient suddenly collapses in grade III or IV shock. A pulse of 95 beats/min may be normal in an elderly patient, but can represent severe vascular compromise in a marathon runner whose resting pulse is 40 beats/min.

Medications (especially beta-blockers which slow down the pulse) may mask the normal responses to shock, such as tachycardia. The patient's previous medical history should always be considered during the assessment of shock. Patients with ischaemic heart disease, cerebrovascular disease and pregnancy are less able to cope with the effects of shock.

Treatment Principles

Attention to simple, competently performed procedures executed in the shortest period of time and accompanied by rapid, safe evacuation of the patient to hospital is the key to success in the pre-hospital management of shock.

The concept that a patient can (or should) be 'stabilized' at the scene before transfer to hospital is dangerously wrong. Except where delays are unavoidable because of geographical or environmental problems or entrapment, the delivery of the patient to hospital must never be delayed by interventions such as intravenous access or volume replacement.

Airway and breathing (A + B) on scene

The primary objective in the management of shock is to restore tissue perfusion, with the delivery of adequate oxygen and other metabolites. It should be recognized that only the start of this process will occur before the patient reaches hospital and that this phase of resuscitation is only the beginning of definitive treatment, which may require surgery or other interventions in hospital.

All shocked patients require the highest possible concentration of inspired oxygen delivered to the lungs. Except where a patient is known to have severe chronic obstructive pulmonary disease (COPD), every shocked or potentially shocked patient should be given high-flow oxygen by a face mask. Even in cases of COPD and severe trauma the injured tissues require oxygen – a patient who truly has 'hypoxic drive' and stops breathing can be ventilated. Clearance and maintenance of a patent upper and lower airway as detailed in Chapters 5 and 6 are mandatory. This may require the patient to be intubated and positive pressure ventilation commenced. Factors impeding ventilation, such as pneumothorax, haemothorax or gastric dilatation, will require specific correction.

High-concentration oxygen saves lives

Where there is an overt source of blood loss, such as an open wound, elevate the affected part and apply direct local pressure. In general, clamping or tying off arterial bleeding points and the application of tourniquets are contraindicated as these interventions can cause additional damage. Limbs with long bone fractures should be splinted (see Chapter 27). Splintage not only reduces the pain experienced by the patient but also reduces blood loss from fracture sites by up to 50%. Unless splinted, of course, a leg with significant long bone fractures cannot be elevated!

Vascular access to the circulation is achieved by the insertion of two large-bore intravenous cannulae into accessible peripheral veins (see Chapter 6). In many shocked patients, vascular access is difficult because of the combination of hypovolaemia with collapsed veins, venoconstriction and the problems of performing the technique in adverse conditions where cold, movement and poor lighting render the task difficult. In such situations, do not waste time attempting to achieve vascular access – this will only delay the delivery of the patient to hospital. If necessary, further attempts can be made in the back of the moving ambulance.

Circulation (C) *en route*

Although popular in the 1970s and 1980s in North America, the use of MAST, military anti-shock trousers or the pneumatic anti-shock garment (PASG) for lower limb or pelvic fractures or for hypovolaemic shock (Figure 20.1) has not been shown to improve mortality or morbidity rates. Their use is rarely indicated (see Chapter 27).

Except in unusual circumstances, there is no merit in taking blood samples from the patient before reaching hospital. The

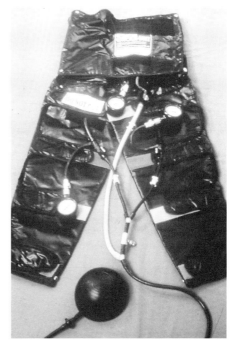

Fig. 20.1   *The MAST military anti-shock trousers*

difficulties of patient identification, labelling and the dangers of potential mismatched blood transfusion almost always exceed the potential benefits. An exception to this rule may be where a patient is trapped and full identification of the patient can be made both for the purpose of blood sampling, and subsequently if blood or other products are delivered to the scene for on-site management. However, even in this situation it is probably better to use universal donor (O Rh negative) blood rather than relying on the delays involved in blood grouping, cross-matching and then sending type-specific blood to the scene.

Although it is the source of much debate, the arguments for choices of intravenous fluid used for volume restoration in shocked patients are based more on dogma than sound clinical evaluation. What is not in doubt is that, if fluids are given, they must contain sodium ions. This apart, a bewildering array of fluids for volume restoration are available, including crystalloids, colloids (Figure 20.2) and both iso-oncotic and hyper-oncotic solutions.

It is standard practice in the UK to start intravenous volume replacement with isotonic crystalloid solutions such as 0.9% (normal) saline or sodium lactate (Hartmann's or Ringer lactate) solution. Despite the theoretical advantages of Hartmann's solution, no difference has been shown in terms of clinical efficacy. Both are cheap, easy to use, have long shelf-lives and do not cause anaphylactic reactions.

Colloid solutions available in the UK include gelatin solutions such as Haemaccel or Gelofusine, starch solutions such as

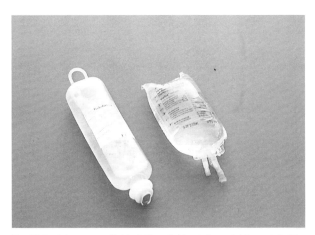

Fig. 20.2 Intravenous fluids: left, colloid solution; right, crystalloid solution

hetastarch, dextran solutions such as dextran 70, and human plasma components such as 4.5% albumin and plasma protein fraction (PPF). All of these solutions are significantly more expensive than crystalloids. They all also have a small but recognized risk of anaphylactic reaction. Gelatin solutions, albumin solutions, PPF and any other blood products cannot be given to patients with certain religious beliefs such as Jehovah's Witnesses. In the restoration of hypovolaemic shock, colloids are relatively more efficient volume for volume than crystalloid solutions. For crystalloids, a ratio of 3:1 for volume replacement to blood loss is normally required to reach an appropriate haemodynamic end-point. For colloid solutions the ratio is nearer to 1:1. In addition, the colloid will stay within the circulation for a longer period.

The exact choice of fluid and its infusion rate depend upon the clinical situation. Most patients with grade I haemorrhage who require volume replacement will only require crystalloid solutions. Patients with greater losses are commonly given crystalloid for the first 1000 ml of replacement, and then colloid solutions are given in addition. Individual regimens should follow local protocols.

Irrespective of the initial choice of fluid administered, for patients with continuing haemorrhage there will come a point at which the oxygen-carrying capacity of the circulating blood is impaired simply because there is insufficient haemoglobin available. Some form of red cell product will then be required. Depending upon local blood transfusion practice and product availability this may be in the form of packed red cells or (occasionally) fresh whole blood. In hospital the maintenance of a haematocrit at or around 30% is considered optimal, by judicious transfusion of red cells, colloid blood substitutes and crystalloid solutions.

All fluid given should be warmed to 37 °C to prevent the adverse effects of rapid infusion of cold fluid into a shocked patient. Boluses of cold fluid reaching the central circulation can cause cardiac arrhythmias, impair myocardial contractility and hence cardiac output, and impede normal blood coagulation. A number of studies have suggested that the pre-hospital administration of fluids to shocked patients may increase both morbidity and mortality rates. The reasons for this apparent paradox are multifactorial. Firstly, where bleeding cannot be controlled, increasing the patient's blood pressure by rapid infusion of fluid may dislodge the newly formed and fragile clots in traumatized blood vessels, and aggravate the bleeding. Secondly, the expansion of the circulation with crystalloid or colloid dilutes the circulating coagulation factors and impairs the ability to initiate the coagulation process.

For these reasons some authorities have stated that intravenous fluids should never be given except where there will be unavoidable delay in the patient reaching hospital. It is clearly appropriate to give fluids when the patient is trapped or transfer times are prolonged, but even so the systolic blood pressure should be maintained at no more than 100 mmHg. This will minimize the bleeding due to the mechanisms given above.

> **In hypovolaemic shock maintain the systolic blood pressure at 90–100 mmHg**

This area of controversy is of central importance to the pre-hospital management of patients with hypovolaemic shock. There is at present insufficient evidence to recommend that pre-hospital volume replacement is contraindicated, it is, however, necessary to stress two points – firstly, these procedures must *never* compromise the rapid delivery of the patient to the nearest appropriate hospital, and secondly, the performance of simple measures for airway control, oxygenation, applying pressure to bleeding points and splinting of long bone fractures are likely to be of greater value than more complex, time-consuming and potentially disadvantageous procedures.

CARDIOGENIC SHOCK

Shock is inadequate tissue perfusion: this can also be caused by failure of the pump mechanism. This is cardiogenic shock.

Cardiogenic shock may be caused by failure of the heart muscle owing to ischaemia of the myocardium, myocardial infarction or contusion. Rupture of the heart following ischaemia or penetrating trauma will also result in cardiogenic shock, exacerbated by compression of the heart caused by blood within the pericardium (*cardiac tamponade*). Management of cardiac tamponade due to trauma is considered in Chapter 23. Massive pulmonary embolism prevents normal cardiac function and will also produce cardiogenic shock.

Causes of cardiogenic shock

- Heart muscle (myocardial) dysfunction
    ischaemia
    infarction
    contusion
- Cardiac tamponade
    trauma
    post-infarction

- Pulmonary embolism

The most common cause of cardiogenic shock is myocardial infarction producing cardiac muscle or valve rupture. This results in a mortality rate greater than 90%.
Cardiogenic shock due to tamponade responds to aspiration of blood from the pericardium. This must be performed by an experienced doctor and is best performed in the accident and emergency department rather than delaying departure from the scene. Vigorous fluid resuscitation (see Chapter 23) will also be required in hospital – mortality has shown to be increased where intravenous fluids are given pre-hospital following penetrating cardiac injury. Other causes of cardiogenic shock require only oxygen therapy and immediate evacuation for definitive treatment.

SEPTIC SHOCK

Septic shock results from the action of substances (mediators) released from cells as a consequence of severe infection (usually bacterial). Dilatation of blood vessels, leakiness of tissue capillaries and a defect of oxygen utilization by the tissues produces shock. The normal regulation of blood flow to organs breaks down. The appropriate treatment for a patient with septic shock is investigation of the source of infection, intravenous antibiotics and intensive supportive care.
Septic shock usually takes some time to develop following the onset of infection. An exception is shock following suspected meningococcal infection (see Chapter 17) when the patient may progress from health to death within a few hours. In this situation benzylpenicillin should be given intravenously or intramuscularly as soon as the diagnosis is made when a doctor is present. All cases of septicaemic shock require oxygen, and IV fluids should be started if the transfer is likely to be delayed. No other pre-hospital treatment is required. Septicaemic shock is rare.

NEUROGENIC SHOCK

Neurogenic shock results from injury to the spinal cord. There is interruption of the nervous mechanism maintaining blood vessel wall tension; as a consequence vessels dilate and peripheral pooling of blood occurs, the effective circulating blood volume is reduced, and shock ensues. Neurogenic shock is therefore not associated with cold peripheries, which are instead warm and well perfused. Additionally, the neurological interruption prevents a compensating tachycardia. *The hallmarks of neurogenic shock are hypotension, warm peripheries and bradycardia.*
Head injury almost never results in hypotension, and shock due to spinal injury is rare. Shock in the trauma patient is far more likely to be due to unrecognized haemorrhage. Management priorities should be directed towards teating hypovolaemia in the shocked patient with a spinal injury.

> Isolated head injuries do not produce shock

ANAPHYLACTIC SHOCK

Anaphylactic shock results from an allergic reaction to a foreign protein such as nuts, bee stings or drugs. The reaction is mediated by immunoglobulins and histamine and results in vasodilation and blood pooling, with reduced effective circulating volume and compensatory tachycardia (compare neurogenic shock). The clinical features and treatment of anaphylactic shock are considered in Chapter 9.

chapter twenty-one:

HEAD INJURIES

The key to management of head injury is to recognize the importance of:

appropriate management of complications
early surgery where indicated

The treatment has to be prompt and specific to the needs of the injured brain.

ANATOMY

The brain is a soft, spongy organ with three main parts (Figure 21.1):

1. The right and left *cerebral hemispheres* forming the cerebrum. The cerebral hemispheres have different lobes. They are concerned with higher functions which include motor and sensory functions such as vision.
2. The *cerebellum* acts as a control centre. It is responsible for balance and coordination.
3. The *brain stem* consists of the midbrain, pons and medulla. The medulla is continuous with the spinal cord. Vital centres controlling cardiac and respiration function are in the lower brain stem.

Various nerves arise from the brain as *cranial nerves*, and from the spinal cord as *peripheral nerves*. These nerves supply motor and sensory function to various parts of the body.

Damage to nerve cells is permanent and recovery of central nervous system damage is not possible. Peripheral nerves do have some powers of recovery.

The cerebral hemispheres are responsible for motor and sensory function as well as vision and hearing. They are also responsible for the independent thought processes. The cerebral hemispheres have multiple folds which enlarge the surface area. The female brain is smaller and weighs less than the male brain, and therefore is more compact for similar function.

The midbrain has many pathways and cross-linkages. It tapers down to the brain stem, becoming continuous with the spinal cord. Because of its shape, swelling and increased intracranial pressure cause compression of the brain and tend to push it through the large hole in the base of skull, known as the *foramen magnum*.

The brain itself has a good blood supply, both internally and externally. However, some arteries are 'end arteries', and there is no other collateral supply to that area of the brain. Any damage to these arteries, in disease or injury, will lead to ischaemia, infarction and death of that area of the brain.

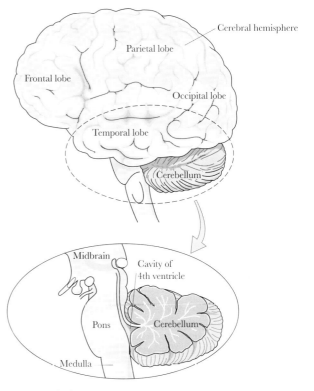

Fig. 21.1 *The brain*

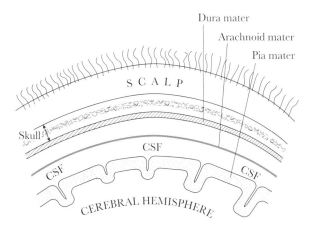

Fig. 21.2 *The coverings of the brain*

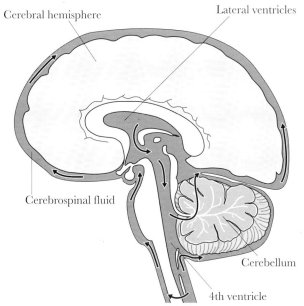

Fig. 21.3 *The flow of cerebrospinal fluid (arrows)*

The coverings of the brain are known as the *meninges* (Figure 21.2). The innermost of these is the *pia mater*, a thin film adherent to the brain surface. Outside this is the *arachnoid*, and surrounding the whole brain is the thick, rigid layer of fibrous tissue known as the *dura mater*. Between the pia mater and the arachnoid is a fluid-filled space in which there is cerebrospinal fluid (CSF). The brain is suspended, or floats, in this fluid, which acts as a shock absorber.

The cerebrospinal fluid is produced inside the brain from the choroid plexuses, mainly in the large lateral ventricles. The ventricular system and various passages (Figure 21.3) can be damaged by natural disease or by injury. This can produce internal swelling of the brain, known as *hydrocephalus*. Hydrocephalus causes a raised intracranial pressure, the treatment of which is CSF decompression through special catheters or shunts. From time to time these become blocked, leading to an altered conscious level. Such patients require emergency treatment.

Reflections of the dura mater form thick, fibrous folds known as *falces*, which are firmly attached to the skull. Running from front to back is a vertical fold between the two cerebral hemispheres – the *falx cerebri*. At 90 degrees to this is a transverse horizontal fold separating the cerebral hemispheres and the cerebellum. This partially surrounds the rear of the brain and is called the *tentorium cerebelli*. These fibrous folds act as baffles and hold the brain in position while it is suspended in the cerebrospinal fluid. However, in injury there can be mechanical distortion and brain damage. Large venous sinuses lie between the dural layers, and bleed if torn.

The skull itself is a rigid box. The cranium is an expanded dome and the wall of the skull is of an even thickness. In some people it can be thin and more prone to injury. The base or floor of the skull is tiered with numerous ridges and bumps. Any twisting or deceleration injury can cause damage to the undersurface of the brain against these bumps and ridges. Parts of the skeleton of the face and skull have much thinner bone. Above the nasal passages is a thin *cribriform plate*, which communicates with the base of the skull. The middle ear is also close to the base of the skull. With basal skull fractures damage to the cribriform plate and middle ear allows leakage of cerebrospinal fluid and blood from the nose or ears.

The skull itself is covered by the scalp, which consists of skin and a fibrous membrane, the *galea*. There is a potential space between the galea and the skull. If bleeding occurs into this space it can produce a large scalp haematoma. The scalp has a good blood supply and bleeds readily, so a large volume of blood can be lost following injury; this is unlikely to cause the symptoms and signs of hypovolaemia, except in children and the elderly (Fig 21.4)

PHYSIOLOGY

One of the important features of the central nervous system is that it has no stores for oxygen, glucose or other substances required for cell metabolism. If the blood supply is interrupted, depriving the brain of oxygen, consciousness is lost within 15–20 seconds. The brain cells will then die within 3–4 minutes. Any retention of carbon dioxide as a waste product of metabolism will retard brain function and aggravate the effects of hypoxia, or lack of oxygen. A supply of glucose is also essential for normal brain function.

The brain is particularly sensitive to increased pressure – nerve cells do not tolerate high pressure well.

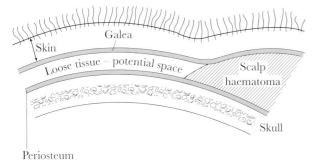

Skin
Galea
Loose tissue – potential space
Scalp haematoma
Skull
Periosteum

Fig. 21.4 *Layers of the scalp*

PATHOPHYSIOLOGY

Damage and abnormal function of the brain can occur in two ways:

generalized brain injury
localized brain injury

Damage to the brain is a frequent occurrence. The brain injury sustained at the time of the accident is known as the *primary injury*, and it is something that the paramedic cannot treat once it has occurred. What can be minimized is the *secondary brain injury*; this is due to complications following the original trauma. Injuries to the brain are traditionally divided into:

blunt injuries
penetrating injuries

Blunt injuries are caused by a variety of forces, primarily direct contact, for example from a hammer blow, causing force to be transmitted to the brain beneath the skull. Associated with this are other dynamic forces related to twisting or *shearing* of the brain inside the skull. Such forces are liable to tear or squeeze the brain cells. The damage to the brain is usually caused by the rough projections on the skull base, or torn by the folds of the falx.

Skull Fractures

Blunt injuries can cause fractures of the skull. Such fractures are common, and although they are not necessarily significant

Table 21.1 Risk of intracranial haematoma

Conscious level	Skull X-ray	Risk of intracranial haematoma
Normal	Normal	1 in 5000
Normal	Fracture	1 in 32
Altered	Normal	1 in 120
Altered	Fracture	1 in 4

injuries they reflect the degree of violence to which the brain has been subjected. Damage to the brain is demonstrated by an altered conscious level. A significant point about skull fracture is its relation to intracranial bleeding. The combination of a fracture of the skull *and* loss of consciousness increases the chance of intracranial bleeding from 1 in 5000 to 1 in 4 (Table 21.1).

Linear skull fractures require no specific treatment. The emphasis for treatment is on the underlying brain injury. A more severe form of fracture is where the bone is depressed, but surgical treatment will only be required if there is pressure on the brain. This pressure may lead to epilepsy.

Leakage of cerebrospinal fluid from the nose or the ears is diagnostic of a basal skull fracture, as is bleeding from the ears. As there is an open communication with the exterior, there is a clear channel for infection.

Other features of a basal skull fracture are black eyes: tracking of blood around both eyes gives the appearance known as 'panda' or 'raccoon' eyes. Swelling and bruising behind the ear over the mastoid process also indicates leakage of blood from a fractured base of skull. This is known as Battle's sign.

Signs of basal skull fracture

- CSF leakage from nose (rhinorrhoea)
- CSF leakage from ear (otorrhoea)
- Panda (raccoon) eyes
- Battle's sign
- Bleeding from the ears

Very severe open injuries may expose the brain. Moist non-adherent dressings are needed to cover the area, to stop the brain tissue drying out.

Localized Brain Injury

Localized brain injuries consist of:

- Bruising or contusion
- Intracranial haemorrhages
- Lacerations and penetrating injuries

Contusion

A contusion is a bruise. It can be small or large, localized or involve a large area of the brain. Most cerebral contusions present with a period of concussion. It is important to realize that patients do not remember the duration of coma. This history is obtained from the observers. For this reason it is essential that all information about loss of consciousness is documented on the patient's report form. Because of the inflammatory response, there will be a secondary injury around the area of bruising with a collection of fluid causing localized swelling. The secondary oedema around a contusion may cause further deterioration. Modern management of such injuries is non-surgical, but includes monitoring of the intracranial pressure.

Intracranial bleeding

Intracranial haemorrhage may be:

- Extradural
- Subdural
- Intracerebral
- Subarachnoid

It is usually caused by tearing of veins or arteries. Damage to the middle meningeal artery can cause an *extradural haemorrhage* – bleeding between the skull and the dura mater. It is not a common injury, occurring in less than 1% of head-injured patients, but it can be rapidly fatal. An important feature is that if treated in the optimum time, ideally within 2 hours, patients may make a complete recovery. Delay beyond 4 hours will significantly alter the degree of recovery (Figure 21.5).

An extradural haematoma characteristically presents as a loss of consciousness (initial concussion), following which the patient may recover, be alert and talkative, or have an improved Glasgow Coma Scale rating. The patient then lapses into unconsciousness as the intracranial pressure increases. For this secondary loss of consciousness treatment has to be surgical, and must be prompt. Often there is weakness on the opposite side of the body to the head injury, with a dilated and fixed pupil on the same side as the injury. The patient is often aggressive, with increasing drowsiness and headache.

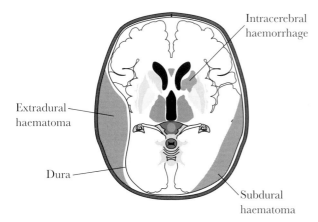

Fig. 21.5 *The anatomy of intracranial bleeding: extradural haematoma, subdural haematoma and intracerebral haemorrhage. A subarachnoid haemorrhage covers the surface of the brain, lying in a thin layer between the arachnoid and the pia mater*

The surgical treatment is to remove the blood clot and seal off the bleeding vessel. If the pressure on the brain is removed and is not prolonged, a recovery rate of 100% can be expected.

Subdural haemorrage – damage to the vessels in the subdural space (between the dura and the arachnoid) – is much more common and accounts for 30% of head injuries. Originally these injuries were thought to have a very poor prognosis. There is increasing evidence that if the patient is operated on within the first 2 hours after injury the survival rate can be as high as 70–80%.

Bleeding may also occur into the tissue of the cerebral hemispheres – *intracerebral haemorrhage*.

Bleeding into the subarachnoid space (*subarachnoid haemorrhage*) produces headache and increasing drowsiness. Once the diagnosis has been made there is no immediate surgical treatment. In pre-hospital care it is extremely difficult to decide which sort of bleeding is causing unconsciousness. The definitive investigation is a computerized tomography (CT) scan. It is therefore important that patients with a significant period of unconsciousness (2–3 minutes or more) are taken to a hospital that has 24-hour CT scanning facilities, and appropriate staff to treat the patient once these scans have been obtained. Only after a scan is performed can a long-term prognosis be given.

Lacerations and penetrating injuries

Lacerations are closed brain injuries, often due to shearing forces causing tearing and haemorrhage within the substance of the brain, producing an intracranial haematoma. This exerts pressure within the substance of the brain, with possible permanent damage. Specialist neurosurgical centres are able to evacuate such haemorrhages and diminish the effects. Such injuries can be devastating and have a high mortality rate.

Brain haemorrhage can also be caused by penetrating trauma, inflicted by a low-velocity implement such as a knife, or by impalement in an industrial or traffic accident.

It is predicted that the degree of violence similar to that seen in North America will increase. In the UK a significant amount of gunshot trauma can be expected in the future. The damage to the brain depends on the size of the bullet and its velocity. In general terms, if the patient is unconscious after the penetrating injury the prognosis is exceedingly poor. Patients who are conscious and talking after such an injury can survive.

Generalized Brain Injury

Diffuse injury

Diffuse injuries, often referred to as *diffuse axonal injury* (DAI), are a principal cause of long-standing coma following head injury. Coma may last days or weeks, and may be permanent. It results from microscopic damage to the nerve cells that are sheared and torn. It is extremely difficult to diagnose such injuries outside hospital. These patients should be assumed to have a treatable lesion until the results of a CT scan and a neurosurgical opinion have been obtained. All significant head injuries leading to an altered conscious level need to be seen in a centre where the proper investigation and treatment facilities are available.

Secondary brain injury

Secondary brain injury (Figure 21.6) is a combination of factors that lead to brain swelling. Because the skull is a rigid box it does not expand (although the sutures and fontanelles do allow a little expansion in the infant under 12 months). Any swelling of the brain within this box causes squeezing and compression. To give an example, if a patient has an extradural haematoma there is a blood clot within the skull. Although the initial injury to the brain is liable to have caused concussion, the patient recovers temporarily (a lucid interval) before deteriorating. The secondary effects are two-fold. Firstly, the underlying area of brain is affected by the injury owing to the inflammatory response, and becomes swollen. This area may be small or large. As the size of the blood clot increases and presses on the surface of the brain, unconsciousness supervenes. The initial effect is pressure on one side of the brain, but if left untreated pressure is applied to the whole brain. As the pressure increases on one side of the brain, part of the temporal lobe extrudes (herniates) into the small space between the brain stem and the tentorium cerebelli. In this space is the third cranial nerve, and as this is compressed the pupil on the same side dilates. As intracranial pressure continues to rise the herniating temporal lobe forces the brain stem against the opposite fold of tentorium, causing the opposite pupil to dilate. This is a pre-terminal sign. An alternative site of herniation is the *foramen magnum*. This is known as 'coning'.

Particular factors that affect the brain's blood supply are:

    lack of oxygen (hypoxia)
    carbon dioxide retention

With hypoxia the brain cells go into an anaerobic metabolism phase. There is damage to the cells, which become swollen. As hypoxia affects the brain as a whole there is generalized swelling – *cerebral oedema*. This swelling results in raised pressure inside the skull – raised intracranial pressure (ICP).

Signs of raised intracranial pressure

- Decreasing level of consciousness
- Increasing blood pressure
- Falling pulse rate
- Decreasing respiratory rate
- Pupillary dilatation

Carbon dioxide retention exaggerates cerebral oedema. When the intracranial pressure equals or exceeds the arterial pressure, blood cannot flow through the brain and so cells will die. The important blood pressure for the brain is not the mean arterial pressure (MAP) alone, but the *perfusion pressure* (PP). The cerebral perfusion pressure is the mean arterial pressure minus the mean intracranial pressure (MICP).

> **Cerebral perfusion pressure is the mean arterial pressure minus the mean intracranial pressure**
> **PP = MAP – MICP**

These pressures can be monitored in hospital. In the swollen brain the ICP is also increased if central venous pressure is increased. Treatment should aim to maintain the cerebral perfusion pressure and keep the patient's arterial pressure near normal limits, and above 100 mmHg in the adult. Hypoxia and hypovolaemia must be corrected. Anything that increases central venous pressure, for example a tension pneumothorax, must also be treated. Nursing the patient slightly head-up with the head in a neutral position will optimize venous drainage from the head.

PATIENT ASSESSMENT

Patient assessment must follow a systematic approach. Since a patient will lose consciousness within 15–30 seconds because of lack of oxygen, the priorities in management are:

1. Protect the airway
2. Ensure delivery of oxygen to the brain

To achieve this there must be an adequate airway (A), uncompromised breathing (B) and adequate cerebral perfusion (C).

The outstanding feature of a head injury is an altered conscious level which will vary from drowsiness or irritability, to lack of response to verbal commands or to pain, and finally to unresponsiveness.

Most patients cannot tell you whether they have been knocked out, and certainly cannot reliably judge the period of unconsciousness. What they will tell you is that they lack memory of an event. This lack of memory is known as *amnesia*. Amnesia can be:

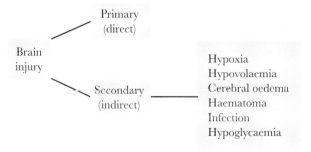

Fig. 21.6 *Primary and secondary brain injury*

1. *Retrograde amnesia* – lack of memory or recall of the event *before* the injury. This can be a period of some minutes, or even an hour or so. It suggests a significant brain injury.
2. *Post-traumatic amnesia* – loss of memory *after* the event. The patient may remember up to the time of a fall, a blow or a traffic accident. The next recall is of a specific location, for example the ambulance, the accident and emergency department or the X-ray department. It is significant to note the length of time the patient has suffered from post-traumatic amnesia.

There are many 'minor' head injuries, where the patient has been knocked out for 1–2 seconds, but then makes a full recovery. The main reason patients are admitted to hospital after a head injury and loss of consciousness is to make sure they do not have a treatable injury, such as an intracranial haematoma that requires surgery. As a result, large numbers of patients are admitted to hospital for head injury observation. These patients are suffering from '*concussion*'.

Any patient who has a witnessed loss of consciousness should be taken to hospital. Patients who have prolonged post-traumatic amnesia of 5 minutes or more should also be observed. Other factors can influence conscious level. These include pre-existing diseases such as epilepsy, where drowsiness is a well-known feature following a grand mal seizure. Alcohol and other drugs will alter the conscious level, and because of the risks involved these patients may need observation, in spite of the fact they have not lost consciousness. Patients who are subject to chronic alcohol abuse can have reduced blood coagulation; they may suffer an insidious intracranial bleed, often without loss of consciousness. These 'regular' accident and emergency patients may end up dying because they have an intracerebral haematoma that is unrecognized because the patient is labelled as a 'drunk'. It is dangerous not to take these patients to hospital, or to discharge them from the accident and emergency department, in spite of the fact they are regular attenders.

> **Never accept alcohol as the sole cause of an altered conscious level**

Another high-risk group are those with blood coagulation disorders, whether inherited (e.g. haemophilia) or secondary to drugs (e.g. warfarin).

Assessment of the head-injured patient assumes the primary survey is carried out with appropriate management for the airway and protection of the cervical spine in every patient who is concussed or who has an altered conscious level. Cervical spine injury is likely in patients who have had a fall from a height of 3 metres or more, or undergone violent deceleration, as in high-speed traffic accidents. Patients involved in a rear-end shunt traffic accident within an urban area, particularly when stationary, rarely suffer cervical spine bony injury.

After the airway, breathing and circulation have been assessed and managed appropriately, the neurological status should be assessed. The general neurological state can be observed by assessing whether the patient is alert (A), responds to verbal commands (V), responds to painful stimuli (P), or is completely unresponsive (U). This is known as 'AVPU':

A > Alert
V > Voice
P > Pain
U > Unresponsive

Glasgow Coma Scale

A more accurate and detailed examination, which is readily repeated by other observers, is the *Glasgow Coma Scale*.

> **The Glasgow Coma Scale is part of the secondary survey**

This will provide a quantitive score, assessing three functions: eye opening, verbal response and motor response.

Eye opening

Eye opening has four responses (Table 21.2).

The painful stimulus should be applied above the neck to ensure that cervical spine injury is not responsible for the lack of response.

Verbal response

If the patient cannot speak it is impossible to carry out this

Table 21.2 Glasgow Coma Scale – eye opening

Response	Score
Eyes are already open and blinking normally	E = 4
Eyes open in response to speech or specific questions	E = 3
Eyes open in response to pain	E = 2
No response	E = 1

Table 21.3 Glasgow Coma Scale – verbal response

Response	Score
Fully oriented; for example, patient can state name, address, date of birth and date and time	V = 5
Confused conversation; patient will not volunteer information, gives lucid answers to specific questions	V = 4
Inappropriate words; patient can produce recognizable words, but at random and not in lucid sentences. May also be exclamatory or swearing	V = 3
Incomprehensible sounds (grunts or groans), but no actual words	V = 2
No response to speech	V = 1

assessment, for example if the patient is intubated. This is relevant and must be documented (Table 21.3).

Motor response

Motor response is assessed as the best response for extremities. It is assessed by the function of the *upper limbs*, assuming no injury to them (Table 21.4).

Overall assessment

The E, V and M scores are added up, giving a maximum total for a normal Glasgow Coma Scale of 15. However, to the specialist a summative score on a Glasgow Coma Scale has little meaning – it is better to use the Glasgow Coma Scale as a means of documenting the patient's condition on a chart. When messages are passed, or when the patient is handed over, the paramedic should state the Glasgow Coma Scale score for each of the components – for example, opens eyes spontaneously (4), responds only to questions (3), and localizes to pain (5), which is more meaningful than an overall score of 12 (Table 21.5).

Other Tests

Motor function can be assessed by testing movements of both the right and left upper limbs and the right and left lower limbs. It is important to record that the patient is not moving the lower limbs spontaneously if spontaneous movement of the upper limbs is present. This is highly suggestive of a spinal cord injury. Similarly, assessment of sensation to each of the limbs is important. In certain instances, for example in a patient who has had a cerebrovascular accident or stroke, loss of feeling and movement on one side of the body indicates an intracranial bleed within the brain on the opposite side – these are known as *lateralizing signs*.

The next part of the neurological examination is assessment of pupil function, documenting the size of the pupil, and their response to light. Normal movements of the eyes should also be recorded.

The patient's vital signs are of great significance, as they provide direct assessments of brain function. These signs include pulse rate, blood pressure and respiratory rate. In hospital the body temperature is also an important brain function.

Knowing the blood glucose level is of value, because hypoglycaemia contributes to secondary brain injury and must be corrected. Recording of blood glucose levels by paramedics is likely to become routine not only in diabetic patients, but also in patients with major head injury.

As time is important in the management of the head-injured patient, paramedics must obtain all this information rapidly and systematically. The assessment of a patient should be completed within 5 minutes, as longer on-scene times will be detrimental. In an untrapped patient the primary survey should take no more than 2 minutes. For the purpose of the primary survey, the 'mini' neurological examination is adequate: this comprises 'AVPU' and an assessment of the pupillary response to light.

> **'Mini' neurological examination = AVPU + pupils**

The assessment *and treatment* of the patient must take no more than 10 minutes. The secondary survey is completed during the ambulance journey to hospital; the performance of the full neurological assessment (Glasgow Coma Scale and lateralizing signs) must not be allowed to delay the patient's transfer to appropriate medical or surgical facilities.

> **Assessment and recording of observations should not delay the transport to hospital**

Table 21.4 Glasgow Coma Scale – motor response

Response	Score
Spontaneously moves limbs to commands	M = 6
Localizes pain by purpose or motion towards the painful stimuli (this stimulus should be applied to the fingernail bed)	M = 5
Withdraws, or pulls away from painful stimuli	M = 4
Abnormal flexion, known as *decorticate* posture	M = 3
Extensor response, known as *decerebrate* posture	M = 2
No movement	M = 1

MANAGEMENT

Attention must be paid to the normal sequence of resuscitation: airway, breathing and circulation (ABC). Appropriate management of these priorities is the basis of the optimal management of head injuries. Thus airway is the first priority, then breathing, followed by circulation. It is important that patient management follows these general guidelines.

Table 21.5 Examples of different Glasgow Coma Scale assessments with identical total scores

	Example 1		Example 2	
Eye opening	3	(speech or questioning)	2	(response to pain)
Verbal response	3	(inappropriate speech)	2	(incomprehensible sounds)
Motor response	3	(abnormal flexion)	5	(localizes pain)
Total score	9		9	

Airway

The primary survey insists on airway assessment and maintenance of the airway first. If simple techniques such as the jaw thrust or chin lift are inadequate, adjuncts such as the oropharyngeal airway should be used. Even with an adequate airway, the patient may have a problem of hypoventilation, i.e. slow or shallow respiratory movements. The effects of hypoventilation can be detected by pulse oximetry and capnography, the first showing low oxygen percentage saturation, and the latter the retention of carbon dioxide in expired air. In a patient who is unconscious and comatose (a Glasgow Coma Scale score of 8 or less), advanced airway support in the form of intubation will be needed. This can be a straightforward procedure if the patient has no gag reflex.

If the patient is irritable, aggressive and has a gag reflex, adequate airway maintenance can be one of the most difficult pre-hospital problems. In hospital this situation is resolved by the intervention of a doctor with skills in intubation, using muscle relaxant drugs. If the patient is trapped or cannot be transported to hospital within 15 minutes, the paramedic must consider calling medical help to the scene. The pre-hospital doctor must be experienced and trained in intubation using muscle relaxants. At the very least advice should be obtained from hospital staff by radio or by telephone. There is no place for sedative drugs in head injury, and they can cause dangerous lowering of the blood pressure.

As well as airway maintenance the patient must be given oxygen. The best method (if the patient is not intubated) is to use a well-fitting face mask, and a high flow of oxygen at 10–15 litres per minute. Oxygen flow rates above 6 litres per minute purge off retained carbon dioxide, reducing accumulation of carbon dioxide and minimizing secondary cerebral oedema. To achieve 90% oxygen supply a reservoir bag and mask must be used.

Breathing

A normal respiratory rate is 10–18 breaths per minute in an adult. A rapid respiratory rate is a sign of hypoxia. Any respiratory rate above 18 breaths per minute should be assumed to be abnormal, indicating that the patient requires oxygen. Slow respiratory rates may be caused by drugs, or by significant head injury.

Unequal chest movements can be due to damage of the chest wall, for example pain from rib fractures, or by a flail chest where there is a detached segment of ribs. A major aggravating factor to a head injury is a tension pneumothorax. As the pressure builds up in the chest cavity there is an increase of central venous pressure, giving further increase of the intracranial pressure and precipitating further cerebral oedema. Relief of a tension pneumothorax as soon as possible by needle thoracocentesis can have a dramatic effect in reducing high cerebral pressures. It also relieves some of the problems related to the hypoxia secondary to the pneumothorax.

Circulation

Head injuries themselves do not cause low blood pressure, with the possible exception of scalp haemorrhage (see example below). An isolated and closed head injury is likely to have the opposite effect. Significant blood loss into the scalp is also a problem in infants who can lose considerable amounts of blood into their relatively loose scalp, even in closed injuries.

Isolated head injuries do not cause shock

A diagnostic problem in head injury management

An 80-year-old woman was knocked off her pedal cycle in the middle of town by a van. She landed on her head and sustained a 15 cm laceration of her scalp. She was noted to have lost blood when she was treated by the ambulance crew at the scene. In spite of pressure dressings to the scalp she continued to bleed. She had no other injuries. In hospital she was confused and disoriented. She opened her eyes to command, was making comprehensible sounds, but her conversation was confused. A diagnosis of dementia was considered. She localized to painful stimuli. Her respiratory rate was 28 per minute, her pulse was 100 per minute and her blood pressure was 95/60 mmHg. The small, spurting arterial vessel in her scalp was secured by a large suture. A rapid infusion of a litre of Hartmann's solution brought her respiratory rate to 22 per minute, her pulse to 88 per minute and her blood pressure to 140/70 mmHg. At that point the patient's confusion settled. She became fully oriented and alert, and was able to give her name, date of birth, her address and her daughter's telephone number, and describe the circumstances of the accident. The uninformed comment that this woman was probably demented was incorrect because she had all the features of hypovolaemic shock. This affected her brain function.

In head injuries patients may lose large volumes of blood from other injuries, such as bleeding into the chest or abdomen, or from multiple fractures. If the patient is hypovolaemic this must be corrected. It is important not to *over*-transfuse patients who have a head injury, as this may cause or aggravate cerebral oedema. Equally, it is important not to withhold fluid in those with blood loss in other areas. Accurate assessment of the blood volume lost, and replacement of that volume, are particularly important in the head-injured patient to maintain good cerebral perfusion. In general it is far more common for patients with associated injuries to be *under*-resuscitated with fluids.

Transfer to Hospital

Once the airway and cervical spine and breathing are stabilized, the patient should be rapidly transported to the nearest appropriate hospital. Circulatory interventions are best attempted in transit. At this stage a Glasgow Coma Scale score can be accurately assessed and can be continually monitored during the journey. An appropriate hospital is one that has a 24-hour accident and emergency department, and access to an available and working CT scanner. Serious head injuries need an intensive care unit and surgeons to deal with any complications that develop. For this reason there is an increased need to use hospitals that have trained trauma teams and rapidly available neurosurgeons. It is not efficient to treat patients by transferring them to the nearest hospital where they may be assessed over a period of 1–2 hours and then require a secondary transfer to a neurosurgical unit. The critical time for surgery may have passed, leading to increased mortality and morbidity rates in head-injured patients.

ADVANCES IN TREATMENT

Over the years it has been recognized that it is dangerous to allow patients with head injuries to become hypoxic. With the increased technical skills of paramedics, better airway maintenance has been achieved using basic and advanced life support techniques. In the future there is likely to be increased use of endotracheal intubation with muscle relaxant drugs being given by appropriately trained staff, who will include specially trained medical as well as paramedical personnel. Adequate oxygenation can be monitored non-invasively by pulse oximetry, and expired air carbon dioxide levels can also be monitored (capnography or end-tidal CO_2 monitoring).

One technique that is used to 'shrink' the swollen brain is hyperventilation, either manually or with an automatic ventilator. On its own this may not be as successful as was originally thought, possibly because of an excess of free oxygen radicals – these are unattached oxygen molecules in the biochemical system, which cause cell damage. New drugs becoming available act by mopping up these free oxygen radicals. Some of these drugs, such as acetylcysteine, seem to have a protective effect on the brain.

Because of the success of pre-hospital care by paramedics and immediate care doctors in maintaining the airway, providing oxygen and maintaining a normal blood pressure, and by careful attention to pre-hospital times, patients are arriving in hospital in a much better condition. Allied to this are significant advances in the management of head injuries within neurosurgical units. Intracranial pressure monitoring is the norm in the UK, and there is now the recognition of the need of the brain for glucose and other energy sources. Brain *function* can be monitored with sophisticated techniques such as the positron emission scan, which identifies the actual levels of glucose being circulated to all parts of the brain. Patients with significant brain injury need to be treated in these specialized centres.

The implication of these developments and their effects on outcome is that paramedics will have the responsibility of transporting a head-injured patient to the most appropriate unit for that patient's injury. It is of paramount importance that the paramedic pays attention to the basic management of the patient, that is the provision of a clear airway, good oxygenation, protection of normal breathing and treatment of any complication. Any hypovolaemia should be corrected by fluid replacement, and continuing assessment of the patient's disability or neurological state is required throughout the transfer to hospital.

The greatest advance for recovery of the injured brain has been attention to detail in the pre-hospital phase. The sophisticated skills of the modern neurosurgeon will not be effective unless the paramedic adheres to these basic principles.

chapter twenty-two:

FACIAL INJURIES

Facial injuries occur in isolation or in association with multiple trauma. The management of such injuries usually occurs during the secondary survey and forms part of the detailed assessment of the trauma patient. However, severe facial injuries may compromise the airway and induce haemorrhage, and both of these problems should be treated as part of the primary survey.

Airway problems arise from:

- Inhalation of foreign bodies
- Posterior impaction of the fractured maxilla
- Loss of tongue control in a fractured mandible
- Intraoral tissue swelling
- Direct trauma to the larynx
- Haemorrhage

Haemorrhage from facial fractures may produce :

1. Hypovolaemic shock
2. Airway obstruction

Two per cent of facial injuries have associated cervical injuries, and the patient's cervical spine should *always* be protected using a semirigid collar, sandbags and tape until adequate radiographs confirm the absence of injury. Severe facial injury may necessitate advanced airway procedures such as cricothyroidotomy (Chapter 5).
Facial injuries can be conveniently divided into soft tissue injuries (including the eye) and hard tissue injuries (teeth and bone).

ANATOMY OF THE FACIAL SKELETON

Mandible

The mandible or lower jaw articulates with the rest of the skull at the *condyles*. The thin *neck* of the condyle is connected to the

ramus of the mandible and this to the *body*. The teeth are held in the bone in the dentoalveolar region.

Maxilla (Figure 22.1)

The upper jaw also supports teeth in the dentoalveolar bone and is closely related to the bones that form the orbit and nose. Lying behind the front wall of the maxilla is the air-filled *maxillary sinus*.

Orbit and Zygomaticomaxillary Complex

The *zygoma* or *malar bone* forms part of the outer margin of the orbital rim and gives the face a cheek prominence. The bone forming the eye socket is very thin and is divided into the floor, the roof and the medial and lateral walls. The lower rim (infraorbital margin) is formed partly by the zygoma and partly by the maxilla. The upper rim (supraorbital margin) is part of the frontal bone of the skull. The eye is contained within the bony orbit and is surrounded by the extraocular muscles and periorbital fat..

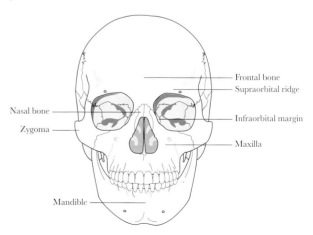

Frontal bone
Supraorbital ridge
Nasal bone
Infraorbital margin
Zygoma
Maxilla
Mandible

***Fig. 22.1** The facial skeleton*

Nasal Complex

The nose consists of a bony part articulating with the frontal bone and maxilla, and a cartilaginous framework. The thin *ethmoid bone* forms the medial aspect of the orbit. The ethmoids contain air-filled sinuses and are closely related to the nose and the frontal region of the brain.

Blood Supply to the Face and Scalp

The blood supply to the face and scalp is excellent and soft tissue wounds may bleed profusely. The *facial artery*, a branch of the external carotid artery, supplies the tissues of the face and there is considerable cross-over from one side to the other. The same applies to the vessels supplying the scalp. In addition the terminal branches of the *maxillary artery*, and the anterior and posterior *ethmoidal arteries* contribute to the midfacial blood supply and can be responsible for life-threatening haemorrhage. Control of massive facial bleeding is discussed below.

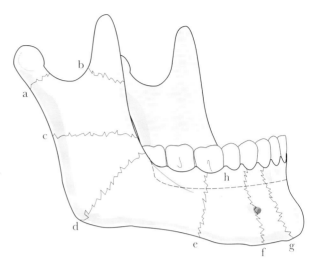

Fig. 22.2 *Mandibular fractures: a, condyle; b, coronoid; c, ramus; d, angle; e, body; f, parasymphysis; g, symphysis; h, dentoalveolar*

CLASSIFICATION OF FACIAL INJURIES

Facial injuries can be grouped into soft tissue injuries (including the eye), and hard tissue injuries which may involve teeth or bone.

Soft Tissue

Soft tissue injuries may be divided into superficial cuts and grazes, lacerations and penetrating wounds. There may be loss of tissue or degloving injuries, as seen for example in the lower labial sulcus (groove behind the lower lip) when the skin over the chin is forcibly pushed backwards.

Eye injuries may be divided into:

- Foreign bodies
- Penetrating injuries
- Chemical injury

Hard Tissue

Teeth

Teeth may be loosened, partially extruded or completely avulsed (extracted). They may be fractured at the level of the crown or lower down on the root. Fractures involving segments of tooth-bearing bone may occur and are known as *dentoalveolar fractures*.

Bone

It is convenient to consider the fractures of the facial skeleton according to the anatomical areas described before. Facial fractures can occur on one side (unilateral) or both sides (bilateral), and combinations are frequent.

Fractures of the mandible A patient with a fractured mandible (Figure 22.2) will give a history of recent trauma to the jaw. For example, a patient who has sustained a blow to the right side of the jaw may have a fracture through the right angle and/or a fracture of the left condylar neck. The patient may complain of pain and swelling over the site of the injury and be unable to open the mouth fully. A number of teeth may have been lost or displaced and the patient may have difficulty in putting the teeth together properly (abnormal occlusion). Examination of the face may reveal a step deformity along the line of the lower jaw. Intraoral inspection may show lacerated and bleeding gums and loose teeth. Gentle manipulation of the jaw across the fracture line can be painful but will help in diagnosis. Bruising underneath the tongue usually occurs adjacent to the fracture line.

Fractures of the maxilla A patient with a fractured upper jaw (Figure 22.3) is likely to have sustained high-impact trauma to the face. Gentle manipulation of the maxilla will reveal mobility of the upper jaw and the patient may have a 'dish-face' deformity. Marked swelling is a feature of the Le Fort II and Le Fort III fractures and may be accompanied by bruising around the eyes. Again, the patient may complain that the teeth do not meet properly and indeed the mouth may be gagged open.

Orbital and zygomaticomaxillary complex fractures Fractures in this region are of particular concern because of

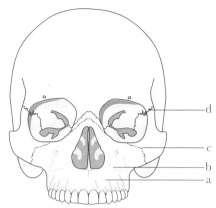

Fig. 22.3 *Maxillary fractures: a, dentoalveolar; b, Le Fort I (low level); c, Le Fort II (pyramidal); d, Le Fort III (high level)*

the potential damage to the eye. Trauma to the cheek can produce marked periorbital swelling and bruising. A step deformity may be felt along the infraorbital margin and there may be flattening of the cheek. Swelling of the eyelids may make examination of the eye more difficult, but it is important that any globe injuries are not missed. Gentle pressure on the eyelids for a few minutes will disperse the oedema and allow a full examination of the eye. Subconjunctival haemorrhage can indicate a fracture of the zygoma.

The patient may complain of double vision (diplopia), and examination of the eye movements should be part of the assessment of the eye. Visual acuity can be objectively measured using a Snellen chart in hospital.

Difficulty in opening the mouth occurs when the zygomatic arch is fractured and restricts the normal movements of the muscles.

Nasal complex fractures Fractures of the nasal bones occur following trauma from the front and from the side. The subsequent deformity reflects the direction of the injury. Nasal fractures can be accompanied by profuse haemorrhage, the management of which is discussed below. Severe midfacial injury may be sufficient to produce disruption of the thin ethmoidal bones. The patient may have a flattened appearance to the bridge of the nose and widening of the distance between the inner corners (*medial canthi*) of the eyes – this is known as hypertelorism.

TREATMENT OF FACIAL INJURIES

Soft Tissue Injuries

Profuse haemorrhage from cuts and lacerations should be stopped during the primary survey. Pressure applied over the wound with a gauze swab held firmly in place may be all that is required. Penetrating injuries should *not* be explored. It is

dangerous to explore neck wounds which should be covered and managed in hospital with arteriography if appropriate.

Foreign bodies should be left in place including those piercing the cheek or penetrating the other intraoral tissues, unless causing airway obstruction.

During the secondary survey a thorough examination of the scalp and face may be made to identify all the soft tissue injuries. These should be cleaned using chlorhexidine solution (chlorhexidine gluconate 0.05%) and covered with a gauze dressing.

The immediate management of foreign bodies in the eye is simply to cover the eye with a non-compressive pad. Similarly, any penetrating foreign bodies must be left *in situ* and no attempt made to remove them. If the globe is disrupted it should be covered with a non-compressive pad. In the event of chemical injury, the eye should be washed with copious amounts (500–1000 ml) of normal saline, sterile water or Hartmann's solution.

Hard Tissue Injuries

Teeth

Loose and avulsed teeth may be inhaled and are a cause of airway obstruction. Denture fragments or poorly fitting dentures can also be inhaled, especially in patients with a decreased level of consciousness. Assessment of the patient's airway and inspection of the mouth are mandatory. Finger sweep to remove foreign bodies and suction should be part of the primary survey (Chapter 4). Well-fitting dentures may be left in place.

In a patient without a head injury, a completely avulsed tooth (usually a front tooth in a child) can be immediately reinserted. The patient should be asked to hold the tooth in position and the advice of a dentist or maxillofacial surgeon sought. Alternatively, the tooth may be placed in a container of milk and transferred with the patient to hospital. Patients with an associated head injury are at particular risk from inhaling foreign bodies and should not be asked to hold their tooth in the inside of the cheek, as has sometimes been advocated. If the tooth is fractured the pieces must be found and taken with the patient to hospital. A chest radiograph may subsequently be necessary if there is any suspicion that a fragment may have been inhaled.

Bone

Posterior impaction of a fractured maxilla A fractured maxilla may cause obstruction of the nasopharynx by backwards and downwards displacement along the slope of the base of the skull. Disimpaction of the maxilla can relieve the obstruction and is performed by placing the middle and index fingers behind the soft palate and pulling forwards (Figure 22.4).

Loss of tongue control in a fractured mandible The fractured mandible may become an immediate airway man-

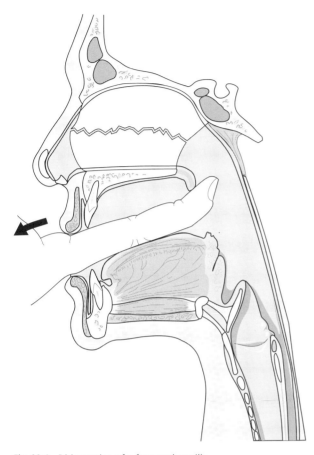

Fig. 22.4 *Disimpaction of a fractured maxilla*

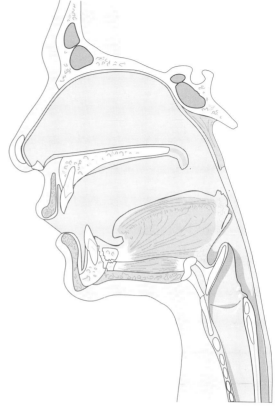

Fig. 22.5 *Loss of tongue support with a fractured mandible*

agement problem when there are bilateral symphysial fractures or extensive bone loss resulting in loss of tongue support. The musculature of the tongue is attached to the genial tubercles in the midline and if this fragment becomes detached the tongue may fall backwards to obstruct the oropharynx. Patients at particular risk from this complication are those with a depressed conscious level who are unable to control their tongue (Figure 22.5).

Immediate management involves pulling the tongue forward and holding it in an unobstructed position. This may be achieved manually or by a large suture (0 gauge black silk) placed *transversely* through the dorsum of the tongue (a large safety pin may even be used) and the suture taped to the side of the face. A transverse stitch is less likely to cut through the tongue when traction is applied.

Haemorrhage control Profuse haemorrhage can result from a fractured maxilla after damage to the terminal branches of the maxillary artery, and from the anterior and posterior ethmoidal arteries. Bleeding can cause respiratory obstruction or

hypovolaemic shock and should be stopped if evident from the mouth and nose. Nasal Epistats (Figure 22. 6) used in

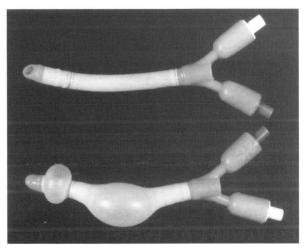

Fig. 22.6 *Nasal Epistats*

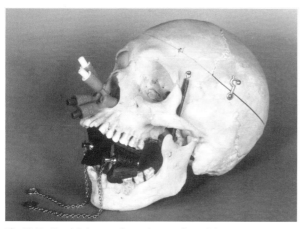

Fig. 22.7 *Nasal Epistat and mouth props in position*

conjunction with mouth props (Figure 22.7) may effectively stop most bleeding, although these would, in general, be reserved for use in the accident and emergency department.

The Epistats are inserted into both nostrils, inflated using normal saline and pulled forward, thus providing a significant compressive force. Nasal bleeding without a facial fracture may alternatively be controlled rapidly with expanding foam packs (Merocel) inserted into the nostrils.

chapter twenty-three:

CHEST INJURIES

Deaths following injuries to the thorax usually result from a lack of oxygen (hypoxia) or lack of circulating blood volume (hypovolaemia). To improve the chances of the patient surviving, you must develop the expertise to recognize and manage these problems and be aware of conditions that require immediate evacuation.

To understand the medical management of thoracic trauma, it is helpful to review the anatomy and physiology of the respiratory system described in Chapter 9.

MECHANISMS OF INJURY

Injuries may be blunt or penetrating. These two types can occur separately or in combination, for example following a bomb blast (see Chapter 28). In all cases, however, the severity of the injury is dependent upon the site of the impact and the energy transferred to the tissues from the causative agent.

Blunt Trauma

In blunt trauma the force can be spread over a wide area. This minimizes the energy transfer at any one spot and so reduces tissue damage. After low-energy impacts, damage is usually localized to the superficial structures. In contrast, following high-energy transfer considerable tissue disruption can be produced with the clinical consequences being dependent upon the organs involved.

Penetrating Trauma

The significance of the local damage following penetrating trauma is dependent on both the site and depth of penetration. However, the degree of injury is also determined by the amount of energy transferred to surrounding tissues (see Chapter 28). It is important to remember that low-energy transfer can still produce significant clinical problems, depending on the site of penetration, e.g. a stab wound to the heart.

Blast Injuries

Following an explosion there is a sudden release of energy which leads to a very rapid rise in pressure in the surrounding air. When this band of high pressure, known as the *shock front* (or *blast wave*), hits the surface of the patient's body, a wave of deformation spreads through all the air-tissue interfaces because of their relative freedom of movement. The extent of tissue damage is directly dependent on both the magnitude and rate of onset of this deformation.

As the deformation mainly affects air-containing organs the lungs and gut are at particular risk, producing damage at the lungs' air-tissue interface and leading to the syndrome known as 'blast lung' (see Chapter 28). If it is extensive the patient becomes hypoxic (see below). High blast pressures can also lead to air emboli which may precipitate sudden death if they obstruct the coronary or cerebral arteries.

Behind the shock front comes a movement of air called the *blast wind*. As this spreads out from the epicentre, it carries with it fragments from the bomb or surrounding debris. Close to the explosion, this material will be travelling at high velocity and can produce high-energy transfer wounds.

In addition to these effects, patients may sustain further blunt trauma from surrounding structures damaged by the explosion, e.g. falling masonry.

PRIMARY SURVEY AND RESUSCITATION

The initial action plan for patients with chest trauma is the same as that described in Chapter 2 – i.e. the airway, breathing and circulation must be assessed and stabilized as quickly as possible. This takes the form of a rapid primary survey and resuscitation, followed by a more detailed secondary survey.

The aim of the primary survey and resuscitation phase is to detect and correct any immediately life-threatening condition. In chest trauma there are five such conditions:

- Tension pneumothorax
- Open chest wound
- Massive haemothorax
- Flail chest
- Cardiac tamponade

Examination

To be confident that these conditions have been found or excluded, it is important that the paramedic develops a systematic way of examining the neck and chest. Ideally, all the clothing covering the thorax should be removed so that a full inspection can be carried out. However, if this is impractical the paramedic will have to adapt to the immediate situation.

The five-point approach to examining the neck and chest

- Inspection of neck and chest
- Palpation of trachea and ribs
- Auscultation of both axillae, top and bottom
- Percussion of both axillae, top and bottom
- Checking the back: inspection, palpation, auscultation and percussion

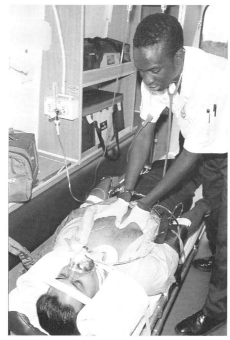

Fig. 23.1 *Palpation of the chest*

Inspection

Assuming the airway has been cleared and secured, inspect the neck for any crepitus, surgical emphysema, tracheal deviation, neck vein distension, bruising and lacerations. The last should only be inspected, and *never* probed with metal instruments or fingers because catastrophic haemorrhage can be precipitated. In all cases formal surgical exploration is required. Once the inspection and palpation has been completed, the neck can then be immobilized in a semirigid collar and the chest examined. Check the respiratory rate, depth and effort at frequent intervals. Rapid, shallow breathing and intercostal or supraclavicular indrawing are all sensitive indicators of underlying lung pathology. Inspect both sides of the chest for symmetry of movement, bruising, abrasions and penetrating wounds.

Palpation

Check the position of the trachea by palpation and note any crepitus or surgical emphysema. Then, starting at the top, palpate the clavicle and each rib to determine if there is crepitus, instability or (in the conscious patient) pain (Figure 23.1).

Auscultation

Listen in both axillae in the upper and lower half of the chest to determine if the air entry is equal. Listening over the anterior chest detects air movement in the large airways which can drown out sounds of pulmonary ventilation, particularly if any secretions are present.

Percussion

If there is a difference in auscultation, the findings on percussion of both sides of the chest should be compared. The most likely findings are either hyperresonance (pneumothorax) or dullness (fluid or contusion) on one side compared with the other.

Checking the back

It is important to assess the back quickly to determine if there is any evidence of a penetrating injury. If there is time, complete the examination by palpation, auscultation and percussion of the posterior aspect of the chest.

All trauma patients have an increased oxygen demand. Therefore, once the airway has been cleared and secured, 100% oxygen should be given at 12–15 litres per minute. The method by which oxygen can be administered depends upon your resources and the clinical state of the patient (see Chapters 4 and 5).

Life-threatening Conditions

Tension pneumothorax

If there is a breach in either the lung or chest wall, then air can be sucked into the vacuum of the pleural space and a pneumothorax created. It is important to remember that the pleural cavity and apex of the lung project above the clavicle. Consequently this can occur following penetrating injuries to the lower neck.

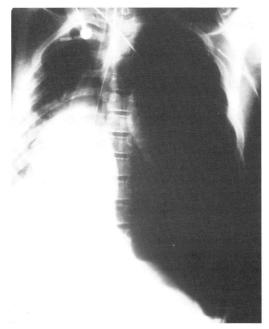

Fig. 23.2 Tension pneumothorax

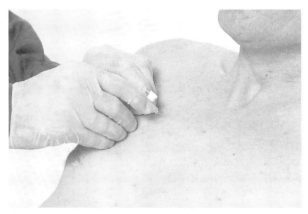

Fig. 23.3 Insertion of an intercostal needle for tension pneumothorax (needle thoracocentesis)

Following trauma, a one-way flap valve may be produced on the lung surface. This allows air to leak into the pleural cavity during inspiration, but obstructs its escape during expiration. With subsequent respiratory cycles, the volume and pressure of air in the pleural cavity increases. This causes the underlying lung to collapse and profound hypoxia to develop. Furthermore, the mediastinum is displaced towards the opposite hemithorax, impeding venous return and diminishing cardiac output. This condition is known as a *tension pneumothorax*, and is fatal if not rapidly relieved (Figure 23.2).

The characteristic signs of a tension pneumothorax are listed below. It is important to remember that this condition can develop rapidly at any stage of the resuscitation. Consequently a high index of suspicion is always required, because patients can die quickly from this condition.

Signs of a tension pneumothorax

- Rapid respiratory rate
- Decreased air entry to the hemithorax
- Hyperresonant hemithorax
- Rapid, weak pulse
- Decreasing level of consciousness
- Deviated trachea
- Raised jugular venous pulse (if no accompanying hypovolaemia)
- Cyanosis (very late)

As an emergency measure a 16 g cannula (Venflon type) connected to a 10 ml syringe should be inserted into the second intercostal space in the midclavicular line on the affected side (Figure 23.3). The aim is to decompress the chest. A rapid release of air confirms the diagnosis, following which the cannula is slid over the needle into the pleural cavity and the syringe and needle removed. The cannula should then be fixed securely in place. Even with this precaution the cannula can become dislodged from the pleural space during transfer of the patient. In such circumstances the patient will deteriorate clinically and a further needle thoracocentesis will be required. Needle thoracocentesis will give the paramedic enough time to transfer the patient rapidly to hospital. However, if this is not possible then a mobile medical team must be summoned so that a chest drain can be inserted. As the paramedic may well have to assist the doctor in such a situation, it is important to be familiar with this procedure.

Tube thoracocentesis (chest drain) Prior to the chest drain being inserted at least one large-bore peripheral venous cannula needs to be in place. Intravenous access must be available should the patient suddenly develop a significant haemorrhage during this procedure. This is most likely to happen if the chest drain releases the tamponade effect of a massive haemothorax. The patient's arm is abducted if possible and the fifth intercostal space palpated, at the level of the nipple in males. If there is an underlying rib fracture then an intercostal space immediately above or below is chosen.

The equipment used for insertion of an intercostal drain is shown in Figure 23.4. Using an aseptic technique, the patient's chest is cleaned. Local anaesthetic solution is injected into the skin and then into deeper structures anterior to the midaxillary line. Finally the needle is directed down onto the sixth rib and local anaesthetic solution is injected onto its periosteum and over its superior surface into the underlying pleura. A 3 cm transverse incision is then made down to the sixth rib, through the anaesthetized area.

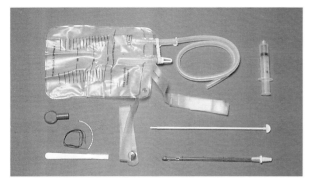

Fig. 23.4 *Equipment for the insertion of an intercostal drain*

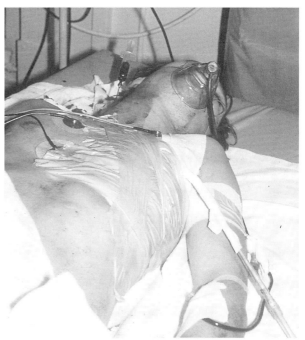

Fig. 23.5 *An intercostal drain* in situ

Using a clamp, the intercostal muscle layers are opened in a cruciate fashion, the pleura above the rib breached and a track formed perpendicular to the skin. The doctor then inserts a finger through the incision and sweeps around the intrapleural space to detect the presence of intrathoracic bowel from a ruptured diaphragm, or lung adhesions. If adhesions prevent the passage of a finger, then a fresh incision should be made in the fourth or sixth intercostal space, just anterior to the midaxillary line.

The chest drain is inserted into the incision and directed, if necessary, with the curved clamp. It is then connected to an appropriate drainage set and the clamps removed. The chest drain must be secured, with both suture and tape. The incision is covered with gauze and tape (Figure 23.5).

Once a chest drain has been inserted, the patient's chest needs to be re-examined to ensure the lung is now ventilating. Kinking, clogging with blood, or displacement of the chest drain may cause a recurrence of the initial symptoms and signs. The insertion of a chest drain should be done by trained staff because it can give rise to several complications if it is performed incorrectly. The main complications are:

- Bleeding
- Damage to the intercostal vessels and nerves
- Lung and mediastinal injury
- Damage to abdominal organs and vessels
- Infection
- Allergic reactions

Open chest wound

An open chest wound will automatically produce an open pneumothorax on the same side. In addition, if the wound is greater than two-thirds the diameter of the trachea then air preferentially enters the chest through this hole during inspiration ('sucking' chest wound). This causes failure of ventilation of the lung which eventually collapses. A particularly danger-ous situation is when the wound or an inadequately applied dressing acts as a one-way valve and air can enter the chest via the hole but not escape: this gives rise to a tension pneumothorax. The immediate management of an open chest wound is to apply a sterile dressing, sealed on three sides. Air can then escape via the free edge during expiration, but cannot enter through the wound during inspiration because the dressing is sucked against the wound. The primary survey can then be completed and the patient transferred to hospital where a chest drain is inserted via a freshly created incision. If a tension pneumothorax develops, any occluding dressing must be removed, thereby opening the wound and allowing air to escape. This is more effective than simply inserting a cannula into the chest because the hole will be wider than the cannula and so will produce a more rapid decompression.

Massive haemothorax

When blood collects in the pleural cavity it is called a haemo-thorax. Following trauma this is usually caused by tearing of vascular structures. A massive haemothorax is defined as the presence of more than 1.5 litres of blood in the chest cavity; it usually results from laceration of either an intercostal vessel or the internal mammary artery.

The physical signs are listed below. Many of these patients will require early surgery if they are to survive. In the meantime you should continue to resuscitate the patient with colloid or blood (if available), complete the rest of the primary survey and rapidly transfer the patient to hospital.

Signs of a massive haemothorax

- Decreased air entry on the affected side
- Dull percussion note over the affected side
- Shock, grade II or III (Chapter 20)
- Jugular venous pulse usually low

Flail chest

Flail chest occurs when two or more ribs are fractured in two or more places, or when the clavicle and first rib are fractured

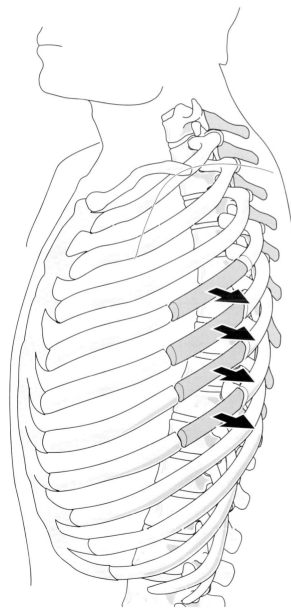

Fig. 23.6 *Flail chest*

(Figure 23.6). Normally the chest moves out during inspiration and in with expiration. When a rib is fractured in two places the middle section can move independently from the relatively fixed end pieces and tends to be drawn in during inspiration and pushed out in expiration. This is known as *paradoxical movement*. Shortly after trauma, this type of movement will only be evident if there is either a large flail chest (over five ribs) or a central flail (multiple bilateral costochondral fractures with a flail sternum). More commonly the spasm of the chest wall musculature is sufficient to splint the flail segment and mask paradoxical movement. However, this spasm leads to an increased energy expenditure for breathing. Consequently, after a time the intercostal muscles become fatigued and the abnormal chest movement becomes apparent. A flail segment can be a life-threatening condition, mainly because of the underlying pulmonary contusion (see later) which adds greatly to the hypoxia already produced as a result of the impaired breathing.

These patients must be managed in such a way that their hypoxia is corrected. In the majority of cases this will require immediate evacuation so that high-flow, warm, humidified oxygen can be administered. While awaiting this, continue to monitor the patient for signs indicating either the development of a tension pneumothorax or that intubation and ventilation are required to prevent further deterioration. These warning signs include:

- Exhaustion
- Respiratory rate greater than 30/minute
- Significant associated injuries of the abdomen and head
- Pulse oximeter reading of 85% on air
- Pulse oximeter reading of 90% with supplemental oxygen

Manual immobilization of the flail segment by direct pressure may be beneficial.

Cardiac tamponade

The heart is covered with a tough, elastic fibrous sac called the *pericardium*. A small collection of blood within the pericardium will constrict the heart, compromising ventricular filling and hence cardiac output. Paradoxically, the jugular venous pulse (JVP) may be raised because of the impaired venous return to the right side of the heart. This condition is known as *cardiac tamponade* and usually follows penetrating chest wound within the anatomical area indicated in Figure 23.7.

In all cases an urgent thoracotomy is necessary if the patient is to survive: rapid transfer to hospital is essential.

Monitoring the Patient

At the end of the primary survey and resuscitation phase it is essential that the life-threatening problems involving the airway, breathing and circulatory systems have been identified and managed appropriately. A policy of continual vigilance is essen-

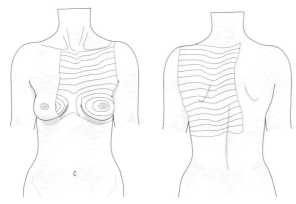

Fig. 23.7 *Penetrating wounds in the area indicated may result in cardiac tamponade. From Landon, B, Driscoll, P and Goodall, J (1994) An Atlas of Trauma Management: The First Hour, with permission from Parthenon Publishing Group*

tial in patients with thoracic trauma because serious problems may not only be present immediately, but may develop at any time during resuscitation or transfer. If a patient's condition does deteriorate, then a reassessment must be carried out beginning with the airway in the manner described in Chapter 2 and continuing with assessment of the breathing and circulation.

When available, an automatic blood pressure, pulse oximeter and ECG monitor can be used for frequent measurements of the patient's vital signs. The absence of these devices or their unreliability during transportation will require the person in charge of the patient to record and document the patient's respiratory rate, blood pressure, pulse, skin perfusion and conscious level.

SECONDARY SURVEY

The secondary survey involves a detailed head-to-toe examination as described in Chapter 19.

Acceleration and deceleration forces can produce extensive intrathoracic injuries.

Potentially life-threatening thoracic conditions

- Pulmonary contusion
- Cardiac contusion
- Ruptured diaphragm
- Dissecting aorta
- Oesophageal rupture
- Ruptured bronchi

Clues to the existence of these injuries are given by the presence of marks on the chest wall which should lead you to consider particular types of injury. For example, the diagonal seat-belt bruise may overlap a fractured clavicle, a thoracic aortic tear, pulmonary contusion or pancreatic laceration.

Unlike the thoracic problems detected during the primary survey, these conditions cannot be immediately corrected or their presence easily confirmed. This is true whether you are working in the accident and emergency department or in the field. Their discovery does indicate the need for urgent evacuation for specialized surgical treatment. Therefore, knowledge of the mechanism of the injury and a detailed physical examination are essential for early detection of these conditions.

During the secondary survey, the chest wall must be inspected more closely for bruising, signs of obstruction, asymmetry of movement and wounds. Palpate the sternum and each rib. The presence of any crepitus, tenderness or subcutaneous emphysema must be noted. If feasible, auscultation and percussion of the whole chest should be done to determine if there is any asymmetry between the right and left sides of the chest.

Examination of the back of the chest is important but it will require sufficient people to enable the patient to be log-rolled safely onto his or her side. In the accident and emergency department this procedure is usually deferred until the end of the secondary survey when the whole of the back (i.e. head to heels) is examined. However, if there is evidence of a posterior penetrating injury, e.g. blood staining on the clothing or floor, then the victim's back *must* be inspected at the earliest opportunity. *In doing so as much care as possible must be taken in stabilizing the vertebral column*, especially in patients with neurological deficit or pain over the spine, or where there is blunt injury anywhere above the level of the clavicles.

Life-threatening Conditions

Pulmonary contusion

Pulmonary contusion represents one of the most common causes of death following thoracic trauma, and usually follows a blunt injury in which energy is transmitted to the underlying lung tissue. It results in an increase in the permeability of the small pulmonary capillaries leading to fluid collecting both inside the alveoli (alveolar oedema), as well as in the surrounding connective tissue (interstitial oedema). As a result, the affected lung area becomes more stiff (or less compliant), and less air is drawn into the lungs with each breath. This, in turn, leads to further hypoxia and additional tissue damage.

As the lungs become 'stiff', the effort required by the patient to inflate them increases. The tidal volume decreases, and initially the respiratory rate increases to try to maintain alveolar ventilation. As the patient becomes exhausted from the increased effort of breathing, the respiratory rate falls and ventilation is reduced leading to progressive hypoxia. In addition, infection frequently develops in the contused area at a later stage if the patient survives.

On examination respiration is often rapid and shallow, and there may be tenderness or marks on the chest wall due to the original injury. Overlying fractured ribs may be present, but in children the natural elasticity of the chest wall may prevent this. Auscultation can be normal. As the disease process develops the respiratory distress increases and ventilation becomes progressively more difficult. However, *the most significant sign is slowing of the respiratory rate*, suggesting that the patient is exhausted.

The risk of pulmonary oedema resulting from overtransfusion is well recognized in these patients. What is less known is the deleterious effect of undertransfusion. This leads to a fall in the cardiac output and, in turn, a reduction in the pulmonary perfusion. The hypoxia that results leads to further damage to the alveolar membrane and the process becomes self-perpetuating. Invasive monitoring (using a Swan-Ganz pulmonary artery catheter) is usually required to determine the appropriate fluid requirements. If this condition is identified in the field, immediate transfer to hospital is necessary. In the meantime the paramedic should manage the patient in the manner described for a flail chest to optimize oxygenation and reduce the work of ventilation.

Cardiac contusion

In cardiac contusion there is bleeding into the wall of the heart following blunt trauma to the chest. It can lead to myocardial dysfunction or, occasionally, coronary artery occlusion giving rise to further myocardial damage.

On examination the patient may have sternal bruising and tenderness due to the force of the impact. There is also an association between cardiac contusions and fractures of the sternum, or wedge fractures of the thoracic vertebrae. Should the contusion be significant then the patient may develop arrhythmias (an abnormal pulse), heart failure or hypotension which do not respond to resuscitation.

Ruptured diaphragm

Ruptured diaphragm can result from either blunt or penetrating trauma. In the latter case 75% are associated with intra-abdominal injury. The reason for this is that during expiration, the diaphragm is elevated and the lower seven ribs overlie the abdominal cavity. Therefore a penetrating wound in this area may enter the peritoneal cavity as well as causing pulmonary injury. Furthermore, a fracture of these ribs can be associated with injury to the underlying liver (10%) and spleen (20%).

> **Injuries between the nipple line and the umbilicus should be considered an indicator of potential underlying chest damage as well as abdominal damage**

On examination of the patient, suspicion should be raised if a wound is found between the fifth and the twelfth ribs. The patient may be breathless and have decreased breath sounds over the lower aspect of the affected side. Occasionally bowel sounds can be heard on auscultation of the chest.

This condition requires early surgical treatment. If it is suspected, immediate evacuation is required.

Disruption of the thoracic aorta

In patients who have sustained rapid deceleration (e.g. a fall from a great height or a car crash at high speed), movement occurs between the fixed and mobile parts of the thoracic aorta. If only the inner two layers of the aorta are torn, blood escapes but is contained by the third outer layer (10% of cases). If this outer layer is also breached in the injury then the patient rapidly exsanguinates at the scene of the incident (90% of cases). In the 10% who survive the initial accident, only around 500 ml of blood will be lost from the systemic circulation. Consequently the patient will not demonstrate the characteristic signs of shock (providing there are no other sources of haemorrhage). Variable signs which may be present are hoarseness of the voice (caused by pressure on the recurrent laryngeal nerve from the expanding haematoma), upper limb hypertension, and pulse differences between upper and lower limbs.

If these patients are to survive then the aorta needs to be surgically repaired before the outer layer ruptures. Time is crucial, because half the immediate survivors will die each day if no operation is performed. Therefore *immediate transfer to hospital is required if this condition is suspected*.

Oesophageal rupture

Following a severe blow to the epigastrium, gastric contents are forced into the lower oesophagus and may tear it. Penetrating trauma can also rupture the oesophagus at any level, and is likely to be associated with injuries to neighbouring structures.

On examination the patient has a degree of shock and pain greater than that due to the apparent injuries. Surgical emphysema in the neck and upper chest may develop with time. Suspicion should be further raised if there is a left pneumothorax (or pleural effusion) without a history of left chest trauma or fractured ribs on the left side.

These patients will require further investigations and in almost all cases a surgical repair.

Ruptured bronchi

The main bronchi are firmly anchored and so are unable to move when the body is subjected to rapid deceleration forces. A tear can be partial or complete and is associated with a high mortality rate (30%), owing to the other injuries which occur following rapid deceleration.

On examination there may be haemoptysis, surgical emphysema, a pneumothorax and overt signs of a chest injury. If intubation of the trachea is attempted (for another reason), then it may be technically difficult or impossible to perform.

As these patients require the expertise of a thoracic surgeon for their definitive management, immediate evacuation from the scene of the incident is required.

Non-life-threatening Conditions

Thoracic injuries that are not life-threatening conditions are listed over.

Non-life-threatening thoracic injuries

- Simple or closed pneumothorax
- Fractured sternum
- Fractured ribs
- Surgical emphysema

Simple or closed pneumothorax occurs when air enters the pleural space through a tear in the lung secondary to blunt trauma. The most likely agent is the sharp end of a fractured rib. Simple pneumothorax may be difficult to detect clinically, requiring an X-ray for diagnosis. The clinical signs are reduced expansion, air entry and breath sounds, and hyperresonance to percussion, although these will vary according to the size of the pneumothorax. *The trachea is not deviated.*

Fracture of the sternum (see Chapter 25) is common in frontal impacts and may be associated with seat-belt injuries; localized pain and tenderness is characteristic.

Fractured ribs (see Chapter 25) are common and may be due to both direct and indirect forces. Although not life-threatening, they are extremely painful, and each individual fracture can be associated with the loss of 150 ml of blood. The pain from rib fractures can be improved by manual stabilization and patient positioning.

Surgical emphysema results from leakage of air into the subcutaneous tissues; it may result from either penetrating chest injury or more commonly blunt trauma. Severe surgical emphysema is associated with major airway disruption; minor surgical emphysema is not a life-threatening problem.

TRANSFER

Transfer is a particularly dangerous time for the patient, therefore great care must be taken to anticipate and minimize any potential problems. Where other injuries permit, the patient should be transferred sitting up.

Assessment

Oxygen should be provided during transfer and all cannulae, tubes and drains must be secured with the knowledge that if they *can* fall out, they *will* fall out!

Monitoring

Monitoring will ensure that ventilation and tissue perfusion is adequate. As a minimum, an ECG monitor, automatic blood pressure recorder and pulse oximeter are essential.

Analgesia in Chest Injuries

Nitrous oxide and oxygen inhalation (Entonox) is contraindicated in chest injuries not only because it will reduce the inspired oxygen to 50% but also, and most importantly, because nitrous oxide will diffuse rapidly into a simple or potential pneumothorax to produce a life-threatening tension pneumothorax.

Entonox is contraindicated in chest injuries

Transfer Personnel

During transit, the patient should be accompanied by a person trained to monitor and intervene should any problems arise. *Where possible, radio contact should be maintained between the ambulance and the receiving hospital.*

SUMMARY

Fatalities in patients with chest trauma commonly result from easily correctable hypoxia or hypovolaemia. The management of these patients therefore follows the standard 'ABC' principles. In the majority of cases, immediate transfer to hospital will be required, or help from a mobile medical team if the patient cannot be moved.

FURTHER READING

American College of Surgeons Committee on Trauma (1993) *Advanced Trauma Life Support Course for Physicians*. Chicago: American College of Surgeons.
Driscoll P, Gwinnutt C, Jimmerson C & Goodall O, eds (1994) *Trauma Resuscitation: The Team Approach*. London: Macmillan.

chapter twenty-four:

ABDOMINAL AND GENITOURINARY TRAUMA

In the UK the incidence of life-threatening abdominal and genitourinary trauma is low, accounting for just over 1% of all trauma admissions to hospital. Nevertheless, serious injury is often overlooked, particularly in the pre-hospital setting, and this results in an unacceptably high rate of morbidity and mortality. To illustrate this point, in the USA abdominal trauma is the second leading cause of preventable death. This is not due to failure to provide an acceptable standard of care. Physical signs immediately after trauma are often subtle and may even be absent initially. Signs, even when present, may be masked owing to multiple injuries. An associated head injury with alteration in conscious level or intoxication by drugs or alcohol may cause particular difficulty with diagnosis. A high index of suspicion is therefore mandatory, particularly if the mechanism of injury points to the likelihood of abdominal or genitourinary injury. In the UK the majority of injuries are the result of blunt impact following road traffic accidents, and trauma to multiple systems is the rule rather than the exception. Penetrating injury by knife, bullet or fragment, while still rare, is on the increase, particularly in urban areas.

ESSENTIAL ANATOMY

Failure to appreciate the physical extent of the abdominal cavity and the diversity of its contents is an important factor in missed or neglected injury. This is particularly important for pre-hospital personnel who have to assess patients under arduous conditions and at a time when objective signs may be absent or subtle in presentation. The abdomen has three distinct regions, the true peritoneal cavity, the retroperitoneum and the pelvis (see Chapter 15). The true peritoneal cavity has two compartments – intrathoracic and abdominal. The intrathoracic abdomen is an extensive area hidden under the lower ribs, comprising the diaphragm, liver, spleen, stomach and transverse colon. The extent of the compartment varies with respiration – in full expiration, the diaphragm may rise to the fourth intercostal space. This is important because vital structures such as the liver are at risk following lower thoracic injury, particularly penetrating injury. In the pre-hospital setting, if a wound is noted over the lower chest (below the nipple in the male) the paramedic should assume intra-abdominal injury and give a high priority to transfer to hospital, even in the absence of physical signs on abdominal examination. Obvious fractures of lower ribs also put abdominal viscera at risk and should heighten suspicion even in the absence of signs. The abdominal compartment contains the soft organs of digestion, the small and large intestines. It is a vulnerable area, protected anteriorly only by the muscles of the abdominal wall. Lying behind the abdominal compartment is the retroperitoneal space containing major blood vessels such as the inferior vena cava and the aorta, genitourinary structures, reproductive organs, pancreas and segments of the intestinal tract including part of the duodenum and colon. This is a notoriously silent area following serious injury – physical signs are masked or may be absent during the 'golden hour'. The pelvic region contains the bladder, rectum and major vessels in both sexes – in the female the uterus and vagina are present. Although protected by the bony pelvis, intrapelvic structures are prone to injury, particularly in association with pelvic fractures or penetrating injury.

MECHANISMS OF INJURY

Two mechanisms of injury exist – blunt and penetrating. Patients may present with combined injury associated with both mechanisms, a particular feature of injury following terrorist explosions or acts of war. In the majority of instances, injury results from blunt impact following a road traffic accident, sporting accident, fall or industrial accident.

Blunt Injuries

Blunt impact results in definable injury patterns, as follows.

Compression

Sudden, violent compression of the abdominal wall may dramatically raise intra-abdominal pressure leading to rupture of a bowel loop. An incorrectly fitted seat-belt is a common factor in these injuries.

Crush

Direct crush injuries occur when a viscus is injured by directly applied pressure. A common event is rupture of the retroperitoneal portion of the duodenum in bicycle accidents – the duodenum is compressed between a handlebar and the lumbar spine. The pancreas and liver are also readily injured in this way.

Shear

Shear force injuries occur when force is applied tangentially across vascular pedicles; structures at risk include the spleen, liver and small bowel mesentery. These injuries are commonly associated with sudden deceleration.

Collision

Collision injuries result typically from impact of a motor vehicle on a pedestrian. The pattern of injury will depend on the size of the victim – bumper (fender) impact on an adult usually involves the limbs and abdominal injury is relatively uncommon, but in a child the torso takes the brunt of the force and abdominal and chest injury should be assumed in the pre-hospital setting.

Ejection

Ejection from a vehicle can result in multiple injuries, including damage to the cervical spine, depending on how the casualty lands – the torso is a large target and the likelihood of abdominal injury under these circumstances is high.

Types of blunt injury

- Compression
- Crush
- Shear force
- Collision
- Ejection

Evaluation of blunt injuries

Injury from more than one mechanism is not uncommon and may on occasion be suspected from an inspection of the accident scene, referred to as 'reading the wreckage'. A head-on collision with a poorly restrained driver may result in compression injury to a bowel loop, if the driver strikes the steering column; direct injury to the abdomen (or chest) may occur and deceleration may result in tearing injury due to shear forces. The paramedic assessing the victim should not be overly concerned with making these deductions; what is important is that an injury has taken place and that the victim has a high priority for transfer to an appropriate hospital. Decision-making will be based on a high index of suspicion knowing the mechanism of injury, and supported by physical assessment (discussed later).

Penetrating Injuries

Penetrating injury is on the increase throughout the developed world and is already a particular feature of trauma in some UK inner cities.

Intra-abdominal penetration may be obvious, for example with a wound clearly visible in the anterior abdominal wall. However, penetrating objects, bullets, fragments, knives or damaged vehicle parts can reach the abdomen from the lower chest, the back, flanks, buttocks and perineum. In the case of bullets and missile fragments, the entry site may be *anywhere*, as they may travel unpredictable distances and readily deflect from their original line of flight. Be particularly wary about discounting torso penetration in any case involving ballistic missiles. Penetration into the abdominal cavity by whatever mechanism is a serious matter – the morbidity and mortality rates are high, particularly if there is a delay in recognition that injury has occurred.

Energy Transfer Factors

It is now conventional to describe penetrating injury in terms of injury caused by laceration and crushing in the path of the missile, and in terms of energy transfer to surrounding tissues (see Chapter 28). Penetration by sharp objects in road traffic accidents and stabbings, and wounding by low-velocity (usually handgun) bullets, typically result in *low-energy transfer* with the injury confined to the wound track. The outcome therefore depends on which structures lie in the path of the penetrating object. In contrast, penetration by high-velocity missiles from modern assault rifles and exploding devices is associated with *high-energy transfer*, raising the possibility of injury occurring remote from the track. In practice, this *is* rare in the UK and should not alter pre-hospital decision-making. However, low-velocity missiles may still produce high-energy transfer wounds, and vice versa. The initial assessment and resuscitation system for such patients is in no way different from resuscitation in any other trauma situation (see Chapter 28).

RECOGNITION OF INJURY

Serious trauma to abdominal structures is readily missed even in a well-equipped resuscitation room. This is particularly so following blunt impact. As many as 20% of patients with significant intra-abdominal bleeding reveal little or nothing in the way of physical signs. How, then, is it possible to avoid overlooking trauma in the challenging pre-hospital environment? The attending paramedic may have to rely on an intelligence-gathering exercise, with information gleaned from the mechanism of injury (see above), a history from the patient if possible or from others at the scene, and information from an initial clinical assessment or primary survey of the patient.

Event History

The event history may be provided by the patient, other victims or bystanders. It is frequently unavailable. A clear history from the patient is the ideal. Ask what happened. Enquire about pain, points of impact or wounds. Ask also if pain is present in the shoulders or back – referred pain from these sites may give clues to the presence of intra-abdominal bleeding or faecal spillage. Other questions may yield clues: if the patient was fully conscious and alert after the impact, but now has an altered conscious level or is unresponsive, one of the reasons may be occult intra-abdominal bleeding. Remember that head injury, drugs or alcohol, and the absence of witnesses may mean no event history is obtainable (see Chapter 18).

Initial Clinical Assessment

Start by being suspicious. Accurate assessment may be difficult because of the environment or because of entrapment. Within the limits imposed the approach should be that described in Chapter 19. There is no point in looking for signs of abdominal trauma if the airway remains in jeopardy. In the primary survey, the first indication of abdominal trauma typically arises during assessment of 'C' (circulation) of the 'ABCDE' system, when shock is found and no obvious cause is present – this is known as shock of unexplained aetiology. Another clue may be when the extent of shock is out of proportion to the observed injuries. If shock is not a particular feature and the patient is readily stabilized, the secondary survey may reveal tenderness, rebound tenderness or even rigidity. In particular, the paramedic should:

- Expose the abdomen as far as possible
- Inspect or look at the abdomen, including flanks, lower chest and pelvic region
- Palpate or feel the abdomen, including the flanks and as much of the back as possible
- Auscultate the abdomen – although this may be impractical

Wounds, bruises or abrasions should raise the level of suspicion – *remember, the paramedic is not concerned with establishing a specific diagnosis, and only needs to assess the likelihood of injury being present and arrange expeditious transport to hospital.*
The secondary survey assessment is only indicated for stable patients. Patients exhibiting shock should be taken immediately to hospital.

Pathophysiology

It may be helpful to look briefly at the pathophysiological consequences of some intra-abdominal injuries. Irrespective of the mechanism of injury, it is safe to assume that solid organs (such as liver and spleen) and vascular structures bleed, while the soft digestive organs will leak bowel contents. Bleeding, if significant, will lead to haemorrhagic shock whose onset may be rapid, dramatic and obvious; while leakage of bowel contents leads to faecal peritonitis and finally septicaemia whose onset may be more gradual and less obvious in the pre-hospital setting. Of course, both phenomena may be present and this is not unusual. Under these circumstances, signs of haemorrhagic shock present first and may mask evidence of early peritoneal soiling.

Genitourinary Trauma

Genitourinary trauma is virtually inextricable from abdominal trauma and the two are normally considered together. In general, patients suffering genitourinary trauma are managed as abdominal trauma victims. However, there are a number of points worthy of emphasis. Because the kidneys and ureters lie in the retroperitoneal space, injury is often silent and easily missed. Haematuria is *not* a constant feature. Take particular heed of patients with blunt or penetrating injury to the back and flanks, and regard bruises, contusions or areas of tenderness as significant. Injuries to the lower urinary tract may involve bladder, urethra and external genitalia and are usually more obvious, provided they are looked for. Blood at the external urinary meatus or an inability to pass urine are clear signs of injury. The lower urinary tract is also vulnerable to injury following pelvic trauma. There is little to be done in the pre-hospital setting apart from injury recognition, understanding the implications and transporting the patient to hospital as a priority.

Pelvic Fractures

Pelvic fractures are common components in multisystem injury and they should be particularly looked for. The extent of injury varies from an uncomplicated single bone injury to multiple fractures which disrupt the pelvic ring and render it unstable. The more severe pelvic fractures are usually associated with high-speed impact and should therefore be suspected from the history and mechanism of injury. From a paramedical perspective these are critical injuries to recognize. Unstable, complex pelvic injuries are associated with a very high mortality rate, principally due to uncontrolled haemorrhage.
Physical examination and extrication should be handled with great care. Stabilization of an unstable pelvis is difficult in the pre-hospital setting and it is reasonable to consider the application of military anti-shock trousers (MAST) as a splinting device. Initial management may involve massive fluid volume

replacement and should be started as early as possible. The nature of the fluid used is not critical – starting early and giving enough is! Rapid transportation to hospital is of paramount importance. Large volumes of whole blood are typically needed and some patients will continue to haemorrhage until the pelvis is stabilized by application of an external fixator.

Abdominal Trauma in Pregnancy

Trauma in pregnancy is dealt with in Chapter 49 and is not covered here in detail; however, some points specific to abdominal trauma are worth emphasizing. Remember that the pregnant uterus remains inside the protection of the bony pelvis until the 12th week of gestation and pregnancy therefore may not be obvious, particularly in an unconscious patient. After 12 weeks the uterus rises above the pelvic brim and is palpable. *The possibility of pregnancy should always be considered in a woman of childbearing age* and should be actively sought. The best possible care for the fetus is optimal care for the mother, and this must be the aim. Trauma to the abdomen in later pregnancy when the uterus is thin-walled may result in uterine rupture or placental abruption associated with significant blood loss. Signs of shock should be evident in the primary survey and appropriate action taken. Shock management must be prompt and vigorous and

the patient quickly transported to hospital. Remember the problem of postural hypotension which may require manual displacement of the uterus to the left, elevation of the right hip, or, if a spine board is available, turning the spine board and patient onto the left side during transportation.

> **The outcome for the fetus depends on how well the mother is managed**

RESUSCITATION IN THE PRE-HOSPITAL SETTING

The measures appropriate to treat patients with abdominal injuries are outlined in Chapter 19. It is important again to emphasize the need to transfer patients to the ideal setting of a modern hospital where management can be optimized. However, in certain circumstances, for example entrapment, a prolonged period of pre-hospital management may be unavoidable. Be guided by the system outlined in Chapter 19 – it provides an approach to trauma life support appropriate for all casualties.

chapter twenty-five:

BONE AND JOINT INJURIES

The human skeleton consists of over 200 bones (Figure 25.1). The functions of this skeleton include:

- Support for the numerous organs of the body
- Protection for vital organs such as the brain
- A frame which in conjunction with the muscular system allows locomotion

ANATOMY

Bones and joints can only rarely be considered in isolation. In the extremities they are intimately related to the muscles, nerves and blood vessels of the limb. The thoracic cage and vertebral column are related to the body organs of the thorax, abdomen and pelvis. Injury to the bones and joints invariably results in injury to the soft tissues.

Bones have an outer layer of compact bone called the *cortex*, which is relatively thin. The cortex is surrounded by a layer called the *periosteum*. This has been likened to the 'skin' of the bone, and contains cells that are able to divide and mature into osteoblasts which in turn form new bone. The inner layer of bone, the *medulla*, has a lattice structure of trabeculae. It contains fat and (in certain bones), the bone marrow.

Bones can be divided into groups, depending on their anatomical structure. *Long bones* include the humerus of the upper arm and the femur of the upper leg. The different parts of a typical long bone are shown in Figure 25.2.

Flat bones include the mandible and parts of the skull, which are shaped according to their function.

The soft tissues of the limb comprise:

- Vascular structures, such as arteries, arterioles, capillaries, venules, veins and lymphatics

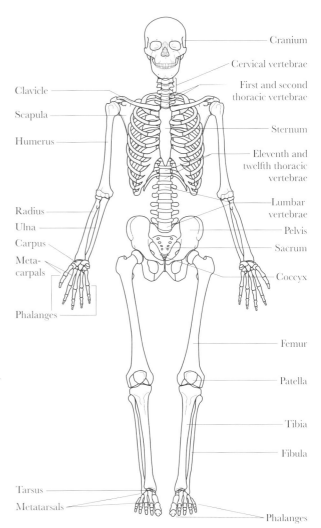

Fig. 25.1 The bony skeleton

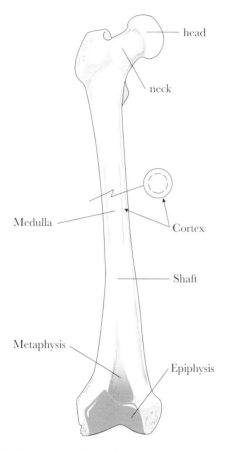

- head
- neck

Medulla

Cortex

Shaft

Metaphysis

Epiphysis

Fig. 25.2 *The anatomy of a long bone*

- Neurological structures, such as nerves (sensory, motor or mixed) and sense organs
- Muscular structures, such as muscles, tendons and ligaments
- Other soft tissue structures, such as fat , connective tissue and skin

The bones are connected to each other by articulations or joints which can be of varying type and structure. Joints can be classified as:

- Fibrous – such as the joints between the individual bones of the skull; there is little or no movement possible at such joints
- Synovial – movement can occur at these joints which have a capsule lined with a membrane called the synovium; under normal circumstances these joints contain a small quantity of synovial fluid

Joints rely on a soft tissue capsule, ligaments and to a lesser extent the tendons and muscles which cross them for their structural stability. Injury to these soft tissues may result in either dislocation or subluxation of the joint.

MECHANISM OF INJURY

Fractures

Fractures occur when the force applied to a bone exceeds its tensile strength. This can be a large force applied to a normal, healthy bone, or a moderate or even trivial force applied to a weak bone.

The deceleration forces applied to bone during a road traffic accident or a fall from a significant height can be enormous and will fracture even the healthiest bone. Bones may become weak as a result of a loss of calcium, e.g. in osteoporosis or perhaps owing to a structural abnormality such as a cyst or a tumour. Such a diseased bone may fracture even after a minimal injury, for example a simple fall in the home.

The characteristics of the force applied to the bone lead to different patterns of fractures.

Classification of fractures

Fractures may be classified in several ways.

Open and closed injuries Injuries may be *closed* (simple) if the skin and soft tissues overlying the injury are intact, or *open* (compound) if they are not (Figure 25.3). If the fracture is closed then there can be no direct contamination of the fracture site. An open fracture exists where there is a wound overlying the injury. The skin and soft tissues may be breached from the outside, perhaps from abrasion on the road surface, or a penetrating object or projectile (*compound from without*). Alternatively, open wounds may be caused directly by the ends of the fractured bone penetrating the skin (*compound from within*). The wound contamination is likely to be greater in the first category. If the fracture is open, then direct contamination may occur from clothes, street debris, bacteria (e.g. *Staphylococcus aureus*), and spores (e.g. *Clostridium tetani* which can lead to tetanus). An open fracture of a bone may lose twice as much blood as its closed counterpart.

One of the most important aims in the initial pre-hospital management of fractures is to prevent the conversion of a closed fracture into an open fracture.

Fracture anatomy After a bone has been fractured the fragments may remain in their normal anatomical relationship to one another (undisplaced), or their relative positions may change (displaced). The fragments can lie at an angle, or the ends of the bone can lose all contact with each other (offended). One fragment may rotate with respect to its normal position (malrotation). Muscle spasm may shorten the limb,

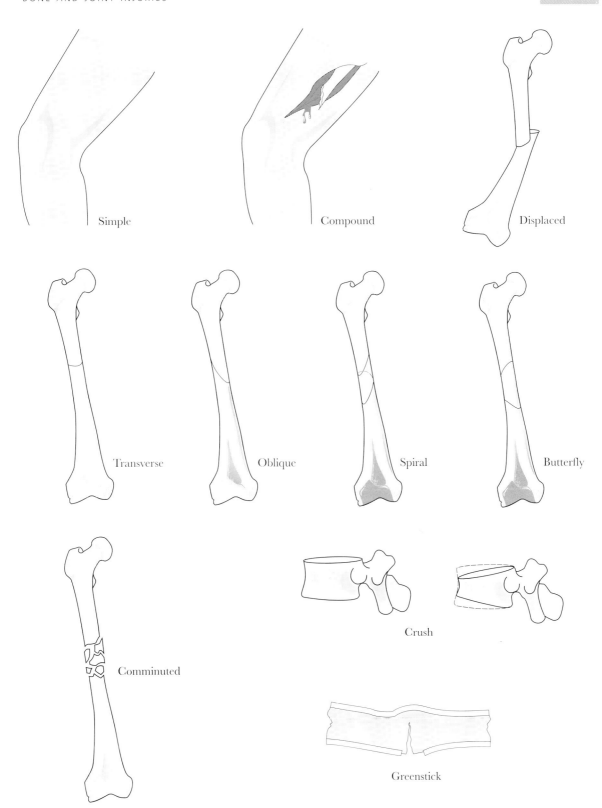

Fig. 25.3 Classification of fractures

leading to overlap of the ends of the bone, and may also lead to an increase in blood loss.

The combination of the mechanism and severity of injury, and the strength of the patient's bony skeleton, will lead to the bone breaking in different ways (Figure 25.3). When the shaft (diaphysis) of a long bone such as the tibia or humerus fractures it may do so in a simple *transverse* pattern. If the mechanism of injury includes a rotational force then the fracture may be *oblique* or even *spiral*. If this leads to the separation of a fragment of bone then this is known as a *butterfly fragment*. If the bone shatters into many pieces the fracture is said to be *comminuted*. Falls from a height or rapid vertical deceleration may lead to a *compressed* fracture, typically seen in the vertebral body. This fracture pattern may also be seen in the elderly patient with osteoporotic bone after only minimal injury, or it sometimes occurs spontaneously. Flat bones such as the skull may have simple *linear* fractures. If a complete section of bone becomes detached then it may be pushed inside the skull cavity towards the brain – a *depressed* fracture.

Fractures in children

Fractures in children need special consideration. The mechanism and precise type of injury may differ from those of adults. They should, however, be assessed and treated in the same way as similar fractures in adults. Children's bone is growing, and generally speaking the younger the patient, the more quickly the bone will heal.

Epiphyseal fractures The bones of a child have special growth plates or *epiphyses* to enable longitudinal growth. These plates consist of cartilage which divides and is then converted to bone. They are a potentially weak area in the bone and are subject to shear fractures. The fall on the outstretched hand that will produce a fracture of the distal radius in the elderly adult will lead to a fracture of the distal radial epiphysis in a skeletally immature child.

Greenstick fractures The bone of a child is not as brittle as that of an adult. Forces on that bone may cause an incomplete fracture. If one cortex of the bone is disrupted this is known as a 'torus' or buckle fracture. If one cortex and medullary bone are fractured but the other cortex is buckled but intact, the injury is known as a Greenstick fracture (Figure 25.4). Anyone who has attempted to snap a wet twig will understand how this name was derived.

Dislocations

Dislocations may occur when similar forces are placed on joints, but the soft tissue structures fail before the surrounding bone fractures.

There are some injuries where fracture and dislocation occur at the same time, e.g. posterior dislocation of the hip with a fracture of the posterior lip of the acetabulum (hip socket).

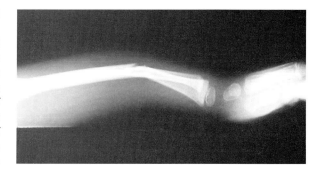

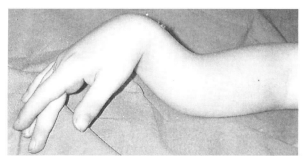

Fig. 25.4 *A greenstick fracture of the radius*

GENERAL EXAMINATION

The principles of the initial assessment and treatment of life-threatening conditions have been outlined earlier in this book. It is essential that the patient has a primary survey and that immediately life-threatening problems are recognized and treated. The majority of fractures and dislocations are not immediately life-threatening, but exceptions include fractures of the pelvis, multiple closed fractures or compound fractures of long bones, where serious haemorrhage may occur. Fractures of the skull and face may lead to airway obstruction or be associated with life-threatening neurological injuries. Fractures may coexist with injuries to the vital thoracic or abdominal organs.

Limb-threatening injuries are much more common. Many fractures and dislocations can lead to lifelong disability and thus are very important for the individual patient. Correct identification and treatment of such injuries will prevent further damage and reduce long-term disability. Injudicious handling of such injuries may result in increased long-term morbidity.

Fractures, particularly of the limbs, are usually obvious and cause the patient great discomfort. Life-threatening chest, head and abdominal injuries may not be so obvious. It is essential to avoid the temptation to concentrate on the most obvious injuries. Only when life-threatening injuries have been excluded or treated should limb injuries be assessed. The multiply injured patient may require immediate transfer to hospital *without* full assessment or treatment of such injuries. These decisions ('judgement calls') in the field can be difficult, but a common-sense approach based on a proficient primary survey is above criticism.

Examination of bones and joint must be systematic if injuries are to be identified. The system advocated by Apley is simple and easy to master, and can be applied in the pre-hospital setting: this is the *'look'* – *'feel'* – *'move'* system.

- **Look** – the part should be inspected for swelling, deformity and overlying wounds. Are there any pre-existing scars? Compare with the normal side
- **Feel** – is the injured part painful, and if so, where? Is there any protective muscle spasm? Are the pulses distal to the injury intact?
- **Move** – can the patient move the injured part? If there is a fracture then the sensation of grating of the bone ends may be experienced ('crepitus'). *This is extremely painful for the patient and deliberate attempts to elicit crepitus should be avoided*

It is essential that all patients who have sustained limb injuries are assessed for vascular injury. The palpation of a distal pulse alone is not sufficient. In the early phase of a compartment syndrome the arterial pressure may be sufficient to produce a pulse, while the tissue pressure is such that there is no effective perfusion of the cells. It is important to assess capillary refill in order to assess tissue perfusion. The nail bed is compressed for 5 seconds. The pressure is released and the time taken for the return of the normal pink colour is measured. If this is greater than 2 seconds (approximately the length of time it takes to say 'capillary refill') then tissue perfusion is abnormal. The capillary refill test is best performed in good light and a warm environment.

A neurological assessment of sensation and muscle power should be made in order to determine any nerve damage.

GENERAL TREATMENT CONSIDERATIONS

Priorities

Life-threatening conditions must be sought and treated where necessary. Perform a primary survey, and treat life-threatening injuries before treating any fractures or dislocations. The priorities in fracture management are:

- Safety
- Airway and cervical spine control
- Breathing
- Circulation and haemorrhage control
- Disability
- Exposure

The patient's history of tetanus immunization must be elicited, along with the features of the 'AMPLE' history (see Chapter 7). All patients who have sustained a long-bone injury should be given oxygen via a Hudson mask with a non-rebreathe valve and a reservoir bag at a rate of 15 l/min.

> All patients who have a long-bone injury require oxygen

Unnecessary delay at the scene must be avoided. The more serious the injury, the more important this is. If pre-hospital treatment is contemplated, will it stabilize or improve the patient's condition? If not, then early evacuation to hospital is imperative. If a patient is less than 20 minutes' journey from an appropriate hospital and is not trapped, an intravenous infusion should not be attempted at the scene, but performed *en route* to hospital.

A succinct history, including the mechanism of injury, and brief but accurate records will ensure efficient transfer of the patient to the care of hospital staff.

Analgesia

Pain relief (analgesia) is of prime importance. It can be justified on humane grounds alone, but there is an increasing amount of evidence that adequate pain relief lessens the potential serious complications from major injury.

> Splinting a fracture or dislocation to prevent movement of the injured part is one of the best and simplest forms of pain relief

Most ambulances carry a 50/50 mixture of oxygen and nitrous oxide (Entonox, popularly called 'laughing gas'). It is used as the basis for pain relief in most gaseous anaesthetics administered by anaesthetists in hospital. It has excellent pain-relieving properties and if used properly will be sufficient for most situations out of hospital. It should *not* be used if there is any suspicion of a pneumothorax. It is best avoided in head injuries. It is excellent for fractures and dislocations sustained as sports injuries.

An increasing number of ambulance services are carrying non-steroidal anti-inflammatory drugs in an injectable form. It is still unclear whether these are an effective adjunct to pre-hospital treatment.

The types of analgesic agent carried and the indications for their use are variable, and beyond the scope of this chapter. Close study of local rules and protocols, and adequate practical training, are essential before the paramedic administers any analgesia to a patient.

Compound Fractures and Serious Wounds

Infection of a fracture is a disaster for the patient. Osteomyelitis can be controlled, but rarely cured. Good wound care starting at the scene of an accident will help reduce the incidence of this complication of compound fractures.

The fracture must be stabilized to avoid further damage to the soft tissues. Some form of manual immobilization or splinting is required. Traction splinting will reduce blood loss, but must not be applied excessively if traction injuries to the nerves are to be avoided.

The wound should be covered in a sterile dressing, soaked in 0.9% saline or aqueous iodine solution. Life-threatening bleeding should be controlled by direct pressure.

Splinting

Adequate splintage of a fractured limb (Figure 25.5) will result in analgesia, reduce blood loss, and will decrease the chances of further damage occurring to the soft tissues during transfer to hospital.

There is no substitute for practical experience of splintage tech-niques, which cannot be learned from a book. Generally splin-tage can be divided into two categories: simple splintage, and traction splintage.

Simple splintage

Simple splintage of the lower limb may be achieved by secure-ly fastening the injured part to the opposite uninjured leg using triangular bandages, or a purpose-built splint. Alternatively, the limb may be placed in a box splint which should be well padded, and should be of the appropriate size for the injured limb. Vacuum splints can also be effective. With the injured upper limb it is often sufficient to immobilize using a simple broad arm sling, or allow the patient to support the arm with the uninjured hand.

Traction splintage

Traction splintage is generally employed for femoral fractures. The first traction splint, the Thomas splint, was used extensive-

A

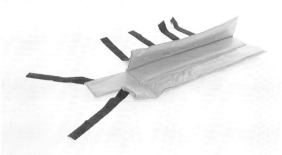

B

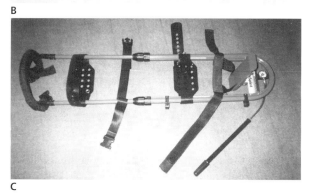

C

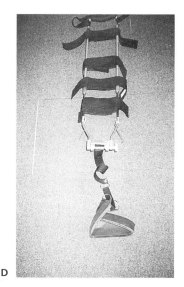

D

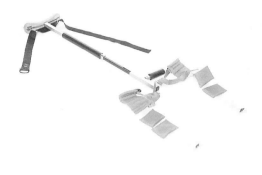

E

Fig. 25.5 Types of splint. A, inflatable splint; B, box splint, C, Donway splint, D, Hare splint; E, Sager splint

ly in the first World War and slashed the mortality rate from open fractured femurs from 80% to 20%. Modern day traction splints work on the same principle of traction at the ankle and counter-traction via a ring at the ischial tuberosity, except for the Sager splint (a padded T-bar that fits between the legs) which exerts counter-traction on the symphysis pubis. The principle is to reduce the fracture and overcome the deforming force of the surrounding muscles which are in spasm. The restoration of the normal length and shape of the limb also has the advantage of reducing blood loss (by up to 20–30%). Splints that apply traction to one (e.g. Hare, Donway, Trac-III) or both lower limbs (e.g. Sager) are effective. They can be time-consuming to apply, particularly if used infrequently. Familiarity with the splint used locally is essential. These splints are discussed in more detail in Chapter 27.

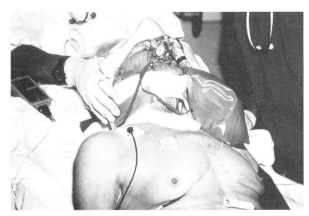

Fig. 25.6 *Cervical spine immobilization*

BONE AND JOINT INJURIES IN SPECIFIC REGIONS

Skull, Facial Skeleton and Cervical Spine

Head injuries are discussed in Chapter 21. Patients who have sustained a fracture to the skull or facial bones have sustained a serious head injury and must be treated with extreme caution. The airway may be compromised either directly owing to instability of the facial skeleton (e.g. an unstable fracture of the mandible) or owing to secondary factors such as swelling, bleeding or unconsciousness. All head injuries should be assessed for injury to the cervical spine. These are not always symptomatic, and an altered level of consciousness may make clinical evaluation unreliable or impossible.

> There is a 5% chance of significant cervical spine injury in the unconscious patient

The airway must take priority, but all reasonable precautions to prevent cervical spine movement must be taken until a radiological and clinical assessment has been made at the hospital. A rigid cervical collar is the minimum requirement. Additional immobilization techniques will be required (Figure 25.6). A blanket placed under the head and rolled at each side, combined with secure tape applied to the stretcher or bed and the patient's forehead, will provide further security. A full spinal immobilization splint such as a Russell Extrication Device or Kendrick Extrication Device combines immobilization of the cervical spine and other areas of the vertebral column during extrication and transport to hospital (see Chapter 27). Neck braces which are combined with immobilization on a spinal board effect the most secure immobilization when properly applied (for example, the 'head box'). It must be remembered that pressure necrosis of the skin and soft tissues can be caused by even short periods on a spinal board. This is particularly true in the patient with compromised sensation, which may be a direct result of spinal injury.

Scoop stretchers are invaluable when transferring patients from the floor to a stretcher or bed. They can be adjusted to the correct length, and then divided longitudinally to allow the stretcher to be slid under the patient with minimal movement from either side before they are reconnected and the patient lifted to safety. It should be noted that they should only be used for short periods and they are designed to transfer the patient from floor to spine board. They should then be removed unless the distance to hospital is minimal.

The prevention of pressure sores by good patient care starts with the ambulance crew at the scene, and is continued during transport to hospital, in the accident and emergency department, the operating theatre and on the ward. Patient's clothing must be checked for sharp or lumpy objects such as coins or wallets as these will quickly lead to the development of pressure sores in the immobilized patient. This is particularly important in the unconscious patient.

The Upper Limb

The upper limb is suspended from the trunk by the clavicle, scapula and various muscles which include the deltoid. Forces from the distal parts of the limb are transmitted to the trunk via these bones and the muscles and ligaments which are attached to them. Following a fall the whole of the upper limb must be examined and this includes the sternoclavicular joint, the clavicle, the acromioclavicular joint and the scapula.

Fractured clavicle

Cause A fractured clavicle can be caused by a fall on the outstretched hand, or a direct blow. The forces transmitted up the upper limb may indirectly result in a fracture. Typically the fall occurs from a bicycle, a horse, or a tree in children, or from a motorcycle in adults.

Signs and symptoms Pain occurs at the site of the fracture whenever the upper limb is moved. The patient often supports the injured arm at the elbow in an attempt to reduce movement of the limb. There is usually swelling at the site of the fracture, which typically occurs at the junction of the outer (lateral) third and inner (medial) two-thirds of the bone. There may be a wound associated with the fracture.

Treatment The upper limb should be immobilized in a broad arm sling.

Potential problems Usually this is a straightforward injury to treat. The sling will often control the pain as it prevents movement at the fracture site. As with all limb injuries there is a chance of damage to important vascular and neurological structures close to the fracture site. The subclavian artery and vein are in close proximity to the clavicle, and although injury is rare it can be serious. Similarly the nerves that supply the upper limb may be injured, particularly when the fracture has been caused by direct rather than indirect force. Direct injury to this region may also result in chest injury, and the assessment must not be confined to the clavicle.

Fractured scapula
Cause A fractured scapula is usually due to a direct blow, most commonly after a fall from a motorcycle, from a blunt weapon during an assault, or accidentally during a sporting event with a stick or bat (e.g. a hockey stick). The scapula is surrounded by muscle and this is an unusual injury, considerable force being required.

Signs and symptoms Pain occurs over the site of the fracture, and may be made worse with movement of the upper limb.

Treatment Immobilization of the upper limb in a broad arm sling will reduce the discomfort.

Potential problems There may be associated injuries to the thoracic cage and ribs, and these need careful examination.

Dislocation of the sternoclavicular joint
Cause Dislocation of the sternoclavicular joint may be caused by a fall on the outstretched hand or by direct injury to the anterior aspect of the shoulder, levering the medial end of the clavicle away from its usual articulation with the manubrium of the sternum.

Signs and symptoms There is pain localized at the medial end of the clavicle, made worse by movement of the upper limb. There may be swelling and deformity over the sternoclavicular joint.

Treatment The vast majority of these injuries are subluxations or partial dislocations. They are best treated in a broad arm sling.

Potential problems Occasionally there is severe displacement. If the medial end of the clavicle has been dislocated posteriorly then the major vessels are in danger of injury. Examine the patient for signs of chest injury and shock. *If there is evidence of shock treat this as a severe, potentially life-threatening injury and evacuate to hospital immediately.* If you are able to gain intravenous access on the way to hospital then do so, but do not cause unnecessary delay.

Occasionally posterior dislocation of the sternoclavicular joint may produce airway obstruction: the clavicle should be pulled forwards, as a matter of urgency

Dislocation of the acromioclavicular joint
Cause Acromioclavicular joint dislocation occurs with a fall onto the point of the shoulder. It is a common injury in rugby football.

Signs and symptoms There will be pain situated at the lateral end of the clavicle, made worse by attempting to carry any weight with the affected arm. This injury will result from partial or complete disruption of ligaments between the clavicle and the acromion, and in severe cases also the ligaments between the clavicle and the underlying coracoid process of the scapula. There will be a variable amount of local swelling and usually a step is visible between the lateral end of the clavicle and the acromion (this is the expanded anterolateral process of the scapula which forms a bony roof over the shoulder joint and muscles, and normally articulates with the clavicle).

Treatment The upper limb should be immobilized in a broad arm sling.

Potential problems The mechanism of injury should lead to a high level of suspicion of associated injuries to the cervical spine and nerves in the brachial plexus.

Anterior dislocation of the shoulder
Cause Anterior dislocation (Figure 25.7) is usually caused by forced external rotation of the glenohumeral joint (the joint between the humerus and the glenoid process of the scapula). Typically this results from a fall or a mis-timed rugby tackle. If the shoulder has previously been dislocated then less force is required to produce a recurrent injury. Arm wrestling is another cause. Occasionally patients are able to dislocate their shoulder as a 'party trick'; they usually have a chronically unstable joint which dislocates without pain.

Symptoms and signs The acute injury gives rise to severe pain at the site of dislocation and protective spasm of the deltoid muscle. The patient will be supporting the forearm with the elbow flexed. The shoulder will look abnormal (square contour) compared with the other side, with a loss of the usual rounded contour. The lateral edge of the scapula may well appear prominent. It is important to assess the sensory portion

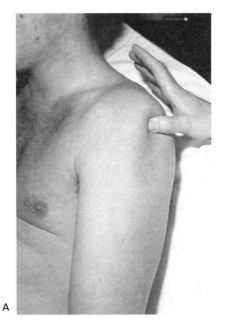

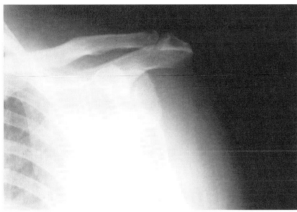

Fig. 25.7 Anterior dislocation of the shoulder: A, clinical appearance; B, X-ray

of the axillary nerve which provides sensation to the 'regimental badge' area of skin on the lateral aspect of the proximal arm. The axillary nerve winds around the neck of the humerus and may be damaged either during the dislocation of the shoulder or its reduction. The motor portion of the axillary nerve is important because it supplies much of the deltoid muscle.

Treatment Treatment should be directed at immobilizing the upper limb during transfer to hospital for relocation of the joint. An acceptable method is to allow the patient to sit upright and support the arm, perhaps resting it on a pillow. The sooner the joint is relocated the better, and at a sporting event there may a doctor present who is able to achieve this at the venue. Otherwise the patient requires assessment in the accident and emergency department. In general, it is recommended that the

shoulder is X-rayed before reduction, to exclude a fracture dislocation that requires surgical reduction.

Potential problems The longer the joint is dislocated, the more permanent damage is done to the articular surface of the bone and to the soft tissues. Damage to the axillary nerve has been mentioned above, but *all* the nerves of the upper limb can be at risk. Damage to the major blood vessels may occur and proper examination and re-examination of the distal limb circulation is essential. Severe fractures and fracture-dislocations of the surgical neck of humerus may mimic simple anterior dislocation.

Posterior dislocation of the shoulder

Cause Posterior dislocation may be caused by a fall on the outstretched hand with the arm internally rotated or a direct blow to the anterior aspect of the shoulder. An electric shock, epileptic fit or chronic muscle spasticity such as is seen in cerebral palsy can also cause posterior dislocation.

Symptoms and signs These are similar to those of anterior dislocation, with pain, swelling and local deformity.

Treatment The arm should be immobilized and the patient transported to hospital.

Potential problems The nerves in the brachial plexus are particularly susceptible to damage due to pressure of the humeral head. Recognition and early relocation are essential. The X-ray changes are very subtle, and this injury can be easily missed in hospital.

Inferior dislocation of the shoulder

Cause Inferior dislocation is extremely rare but can follow a violent convulsion or an electric shock.

Symptoms and signs The arm is held extended above the head, and the injury is extremely painful. The condition is often bilateral.

Treatment Provide analgesia and support during the transfer to the hospital.

Potential problems Fitting the patient onto the stretcher may be difficult.

Fracture of the proximal humerus

Cause A fracture of the proximal humerus (Figure 25.8) may occur through a fall onto the outstretched hand, or a direct fall onto the upper arm, particularly in elderly patients and those with osteoporosis. The fracture can occur in younger patients in violent injuries.

Symptoms and signs There is pain at the upper end of the

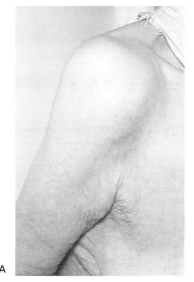

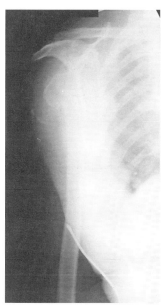

Fig. 25.8 *Fracture of the humerus: A, clinical appearance; B, X-ray*

arm. The patient will usually be supporting the arm at the elbow with the other hand. There may be obvious deformity. Swelling is almost immediate, but the severe bruising which accompanies this injury may not be apparent for several days and can track distally down the lateral aspect of the arm. In the younger group of patients who have sustained this fracture as a result of extreme violence care should be taken to fully assess for life-threatening injuries.

Treatment The arm is supported in a broad arm sling initially. Once the diagnosis has been confirmed in the accident and emergency department, the sling should be changed to a 'collar and cuff'. This allows the weight of the arm to apply traction to the fracture and tends to reduce the fractured bone into its normal anatomical position.

Potential problems As with all fractures, the surrounding nerves and blood vessels can be injured directly at the time of the fracture.

Fracture of the shaft of the humerus

Cause The shaft of the humerus may be fractured through direct injury such as a fall onto the arm, or a blow from a blunt weapon. Indirect force can cause these fractures, although the fracture pattern may be different. A fall onto the outstretched hand often results in internal or external rotation at the shoulder – the forearm acts as a long lever and thus the humeral shaft is subjected to significant rotational forces. A spiral fracture is therefore common.

Symptoms and signs The arm is painful and may be supported at the elbow by the other hand. There may be obvious angular deformity, but rotational malalignment is not always obvious. There may be significant swelling and bruising. It is essential to examine the distal portions of the limb to exclude vascular and neurological injury.

Treatment The arm should be supported in a broad arm sling.

Potential problems The radial nerve runs in a groove, closely applied to the humeral shaft posteriorly. It may be damaged directly, or secondarily due to swelling (*compartment syndrome*). Loss of radial nerve function may lead to weakness of the muscles that extend the wrist, i.e. the patient will demonstrate 'wrist drop' (inability to extend the wrist). The arterial blood supply to the upper limb is via just one vessel at this point, the brachial artery. This artery may suffer direct injury, or may be constricted owing to a compartment syndrome.

Treatment The arm should be immobilized in a broad arm sling.

Supracondylar fracture of the humerus

Cause Supracondylar fractures of the distal portion of the humerus just proximal to the elbow joint are common in childhood. They are typically caused by a fall onto the outstretched hand. The fractures can range from an undisplaced crack, to a completely displaced injury with vascular and neurological damage.

Symptoms and signs There is pain at the elbow after a fall. The child will support the elbow with the other hand. There may be obvious swelling and deformity. There may be serious interference with the blood supply to the distal part of the limb.

Treatment The arm should be immobilized in a broad arm sling in slight extension. Constant evaluation of the distal circulation is essential. If the circulation is compromised the elbow should be extended (straightened).

Potential problems The brachial artery can be kinked over the bone ends, trapped between the bone ends, or directly damaged by the fracture. If the circulation to the distal forearm is not restored then there is real danger of Volkmann's ischaemic contracture (the death of all the muscle in the forearm), leaving a contracted, painful, useless arm. This can also be the result of compartment syndrome caused by swelling after this injury. Volkmann's contracture is a serious injury which often leads to long-term disability.

Fracture of the radial head

Cause Fracture of the radial head is caused by a fall on the outstretched hand.

Symptoms and signs There is pain over the lateral aspect of the forearm just distal to the elbow joint. There is often pain on rotation of the forearm (pronation and supination) and the elbow cannot be fully extended.

Treatment The arm should be placed in a broad arm sling. Once diagnosis has been confirmed at the accident and emergency department this may be replaced by a collar and cuff.

Potential problems The distal circulation should be assessed, but this injury rarely leads to complications.

Fracture of the olecranon

Cause Fracture of the olecranon (Figure 25.9) can result from a fall directly onto the elbow, or from violent contraction of the triceps muscle in an attempt to extend the elbow against resistance.

Symptoms and signs The elbow is very painful and there is considerable swelling. If the triceps tendon is still attached to the distal part of the ulna then it will still be possible to active-

ly extend the elbow, although this will be very painful. If the attachment has been pulled off, or is solely to the proximal fragment, then there can be no active extension of the elbow.

Treatment The arm is immobilized in a broad arm sling. The distal neurological and vascular status is monitored.

Potential problems The swelling may cause vascular insufficiency and compartment syndrome. There is a potential for damage to the nerves that cross the elbow joint. This is particularly true for the ulnar nerve which is closely applied to the medial side of the joint in the ulnar groove. Damage may lead to altered or lost sensation of the palmar surface of the small and ring fingers of the hand. It may also lead to loss of function of the small muscles of the hand with the exception of those that move the thumb.

Dislocation of the elbow

Cause Elbow dislocation is caused by a fall on the outstretched hand. This injury may be associated with fractures of the distal humerus and/or the proximal radius and ulna.

Symptoms and signs There is obvious deformity and gross swelling, and the injury is usually very painful. Little movement is possible and attempts to do so are exquisitely tender. There is significant risk of vascular compromise due to swelling and neurological damage due to the stretching of the nerves at the elbow.

Treatment The elbow should be immobilized in a well-padded splint. The distal circulation and neurological status require constant assessment.

Potential problems The potential for vascular and neurological complications is high and the patient is best served by rapid transfer to hospital to enable early reduction of the dislocation.

Fractures of the shafts of radius and ulna

Cause Falling on an outstretched hand may cause a fracture of both forearm bones, the radius and ulna (Figure 25.10). Direct injury such as a fall onto the forearm or a direct blow may also fracture both bones, but it is possible to fracture one or the other in isolation. If one bone is fractured there is often an associated dislocation of the proximal or distal joint between the radius and ulna. Children may fracture the radius and ulna in the midshaft region, or they may sustain a fracture involving the growth plate of the bones (epiphyseal injuries — see below).

Signs and symptoms The forearm is painful and is supported by the other hand. There may be an obvious angular deformity.

Treatment The arm requires immobilization, which is best achieved using some form of splintage. However, if this is

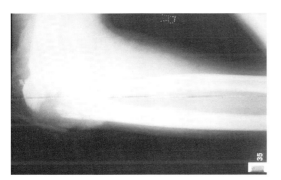

Fig. 25.9 *Fracture of the olecranon*

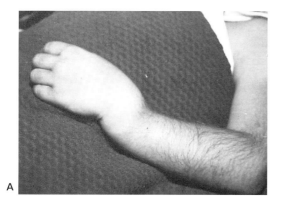

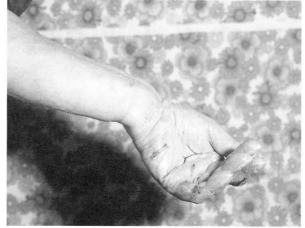

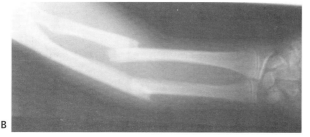

Fig. 25.10 *Fractures of the radius and ulna: A, clinical appearance; B, X-ray*

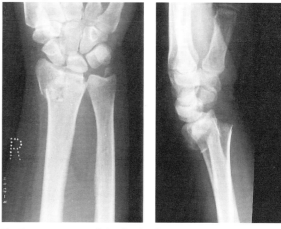

Fig. 25.11 *Fracture of the distal radius: A, clinical appearance; B, X-ray*

difficult to apply because of angulation or discomfort, then a broad arm sling may be appropriate. It is important that the sling prevents movement at the fracture site. It is also essential to ensure that it does not compromise the circulation because it is too tight. It is almost impossible to apply a splint single-handed, and attempts to do so may cause the patient unnecessary discomfort and may even increase the soft tissue damage at the fracture site.

Potential problems There is the ever-present possibility of circulatory compromise with these fractures and the distal portion of the limb must be regularly assessed. The skin and soft tissues directly overlying the fracture may be placed under tension if there is significant angulation. This may cause local skin ischaemia and necrosis. There is a real danger that closed fractures may become open if the forearm is not immobilized.

Fractures of the distal radius
Cause Fracture of the distal radius (Colles' fracture, Figure 25.11) is caused by a fall on the outstretched hand (FOOSH). This is particularly common in the elderly with osteoporotic bone. The younger age groups can also sustain fractures of the distal radius. With children the injury is usually through the soft cartilage of the growth plate of the bone, or 'epiphysis'. Young adults with mature bone may also sustain a fracture of the distal radius, but this is usually due to a highly violent injury such as a road traffic accident or serious fall, and should be taken

very seriously. This last group will often sustain fractures that extend into the surface of the wrist joint and are often displaced. The wide diversity of injuries illustrates why each distal radius fracture should be treated individually, and not just dismissed as a Colles' fracture.

If the patient falls onto the back of the wrist with the forearm supinated then the distal fragment of the fracture may be displaced towards the palmar (volar or ventral) surface. This is often known as a *Smith's fracture*.

Symptoms and signs There is pain and swelling at the wrist. If the distal fragment has been displaced dorsally there is said to be a 'dinner fork' deformity. If there is volar displacement of the fragment there is said to be a 'garden spade' deformity. There may be symptoms of nerve injury in the palm of the hand. The median nerve is situated in the midline of the wrist and enters the hand via the carpal tunnel. It supplies sensation to the palmar surfaces of the thumb, index and middle fingers and supplies the motor branches to the small muscles of the thumb. It may sustain a direct damage at the time of fracture, or it may be compressed within the carpal tunnel owing to swelling, or displacement of the fragments of the bone. The ulnar nerve may also be affected in fractures of the distal radius, but less frequently than the median nerve. The ulnar nerve supplies sensation to the little and ring fingers, and motor branches to the remainder of the small muscles of the hand.

Treatment The distal radius must be immobilized. A broad arm sling may be sufficient in some cases, but in injuries caused by violence a splint should be applied. The sensation and circulation to the hand and fingers must be monitored.

Potential problems The nerve injuries outlined above may cause symptoms. The hand must be examined to exclude vascular damage. If there is massive swelling then the hand and wrist should be elevated after the fracture has been immobilized.

Fractures of the carpal bones
Cause Fractures of the carpal bones are caused by a fall on the outstretched hand. Scaphoid fractures (the most common) are caused when the wrist is forced into hyperextension.

Symptoms and signs The wrist is painful. There may be no significant swelling.

Treatment The arm should be placed in a broad arm sling.

Potential problems If fractures of these bones are missed and not immobilized in plaster, the fracture may fail to unite and the patient will be left with a stiff wrist.

Fractures of the metacarpals and fingers
Cause Injuries to the metacarpals and fingers are usually caused by direct falls or blows.

Symptoms and signs The injured bone will be painful. There will be considerable swelling on the dorsum (back) of the hand. The palmar skin is firmly attached to the bony skeleton of the hand to allow good grip, but the dorsal skin is loose, and thus bruising and swelling track dorsally. There may be obvious bony deformity. The fifth metacarpal is most commonly broken, often as a result of a punch.

Treatment The hand should be elevated in a high arm sling.

Potential problems The blood supply to the digits may be compromised, either directly as a result of the injury, or secondary to swelling. *It is of paramount importance that rings and jewellery are removed from an injured hand as soon as is practicable. This applies to rings on uninjured digits because they will subsequently swell in any hand injury.* If it is not possible to remove them pre-hospital then their presence must be communicated to the staff in the accident and emergency department so that arrangements can be made to cut the rings off. Failure to remove rings may lead to swelling, circulatory compromise and even death of the digit.

Dislocation of the fingers
Cause Finger dislocation is usually caused by direct injury, for instance by a cricket ball.

Symptoms and signs There is obvious deformity of the joint, which is painful.

Treatment It is often said that these dislocations should be reduced quickly, without anaesthesia. This cannot be recommended. Relocation of these joints is not always straightforward, and there may be a fracture associated with the dislocation. It is better to transport the patient to the accident and emergency department where a fracture can be excluded by X-ray, and reduction performed painlessly under a ring block or other regional anaesthesia.

The Thoracic Skeleton

The injuries to organs within the chest have been outlined in Chapter 23. The following describes the bony injuries that may affect the thoracic cage.

Fractures of the ribs and flail chest
Cause Rib fractures are usually a result of direct trauma. They may be multiple.

Symptoms and signs The rib is painful. Clearly it is not possible to stop moving the injured rib without stopping breathing. Thus tenderness is experienced with each inspiratory and expiratory movement. If there have been fractures of more than one rib in more than one place then a segment of the thoracic cage may move independently of the main chest wall. This is referred to as a *flail segment* (flail chest). A flail segment will exhibit paradoxical movement, that is it will move in the *opposite* direction to the rest of the chest wall. This has significant consequences for the ventilation of the underlying lung (see Chapter 23). Patients with significant chest injuries will have an abnormal respiratory rate (usually high). This is one of the most important factors in the assessment of a severely ill patient. It is also the observation which is most usually omitted by pre-hospital care professionals, ambulance staff and doctors alike!

Record the respiratory rate and monitor changes

A fractured rib may result in blood loss of up to 150 ml. Multiple rib fractures may therefore be a significant contributory factor in hypovolaemic shock.

If the facilities for monitoring the percutaneous oxygen saturation (SpO_2) are available they should be used.

Treatment The patient must be given high-flow oxygen (15 l/min) through a mask with reservoir bag. Large flail segments may be treated by lying the patient on the injured side (remembering the cervical spine precautions) or by strapping the chest. If strapping is applied it should not be circumferential so as to restrict movement at the uninjured chest wall. In an emergency, stabilizing a flail segment with your hand can be life-saving. If the patient is shocked then an intravenous infusion should be started, but this must not delay transfer to hospital.

Fractures of the sternum

Cause Fractures of the sternum are characteristically caused when the chest strikes the steering wheel in a decelerating vehicle. The correct use of seat-belts, and more recently the deployment of air bags during an accident, will prevent many of these injuries.

Symptoms and signs There is pain in the anterior aspect of the chest. There may also be symptoms and signs of other significant chest injury (see Chapter 23).

Treatment Assume that there is also myocardial contusion. Give the patient oxygen by face mask (15 l/min through mask with reservoir bag). Monitor pulse, blood pressure, respiratory rate, ECG and oxygen saturation. Obtain intravenous access, either at the scene if this causes no delay, or on the way to hospital.

Potential problems The main problem with these fractures is not the bony injury, but contusion or bruising of the heart which lies just posterior to the sternum. This injury requires careful cardiac monitoring and observation in hospital. If cardiac arrhythmias occur they require urgent treatment.

Fractures of the thoracic and lumbar spine
These injuries are described in Chapter 26.

The Pelvis

Pelvic fractures can be relatively minor, or they can be life-threatening. A good history of the mechanism of injury is essential. The anatomy of the pelvis is shown in Figure 25.12.

MINOR PELVIC FRACTURES

Fractures of the pubic ramus
Cause The cause of a fracture of the pubic ramus is usually a fall, particularly in an elderly patient.

Symptoms and signs The patient will complain of pain in the hip. Careful elucidation of the site of the pain will reveal

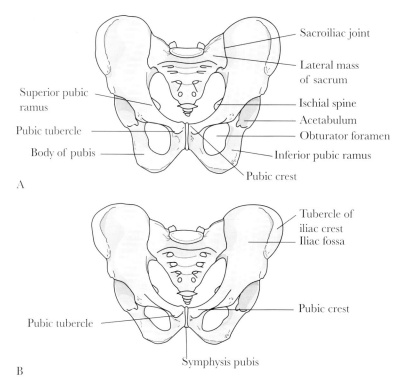

Fig. 25.12 Anatomy of the bony pelvis: A, male; B, female

that it is in fact groin pain. There is no external rotation or shortening of the leg. The patient is usually unable to walk. The injury is frequently confused with fracture of the femoral neck.

Treatment The patient requires supportive treatment and transfer to hospital.

Avulsion fracture of the pelvis

Cause Many powerful muscles have attachment to the pelvis (e.g. the hamstring muscles). Strong contraction of these, perhaps during sporting activity, may lead to an avulsion fracture (where the muscle inserts onto bone a small fragment of bone is pulled off).

Symptoms and signs The patient experiences acute pain after a muscular effort, and may be unable to stand or walk. The symptoms are similar to those of a severe pulled muscle.

Treatment The patient will need analgesia and should be transferred to hospital for assessment.

Major pelvic fractures

Cause Major pelvic fractures are usually caused by severe violence. Falls directly onto the pelvis or force transmitted down the femoral shaft are the usual causes; direct injury by a heavy weight falling on the pelvis can also be responsible. The pelvis can be considered as a ring and usually fails in at least two places. The fracture pattern is dependent on the mechanism of injury.

Symptoms and signs The patient will be in pain. There may be a leg length discrepancy in pelvic fractures with a vertical shear fracture. Major blood vessels lie on the inner pelvic surface anterior to the sacroiliac joint, and pelvic fractures can be complicated by life-threatening haemorrhage. The patient must be examined and assessed for signs of hypovolaemia. The pelvic organs are also at risk of severe injury. The male patient may have blood at the tip of his penis and swelling of the scrotum as a result of rupture of the urethra. The pregnant woman will be susceptible to uterine rupture or detachment of the placenta (abruptio placentae). She will also mask the signs of hypovolaemia because she has a proportionately greater blood volume in pregnancy.

Treatment The patient should be administered high-flow oxygen (15 l/min through a mask with reservoir). Haemorrhage can be fatal and an external fixator may need to be applied as an emergency at hospital (Figure 25.13). Although intravenous infusion and transfusion are essential pre-hospital care, it is unlikely that the paramedic will be able to keep up with the blood loss. Any delay is thus detrimental to the patient, who must be transported to hospital quickly. If it is possible the pelvis should be stabilized during transfer. This may be achieved using a Russell Extrication Device (RED) splint *reversed* so that the back

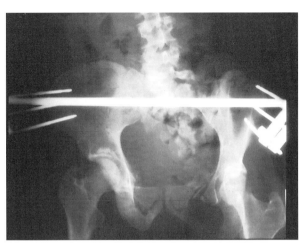

Fig. 25.13 *Pelvic external fixation and fracture*

and sides stabilize the fracture from the front; alternatively military anti-shock trousers (MAST) can be used.

Potential problems Severe hypovolaemic shock may lead to electromechanical dissociation and death. The patient may also have sustained other life-threatening injuries which must be identified and treated.

Acetabular fractures

Cause The acetabulum is the bony socket of the hip joint. It is part of the pelvis. Fractures usually occur when force is transmitted indirectly from the femoral shaft. This is a high-violence injury and follows a road traffic accident or a fall from a height. The exact injury will depend on the position of the femur. If the hip is flexed or extended then it will usually dislocate, perhaps fracturing the rim of the acetabulum. However, if the hip is in neutral then the force is transmitted directly to the acetabulum which will fracture.

Symptoms and signs The patient will be in pain which is made worse by any attempt to move the leg. The leg may be short, adducted and internally rotated (see dislocated hip, below). There may be extensive haemorrhage and thus the patient may show signs of shock.

Treatment The patient should be administered high-flow oxygen (15 l/min through a mask with reservoir). An intravenous infusion should be started if this does not delay transporting the patient to hospital. The injured leg should be supported by splinting it to the other leg.

Potential problems The patient may have sustained other life-threatening injuries which must be identified and treated. If there has been displacement of the femoral head into the pelvis then there may be severe haemorrhage and damage to other pelvic organs.

The Lower Limb

All fractures of the femur and tibia are major injuries and require thoughtful management. The patient requires high-flow oxygen, adequate splintage and analgesia, and should be expeditiously transferred to hospital with an intravenous infusion started *en route*.

Fractured neck of the femur

Cause Fracture of the neck of the femur occurs in the elderly population. A fall or twisting injury may result in this injury. Some children (often overweight adolescents) have a condition where the upper femoral growth plate slips. Minor trauma in these children may precipitate a complete slipped epiphysis which has similar signs and symptoms to fractured neck of femur.

Symptoms and signs The hip is painful. There may also be referred pain to the knee of the same side. The leg may be shorter than the normal side and may lie in external rotation (Fig 25.14). All movements of the hip joint cause pain. It is often the case with the elderly person who lives alone that the patient has been lying on the floor for some time since the injury. This increases the possibility of chest infection, pressure necrosis to the skin, and hypothermia. The elderly patient may have had some medical event to cause the fall in the first instance (e.g. myocardial infarction).

Treatment The leg should be immobilized during transfer to hospital. This is best achieved by using some form of strap or bandage to tie the injured leg to the normal one. The possibility of medical conditions or other injuries should not be forgotten.

Potential problems Access to and egress from the patient's home may be a problem. The police may be required to effect an entry. There may be difficulty getting the patient out once immobilized on a stretcher. The patient may require airway support and a primary survey is mandatory. Oxygen should be administered and if there is any suspicion of a fall with head injury, however minor, the cervical spine should be immobilized. Dehydration may require urgent treatment with intravenous infusion. Precipitating cardiac events may have led to left ventricular failure in which case intravenous infusion may worsen rather than improve the patient's condition. Hypothermia may lead to cardiac dysrhythmias. The patient should be kept warm, and the pulse, blood pressure, oxygen saturation and ECG monitored.

Dislocation of the hip

Cause Hip dislocation is caused by a high-energy injury. Typically the knee is struck when the hip is flexed, e.g. on the dashboard of a car in a high-speed road traffic accident. Posterior dislocation is the norm, and there is often an associated fracture of the lip of the acetabulum (see above). If the hip

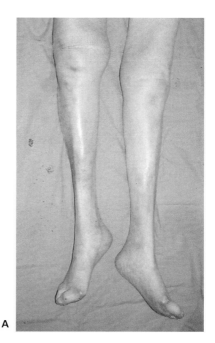

A

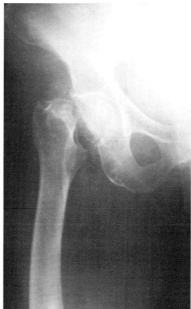

B

Fig. 25.14 *Fractured neck of femur: A, clinical appearance – note the shortened and externally rotated leg; B, X-ray*

is in the extended position at the time of injury an acetabular fracture is likely. Hip prostheses are particularly vulnerable to dislocation.

Symptoms and signs The hip is painful. There may be referred pain down the thigh and in the knee joint. The hip is held flexed and adducted, and the leg is internally rotated. There may be associated sciatica. The mechanism of injury is such that other life-threatening injuries are extremely likely, and examination should identify these urgently.

Treatment The patient should be given oxygen (15 l/min through a mask with reservoir). Cervical spine immobilization will be required. The vital signs should be measured and recorded, and appropriate treatment for other injuries instituted. An intravenous infusion should be started. It is not possible to place the femur in the normal position until reduction is performed under anaesthesia. Attempts to reduce the dislocation without anaesthesia will be fruitless, extremely painful and delay the patient at the scene. The injured leg should be immobilized by securing it to the uninjured side and the patient transported to hospital as soon as possible. The distal circulation should be monitored. Analgesia will certainly be required. If the patient is trapped then medical assistance should be requested. Intravenous drugs will probably be required in addition to Entonox, if the patient is responsive.

Potential problems The mechanism of injury is such that the patient may have multiple injuries. There is considerable disruption to the muscles and soft tissues around the hip joint, leading to haemorrhage. The patient must be monitored and treated for hypovolaemic shock where appropriate. Good analgesia is essential. The head of the femur will compress the sciatic nerve as it leaves the pelvis. This may lead to temporary or permanent damage. If the displacement of the joint is significant then the femoral vessels may become kinked and the distal circulation threatened. It can be difficult to extricate a patient with this injury, even if the vehicle damage is minimal, and good liaison with the fire and rescue services will be essential.

Fracture of the shaft of femur

Fracture of the shaft of the femur is always a major injury.

Cause Fractures of the femoral shaft are usually the result of high-energy injury, such as a road traffic accident or a fall from a height.

Symptoms and signs The exact symptoms and signs will depend on the level of the fracture. There will be pain, and usually swelling at the site of the injury. There is often some degree of deformity, which may be rotational or angular. The leg may be short. The distal circulation may be compromised. Other coexistent life-threatening injuries should be identified and treated.

Treatment The patient should receive high-flow oxygen (15 l/min through a mask with reservoir). An intravenous infusion should be started particularly if there is a delay before the patient can be transferred to hospital. Analgesia will be required – a regional nerve block (femoral nerve block) and intravenous analgesia administered by an immediate care doctor are often indicated. Some form of splintage is required: the best splintage will be afforded by a traction splint (see Chapter 27), but if this is not easily applied or unavailable then a long leg splint (box splint, lollipop splint) or splinting to the other leg will suffice.

Potential problems Hypoxia must be avoided. Other major injuries must be identified and treated. A femoral fracture may lose up to 1500 ml blood. This may be doubled in a compound injury. Monitor the signs of shock and treat with infusion. Remember that the infusion volumes achievable in hospital are far greater than those at the roadside. Minimal delay is essential. It may not be possible to immobilize a badly displaced fracture without manipulation. This should be performed with intravenous sedation and analgesia in conjunction with an immediate care doctor.

Fractures of the patella

Cause Fracture of the patella (knee-cap) may be sustained in a number of ways. The knee may strike the dashboard in a road traffic accident, or it may strike the floor in a fall. In both these situations, remember the association between fractured patella, fracture of the femoral shaft, fracture of the acetabulum of the pelvis and posterior dislocation of the hip. Alternatively, a heavy object falling on the knee may cause a patella fracture, as may violent contraction of the quadriceps tendon (which may occur for instance when a footballer kicks at the ball, expecting some resistance due to the mass of the ball, but misses, allowing unresisted contraction).

Signs and symptoms The knee is painful and swollen. There may be a laceration or abrasion over the patella. If the fracture is displaced, it is possible to feel the gap between the ends of the bone. The extensor mechanism of the knee consists of the quadriceps tendon superiorly, the patella, and the patella tendon inferiorly. The latter attaches to the tibia at the tibial tubercle which can be felt 4–5 cm below the patella. If any of these soft tissue or bony structures are disrupted then the knee cannot be extended.

Treatment The leg should be placed in a well-padded, long leg splint.

Potential problems A careful history will ensure that potentially serious associated injuries can be identified and treated.

Dislocation of the patella

Cause The patella may dislocate with minor trauma. The patient will often have experienced this injury previously.

Symptoms and signs The patella always dislocates laterally (Figure 25.15). The acute injury is usually painful. The knee

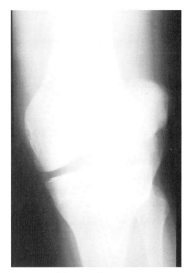

Fig. 25.15 *Dislocation of the patella*

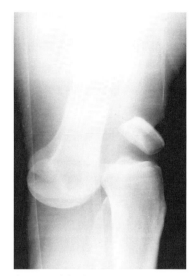

Fig. 25.16 *Dislocation of the knee*

appears abnormal with the patella located over the lateral femoral condyle. There may be swelling (effusion) inside the joint. The patient will not be able to move the joint.

Treatment Analgesia with Entonox may be sufficient to allow relocation of the patella. The important manoeuvre is to extend (straighten) the knee while pressing the knee cap medially. It will be very difficult to reduce while the knee is flexed (bent). If one attempt fails then the leg is placed in a long leg splint and the patient transported to hospital. If the patella is successfully relocated, hospital consultation is still required as the patient will need orthopaedic follow-up.

Potential problems This condition can be extremely painful and the patient may not tolerate a splint.

Dislocation of the knee

Cause Dislocation of the knee (Figure 25.16) is a serious injury which inevitably means that the majority of the ligaments of the knee have been disrupted. The vessels and nerves to the distal portion of the limb are frequently compromised. Surprisingly, this injury may result from a comparatively trivial event.

Symptoms and signs The knee will be painful and swollen. There may be significant angular deformity of the joint, although elastic recoil may have returned it to an anatomical position. The disruption of the ligaments and capsule render the joint unstable. There is a serious possibility of vascular and neurological deficit to all structures below the knee.

Treatment The vascular status must be assessed and monitored. The leg should be placed in a long leg splint.

Potential problems The joint is unstable and may have few ligamentous and capsular attachments remaining. Re-dislocation of the joint may further damage the vascular and neurological structures. When placing the leg in the splint, support the limb above and below the knee.

Soft tissue and ligament injuries to the knee joint

Cause Injuries to the ligaments of the knee joint are common, and are frequently sustained during sporting activities such as football, rugby and skiing. Damage to the menisci of the knee (commonly known as 'cartilages') can occur in isolation or in concert with such ligament injuries.

Symptoms and signs The knee will be painful. It may swell immediately (if there is bleeding into the joint, a *haemarthrosis*), or over the next 12–24 hours (an *effusion*). It is important to ascertain the exact mechanism of injury as this will help the medical staff make the diagnosis.

Treatment The leg should be immobilized in a long leg splint until a fracture has been excluded in hospital. The distal circulation should be assessed and monitored.

Potential problems The joint may be potentially unstable when severe ligament disruption has occurred and dislocation of the knee may be possible.

Fractures of the tibial plateau

Cause Fracture of the tibial plateau is caused by a large valgus force (the lower tibia is forced away from the midline) or varus force (the lower tibia is forced towards the midline) (Figure 25.17). This typically occurs when the bumper of a car strikes a pedestrian, or when a skier falls but the bindings on the skis fail to release.

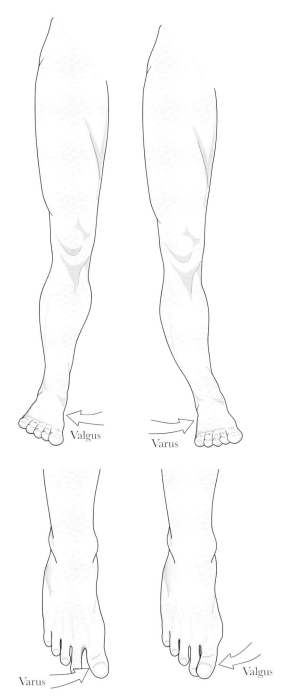

Fig. 25.17 *Varus and valgus forces*

Symptoms and signs There is pain at the knee and often a haemarthrosis (bleeding into the joint). The patient is unable to walk.

Treatment The limb is immobilized in a well-padded splint.

Potential problems Examine the patient for other major injuries. Monitor the distal circulation.

Fractures of the tibial shaft and fibula

Cause Fractures of the tibial shaft and fibula may be caused by direct injury, such as in road traffic accidents and sporting injuries. In some cases of direct injury either the tibia or fibula may be fractured in isolation. Longitudinal compression as a result of a fall may also lead to these fractures. They may also result from indirect torsional forces caused by rotation transmitted from the foot, or from the upper body if the foot is fixed. Finally the tibia may fracture as a result of completion of a pre-existing stress fracture.

Symptoms and signs There is localized pain and swelling. There may be angular or rotational deformity. The distal circulation may be compromised.

Treatment The patient should be given high-flow oxygen. This is often omitted, particularly in the young athlete. However, these injuries are serious and should be treated with the same respect as a fracture of the femur. Hypoxia is common after tibial fractures and must be avoided. Similarly, there may be considerable haemorrhage. The patient must be examined for circulatory shock, and subsequently monitored. An intravenous infusion should be started without causing undue delay in transferring the patient to hospital. The injured limb should be immobilized in a long leg splint. It may be necessary to reduce the fracture before immobilization is possible and therefore good analgesia is required. In certain circumstances it may be necessary to ask for medical assistance to allow intravenous analgesia and sedation before this can be achieved and the patient safely immobilized. Only then should the limb be subjected to gentle longitudinal traction to reverse any shortening caused by muscle spasm and overlap of bone. Once the limb is extended to its normal length the fracture is reduced to its anatomical position. Excessive traction must be avoided as this may lead to secondary injury to the vessels and nerves. Accurate fracture reduction will reduce the amount of haemorrhage at the fracture site and from the soft tissues.

Potential problems The tibia is a subcutaneous bone. It is easy to convert a simple fracture to a compound fracture by careless handling of the limb: this is inexcusable. The vascular supply of the lower parts of the limb may be compromised in several ways. Firstly, the vessels may have been directly injured at the time of the fracture. They may also sustain injury if the sharp bone ends of a displaced fracture are not effectively immobilized. The vessels may be trapped within the fracture site, and rough handling during fracture reduction may make this worse.

Compound injuries of the tibia are not uncommon,

particularly after motor-cycle accidents (Figure 25.18). These are potentially limb-threatening injuries; there is significant soft tissue damage and sometimes loss as a result of the primary injury. Wounds are often seriously contaminated.

There is a significant risk of compartment syndrome following fracture of the tibia. The muscles of the lower legs are enclosed in tough fibrous sheaths. There are four compartments: antero-lateral, medial, superficial posterior and deep posterior. If bleeding occurs into these compartments, or if there is signifi-cant swelling following a soft tissue injury, then the pressure within the compartment will rise. The risk is highest when there is a closed fracture, or a soft tissue injury such as a muscle haematoma following a kick. As the pressure rises, perfusion of the tissues and cells decreases and they are starved of oxygen. The pressure in the arteries may be high enough to allow con-tinued flow into the compartment, making the situation worse. *The presence of a palpable distal pulse does not guarantee that the tissues*

are adequately perfused. The capillary refill test must be performed to allow a more complete assessment of the vascular status of the tissues.

Fractures and dislocations of the ankle

Cause The anatomy of the ankle joint is shown in Figure 25.19. The exact pattern of fracture depends on the mecha-nism of injury, but the pre-hospital treatment is identical regardless of the fracture type. The typical history is of 'going over' on or 'twisting' the ankle, which may be combined with a fall down a kerbstone or step. These injuries are also common on the sports field. The ankle may be trapped by the foot pedals in a motor vehicle, or a fall may lead to a fracture or dislocation (Figure 25.20) of the ankle.

Symptoms and signs The ankle is extremely tender over the fracture site, and swelling occurs rapidly. Any attempt at walk-ing is very painful. There may be associated deformity. Distal nerve or vessel injury may occur.

Treatment The ankle should be immobilized in a well-padded splint – this will probably require analgesia. The neurological and vascular status of the foot must be carefully monitored. If the ankle is dislocated it requires urgent relocation. With an unstable injury, the act of splinting the joint may lead to reduction. However, reduction often requires sedation and intravenous analgesia. Unless it is impossible to effect early evacuation to hospital, this should be performed in the accident and emergency department. If rapid evacuation is not possible the services of an immediate care doctor may be needed.

Potential problems If there is significant deformity following this fracture then the skin overlying the joint can become tight-ly stretched over the bony fragments. This will quickly lead to pressure necrosis and death of that skin. Penetration of the skin converting a closed to an open injury must be avoided.

At times it can be difficult to distinguish between a fracture and a sprain of the ankle. Typically the pain and swelling of a sprain to the anterior talofibular ligament are distal and anteromedial to the lateral malleolus. Careful examination will show that there is no bony tenderness in such circumstances. However, the consequences of encouraging weight-bearing on a fractured ankle mistakenly believed to be a sprain can be significant, and so if there is any doubt in the diagnosis it is best to treat these injuries as fractures until they have been assessed at hospital.

Fractures of the talus and os calcis

Cause The talus is situated between the lower tibia (and forms part of the ankle joint) and the os calcis (heel bone). Both these bones are vulnerable to fracture as a result of falls from a height. They can also fracture when struck or trapped by foot pedals in a motor vehicle.

Symptoms and signs There is pain on attempts to walk or

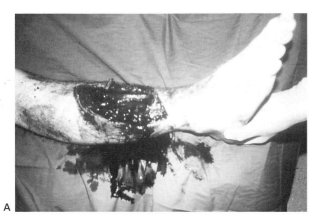

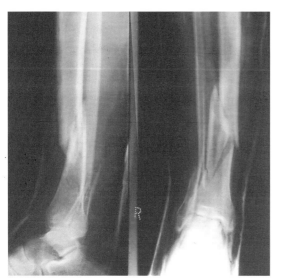

Fig. 25.18 A compound fracture of the tibia: A, clinical appearance, B, X-ray

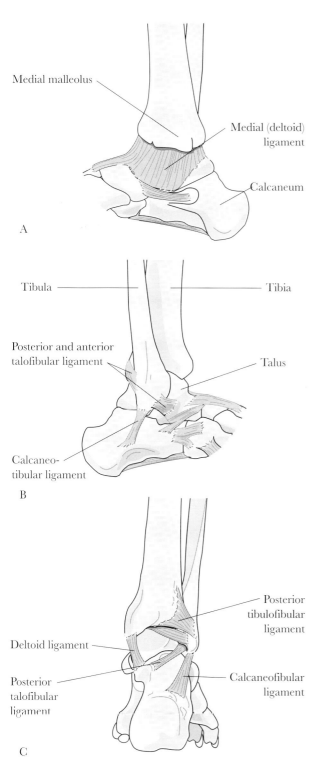

Medial malleolus

Medial (deltoid) ligament

Calcaneum

A

Tibula

Tibia

Posterior and anterior talofibular ligament

Talus

Calcaneo-tibular ligament

B

Posterior tibulofibular ligament

Deltoid ligament

Calcaneofibular ligament

Posterior talofibular ligament

C

Fig. 25.19 *Anatomy of the ankle joint: A, medial view; B, lateral view; C, posterior view*

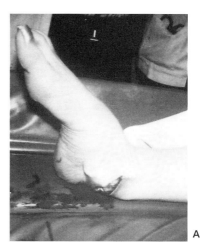

A

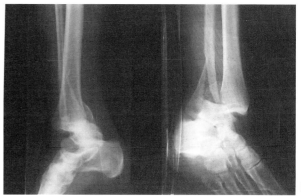

B

Fig. 25.20 *Fracture of the ankle: A, clinical appearance; B, X-ray*

on direct palpation. There may be significant deformity if these fractures are associated with dislocation of either the ankle or the midfoot joints.

Treatment The ankle and foot should be placed in a well-padded splint and elevated. The circulation to the foot should be monitored and the neurological state assessed.

Potential problems The mechanism of injury usually causes associated injuries. A fall from a height may produce fractures of the os calcis, talus, femoral neck, acetabulum and vertebrae and a thorough secondary survey is mandatory, but this will often be deferred until the patient arrives in hospital.

Dislocations of the midfoot

Cause Midfoot dislocations result from a fall from a height, landing on the foot with the toes pointing downwards.

Symptoms and signs The deformity is usually obvious, although it may be obscured by the footwear, and swelling will occur quickly. There may be associated vascular injury, either directly or indirectly, because of a compartment syndrome.

Treatment It is unlikely that the paramedic will be able to relocate the dislocation at the scene because of the pain. The foot should be placed in a well-padded splint and elevated, and the patient evacuated to hospital. The circulation to the distal part of the foot must be assessed and recorded.

Potential problems Do not forget the possibility of other associated severe injuries.

Fractures of the metatarsals and toes

Cause Fractures of the metatarsals and toes can be caused by direct blows, falls, and even by overuse (e.g. the 'march fracture' of the second metatarsal seen in army recruits unused to marching in boots). Overuse injuries will rarely present to the ambulance service as an emergency.

Symptoms and signs There is pain over the fracture which is made worse when attempting to walk. The foot swells dorsally (the top surface), an analogous situation with hand injuries.

Treatment The foot should be elevated. A splint is not always required, but when used it should be well padded.

Potential problems The main problem is swelling which may compromise the circulation, particularly of the digits.

Traumatic Amputation

A definition of major trauma is '. . . when the patient arrives at the hospital in more than one ambulance'!

There are many misconceptions about the best way in which to preserve an amputated extremity. Traumatic amputation can range from a relatively minor fingertip injury to a life-threatening avulsion of a limb (Figure 25.21). Recent improvements in microsurgical techniques have increased the possibility of reimplantation of the amputated part.

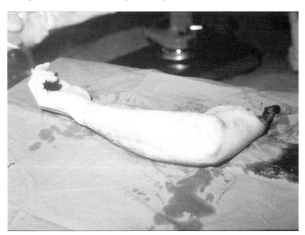

Fig. 25.21 *A traumatic amputation*

In order to minimize the damage to the amputated part, and thus improve the chances of successful surgery, the following steps should be performed.

1. The time of amputation should be recorded.
2. The amputated part should not be placed in water or directly in ice, as this can cause further cellular damage.
3. The amputated part should be securely wrapped up in a sealed plastic bag, which should be placed in a second bag, and the double-wrapped part kept cool. It is safe to place the part in an ice–water mixture after wrapping it in this way as direct contact is avoided.
4. If the patient is still trapped then the part should be clearly labelled, and sent to the receiving hospital after discussion with the medical staff who will be receiving and treating the patient.

However damaged the amputated part is, it should always be transported to hospital with the patient. Even if reimplantation is not possible, use of the skin for grafting may be considered.

COMPLICATIONS OF FRACTURES

Complications of any injury can be divided into immediate, early and late. It is not always appreciated that the quality of care given in the immediate period will influence the complication rate at *all* stages of the rehabilitation from injury. For instance, good care of a compound fracture at the scene of injury may, in conjunction with correct treatment in the hospital, prevent the long-term sequelae of osteomyelitis. Bad immediate care can be life-threatening or limb-threatening.

Immediate Complications

A simple fracture may be converted to a compound fracture by injudicious handling of the injured part. This will increase the chance of long-term complications and must be avoided. The deformity that occurs at the time of injury and any subsequent movement at the fracture site may lead to vascular damage. Such damage in the immediate phase is usually due to direct vascular injury, but at later stages indirect compromise such as compartment syndrome may result from swelling.

The direct result of the injury may also lead to neural damage. Nerves can sustain damage due to hypoxia if their blood supply is interrupted. This may be a result of direct or indirect vascular injury, or simply as a result of prolonged hypotension secondary to hypovalaemic shock.

Early Complications

Compartment syndrome has been mentioned earlier. Swelling of an injured limb or digit may lead to a situation where there is no tissue perfusion because no blood flow occurs in the capillaries. In the early stages there may be a palpable peripheral pulse but this alone is not a foolproof guide to the state of a limb's circulation. The consequences of compartment syndrome can be devastating, with the death of or injury to all the muscle groups, leaving a useless, contracted, painful limb.

Infection of a fracture is a similar disaster. Compound fractures are far more likely to become infected. Infection of bone is almost impossible to cure and the patient is committed to life-long misery with episodic relapse. If a fracture does become infected it is far less likely that it will properly unite. A compound wound must be covered as soon as is practical, and preferably with dressings soaked in aqueous iodine solution. *Conversion of a simple to a compound fracture must not be allowed to happen.*

Fat embolism is a rare condition which is still poorly understood. It can occur even after minor fractures, but the incidence seems to be greatest in the case of poorly immobilized long-bone fractures. Fat globules appear in the brain and other tissues. These may be due to a chemical change resultant from factors released due to the injury itself, rather than fat globules transported from the bone marrow direct. The consequences of fat embolism are far worse if there is coexistent hypoxia, so all fractures of long bone *must* be treated with oxygen to minimize hypoxia.

Late Complications

Infection of the bone, or *osteomyelitis*, is a complication which lasts for the patient's lifetime. Although there may be long periods when infection is dormant and the patient is symptom-free, there will always remain a possibility of recrudescence of the infection. Steps to reduce the chances of acute infection of a fracture start at the scene of the injury, and are of vital importance.

Non-union is the failure of a fracture to heal. There may be no new bone production, or there may be massive new bone production, but the functional outcome is the same. If a fracture is slow to unite then the patient must be investigated for infection as this is one of the most common causes of the condition.

Malunion describes a fracture that has united, but in the wrong position. The effects of this vary. The mobility of a normal shoulder and elbow may compensate completely for a mal-united humeral shaft fracture. Conversely, the forearm bones which rotate around each other during pronation and supination may be adversely affected by only minimal degrees of angular malunion. The accurate positioning of the ends of fractured bones is one of the highest priorities in fracture management.

Arthritis will occur early in a joint that has sustained a displaced fracture of the joint surface. The displacement only needs to be 1 mm before there are massive changes in the stresses placed on the articular cartilage. Point loading occurs and the joint rapidly wears out. This explains the importance of the accurate fixation of fractures involving the joint.

FURTHER READING

Apley AG & Solomon L (1993) *Apley's System of Orthopaedics and Fractures.* Oxford: Butterworth.

Eaton CJ (1992) *Essentials of Immediate Medical Care.* Edinburgh: Churchill Livingstone.

McRea R (1989) *Practical Fracture Treatment* 2nd edn. Edinburgh: Churchill Livingstone.

Peterson L & Renstrom P (1986) *Sports Injuries – Their Prevention and Treatment.* London: Martin Dunitz.

chapter twenty-six:

SPINAL INJURIES

This chapter is concerned with injuries to the vertebral column that produce (or have the capacity to produce) injuries to the spinal cord. There are around 500 new spinal cord injuries in the UK annually, comprising about 5% of total neck and back injuries. While relatively rare (2–3 cases per health district per year), their significance lies in the failure of the central nervous system to regenerate.

Spinal cord injury may either be complete (i.e. with no motor or sensory function below the level of injury) or incomplete (i.e. with partial preservation of sensory or motor function, or both). The incomplete cord injury has the capacity to recover in whole or part. Equally, however, it is susceptible to further injury through improper management. Complete lesions do not recover. Since 1980 the proportion of cord injuries that are incomplete has increased from under 50% to over 60%. This is partly a result of seat-belt legislation leading to reduced high-velocity blunt injuries, but much is through improved standards of patient handling and management. It has been estimated, however, that 75% of spinal cord injuries are incomplete at the moment of primary injury; so there is room for further improvement. The increase in the number of patients with an incomplete cord lesion does mean that the presentation of such patients will include some partial cord function and the attendant must be capable of recognizing this, rather than regarding incomplete function as evidence of a lack of injury.

In 50% of cases, moreover, there are associated injuries which also may require their own urgent management. Therefore, the responsibilities of those attending are threefold:

- To avoid death or disability from associated injury
- To prevent neurological deterioration or production of a neurological injury
- To prevent complications of spinal paralysis

The first two tasks are interrelated in so far as a secondary injury to the spinal cord is not exclusively due to additional movement of the vertebral column with further mechanical injury during handling. It also arises as a result of an hypoxic injury to the spinal cord through inadequately managed disturbances of ventilation and circulation. Thus, there are two parallel approaches to the stabilization of a patient with a spinal cord injury: the biomechanical stabilization of the vertebral column, and the stabilization of the pathophysiological changes to which the damaged spinal cord will be exposed.

The major source of deterioration is a lack of recognition of the potential for a spinal cord injury. It is these cases where the patient is either sat up or stood up, or is transported sitting or standing. It is important, therefore, to have a high index of suspicion based on the mechanism of injury and thereafter to manage the patient as if there was a spinal cord injury even if ultimately no such injury is discovered.

ANATOMY AND PHYSIOLOGY

The spinal column is made up of 33 vertebrae: 7 cervical, 12 thoracic, 5 lumbar and the remainder fused into the sacrum and coccyx (Figure 26.1). The first and second cervical vertebrae are specialized and are known as the *atlas* and the *axis* (Figure 26.2). Movement of the head anteroposteriorly normally occurs at the atlanto-occipital joints, and rotation of the head takes place between the first and second vertebrae about the odontoid peg. Fractures of these two vertebrae result in a widening of the canal rather than narrowing. However, fracture through the odontoid together with tearing of the ligaments that attach it to the atlas leaves a freely moving body that can cause considerable cord damage. If this occurs then neurogenic respiratory arrest followed by cardiac arrest is possible. Injuries to the first two cervical vertebrae are often associated with severe craniofacial trauma.

The remainder of the cervical vertebrae follow the normal vertebral pattern. Anteriorly lies a large load-bearing mass, the vertebral body, and the body of each vertebra is separated from the next by an intervertebral disc. The spinal canal is formed by

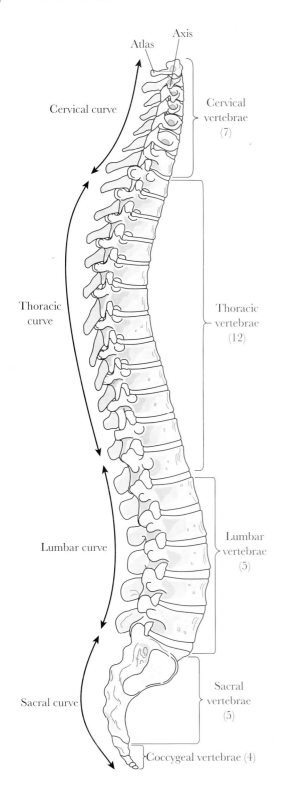

Fig. 26.1 *The spinal column*

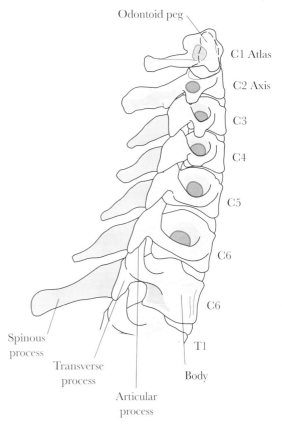

Fig. 26.2 *The cervical spine*

backward projections (pedicles) and the posterior part of the arch comprises the two laminae. Acting as muscle attachments are the three processes, the posterior spinous process and two transverse processes. Each vertebra has two articular processes superiorly which interlock with the inferior articular processes of the vertebra above, and likewise that vertebral body's inferior articular processes articulate with the superior processes (facets) of the vertebra below (Figure 26.3).

Injuries to the vertebral column can arise either by a movement of one vertebral body on another, thereby narrowing the canal, or by the vertebral body being sufficiently disrupted to allow fragments to be retropulsed into the spinal canal, causing compression.

The areas substantially at risk are the cervical spine, the thoracolumbar junction and the lumbar spine. This is partly because the natural curve of the spine in these areas is lordotic, partly because the associated muscles are weaker, and finally because in the dorsal (thoracic) spine the vertebrae articulate with the ribs (which in turn articulate with the sternum) – if the rib cage and sternum are intact, the chances of a biomechanically unstable vertebral fracture are low. Conversely, the incidence of coincident sternal fracture and vertebral fracture in motor vehicle accidents is high.

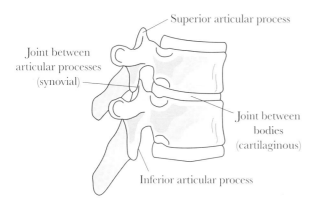

Fig. 26.3 *Thoracic vertebrae*

Movement of one vertebral body on another is prevented by strong ligaments anteriorly and posteriorly. If the posterior ligaments are ruptured by forced flexion of the spine it may then be possible for the vertebra above to move anteriorly. Likewise, a forced extension injury tears the anterior ligaments and it is then possible for the superior vertebra to glide posteriorly upon its inferior neighbour. In the process, damage may occur to the facets, or to the anterior part of the vertebral body, or to the posterior elements (Figure 26.4).

A combined anterior and posterior ligamentous injury is fortunately rare: with this injury, movement may occur despite the best immobilization techniques. Where there is only one ligamentous tear, it is unlikely that further neurological damage will occur if spinal immobilization procedures are followed.

Compression is the usual mechanism that causes retropulsion of the vertebral body. Minor degrees of compression may damage the periphery of the body, but in the more severe 'burst' injury the vertebral body fractures into fragments that can retropulse into the spinal canal.

In addition to the above mechanisms, damage to the cord may be caused by rotational forces producing ligamentous and bony damage, or by a laterally applied force. A lateral force may occur in 'side-swipe' injuries from motor vehicles. In any high-velocity impact where there is flexion and hyperextension, there may be also a rotatory component. The final mechanism is distraction, which occurs either as the result of hanging or by overdistraction of the injured spine by health-care attendants.

Spinal Cord Anatomy

The spinal cord (neuraxis) extends from the foramen magnum to L1 in the adult, and to L3 in children. The bottom end of the spinal cord is termed the *conus medullaris* (conus). The nerve roots below L1 hang down inside a sac (theca) that surrounds the whole neuraxis, and are bathed in cerebrospinal fluid. These nerve roots collectively are known as the *cauda equina*. Injuries to the cauda equina, as to the spinal cord, will cause

paralysis and sensory loss and injury to the autonomic nervous system serving the bladder, bowel and sexual function (Figure 26.4).

The nerves of the spinal cord itself are arranged in a common pattern (Figure 26.5). Posteriorly lies the point of entry of the sensory roots and anteriorly the exit of the motor roots. There are reflex connections (reflex arcs) between these roots which allow for reflex movements. However, the outflow is regulated by descending bundles of fibres (tracts) coming down the spinal column from the brain, and sensory input is transmitted to the brain through ascending tracts. Since the left half of the brain controls the right half of the body, and the right half of the brain controls the left side, the ascending and descending fibres have to cross the midline in their journey down the neuraxis. The point of cross-over, however, varies between motor tracts and sensory tracts – and indeed within the sensory tracts themselves the point of cross-over is different for each type of sensation (vibration, pain, temperature and light touch) (Figure 26.6).

The organization of the ascending and descending tracts share one similarity – those areas subserving the hands are in the most central part of the cord, with the areas for the arms lying further out, and the areas for the legs being the furthest out on the periphery of the spinal cord (Figure 26.7).

Sensory nerves (touch, pain and temperature) lie in the antero-lateral part of the cord, while nociceptive stimuli (concerned with knowing where a patient's own limbs are in space) are transmitted posteriorly.

The significance of this is that discrete anatomical lesions produce specific patterns of sensory and motor change. Unless one is aware of the neuroanatomy these symptoms can occasionally be mistaken as being the effects of hysteria or 'shock'.

Physiology of the Spinal Cord

Anatomic transection of the cord is rare. The majority of mechanical injuries are produced by disruption caused by compression of the cord or the nerve roots of the cauda equina. Whether injury is complete or not will depend, in mechanical terms, upon the severity of the compression force produced.

However, this is not the only factor at work. Damage may be caused (as in head injury) by secondary hypoxic damage to the cord, either by permitting the patient to become hypoxic, or as a result of reduced blood flow to the spinal cord.

The blood flow to the spinal cord is derived from two major inputs. Firstly, each segment has its own vessel. Additionally, the blood supply of the dorsolumbar (thoracolumbar) cord is provided by a number of vessels collectively known as the *artery of Adamkiewicz*; the blood supply of the cervical spinal cord is derived from the anterior spinal artery, which in turn derives from the two vertebral arteries. There is a zone at the lower limit of the territory of the anterior spinal artery and the upper limit of the territory of the artery of Adamkiewicz where vascular injury is particularly likely. Neglecting to secure the circu-

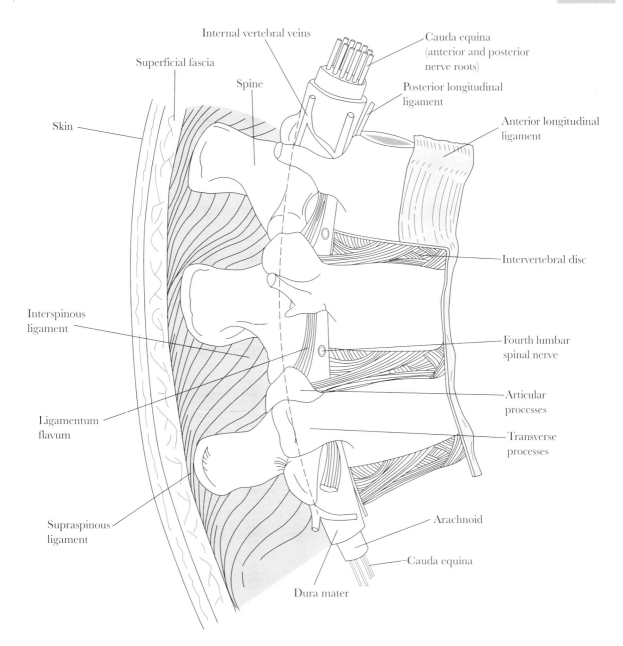

Fig. 26.4 *Ligaments of the spine*

lation can convert a person who would otherwise be paraplegic into somebody who is tetraplegic. The risk is, however, not solely anatomical. It depends on the microcirculation and the changes that are associated with a spinal cord injury. In cervicothoracic lesions the sympathetic nervous system (which travels in the spinal cord between T1 and L1) is interrupted. This causes a general vasodilation, with a fall in blood pressure even when the patient is lying flat. The hypotension is considerably more pronounced if the patient sits or stands up, because it is the vasomotor tone and the muscle pump in the legs (neither of which are then functioning) that maintain the perfusion pressure. In the uninjured person with an intact nervous system the blood pressure can fall and rise while the blood flow to the brain and spinal cord remains constant. This is known as *autoregulation* and explains why a person who faints is not quadriplegic (all limbs paralysed), paraplegic (lower limbs paralysed) or hemiplegic (limbs on one side paralysed) on recovery. When the neuroaxis is damaged there is a failure of autoregulation and

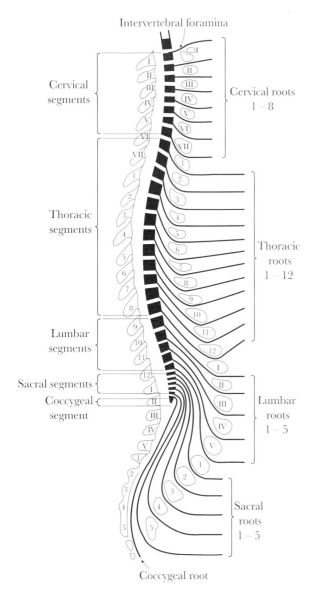

Fig. 26.5 *The spinal cord. From Lindsay, Kenneth W (1991) Neurology and Neurosurgery Illustrated, with permission from Churchill Livingstone*

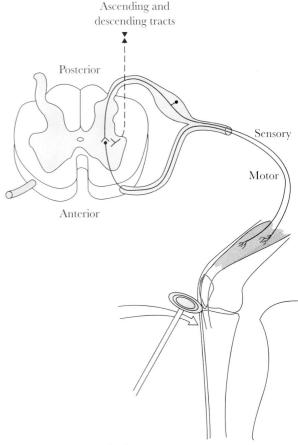

Fig. 26.6 *Nerve roots and reflex arcs*

the spinal cord blood flow directly mirrors the blood pressure. Thus, a fall in blood pressure *will* produce a fall in blood flow in the damaged area of the cord, and an area of spinal cord already compromised by a compressive force will have an hypoxic insult as well.

Three elements therefore contribute to spinal cord injury:

> biomechanical movement
> hypoxia
> underperfusion

The tendency in treating spinal cord injury has been to dwell on the mechanical factors alone and avoid moving the patient at all, placing the cord at risk of hypoxia, underperfusion, or both.

DIAGNOSIS

The symptoms and signs of spinal injury are related to disruption of the spinal column (the bones, ligaments, and muscles) and disruption of the spinal cord. Bone injury causes pain, tenderness, swelling, bruising and an irregularity in the spine on palpation (a 'step'). Pain is prominent when there is a dislocation. However, pain from a spinal injury may be masked by more severe pain elsewhere. Superficial bruising is rare and is usually a late sign. When muscles are disrupted and bleeding occurs, an intramuscular haematoma forms which is usually not apparent on the surface. A step, if found, is a useful sign but it is present in only 10% of cases. The feeling of being 'severed in two' (agnosognosia) occurs in only 4%.

Motor symptoms and signs may be confined either to the proximal or to the distal muscle groups – the screening test of ask-

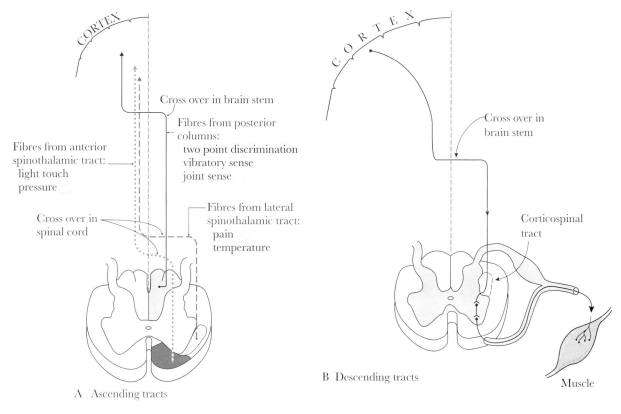

Fig. 26.7 *Ascending (A) and descending (B) pathways*

ing the patient to move fingers and toes is insufficient to exclude motor involvement. Many of the patients who deteriorate do so because their injury is not recognized and they are allowed to sit or stand up during their management. There are two principal reasons for missing the injury. Firstly, the local (spinal column injury) signs traditionally described in textbooks are frequently not present; secondly, the textbook descriptions of spinal cord injury have often been confined to those of a complete spinal cord injury.

Difficulty in interpreting the motor symptoms and signs is common in the specific partial cord injury syndromes. The first of these is the *central cord injury*. From the anatomical description above it will be appreciated that with a central cord injury the legs may be little affected, the arms more seriously affected and the hands most affected of all. This injury is produced by hyperextension. It is a common pattern of injury in the elderly with existing osteoarthritis in the spine. The osteophytes on the back of the vertebral body (outgrowths of bone resulting from the osteoarthritis) often press against the spinal cord before the accident without producing symptoms. A minor fall in the home, for example, where the head and face first hit a piece of furniture will produce an extension injury which has disproportionately severe effects.

The second pattern of partial cord injury is the *rotational* or '*side-swipe*' injury. This, incidentally, is also produced by stab wounds to the spine. The clinical picture is of a modified hemisection of the cord – the patient loses motor function on one side, and loses pain and temperature sensation as well as the ability to recognize light touch on the other. This odd picture is because of the different levels at which the motor and sensory tracts cross over from one side of the cord to the other. In addition, the posterior columns may be affected. In brief, weakness occurs down one side with numbness on the opposite side. The risk with this injury is that the patient will be misdiagnosed as 'hysterical'.

The sensory disturbances are even wider in their spectrum. They include:

- 'Pins and needles' sensation
- Electric shock-like pain at the moment of impact with no other indicator that injury has taken place
- Disturbances of proprioception, where the patient feels he or she is still in the same position as at the moment of impact, despite clearly now lying in another
- Burning pains throughout both arms or both lower limbs

The upper limb variant of this is frequently seen in motor vehicle deceleration accidents. In the lower limbs burning pains are associated with 'hyperpathia' (touch registers as pain), seen most frequently in conus injuries. The result is that touching or moving the patient's legs during extrication produces severe pain, and there is a real risk that these patients are misdiagnosed as hysterical or histrionic.

Finally, minor degrees of sensory or motor loss are frequently described by patients either in terms of 'clumsiness', 'stiffness' or 'heaviness', and such complaints must always be treated seriously. Because of the diversity of symptoms and signs in spinal injury, the management of patients with potential spinal injury requires particular attention to the history and mechanism of injury. Patients who have congenitally abnormal spines, or diseases such as ankylosing spondylitis or central cord syndrome seen in the elderly, do not require the same degree of force to produce a cord injury as those with a normal spine.

Causes of Spinal Cord Injury

The principal causes of spinal cord injury are as follows:

- Motor vehicle accidents
- Falls
- Gymnastics and trampolining
- Rugby football
- Horse riding and hunting
- Skiing
- Hang-gliding
- Aquatic injuries
- Weight falling on the back

Motor vehicle accidents

Fifty per cent of all spinal injuries are still produced by motor vehicles and half of these occur to people on motor-cycles. The motor-cyclist's injury depends on the attitude of the head on falling, and characteristically produces compression-flexion or extension with rotation. In motor vehicle accidents the unsecured person can be thrown out of the vehicle either through a door or through the windscreen. A person who is restrained can still have a deceleration injury, particularly to the cervical spine; roll-over accidents or underrunning a larger vehicle can produce a compression injury, and in vehicles where there are no rear seat-belts the unrestrained back-seat passenger can injure the restrained front-seat passenger *en passant*, as the back-seat passenger is thrown through the windscreen (the 'flying granny' syndrome). The deceleration injury (whiplash injury) is a combined injury of flexion followed by extension. Vertebral column injury or spinal cord injury can occur in either phase, and on some occasions the vertebral column injury has occurred as the head and neck move in one direction and the cord injury as they move in the other.

Dorsal (thoracic) spine injuries commonly occur in association with injuries to the chest wall (ribs and sternum). Dorsolumbar injuries are more common when a lap strap only rather than a conventional seat-belt is worn.

Falls

Falls may be from a height onto the feet, or a result of jumping (including parachuting). The injuries are usually at the dorsolumbar junction. Remember that there may have been a medical condition causing the fall in the first place.

Rugby football

Injuries result either from scrum collapse or tackles.

Horse riding

Horse riding is the one cause of spinal cord injury where there is a female preponderance. All other causes have male preponderance of 5:1.

Aquatic injuries

Aquatic injuries are principally diving accidents. There is a compression force, and either a flexion or extension force depending on the attitude of the head. There are additional problems – the patient may float to the surface face down and be at risk of inhaling water and drowning; also diving accidents are frequently associated with alcohol excess, not only on the part of the victim but also of the victim's companions, and there is therefore a delay in recognition which makes the risk of inhalation much greater. If airway destruction occurs then the patient will have a predisposition to an anoxic injury over and above the mechanical injury.

A more recent cause of spinal injury associated with aquatic activities is neurological decompression sickness. This cause is increasing in importance, not only because the sport is growing in popularity with relatively inexperienced people taking part, but also because people ignore the instruction not to dive on the day they fly home from abroad. The combination of a dive to a depth greater than 30 m and then travelling in an aircraft cabin pressurized to only 3,000 m will produce decompression symptoms and signs. This injury is the only one which is consistently progressive, and also involves the brain and higher function. The effect is that the patient arrives home (often inland, where such symptoms are not recognized) with a progressively spastic ataxic gait and a fatuous and elated manner. Unfortunately, the signs are frequently misdiagnosed as intoxication.

Weight falling on the back

Weight falling on the back was the classical mining injury and does still occur in agriculture and industry. Despite the contraction of the coal-mining industry, there has been a relative increase in the number of such injuries in the mines, attributable to the abolition of central direction of mine safety and fragmentation of the industry.

Associated injuries

Gymnastic injuries, rugby football injuries and diving injuries do not generally produce other mechanical trauma in association with spinal injury. However, with the remainder the incidence of associated major injury is of the order of 50%. These injuries will also need rigorous treatment, often with a higher priority than the spinal cord injury.

> The incidence of associated major injury with spinal cord injury is about 50%

Assessment

Any patient who is unconscious as a result of a head injury (or who could have had a head injury in association with unconsciousness) and any victim of trauma who is unable to give an account of the accident (e.g. through intoxication) must be regarded as having a spinal cord injury until proved otherwise. This also applies to the elderly demented patient and people with learning difficulties, not least as the latter group also harbour abnormalities of the vertebral column. Also at particular risk are casualties who have signs of degenerative or inflammatory joint disease or those who have other skeletal deformities such as dwarfism.

Finally, the circumstances of the injury must not affect management. A fall is a fall is a fall – it does not matter whether a patient is intoxicated or is 'high' on a drug of dependence. The fact that thousands of people who get drunk and fall over do not injure their spines is not an excuse for trivializing the incident. In summary, therefore, raise your index of suspicion. *Think spinal cord injury*. If the situation suggests that there could be a spinal cord injury treat the patient as if there is:

- Do not let the patient get up
- Do not allow others to get the patient up
- Do not get the patient up yourself

The safe position for the patient is supine with the spine in a neutral position.

There are many descriptions of what constitutes an *unstable spinal injury* or a *stable spinal injury* in orthopaedic terms, often cross-correlated with the radiological features and a retrospective calculation of the mechanism of injury. These analyses are of considerable importance to orthopaedic surgeons and paraplegists who have to choose between conservative and operative management, but in practical terms such analyses do not affect the immediate handling. It is important on arrival at an accident to identify or predict factors predisposing to any risk and then proceed on the assumption that the injury is biomechanically unstable, and that a failure to manage the patient properly can and will make the spinal cord injury worse, or produce an injury where none existed before.

Neurological examination at the accident site cannot be detailed. In motor terms, attendants should be looking at voluntary power, for example bending large joints normally. Observe whether the chest wall moves during breathing or whether it is the diaphragm alone (diaphragmatic breathing, see below). Sensory examination may reveal a 'sensory level' below which sensation is altered or lost. The level should be marked on the skin. The following landmarks may be useful: the root of the neck is C4, the nipple line (in the male) is T4, the umbilicus is T10 and the foot (sole) is S1.

IMMEDIATE MANAGEMENT

Causes of deterioration are:

- Mechanical displacement of vertebrae
- Displacement of vertebral fragments
- Hypoxia from underventilation, airway obstruction or lung damage either as a result of associated injuries or from aspiration of vomit
- Underperfusion from reduced cord blood flow which may be due to positioning (e.g. sitting up) or to shock

Because of the risk of anoxic damage and damage from underperfusion airway (A), breathing (B), and circulation (C) must take priority over a cord or a potential cord injury.

Urgency of handling follows these priorities. The problems found in a primary survey are not only life-threatening, but will inevitably make any spinal injury worse. Careful horizontal movement (a 'log roll' if possible) will not produce further permanent damage. Permanent cord damage is produced by thoughtless, uncontrolled movement of the spine, or by applying the force of gravity through the spinal cord.

The patient should be moved as little as possible and there is no place for unnecessary lifts and transfers.

Emergency Extrication

Emergency extrication, that is without the availability of appropriate extrication devices or the assistance of relevant emergency services, is justifiable only when there is an immediate threat to life. An *isolated* spinal cord injury need not be managed in a hurry. Depending on whether the patient is indoors or out, and on the weather, it is perfectly permissible to spend an additional 20–40 minutes organizing a safe removal and transfer from the accident site. Where there are multiple injuries these usually take priority and here the 'golden hour' is of crucial importance if life is to be saved.

Airway

Airway obstruction leads to hypoxia and inevitably to cord deterioration. Airway clearance is therefore vital. Use the technique of jaw thrust or chin lift. It is appropriate initially to attempt to clear the airway with the patient in the position in which he or she is found, but it may be necessary to move the patient carefully into the supine position.

Breathing

Ventilation is often impeded in a thoracic or cervical cord injury. This may be because the patient is breathing using only the diaphragm (the intercostal and abdominal muscles being paralysed), or because of chest injuries and associated pain. Remember that pain from chest injuries may mask the pain from the back injury.

If ventilation is inadequate ventilatory assistance will need to be provided.

Intubation in potential cord injury

There are benefits in intubating the apnoeic and/or unconscious patient in terms of improved airway control, prevention of subsequent bronchial soiling, ease of bronchial toilet and ease of mechanical ventilation.

Against these benefits must be measured the hazards. Neck injury may be associated with laryngeal damage. During intubation the patient may undergo a vagal asystolic arrest. A similar event may occur during endobronchial suction. Both these features are more common if the patient is hypoxic. There may, in addition, be movement of the neck with production of a mechanical cord lesion or the induction of vomiting or reflux during intubation.

If there are good grounds for intubating the patient, the possibility of spinal cord injury should not deter the operator. The roadside respiratory arrest is either neurogenic, or in the aftermath of aspiration or chest injury. A very high cord lesion, i.e. C1 to C3 (the *hangman's fracture*), produces diaphragmatic paralysis. The anatomy of the atlas and axis are such that when these vertebrae are damaged the canal is wider, not narrower. If intubation is needed because of chest injury or aspiration the mechanical risks are more than outweighed by the risks of not securing adequate ventilation. At the roadside the patient, even if unconscious, will still have protective muscle spasm of the neck which will not have been ablated by pharmacological paralysing agents or anaesthetic agents. In addition, spinal cord swelling at that stage will be minimal. For these reasons a paramedic should not fight shy of intubating if valid reasons exist.

Indications for intubation:

- Absence of spontaneous ventilation which is not restarted by airway opening
- Absent or inadequate spontaneous ventilation with evidence of vomiting, reflux or aspiration
- Adequate supine spontaneous ventilation which is associated with problems in airways control
- Adequate supine spontaneous ventilation associated with increasing ventilatory difficulty in association with thoracic or abdominal injury
- The unconscious spinal cord injury patient with isolated head and neck injuries and a progressively deteriorating conscious level

Spinal Cord Injury and Disordered Circulation

Spinal cord injury can be associated with disorders of central circulation, which may cause either a cardiac arrest or a arrhythmia from which a cardiac arrest may follow.

After spinal cord injury the parasympathetic nervous system can be unopposed. While considerable parasympathetic stimulation is required to induce bradycardia or asystole in non-injured humans, in the phase of spinal areflexia the sympathetic nervous system is 'paralysed'. The stimuli required to trigger adverse parasympathomimetic effects are then considerably less. This phenomenon is aggravated by hypoxia and hypothermia. Hypoxia is particularly significant as it may occur temporarily during upper airway suction, attempts at airway insertion, intubation and endobronchial suction through a tracheal tube. The risk rises the further down the airway the stimulus is applied, and tends to be more pronounced the higher the cord lesion.

Pre-hospital management of this bradycardia is the administration of atropine. If the heart rate is below 45 beats per minute, a bolus dose of atropine (500 μg) should be given *before* any of the above interventions are attempted, and should be given in any case if the heart rate falls as low as 40 beats/min. If there is no resting bradycardia the pulse should be monitored during the procedure, and if it falls below 45 beats/min, a bolus dose of atropine should be given.

The acute signs in the limbs are also derived from the suspension of reflex activity in response to a spinal cord injury. Affected limbs are flaccid and areflexic (so-called spinal shock). The suspension of sympathetic drive produces generalized vasodilatation. Thus, even if the circulating blood volume is unchanged there will effectively be underperfusion. However, even in the isolated cord injury, in thoracic and lumbar spinal injuries there can be extensive blood loss into the paravertebral tissues, producing an anatomic blood loss as well as the physiological loss of circulating volume.

Confusion sometimes arises over the term 'spinal shock'. Spinal shock is the phase of areflexia which, depending on the level of the lesion, may also include involvement of the thoracolumbar outflow and thus the sympathetic nervous system. In the latter case haemodynamic changes will follow and these are best termed *underperfusion* or *neurogenic shock*.

In an isolated cervical or thoracic cord injury the 'normal' systolic arterial blood pressure will be found to be around 90 mmHg. At this level, because the vessels are vasodilated, perfusion should be adequate so long as the patient is kept flat. The heart rate may be either slow or normal. A combination of bradycardia and hypotension should always raise the suspicion of spinal cord injury. Where a patient has a normal pulse and apparent hypotension, both spinal cord injury and covert trauma should be suspected. Shock in the patient with multiple trauma must *never* be assumed to be solely due to spinal cord injury. In a patient with *multiple injuries* of which the cord injury is one element, the indications for infusion are the same as for any other polytrauma victim. The amount of fluid infused and the rate of infusion should be sufficient to restore perfusion. In the otherwise young and fit spinal cord injury victim, however, it is only necessary to transfuse to bring the systolic blood pressure to a level of 90–100 mmHg. In the elderly, hypertensive subject a higher blood pressure may be appropriate. The principle is that whatever infusion is required to establish clinically effective perfusion should be provided.

With the *isolated cord injury*, as may occur in a gymnastic or rugby accident, the infusion must be given with extreme care. The acceptable systolic arterial blood pressure is 90–100 mmHg. Because of vasodilatation, so long as the patient is kept flat, perfusion should be adequate. So long as this remains the case cannulation alone or a guaranteed maintenance infusion to keep the vein open is all that is necessary. Where the systolic blood pressure is below 90 mmHg an infusion will be necessary to restore the blood pressure to 90–100 mmHg. *Only 500 ml of intravenous fluid should be given pre-hospital.* This volume is sufficient to compensate for the increased vascular space. Because of the cord damage, however, the circulation is at the limits of vasomotor control. In addition, there is a considerable output of antidiuretic hormone. The result is that it is very easy to over-transfuse a patient – even one who is young – and if a patient is over-transfused it is extremely difficult to correct. This is why the volume infused pre-hospital should be limited to 500 ml, and indeed the total volume for the first 24 hours should not exceed 1500 ml.

Concern about the quantity of fluid infused, however, should not deter the attendant from inserting a cannula or setting up a line while the veins are still easily accessible.

While a head-down tilt can be used temporarily to clear vomit from the airway, continued use of this position on circulatory grounds may cause the abdominal contents to splint the diaphragm and reduce the vital capacity. With associated abdominal injuries and an abdominal cavity filling with gas, blood or both, a secondary ventilatory inadequacy or even arrest may be precipitated.

There are particular problems associated with rescue situations where vertical movement of the casualty may be essential and also in environmental conditions where the cold makes infusion difficult or impossible.

Unconsciousness

There is a high association of head injury with proved spinal cord injuries. The reverse phenomenon, that is to say the association of spinal cord injury with proved head injury, is, however, only 10–15%.

Reviews of significant deceleration motor vehicle accidents have shown that if the patient is alive when the first rescuer arrives the incidence of a grossly unstable biomechanical cervical injury is of the order of 1 in 300.

Two maxims derive from this, and they are not mutually exclusive. The first is that in the presence of a significant head injury, a spinal cord injury should always be suspected. The overall management picture should presume that a spinal cord injury exists until proved otherwise. Until the patient is adequately stabilized, any *necessary* movement must be carried out carefully, with the best immobilization possible under the circumstances. The second maxim is that because of the relative incidences, any movement which is necessary to save life must take priority and must be carried out in accordance with the priorities of primary survey using the greatest care and best endeavours available. To fail to do otherwise will place at risk the 299 patients with a head injury who do not have a grossly biomechanically unstable neck injury, in favour of the one patient who does.

The major risk of unconsciousness is that of aspiration pneumonia induced by inhalation of vomit or refluxed gastric contents. In spinal cord injury there is a greater risk of silent gastro-oesophageal reflux as some of the muscles forming the sphincter between the oesophagus and stomach are disabled. In addition, there is an immediate ileus coupled to gastric stasis. Thirdly, there are no premonitory signs of vomiting-like reflux, which is silent. Lastly, in many of the associated social circumstances the stomach is full, often with alcohol.

The diagnosis of unconsciousness is definitive, while that of spinal cord injury is presumptive. Unconsciousness takes priority: the airway must be maintained and bronchial soiling avoided. In the absence of advanced airway management, the patient will need to be turned on their side. If there is difficulty in maintaining the airway, and there is present or imminent reflux or vomiting an immediate turn onto the side to deal with this problem is essential. The mortality of isolated spinal cord injury is under 1%, but this rises to 40% if aspiration pneumonitis supervenes.

The normal rules for airway protection apply and must not be compromised because there is inadequate assistance or 'packaging' is not yet complete. The attendant must always remember that if a degree of hypoxia is induced which is sufficient to compromise that patient's life then that degree of hypoxia will inevitably render complete an existing incomplete spinal cord lesion.

There are some indicators that a spinal cord injury may coexist in a patient who is unconscious. These indicators are:

- A differential level of responsiveness above and below the level of possible cord injury
- Diaphragmatic ventilation (the cardinal feature of which is that during inspiration the abdominal wall, instead of appearing to recede, balloons out)

- The association of bradycardia, hypotension, and a head injury
- Priapism (sustained erection)

None of these signs is consistently present, and it may be that none is present.

The patient with neurogenic shock will appear warm, pink and well-perfused, with a low or normal pulse despite a low blood pressure.

In the presence of an isolated spinal cord injury, the patient should be lucid. A patient who subsequently becomes unconscious may have an obstructed airway, or be underventilating or shocked in association with previously unsuspected associated injuries, or there may be a deteriorating head injury.

Basic Management Summary

- Always have a high index of suspicion for spinal cord injury
- Remember the history and mechanism of injury
- The patient must not stand or sit up
- Airway, breathing, circulation and unconsciousness require patient movement
- Slow, careful movement is safe
- Careful movement in the horizontal axis preserves life and will also preserve residual cord function

From this list it can be seen that the basic rules are as follows: consider safety, consider the need for resuscitation (primary survey), consider the possibility of a spinal cord injury, control the head and neck position to allow optimal support of the airway, breathing and circulation and lastly, organize the team before embarking on complicated extrication and management procedures. The use of equipment will always require assistance beyond the standard two-person ambulance crew. It may involve summoning ambulance colleagues, making use of fellow emergency service professionals, or even seeking help from the general public. Always ensure that assistants are adequately briefed before a task is undertaken.

SPINAL IMMOBILIZATION AND PATIENT HANDLING

Control of the Head and Neck

Control of the head and neck must be undertaken as soon as possible. Control is secured by immobilizing the base of the skull without exerting a positive traction force. In the unrecognized spinal injury, traction may induce a distraction spinal cord injury secondarily. Although traction is used in the hospital management, it is always tailored in force and direction to the vertebral column injury which has been identified as to its nature and its level. When treating the undiagnosed patient (as occurs at the roadside), traction is contraindicated.

Cervical collars

There are many cervical collars on the market, a few of which are effective and safe, many of which are useless, and a significant proportion of which are dangerous as well. A semirigid collar must be used rather than a soft collar, improvized collar or rehabilitation collar. The only role of an improvized collar is where there are multiple casualties as a marker to indicate suspicion of a spinal cord injury. The collar should restrict flexion, extension, lateral flexion and rotation of the neck, and the resting position of the neck must be in neutral. The collars must be properly stored and the instructions for application rigorously followed. Another person must always control the head and neck while the collar is applied. If a two-piece collar is applied care must be taken not to obstruct the jugular venous outflow (thereby contributing to raised intracranial pressure), and the front piece and the back piece must be individually sized. Lastly, any cervical collar is only a restraint and should be supplemented by manual head control. Manual head control, once applied, should not be removed until a diagnosis is discounted in hospital, clinically and radiographically. During transport in an ambulance there will inevitably be vertical movement and angular velocities as well as acceleration and deceleration. These forces are buffered by the attendant holding the head. A collar alone is not adequate.

Movement at the Accident Site

Movement at the scene is usually:

- *From prone to supine* to maximize ventilation with a conscious patient and place the head in neutral
- *From supine to side* to protect an otherwise unprotected airway or to assist the clearance of vomit
- *From side to supine* once vomit has been cleared, or to intubate or otherwise maintain ventilation of someone whose ventilation is inadequate on their side

Traditionally movement is effected with a 'log roll'. The log roll requires ideally six people and at least five people if it is to be carried out without moving the full length of the spine. Log rolling using three people has been described, but this produces a movement of the dorsal and/or lumbar spine. Equally, in hospital, four people can be used, but this works only where (a) the conditions are ideal and the patient is at the right height, and (b) where the team is highly experienced at the manoeuvre.

Scoop stretcher

For retrieving casualties from the ground, the scoop stretcher is preferable to the long spinal board which requires a log roll procedure. It is almost exclusively a transfer stretcher, though it can be used to remove people from difficult locations – after which they can be transferred to a conventional stretcher or an evacuation mattress. The disadvantage of the scoop stretcher is that it is composed of rigid metal leaves with sharp edges, and can generate pressure sores even in a short journey time – particularly if the patient is underperfused. Once the patient is on the ambulance trolley cot or the evacuation mattress, the scoop stretcher should be removed. It can, however, be positioned under an evacuation mattress to provide greater rigidity for lifting and carrying.

Evacuation (vacuum) mattresses

Whichever type of evacuation mattress is used, the following rules apply. Firstly, it should be tested before the ambulance goes on duty to make sure there are no leaks. Secondly, when laid out it needs to be smoothed flat. Thirdly, once the patient is positioned on it manual contouring is required between the legs and around the head, neck and shoulders. So long as it was laid flat in the first instance, it will protect against pressure sores. The scoop stretcher can be placed underneath it with safety and will add to overall rigidity.

Extrication devices

Extrication devices are based around the design of the short spinal board (Figure 27.21). The designs that are easiest to use have a leading edge which can be applied from either side (and which can be cleared of straps, buckles and other impedimenta so that it can be inserted easily). A minimum of four people are necessary to apply such a device. The ideal device should not 'concertina' during insertion behind the patient. It should *not* be applied before a semirigid cervical collar is in place. There should be an effective cushion component to block out the space between the board and the rear of the collar. All straps should be applied and tightened, except the leg straps in the presence of a fractured femur. Once secured, the patient can be moved in any suitable direction except the vertical. A vertical lift requires the addition of a vertical movement harness. Some devices have what appears to be a handle at the head end. *This must never be used for lifting the patient.*

Long spinal board

The long spinal board has two uses. The first is aquatic rescue: its use is primarily a lifeguard skill, although ambulance service personnel may be required to assist the lifeguards. The second is as part of vehicular extrication. The technique of choice is to bring the device in behind the patient from the rear of the wreckage, and move the patient up the long axis of the spinal board. The spinal board should therefore be rigid, thin, have contoured edges and have a low coefficient of friction both for the undersurface and the top surface.

Helmet removal

It is recognized that the removal of motor-cycle helmets is essential even in the presence of a spinal cord injury. Opening the visor is not sufficient to manage the airway. Ideally every motor-cyclist would wear a *BMW pattern* helmet where the front elements can be hinged away and the helmet removed with relative safety, as with the old-style 'coal-scuttle' helmets before full face helmets were developed. The manual removal of a full face helmet will inevitably move the cervical spine. There is only one way around this, and that is to use a battery-powered reciprocating saw to cut through the face bars, thereby converting a full face helmet into a 'coal-scuttle' one.

General Rules for Equipment

The equipment used today for the management of spinal cord injury is effective, but equally has the capacity to cause mischief in unskilled, unpractised hands. Not only therefore should personnel be trained, but they should also be practised. None of the equipment can be applied by a single person. Even applying a cervical collar or removing a helmet (by whatever means) requires two people. The use of a scoop stretcher requires a minimum of two trained ambulance personnel, with other people assisting by lifting the sides to prevent it bending. The use of the long spinal board, short spinal board and evacuation mattress all require a minimum of four people – six people is optimal. These people need not necessarily be fully trained ambulance personnel – help from other emergency service workers, first-aiders or members of the public may be appropriate. Neurological deterioration is never due to equipment failure, it is due to errors on the part of the people using it.

Pressure Sores

Paralysed patients are at risk from pressure sores because they cannot feel and cannot move. These sores may occur in the usual pressure sites – the bony prominences where only a small amount of tissue interposes between the bone and the hard surface of the stretcher. In the supine position these are the heels, the buttocks, the scapulae and the back of the head. Primary journeys are usually short, and pressure sores are produced at this stage largely by the misapplication of splinting systems, by hard objects in the pockets of the patient such as bunches of keys, and by certain extrication devices. Therefore, clothing should be loosened, including the shoe-laces. Hard objects should be removed from pockets where they are next to the skin. Padding should be placed between the legs. Any additional splintage should be padded. The scoop stretcher, because of its sharp-edged leaves, can produce pressure sores even on a short journey. It should only be used as a transfer stretcher and patients should *not* be left lying directly on it, though they can be left lying on it if cushioned by a vacuum mattress.

Hypothermia

A paralysed person cannot sweat or shiver. Temperature perception is impeded because of sensory impedance, and the control mechanism, stripped of its input and output, also becomes erratic. Patients with spinal injuries must be protected from the cold; they must be kept warm passively by being wrapped up well. During the primary journey this is not usually a problem, but because of the large distances between spinal units, it can be a problem on the secondary journey from the receiving hospital to the spinal unit, for which the ambulance service is also responsible. The problem is likely to arise if, mistakenly, it is thought appropriate to drive an ambulance at 5 miles per hour for the entire distance. Clear directions have now been issued by the Spinal Injuries Consultants in the UK as to how it is possible to move patients at normal road speeds, together with protocols favouring the use of helicopters under certain conditions. In the UK the major problem is hypothermia. However, in hot weather the reverse problem – heat stroke – can also occur. It is also a major problem during aeromedical evacuation of people who may well have been lying out in the sun on the tarmac on some foreign airfield for a long period.

SUMMARY

Spinal cord injury management aims to avoid neurological deterioration, prevent death from acute effects or associated injury, and prevent long-term complications.

It depends first on a high index of suspicion and an ability to make a diagnosis, particularly where the cord injury is incomplete. Deterioration may be produced either by biomechanical, anoxic or vascular mechanisms.

The overall rule is to move patients as little as possible, but correct positioning to protect or maintain the airway, provide adequate ventilation, and maintain the circulation is essential and takes precedence.

Intubation should be undertaken where clear indications exist. An intravenous cannula should always be inserted, but infusion rates and volumes depend on whether the cord lesion is isolated or associated with major multiple trauma. Cardiac arrest may be induced through parasympathetic stimulation and can be prevented with the use of prophylactic atropine. Manual control of the head is crucial and should be instituted at the earliest possible opportunity. The only safe position for the spine is lying in neutral.

In addition, patients should be protected against development of pressure sores and hypothermia. Mishandling is not merely mechanical, it also compromises the spinal cord on a pathophysiological basis. Serial mishandling produces cumulative effects greater than that produced by each element taken individually.

chapter twenty-seven:

PATIENT IMMOBILIZATION AND EXTRICATION

One of the most contentious issues surrounding the pre-hospital management of the injured is the decision whether to stabilize on site or rapidly evacuate to hospital. This management decision will significantly alter the way patients are handled and 'packaged' in preparation for transport to hospital. However, not only should we have the patients' interests and care at heart, but we must also remember the needs and safety of the rescuers and be alert to any risks posed by environmental factors.

It is therefore crucial that decisions about stabilization and evacuation are taken early on in the rescue. The techniques used for stabilization must not be viewed in isolation, but should be part of the total rescue activity and should complement the other treatments used to provide care and comfort to the patient. Whichever technique is used, the method of transport must first be determined, to make sure the equipment needed will fit the vehicle to be used.

In choosing a method of stabilization for the known or suspected injuries, the paramedic must remember the two underlying principles of pre-hospital care: first, do no harm, and second, ensure the patient's comfort.

PRINCIPLES OF IMMOBILIZATION

In the pre-hospital setting the principles of skeletal management are to prevent further injury, ensure neurovascular supply and to make the patient comfortable. Immobilization often helps to reduce further blood loss, and reduces the risk of fat embolism.

The overriding importance of managing the airway, breathing and circulation (ABC) is fundamental to the treatment of any injury. With the exception of cervical spine care, fracture management and extrication follow the primary survey unless a 'snatch rescue' is necessary.

The principles of definitive fracture management are *reduction*, *immobilization* and *preservation of function*. How these principles are applied or modified in the pre-hospital setting, and the equipment available, is considered below.

As nearly every piece of equipment will cover or hide the patient to some extent, it is essential that any local treatment and observations are carried out before the immobilization device is applied. Examination should be as complete as the situation allows and the injuries dictate. Wounds should be photographed using an instant-print camera, and appropriately dressed before immobilization.

Benefit to the Patient

The benefits of immobilization are:

- Pain relief
- Reduction of blood loss
- Prevention of neurovascular damage
- Prevention of fat embolism

Any pre-hospital treatment should always be considered from the standpoint of the patient. Remembering the ABC principles, splinting or extrication devices should in no way produce any airway, breathing or circulation compromise.

The patient should always feel more comfortable after the splint or device has been applied, so that handling becomes easier. This should help to reduce the patient's fear, and as a consequence reduce the circulating catecholamines and their potentially harmful effects (peripheral vasoconstriction with reduced peripheral tissue oxygenation). By correct splinting, bleeding into the tissues may be reduced, thereby lowering the life-threatening risk of hypovolaemia. Fat emboli from fractured long bones will be reduced by early and correct splinting, particularly if combined with oxygen therapy.

FORMS OF SPLINTAGE

Most of the forms of splintage considered in this chapter relate to spinal immobilization, but limb splintage and the pneumatic anti-shock garment (PASG), also known as military anti-shock trousers (MAST), are also considered.

Box Splints

Box splints are simple in design and are often overlooked. They are useful for lower leg and ankle injuries, and are carried by every front-line ambulance (Figure 27.1).

The splint forms an oblong box, open along one side with the other three sides able to be folded in such a way as to form a gutter. There is a foot support at one end. There are adult and child-sized splints.

Application

The injured leg should be exposed and footwear removed (if possible). Appropriate dressings should be applied to any wounds and the ankle straightened. *The peripheral pulses should be checked*.

Remember there may be times when boots or footwear provide a suitable splint for ankle injuries, and in these situations they may be left on.

The leg should be raised and the splint passed underneath the leg. The two sides of the splint are then folded so they fit closely against the leg. The ankle support should hold the foot at right angles. The various Velcro straps are passed over the top of the leg and around the front of the ankle. This arrangement forms a firm support and immobilizes the lower leg effectively (Figure 27.2).

If any strap passes near to an injury, care should be taken that it does not cause pain; if it does, it can be left loose. Once the splint is applied the patient should be re-checked – specifically, the pulses in the limb and the sensation must be noted and recorded.

Some box splints have a side pocket and a long wooden splint can be inserted to form a long leg splint. This together with fracture straps or broad fold triangular bandages and padding can be used to immobilize a fractured femur.

Traction Splints

The primary function of a traction splint is to immobilize the fracture (of a lower limb) in a reduced position. This will greatly aid patient comfort, but more importantly it will prevent further neurovascular damage and reduce the severity of shock by reducing blood loss and pain from the fracture site.

Following a fracture of the femur, if the muscles of the thigh are left without traction they will shorten the leg, causing the bone ends to override, which not only presents a serious potential for neurovascular damage and entrapment, but also increases the radius of the thigh so that it becomes more spherical: this shape has a larger internal volume than a cylinder and so presents a larger space into which blood can escape. Application of traction will restore the cylindrical shape of the

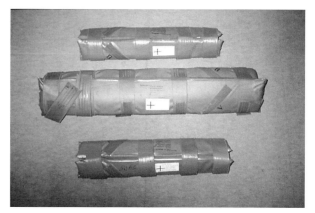

Fig. 27.1 *Box splints*

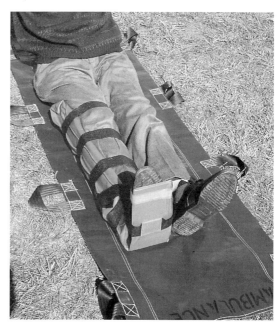

Fig. 27.2 *Leg in box splint*

thigh, reducing its volume and reducing the overall blood loss. It has been suggested that traction splinting also reduces the incidence of fat embolus.

Three types of traction splint are found in pre-hospital care: the Hare or Trac-3 splint, the Sager splint and the Donway splint.

The Hare or Trac-3 traction splint

The Hare traction splint (Figure 27.3) and the Trac-3 traction splint are valuable pieces of equipment. Not only can they be used with traction to maintain a reduced fracture of the lower limb, but they can also be used without traction just for support.

Indications There is some debate about the indications for use of this type of splint and it is wise to check with the local receiving hospital for their views.

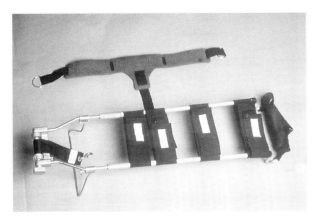

Fig. 27.3 Hare traction splint

Indications with traction

- Closed (simple) fractures of the femoral shaft
- Closed (simple) fractures of the tibia and fibula
- Compound fractures of the femur, tibia and fibula (this is open to debate and local guidance must be sought)

All compound fractures must be surgically explored and cleaned. Therefore the receiving hospital must know that a fracture was compound. If the fracture was reduced at the scene then it is mandatory to ensure that the receiving doctor is completely aware that the fracture was compound (if possible take a photograph using an instant-print camera).

Indications without traction

- Fractures around the knee

Contraindications Contraindications to traction

- Dislocation of the hip
- Fracture dislocation of the knee
- Ankle injuries
- Simple undisplaced fracture of the lower third of the tibia and fibula (better immobilized with a box splint)
- Fractures of the pelvis
- Fractures of the neck of femur (Sager type not contraindicated)

Application Application must be practised regularly. It requires two people to apply the splint correctly. Remember that just because a patient has a fracture which can be dealt with by traction splinting, it does not follow that it is in that per-son's interests always to have a splint put on. There may be other more life-threatening injuries. Remember you do not die from a fracture of the lower limb but you *do* die of a blocked airway. Set up the splint as follows:

1. Give the patient nitrous oxide and oxygen inhalation (Entonox) if required, assuming there are no contraindications to its use (e.g. the presence of a pneumothorax).
2. Expose the fracture site (cut clothes if necessary). Do not remove motor-cycling leathers as these can be dramatically effective in the control of lower limb and pelvic fracture bleeding (see below).
3. Examine the limb thoroughly. Remove the footwear, check pulses distal to fracture together with the colour and warmth of limb; check sensation and motor function distal to fracture – this is the neurovascular examination.
4. Prepare the splint:
    select the appropriate ankle hitch
    place the splint by the good leg and measure for length and adjust accordingly, then lay the splint by injured leg
    check all the straps – these should be open and placed at the correct intervals down the splint
    unwind some of the traction strap
    re-check the splint from top to bottom to make sure all is ready.
5. Dress any wounds if required.
6. Place the ankle hitch under the foot. The foot is straightened and the hitch placed well under the ankle. The side straps are then tightly folded over the ankle (not around the foot) and the rings brought together below the foot. Finally the strap at the bottom of the foot is firmly grasped (Figure 27.4).
7. Manual traction is started with one hand while the other hand supports the leg.
8. The splint is then put in the correct position. Circumstances will dictate to an extent how this is done, but the best method is to roll the patient away from the splint and then slide the splint under the leg. The top padded ring *must* fit under the ischial tuberosity. The patient is then rolled back onto the splint. If the position is still not correct then the patient can be moved down slightly so that he or she is sitting on the padded ring. *Manual traction MUST be maintained THROUGHOUT this procedure.*
9. The top strap is done up: apply padding if required and avoid the external genitalia in males.
10. The traction hook is then put through the 'D' rings and traction taken up, ensuring that manual traction is not released before the splint's mechanical traction is tightened.
11. Traction is applied until the limb is comfortable (to a maximum of 7 kg in adults).
12. Repeat the neurovascular examination.

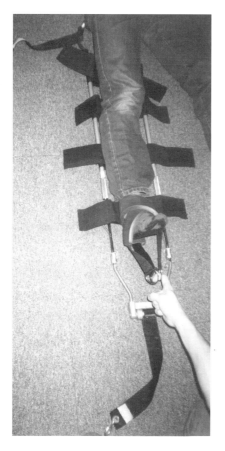

Fig. 27.4 *Manual traction with Hare splint*

13. Elevate the leg by raising the foot stand.
14. Position and tighten the Velcro straps.
15. Cover the leg to keep it warm.

En route *to hospital*

1. The neurovascular examination should be repeated every 5–10 minutes.
2. Check the straps and loosen if required – the leg may swell.
3. Check the tension of traction – as a result of reduced spasm in the muscles tension can be lost.

To release traction The two splints have slightly different release mechanisms. Take up manual traction and then release the mechanical traction having removed all the supporting Velcro straps. The Hare splint has a pull ring which releases the traction suddenly, whereas the Trac-3 has a knob which has to be unwound to release the traction (which is less likely to be accidentally released).

Complications The only real complication that can occur is damage to the neurovascular supply to the leg. This can be

prevented by careful examination of the distal limb function. Absence or change in distal function must be reported to the accident and emergency department. If it is found that the distal pulses diminish or are absent after traction has been applied, firstly check the tightness of the straps in case circumferential occlusion has occurred and then, under manual control, very gently reduce the traction until the pulse returns.

Use of the pulse oximeter can detect alterations in the blood flow if the probe is placed on one of the toes of the fractured leg. However, this can be unreliable.

One problem with a traction splint of this type is that it will extend well beyond the patient's body and therefore handling on a trolley or in a vehicle may be difficult. When treating bilateral fractures two splints are required, and this can make handling very difficult. These problems are not encountered with the Sager splint (see below).

Sager traction splint

The Sager traction splint weighs less than 2 kg and can be used to treat single or bilateral fractures of the lower limb, especially of the femur (Figure 27.5).

It is claimed that the Sager splint can be applied with the patient in any position so long as the leg can be straightened. The great advantage is that the splint does not extend beyond the end of the leg following application, which makes handling and transport easier.

Application

1. Remove the shoe and sock and expose the leg as necessary.
2. Check the distal pulses and sensation in the injured leg.
3. Apply the cushioned end of the splint between the patient's legs, against the perineum and symphysis pubis.
4. Apply the bridle 'S' strap around the top of the thigh.
5. Extend the splint so that the ankle hitch lies between the patient's heels or at the level of the normal heel if the fractured leg has been shortened.

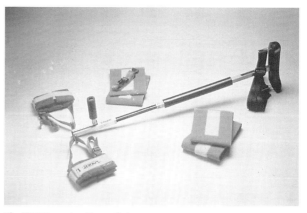

Fig. 27.5 *Sager traction splint*

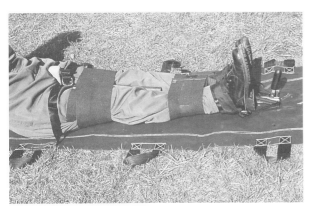

Fig. 27.6 Ankle Hitch on Sager splint

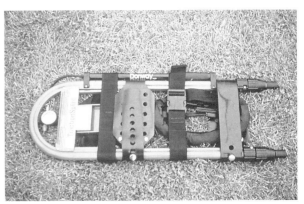

Fig. 27.8 Donway splint

6. Apply the ankle harness beneath the heel and wrap around just above the malleoli, adjusting the cushions on the strap to fit the size of the leg (Figure 27.6).
7. Set the traction (recommended at 10% of the body weight) until the patient is comfortable.
8. Apply the leg cravats.
9. Tighten the bridle around the thigh if necessary.
10. Secure the cravats.
11. Apply the foot binding strap around the feet and ankles in a figure-of-eight.
12. Check the foot pulses following application.

The splinted leg is shown in Figure 27.7.

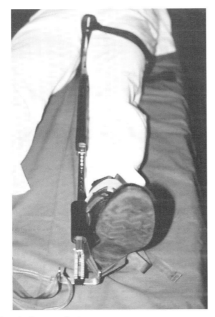

Fig. 27.7 Leg in Sager splint

Remember the ABC priorities before applying the splint. Additional pain relief may be required.

Make out a report form, including photographs if taken.

To release traction Take up manual traction. Remove the cravats and ankle hitch. Along the shaft of the splint there is a small sprung piece of metal which should be lifted, and this will release the tension.

Donway splint

The Donway splint (Figure 27.8) employs a different method to achieve traction. The fractured leg is cradled by the splint with the foot firmly fixed to the ankle support. The top strapping is put around the thigh and then, using the pump provided, the two halves of the splint (lower and upper) are pushed apart by increased pressure (like the slide on a trombone). Once the patient is comfortable the securing screws are tightened; the pressure in the splint is then released through a valve. The leg straps are applied, and (as with other forms of traction splint) the pulses and sensation in the limb must be checked.

Military Anti-shock Trousers

Military anti-shock trousers (MAST), also known as the pneumatic anti-shock garment, are an inflatable garment that surrounds the legs and abdomen and can be inflated to a pressure of 100 mmHg (Figure 27.9).

Indications
Indications for use of the MAST are:

- Splinting of pelvic and lower limb fractures
- Intra-abdominal trauma – tamponade of bleeding vessels

It is no longer recommended for hypovolaemic shock, and there are better alternatives for lower limb fracture splintage.

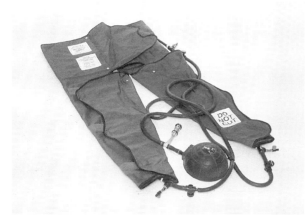

Fig. 27.9 *Military anti-shock trousers*

Method of action

The MAST acts by applying direct pressure to bleeding vessels and splinting of fractures. Investigations have shown that it reduces intra-abdominal haemorrhage. It was originally thought to act by physically squeezing blood from the lower limbs into the central circulation, but later evidence suggests this not to be the case. The mechanism is now thought to be that the MAST increases the peripheral vascular resistance.

The net effect is equivalent to giving a 2–3 unit blood transfusion in an adult. Blood pressure rises, as does cardiac output, stroke volume and mean arterial pressure (see Chapter 10).

Contraindications

Absolute contraindications

- Cardiac failure
- Pulmonary oedema
- Ruptured diaphragm (abdominal compartment only)
- Advanced pregnancy (abdominal compartment only)

Relative contraindications

- Head injury (when isolated injury)
- Uncontrolled bleeding above garment
- Application lasting more than 6 hours

Dangers

The following risks and problems are associated with the use of a MAST:

- Adequate fluid replacement must proceed simultaneously
- Visual examination of covered areas is prevented (photograph injuries first with an instant-print camera)
- Prolonged use (document time of inflation)
- Respiratory embarrassment
- Use by inexperienced personnel and failure to monitor vital signs
- Premature or inappropriate removal

Application

If the use of a MAST is indicated, the garment should be applied as follows, after the patient's vital signs have been recorded.

1. Unpack the MAST and lay them on an ambulance cot or a flat, hard surface.
2. Although it is possible to place the MAST under the patient by rolling, it is much easier to lay the patient onto a prepared MAST. The top of the MAST should be just below the lower border of the costal margin.
3. Check the patient's pockets for any potentially harmful objects, and remove them.
4. The left leg of the MAST is wrapped around the patient's left leg and secured with the Velcro straps.
5. The right leg of the MAST is wrapped around the patient's right leg and secured with the Velcro straps.
6. The abdominal compartment (if it is to be used) is fitted and secured with the Velcro straps.
7. The air tubes are connected and the stopcocks appropriately set ('open').

The fitted MAST is shown in Figure 27.10.

Inflation

Before inflating the MAST, check the patient's vital signs. Inflate the leg compartments first – if possible maintain equality of pressure in each compartment. Inflation should stop when the patient's blood pressure or perfusion has reached acceptable levels; at this point the stopcocks are closed. Remember that the MAST is inflated according to the person's blood pressure reading, *not* according to the pressure reading of the garment.

Continue to monitor the patient's vital signs and adjust the

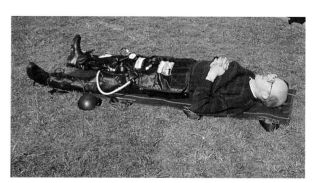

Fig. 27.10 *Patient in MAST*

pressure accordingly. There are safety pressure valves incorporated in the compartments of the garment.
Finally, check the peripheral pulses.

Deflation

Deflation must not be attempted by inexperienced staff

Deflation of the MAST must only take place when definitive surgical facilities for the control of haemorrhage are available; this will either be in the accident and emergency department, or ideally the operating theatre.
1. Before deflation is attempted, one or two large-bore intravenous cannulae must be in place and adequate venous access established.
2. Monitor the vital signs.
3. Start by deflating the abdominal segment, and only when it is completely deflated start to deflate the leg compartments.
4. Reduce the pressure slowly and monitor continually. If the patient's blood pressure falls by 5–10 mmHg, stop deflation, infuse a large volume of fluid, and be prepared to reinflate the MAST.
5. Be prepared for rapid surgical intervention.
6. Deflation may take 20 minutes at least.

Complications

Complications of MAST use are:

- Extreme hypotension, possibly irreversible if inappropriately removed
- Possible association with ischaemic compartment syndrome, tissue damage, metabolic acidosis and respiratory embarrassment
- Exacerbation of:
    cardiac/thoracic vascular bleeding
    pulmonary oedema
    congestive cardiac failure

CERVICAL SPINE IMMOBILIZATION

Cervical spine immobilization may be achieved manually or by the use of a cervical collar.

Manual Methods

Whenever the accident scene or the nature of the injuries suggest the potential for cervical spine damage, as the airway is opened or protected the cervical spine should be immobilized manually. This can be achieved from behind, from the side or from in front of the patient.

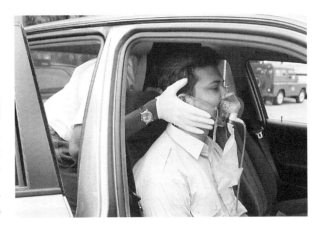

Fig. 27.11 *Manual immobilization from behind*

Behind the patient
From behind the patient, place your palms over the patient's ears. Your little fingers should lie just under the angle of the jaw and your thumbs should be extended upwards behind the posterior aspect of the skull. Adjust your hands so that the patient's ears lie between your fingers. Do not cover the ears: the last thing an anxious patient needs is to be rendered deaf as well!
If the head is not in a neutral position, it should be moved slowly and gently into a neutral position. Having reached a supported neutral position, the neck is held until a more formal support is applied (Figure 27.11). Traction is *not* applied. Move yourself into a comfortable position in order to support your own arms to prevent them from becoming tired.

Side
Place one of your hands behind the patient's head so the occiput lies in your palm. The other hand should support the jaw between your thumb and second finger. Your two hands now hold the neck in a similar way to a cervical collar. The head can be moved into a neutral position (Figure 27.12).

Front
Place your hands over the patient's cheeks so that your fingers pass around the neck and your extended thumbs lie just in front of the ears over the temporomandibular joint. The head may be moved into a neutral position (Figure 27.13).

Cervical Collars

There are a number of different types of cervical collar available. Some are a single piece of equipment, and others come in halves which are joined together around the neck.
The collars have to be sized according to the manufacturer's instructions and then applied correctly while maintaining manual immobilization. *Collars do not completely immobilize the cervical spine* and it is essential to continue manual immobilization until this is replaced by the equivalent of sandbags and tape.

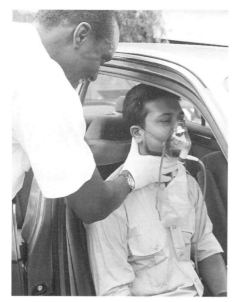

Fig. 27.12 Manual immobilization from the side

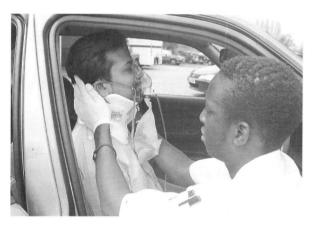

Fig. 27.13 Manual immobilization from the front

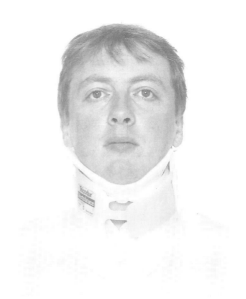

Fig. 27.14 Correctly applied collar (Stiff-neck)

LOG ROLL TECHNIQUE

'Log rolling' is a method of turning patients either to inspect their backs or to help put them on to a long spinal board. To 'log roll' a patient there should be a minimum of four people but more can be utilized if available. The patient should lie with arms by their sides and the palms placed against the legs (Figure 27.15).

The object is to keep the whole spine in alignment, and to achieve this the cervical spine is stabilized and the patient moved with the neck, shoulders and pelvis kept in the same plane.

Remember it is of little use to merely hold on to the collar: the hands have to support the head and should be placed *above* the collar. A correctly applied collar is shown in Figure 27.14.

A correctly sized collar will prevent flexion and extension and to a great extent sideways movement, but will not stop rotation – it is rotation that the rescuer's hands will prevent. Access to the airway and trachea is available at all times through the gap in the front of the collar.

There is some research evidence to suggest that the application of a cervical collar, even when correctly sized, may cause a rise in intracranial pressure (through venous compression), but from a practical viewpoint it is accepted that a correctly fitting cervical collar should be used in the pre-hospital setting when the situation suggests a cervical spine injury.

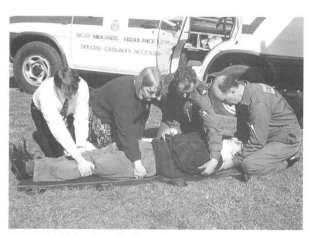

Fig. 27.15 Initial position for 'log roll'

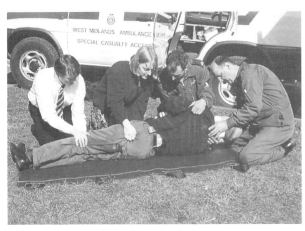

Fig. 27.16 Patient on side during 'log roll'

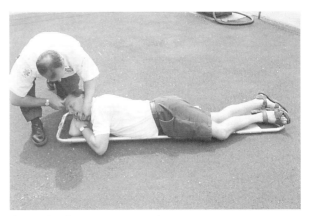

Fig. 27.18 Patient on a scoop stretcher

One person takes the head and this person controls the manoeuvre. The next person grips the patient's shoulder on the opposite side and also the further arm. The third person grips the pelvis, and the fourth person controls the legs. The person at the head calls the instructions and the whole body is rolled over, keeping the spine from twisting. The roll need be only as far as is needed to inspect the back or insert a long board underneath the patient (Figure 27.16).

A fifth person should examine the patient's back, and perform any necessary treatment (for example, dress a bleeding wound). The patient is then rolled back into the supine position.

SCOOP STRETCHER

The scoop stretcher provides a means of lifting a patient onto a trolley or ambulance cot with minimal movement.

The scoop stretcher can be split in half longitudinally and has

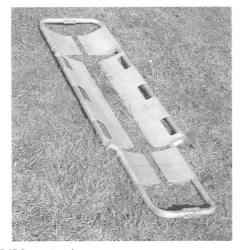

Fig. 27.17 Scoop stretcher

a head cushion. The bottom half can be extended to fit the patient (Figure 27.17).

The scoop should be laid beside the patient and extended to the required length. The patient should be told what is about to happen. The halves are then slid underneath the patient's body from the sides, taking care not to pinch the body as the halves are brought together. The patient may have to be rolled slightly to allow each half stretcher to be slid underneath.

Once the stretcher is in place and the halves are locked together, the head cushion is secured and the patient is lifted onto the trolley or cot. The distance that the stretcher has to be carried should be kept to a minimum, and if rough ground or stairs have to be negotiated, restraining straps can be used to increase the patient's security (Figure 27.18). A spinal board is a much better device for carrying a patient downstairs.

Once the patient is on a trolley the scoop stretcher should be removed to prevent pressure sores developing, unless the transfer time is short and the removal of the stretcher would delay definitive treatment.

The other use of a scoop stretcher is to allow a patient to be turned over. A scoop stretcher is placed underneath the patient, and a second scoop is placed on top, forming a 'sandwich' with the patient in the middle (Figure 27.19). The two stretchers are tied together, and the patient can be lifted and rotated through 180°. The stretchers are then removed.

SPINAL BOARDS

Spinal boards are used to assist in the movement (extrication) of casualties from an accident scene (Figure 27.20). They provide a secure and stable base onto which a patient may be strapped, so providing full spinal immobilization.

Despite the recent concern that patients may develop pressure sores from prolonged use of a spinal board, the boards are still the best form of protection in pre-hospital care. The vacuum mattress (perhaps used in conjunction with a spine board) provides an alternative.

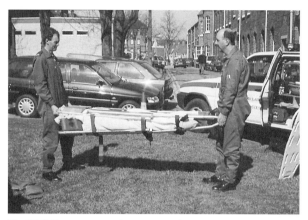

Fig. 27.19 *Two scoops used to turn a patient*

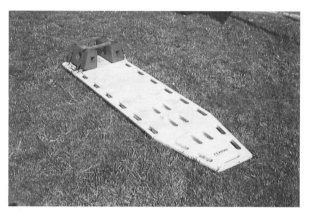

Fig. 27.20 *Spinal board*

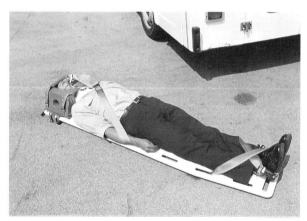

Fig. 27.21 *Patient on a spinal board*

A spinal board may be used to secure and move a person who is on the ground, it may also be used to assist in controlled extrication, or if time is a critical factor the board may be used to rapidly extricate a patient from a vehicle.

The use of a long board requires many hands, and everyone

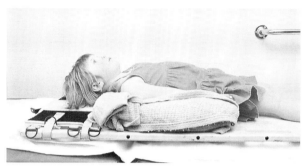

Fig. 27.22 *Padding under child's shoulders*

must be aware of their role because teamwork is all-important. Before using a long board the method of 'log rolling' a patient must be known (see above).

Long Board

A patient may be rolled onto a long board or lifted onto a board using a scoop stretcher.

Depending on the situation of the patient, a cervical collar may be applied before or after placing the patient on the board. Either way, manual in-line cervical stabilization will be required until the patient is secured to the board.

The head should be supported in a head immobilizer ('head box'). The straps on the board are applied according to the manufacturer's instructions (Figure 27.21).

If a child is placed on a long board, because of the relatively larger size of the child's head a pad may be required below the shoulders to prevent any forward flexion of the neck (Figure 27.22).

Rapid Extrication

Access to a patient in a vehicle is obtained either by springing the front door or by removing the roof of the vehicle.

If the roof of the car has been removed, the long board can be slid behind the patient. If the patient is in a front seat, the seat can be reclined as the patient is slid onto the long board and lifted clear. If it is impossible to remove the roof, the front door must be forced open. One person maintains in-line cervical stabilization from the back seat; a second person will apply a cervical collar from the side, while the third brings the long board which is placed on the seat under the patient (Figure 27.23). When room is limited the long board should not be put under the patient until later in the procedure. If time permits a brief assessment should be performed.

The patient's feet and legs are then freed: the first rescuer maintains manual in-line cervical stabilization, while the third rescuer should be beside the patient in the front of the car, ready to lift the patient's legs across the unoccupied front seat. The second rescuer assumes the command of all movements,

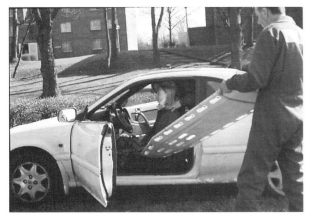

Fig. 27.23 Extrication using a long spinal board

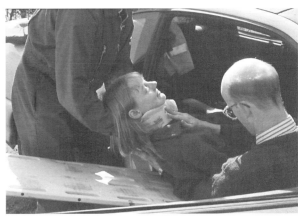

Fig. 27.25 Extrication using a long spinal board

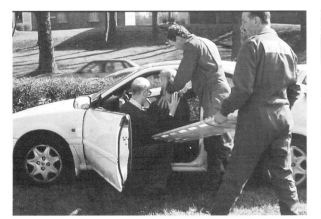

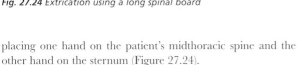

Fig. 27.24 Extrication using a long spinal board

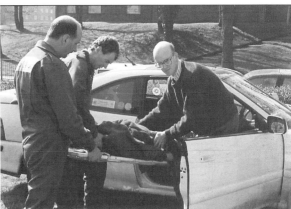

Fig. 27.26 Extrication using a long spinal board

placing one hand on the patient's midthoracic spine and the other hand on the sternum (Figure 27.24).

The second rescuer uses both hands to sense any twisting of the patient's spine, and directs the movement of the patient. The legs are swung onto the seat so that the patient's back faces the open door; this movement should be done in short steps. Depending on the position of the first rescuer, another may have to control the patient's neck while the first rescuer negotiates the door-post.

Once the patient is sitting across the front seat, the long board (if not already in place) is pushed well under the buttocks and the patient is lowered onto the board, then slid in small movements up the board (Figure 27.25).

As the patient is slid up the board rescuer one maintains in-line cervical stabilization; rescuer two's hands are placed in the patient's armpits and the third rescuer steadies the hips, pelvis and legs. Once the patient is on the long board he or she can be carried away from any danger, and appropriate resuscitation started, during which time the patient will be properly stabilized on the long board (Figure 27.26).

VACUUM SPLINTS

Vacuum splints provide rigid support to the body and can be very comfortable. They are bags of polystyrene beads enclosed in tough plastic. The injured limb or the whole patient can be placed onto the splint, which is actively moulded around the injured part. Suction is then applied to the bag, creating a vacuum: the contents take up a rigid form, supporting and splinting the injury.

Vacuum splints can be used to immobilize:

- Limbs (upper or lower)
- The cervical spine, in conjugation with a semi-rigid collar
- Other spinal injuries

The whole body splint (or vacuum mattress) (Figure 27.27) should be laid onto the trolley and the patient is laid onto the mattress, which is secured around the patient's body using Velcro straps or a continuous webbing strap. The mattress is actively moulded around the patient. Care must be taken to support the head as the mattress is moulded around the neck and side of the head. A vacuum is then created inside the mattress using the suction pump provided. The mattress will conform to the patient and provide whole body support. Finally, the valve mechanism is secured and the pump removed. The splint can be removed by opening the valve and allowing air back into the mattress.

A vacuum mattress is a good immobilization device, but a poor lifting device. It will be necessary to place a long spinal board under the vacuum mattress to lift and carry the patient any distance.

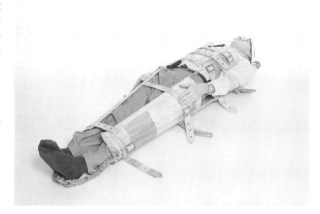

STRETCHERS

The scoop or orthopaedic stretcher has already been described. Sometimes it is appropriate to use a canvas which can be slipped under the patient's body. The canvas can then be lifted in hospital using poles and spreader bars.

Other forms of stretchers which can be used in rescue situations are the Neil Robertson and Paraguard stretchers.

Neil Robertson Stretcher

The Neil Robertson stretcher is constructed in canvas with wood slats sewn into the canvas (Figure 27.28). It has side-straps to fasten the stretcher around the patient's body and rope handles at the head, bottom and sides to help lower or raise the stretcher. The person is placed on the stretcher which is then

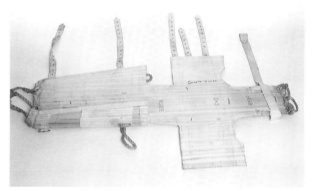

Fig. 27.28 Neil Robertson stretcher

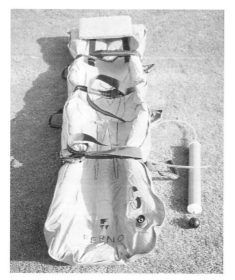

Fig. 27.27 Vacuum mattress

fastened round the body, securing the feet and head to the stretcher. The stretcher can either be carried using the side handles, or poles can be passed through the handles so it can be carried end-to-end.

Paraguard Stretcher

Although the Paraguard stretcher is similar to the Neil Robertson stretcher, there are some significant differences. The Paraguard has a hinge in the middle and can, even with a patient fixed on the stretcher, be bent around obstacles. It has approved lifting points and can be used for helicopter rescue (Figure 27.29).

When unpacked, the Paraguard stretcher should be folded straight and the hinge secured with the metal sleeves. The patient is laid on the stretcher and the corset fitted and secured with the straps. The ankle hitch and head restraints are secured. Once the patient is firmly strapped onto the stretcher it may be moved horizontally or vertically.

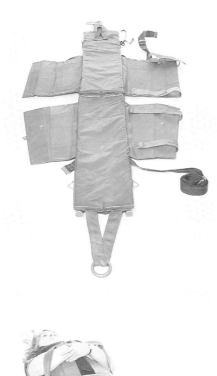

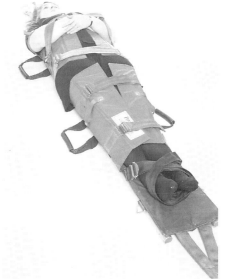

Fig. 27.29 Paraguard stretcher

EXTRICATION DEVICES

There are a number of different types of extrication device available. In current use are the Kendrick Extrication Device (KED), the Russell Extrication Device (RED) and the ED2000. These have replaced the short wooden board, which was always

difficult to use and became increasingly so as car seats became shaped.

These devices have a similar method of application, but each has its own characteristics which must be learnt. The devices are to an extent flexible and can therefore be slipped between the patient and the car seat. Once applied they offer some protection to the spine and allow the patient to be lifted from the vehicle onto a trolley.

The patient must first be assessed, and the cervical spine immobilized manually and with a cervical collar. The extrication device can then be slipped down behind the patient, making sure the various straps do not become caught on any object. While this is being done the cervical spine is immobilized both with a collar and manually. The device is then positioned correctly in relationship to the patient's head and shoulders (Figure 27.30).

The wings of the device forming the chest sides are drawn together with the chest straps which are then tightened, ensuring that this produces no respiratory embarrassment or pain. The leg straps are passed under the patient's legs and then fitted back onto the device. These straps are tightened.

The shoulder straps are placed across the body and fixed to the opposite side of the device. The shoulder straps must not overlap the cervical collar (Figure 27.31). The head straps are applied after making sure that any space behind the head is filled in with the supplied padding. These straps will hold the head and cervical spine firmly, and the person who has been immobilizing the cervical spine can now let go. All straps are checked for tightness and adjusted so they are even (Figure 27.32).

The patient can now be lifted out of the vehicle and placed on a trolley which may have been prepared with a vacuum mattress. The leg straps can be loosened, and if a vacuum mattress is to be used then the extrication device may be removed.

Extrication Chair

The extrication chair (Figure 27.33) is a modification of the scoop stretcher. It is about three-quarters of the length of a scoop stretcher and it does not have the facility to be extended. It not only splits in two longitudinally, but also horizontally.

To use the chair the various joints are undone. This gives four parts, two of which are longer than the others. The two shorter parts are slid underneath the patient and the bottom joint is closed. The patient is now sitting on the bottom of the chair. This can usually be achieved fairly easily by lifting each leg in turn.

The longer parts are now slid behind the patient's back and fixed at the top. The joints between the top and bottom sections of the chair are mobile and can be set to any angle. The two sections are then joined together, which can be a tricky operation.

A head restraint can be fitted using the metal headpiece and the cushion and straps provided. Finally, the middle joints *must* be fixed together with the strap which passes behind the patient

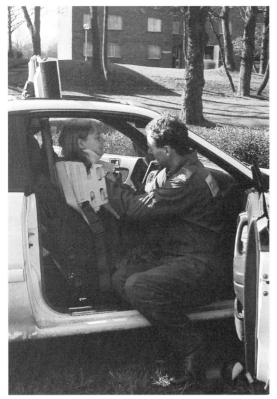

Fig. 27.30 Extrication device in use

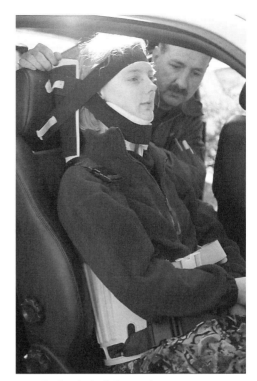

Fig. 27.32 Extrication device being used

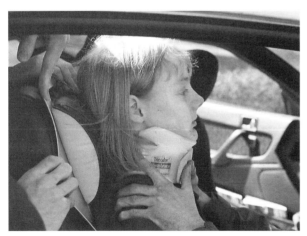

Fig. 27.31 Extrication device being used

hooking onto the two joints, and then passes in front of the patient, returning to the starting point.

The patient is next strapped to the chair using long seat-belt type straps, and can now be lifted with ease onto a trolley. The chair may be removed carefully, ensuring the patient does not move, and with support being provided at all times (Figure 27.34).

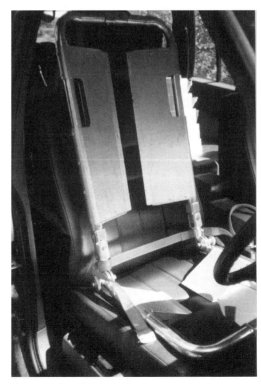

Fig. 27.33 Extrication chair

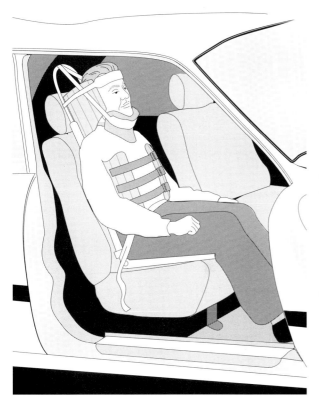

Fig. 27.34 *Patient on extrication chair*

PRINCIPLES OF EXTRICATION

Entrapment is relatively common in high-speed road traffic accidents (RTAs), but can also be encountered in industrial, recreational, aircraft, train, farming or domestic incidents. In dealing with the trapped patient, the pre-hospital worker's role is vital. The time-specific response previously mentioned cannot be applied when casualties are trapped, but the concepts of the 'golden hour' are still important. Therefore the medical priorities must be sorted out at a very early stage.

It is important that early consultation takes place between all the emergency services working at the scene to establish the priorities. It must be appreciated that this involvement should include the hospital staff – firstly to alert them of the pre-hospital problem so that they may be prepared, and secondly to seek their help if extra equipment or skills are required. If a patient is not trapped but has a time-critical injury or the environment is hazardous then the snatch rescue may be needed, with minimal intervention under ABC. Attempts to stabilize the patient may be done in transit.

It must be recognized that if casualties are trapped and have time-critical injuries they may die before being rescued, simply because of the technical difficulties involved in the extrication.

Definitions

Entrapment itself may be:

  actual
  relative

Actual entrapment

Actual entrapment occurs when victims are physically enclosed or held in a vehicle or area by the structure impinging on their body, e.g. a deformed vehicle following an RTA, a roof fall following a mining or caving accident, or building collapse following an explosion or bomb blast where rocks or masonry may be lying on the patient.

Relative entrapment

Relative entrapment occurs when the victim needs help because of their location, the environment or physical injury. For example, a traffic accident victim may have a fractured humerus. It is the pain that immobilizes the patient as well as the fracture. If a few minutes are spent on relatively simple splinting to immobilize the fracture, then the patient may be able to escape from the vehicle unaided.

In other examples injuries, such as a broken ankle, may prevent accident victims climbing out of a cave, or up a cliff. The rescue team may have to use devices such as coastguard equipment or helicopters, not for the sophisticated medical equipment, but as an aerial crane or elevator. Once the rescue has been achieved it may be necessary to release the helicopter for other work and use road ambulances for the hospital transfer.

Management

The basic pre-hospital approach of primary survey, resuscitation and stabilization is even more important when dealing with the trapped patient. The ABC principles apply, and continuing reassessments will be required during the rescue. In a trapped patient, problems created by a missed critical injury cannot be retrieved by early evacuation to hospital.

Preparation

Preparation includes training and a knowledge of the rescue teams and other services. You need to know the equipment they carry and their potential.

Your own equipment must be checked and be up-to-date. The function of all equipment needs to be known. There is nothing worse than having equipment that you do not know how to use, or finding your equipment is incomplete after struggling to reach the accident scene.

Teamwork

Each professional group must recognize their own limitations. The immediate care doctor or the ambulance crew will have some basic rescue equipment. If power-operated tools are required then this part of the rescue should be left to the specialists (the fire service). Equally, these specialists should have a clear understanding of what the medical priorities are. That may mean giving early access to the medical worker to allow stabilization of the casualty: the medical worker can then stand back during the rescue, perhaps monitoring the patient remotely through pulse oximetry and non-invasive blood pressure monitoring..

Clothing

Entrapments can be dangerous to the rescue worker and therefore proper clothing should be worn. This should include a helmet and robust footwear which give protection from sharp metal and glass. Latex rubber or plastic gloves may be easily breached at the scene of the accident because of the many sharp objects and edges found, and once breached no longer protect the rescuer or the casualty from disease. However, hand and eye protection are needed to prevent the potential spread of disease.

Safety

Any entrapment scenario will have its associated dangers. Road traffic accidents, for example, may have the dangers of moving vehicles whose drivers are not concentrating on their driving owing to a morbid interest in observing the accident scene. Industrial accidents may well involve unfamiliar machinery or chemicals. In domestic entrapments risks from falling debris, electricity or gas may exist. The movement and actions of fellow rescue personnel and their associated equipment must not be ignored as a potential cause of additional injury.

Always think safety

Assessment

Assessment begins by looking at the scene and looking at the forces of violence. At the same time the number of casualties involved can be identified. Each casualty's priority should be assessed by airway, breathing and circulation. This may be facilitated by asking other rescue workers with first-aid training to help check that every casualty is breathing. Usually the fire service have plenty of personnel at the scene. Their officers can instruct the crews to see that each casualty has an airway and is breathing (see Chapter 56). This frees the medical workers to perform practical procedures and helps to identify the critical problems.

The assessment of the individual casualty involves talking to the person, examining the injuries and examining the wreckage. At this stage the identification of actual or relative entrapment can be made. The casualty must be protected not only from the dangers found within the accident scene, but also from the effects of the environment, for example from broken glass, fire or noxious fumes. Remember casualties will not be able to escape if they are still physically trapped. The stability of the vehicle or structures such as a building roof is also assessed at this stage. The specialist services should help in stabilizing or gaining access to the area.

Once these early stages of assessment have been completed the patient's 'ABC' can be assessed, followed by 'D' and then 'E'. Often fractures are identified under 'E'. Team discussions can take place on how best to tackle the extrication, allowing for the additional hazards that the environment may pose.

Monitoring

Continual monitoring is essential, usually performed by the ambulance crew who will normally be close to the patient. However, the use of monitoring equipment with electronic read-outs may allow the patient to be monitored at a distance while other aspects of the rescue continue. Electronic blood pressure monitoring, electrocardiography and pulse oximetry are useful, but none of these replaces clinical observation.

Entrapment scenes are often noisy, and electronic equipment can be used without requiring shutdown of the rescue field. Chest auscultation or assessment is almost impossible, so rescue field shutdown is required to enable this procedure to be completed. When there is relative silence, take the opportunity to check the whole patient. The fire service will always help, but do not expect them to stop the rescue unnecessarily.

In a hostile environment a rapid extrication may be necessary. There is little point in unprotected medical or paramedical personnel entering smoky or fume-filled environments such as a coal mine or ship's cargo hold. Their own survival would be put at risk and it would not be possible to treat the casualties. Rescue should be left to specialist crews in protective clothing. In the first instance rapid extrication from a hostile environment is all that can be achieved.

Planning

Dealing with an entrapped patient may take several hours. Early decisions should be made about the method of transportation. If the casualty is going to be trapped for 1–2 hours then the 'golden hour' will be exceeded by the time hospital is reached. If road transport is likely to take some time, air evacuation by helicopter or other means should be considered and requested early.

Snatch rescue

Snatch rescue is the retrieval of the casualty from a difficult environment with minimal stabilization and resuscitation until a place of safety is reached. An example is a person who is in the sea and is drowning. The coastguard or lifeboat service will have to rescue the person before they can protect the airway. Fires and chemical accidents are further examples.

Similar problems occur in mountain and cave rescue and other situations where access is difficult. Because of the location only a minimum of first-aid equipment can be carried to the scene of the rescue.

In civil disturbance or terrorist situations the rescue workers may be under hostile fire. Both rescuers and casualties are at risk. In these situations the airway, breathing and circulation management must be restricted to the basics, safety of all personnel being paramount. Once the casualty is retrieved to a safer area then the primary survey is repeated and more advanced 'ABC' techniques can be achieved.

Working with a trapped casualty is one of the most challenging and difficult areas for pre-hospital personnel: it is noisy, dangerous and difficult, and is not without risk to the rescue worker. Strong team bonds are formed in such rescue situations.

Resource list

Ambulance service The ambulance service has a full range of pre-hospital care equipment, communications and paramedical staff.

Police The police are experienced in scene management, traffic control, escorting ambulances from the scene and sometimes escorting special equipment or staff to the scene. They have special responsibility for the victims pronounced dead.

Fire service The fire service are experienced in scene management, heavy and light rescue and are able to supply large numbers of staff, often for long periods if required. They have a special responsibility for chemical and radiation incidents and the safety of such scenes. The fire service have special rescue units including rock rescue, RTA rescue and radiation and chemical decontamination units.

Medical immediate care schemes Immediate care doctors are experienced in trauma and medical care and can provide rapid assistance to the ambulance technician or paramedic. As only doctors can pronounce a person dead at an accident scene, their presence can release fellow workers to help in some other

aspect of the rescue. Some ambulance services have introduced a protocol for the paramedic to pronounce death.

CONCLUSION

'Casualty packaging' is an art which requires an understanding of injury patterns, a knowledge of equipment and above all teamwork. The removal of the injured person from the accident scene is an often unplanned and nearly forgotten part of the rescue.

There is no argument about the necessity to perform a primary survey before attempting immobilization and the removal of the patient from the scene. Only if a snatch rescue is needed should this principle be altered.

Some methods of immobilization may appear cumbersome and in retrospect (when the casualty's injuries are known) may be regarded as unnecessary, but the paramedic has a duty to prevent *potential* injuries. This does not mean that the paramedic must be obsessive about techniques and manoeuvres, to the extent of losing sight of the needs of the patient and the necessity to reach hospital quickly. Pre-hospital care is a rapidly changing, specialist area and each new technique must be evaluated carefully. All too often techniques may be introduced which have not been fully assessed, and for which there may be little objective evidence of improvement in the welfare of patients.

Priorities in extrication

- Safety
- Airway (with cervical spine control)
- Breathing
- Circulation with haemorrhage control
- Disability
- Exposure

chapter twenty-eight:

BLAST AND GUNSHOT INJURIES

Trauma caused by bomb blast and gunshot is an increasing problem in all developed societies (Figure 28.1). Most paramedics, particularly those working in large urban areas, can expect to manage such patients from time to time. However, it is important to place the injuries caused in context and to reassure medical attendants. Perhaps the most important statement to be made is that victims should be medically managed in the same way as other trauma patients – that is, a period of initial assessment and resuscitation and then transport to hospital. The general approach of primary survey, resuscitation, secondary survey and initiation of definitive care is not altered because of the nature of injury. However, there are other aspects of shootings and bomb blasts which must be noted. The first is the element of danger for paramedical personnel, particularly following a bomb blast. These incidents are controlled by the security services, and approach by medical personnel to victims will be restricted and may be delayed until the area is secure.

There are a number of basic rules governing behaviour which must be followed. These are:

- Do not become a casualty yourself. Do not approach the scene until it has been declared safe – risks of secondary explosions, fire and building collapse are high
- Do not touch objects found in the environment – they may have forensic or other non-medical implications
- Do not disturb obviously dead victims or move body parts
- If there are multiple victims, some form of triage will be necessary so that those most in need are identified, assessed and resuscitated first. This will normally be coordinated by a medical incident officer (in liaison with an ambulance incident officer) already on site (see Chapter 56)
- Care for multiple victims involves teamwork and it may be necessary to summon medical teams to the site – particularly if entrapment of victims is a feature

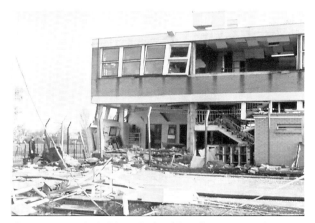

Fig. 28.1 *A terrorist incident: the bombing of Musgrave Park Hospital, Belfast, in 1991*

Blast and gunshot injuries are discussed separately in this chapter, although the victims have much in common, both in the nature of their injuries and in their management needs.

PHYSICAL EFFECTS OF BLAST

Explosives when detonated produce large quantities of gas at very high pressure. At the moment of detonation the explosive substance undergoes compression and chemical decomposition into gaseous products at very high temperature and pressure. A resulting front of high pressure or *shock wave* is formed which is characterized by an instantaneous rise to a peak level. The shock wave then travels through the surrounding environment with a velocity greater than the speed of sound in air. It is the instantaneous rise to peak pressure and the supersonic velocity that distinguishes a shock wave from an ordinary sound wave. As the shock wave or front moves away it declines in velocity (or decays) to ambient levels and then falls below ambient level for a short time, forming a negative pressure component which has little or no biological significance (Figure 28.2).

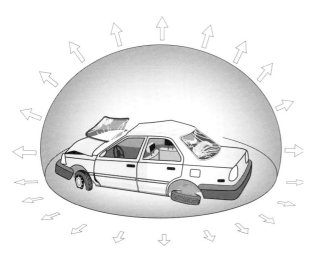

Fig. 28.2 *The shock wave (shock front) — a spherical wave of overpressure expands rapidly from the point of explosion*

Behind the shock front is an area of turbulence defined as the dynamic pressure or 'blast wind'. The forces generated by the dynamic pressure or blast wind can be considerable and have notable biological consequences. The effects of the two phenomena can be simply illustrated. If a shock wave passes through a building with glass windows, the glass will be broken by the shock wave; however, the dangerous showering of glass fragments is caused by the blast wind. Equally, when the shock front causes the collapse or disintegration of buildings, it is the blast wind that converts fragments of the collapsed structures into lethal missiles of varying size, shape and velocity.

The magnitude of an explosion, that is the extent and duration of overpressure and the pressure exerted by blast wind, is determined to a large degree by the type and quantity of explosive used. Another influencing factor is the environment – whether the explosion occurs in an open space or is confined inside a building. Other features of medical significance are the flash from the explosion, the risk of fires developing and the collapse of buildings.

BIOLOGICAL EFFECTS OF BLAST

The biological consequences of an explosion are considerable, and it is customary to divide blast effects into the following categories:

* Primary – Shock wave
* Secondary – fragment injuries (fragmentation)
* Tertiary – blast wind with building collapse
* Burn injury
* Psychological injury

Primary Effects

Primary effects result from exposure of the body to overpressure associated with the shock wave. The most notable effects are in areas of the body where there are air–fluid interfaces. These include the ears, the lungs and the bowel.

The tympanic membrane or eardrum is very susceptible and injury is common. The extent varies from mild vascular congestion of the membrane to rupture with possible disruption of the ossicular chain leading to severe hearing loss. Ear injury is curiously unpredictable following an explosion – the victim's ear must be correctly oriented to the shock wave for significant loading to occur.

Injury to abdominal structures is uncommon in air blasts but is a particular feature of exposure to blast in water. Injuries range from mild contusion of bowel wall to areas of frank perforation with faecal spillage and subsequent peritonitis. It is possible that blast injury to bowel is more common than is realized, and experimental work supports this view. However, injury appears to be mild in most cases of air exposure and is probably of little significance – paramedics should therefore not unduly trouble themselves with overlong abdominal assessments following air explosions, unless of course there are other causes of abdominal trauma, for example perforation by fragments.

The most significant clinical primary effect is contusion injury to the lungs, which may progress in some cases to 'blast lung'. The problem results from widespread pulmonary bruising with resulting haemorrhage into alveolar spaces – the 'haemorrhagic contamination of lung' as described by some blast research scientists. The clinical consequences of this contusion injury is hypoxia caused by a lowering of the partial pressure of oxygen (PaO_2). In addition, the damaged lung continues to accumulate fluid for long periods (24–48 hours), leading to a progressive deterioration if appropriate treatment is not instituted. The clinical presentation in the pre-hospital setting is one of breathlessness; the victim may be in acute distress, refusing to lie down and using accessory muscles of respiration. There may be associated pneumothorax or haemothorax compounding the respiratory distress.

Blast lung is not common, particularly following terrorist explosions. The problem for most bomb victims is one of combined injury caused by penetrating fragments and burns. The overall incidence of true blast lung among bomb blast survivors is under 5%, most recover well and only a very small number present with a progressive, lethal form of the condition. The reason for such a low incidence is clear – casualties close enough to an exploding terrorist device to develop blast lung will usually die from multiple hits by fragments.

An even rarer but striking feature of exposure to blast overpressure is sudden death in individuals with no external signs of injury. This was noted and reported during the blitz on London in World War II. Possible explanations include coronary artery air embolization or cardiac arrhythmias.

Secondary Effects

The most common serious clinical problems facing paramedics after an explosion are the penetrating and non-penetrating injuries caused by fragments. These may arise from the casing of the exploding device, or from the environment, such as pieces of glass, masonry and wood propelled by the blast wind. Size, shape, type of material, velocity and terminal effectiveness vary enormously. Following a car bombing, vehicle parts are generated as fragments and typically produce severe and often lethal injury.

Unlike fragmentation injury in war which is somewhat predictable, injury after a terrorist explosion is very variable. At one end of the spectrum, there are superficial injuries to exposed parts; at the other, multiple, irregular wounds across more than one body system. Widespread contamination by foreign bodies and mixed bacterial species is common to all.

The nature and extent of injuries will depend on many factors; the size of the charge, proximity to the device, the environment and its propensity to generate fragments all play a part. Ballistic aspects of penetrating injury are discussed in the section on gunshot wounds.

Tertiary Effects

Tertiary effects result from gross displacement of the body by the blast wind. The clinical consequences vary from total displacement of an intact body to traumatic amputation and even complete body disintegration. Injury may also be caused by a body being thrown onto a hard or irregular surface. Finally, tertiary injury may result from building collapse caused by the blast winds.

Burn Injury

Burns are a notable feature of blast phenomena and may be caused by flash, flame or both. Flash burns occur at the moment of detonation and particularly affect exposed parts such as face, arms and legs. Although dramatic in appearance, injury tends to be superficial. However, frontal exposure to flash may lead to airway burn with critical consequences (see Chapter 29). Flame burn occurs if the surrounding environment ignites – patterns of injury, immediate management and outlook are as for flame burns under normal circumstances.

Psychological Injury

Over 40% of those involved in incidents such as terrorist explosions may expect to suffer some form of psychological distress in the aftermath period. For the majority of trained personnel, the outlook is very good, particularly if their efforts were successful in reducing morbidity and mortality. Stress counselling ('critical incident stress debriefing') may be very helpful and is now mandatory for many emergency personnel after exposure to a stressful incident such as a bomb explosion.

WOUND BALLISTICS AND MECHANISMS OF INJURY

Before discussing gunshot wounds it is worth considering ballistic injury in general. The field is fraught with controversy, mainly because of disagreement among ballistic scientists, which need not concern paramedical personnel.

Wound ballistics is the study of injury caused by penetrating ballistic missiles. The list of potential wounding agents is prodigious: Table 28.1 is far from complete.

Wounding missiles, irrespective of type, cause injury by penetrating the body and transferring energy to the tissue. Therefore the wounding capacity of a particular missile wound may be defined by:

- The degree of penetration into the body, resulting in laceration and crushing of tissues and structures in its path – the severity or clinical outcome will be determined by the nature of structures in its path: for example, laceration of soft tissue in a forearm will differ in outcome from the same degree of penetration and laceration in the liver or myocardium
- The capacity of the missile to cause injury to structures surrounding and remote from the missile track

Table 28.1 Wounding missiles

Bullets
    Police handgun (many varieties)
    Military handgun
    Military assault rifle (5.56 mm, 7.62 mm)
    Hunting rifle (many varieties)
    Machine gun

Fragments
Primary:
    Natural (fragments from bomb casing, shells and mortars)
    Preformed (claymore mine, etched wire from hand grenades)
    Flechettes (individual darts preloaded into a cargo-carrying munition)

Secondary:
    Masonry
    Glass
    Wood
    Metal

Intrinsic:
    Body parts – typically fragments of bone

The degree of penetration of the missile will be determined by the mass, presenting area of the missile (fragments will usually be large, bullets small), impact velocity and the density of the tissues penetrated.

The capacity to produce remote injury will be determined initially by the efficiency of the missile in imparting kinetic energy (KE) to the tissue. The available KE can be calculated from the formula:

$$KE = \tfrac{1}{2} MV^2$$

Where M is the mass of the missile and V its velocity. There is a critical difference between the *available* KE and the *actual* amount imparted during the wounding. It is important to grasp this principle, as a high-velocity missile with considerable available KE may actually impart very little to the tissue during wounding. The factors that ultimately determine energy disposition or transfer include the impact velocity, tissue characteristics, wound track length and missile characteristics. What should now be obvious is that it is foolhardy to approach any victim of missile injury with preconceived notions concerning wound severity. In particular, the older system of classifying wounds according to known or presumed missile velocity is now considered unsafe. Thus, it must not be assumed that high-velocity or low-velocity missiles produce high-velocity or low-velocity wounds – the terms are misleading and are best abandoned. Most clinicians and ballistic experts now use the terms 'high-energy transfer' and 'low-energy transfer' wounds – the distinction can only be made by surgeons at surgical exploration. This means that medical personnel involved in assessment and resuscitation should be unconcerned by the niceties of wound ballistics – patients with missile wounds are managed in the same way as any other trauma victim – primary survey, resuscitation, secondary survey and initiation of definitive care. There is nothing magical or mystical about missile velocity or ballistic injury.

GUNSHOT INJURIES

In the UK, gunshot wounds are mainly caused by handguns and shotguns. Although patients are now being seen with wounds caused by bullets from military assault rifles and other military automatic weapons, these are still fortunately rare. In civil practice, casualties in a climate of war or conflict present in large numbers in a short time, and present unique problems not dealt with here.

Handguns

Most victims will have single wounds and should present no particular problems. In most instances the wound and its cause should be obvious. However, if there is no event history a gunshot wound may be missed, and indeed this has happened in the resuscitation area of a large London hospital. The approach to assessment, resuscitation and decision-making is as directed in earlier chapters. There are no special rules! Do not come to any decision concerning wound severity based on knowledge, actual or assumed, of the wounding missile or wound appearance. In general, bullet wound entry and exit wounds give very little information on the patient's condition. Assume serious injury in all cases and arrange rapid transfer to hospital.

Remember that bullets may travel an erratic and unpredictable path and may enter several body cavities. A careful primary survey should detect evidence of intrathoracic or abdominal penetration, which is a particularly ominous feature. Deal with thoracic and abdominal problems as directed in Chapters 23 and 24.

Shotguns

Shotguns have a smooth bore and are designed to fire multiple pellets or shot; some fire large, solid lead or plastic slugs. Pellet size varies from large buckshot to small birdshot.

Wound severity varies enormously and depends on range, body region and size of shot. In general wounds tend to be extensive, with heavy foreign body contamination which may include the wadding from the shotgun cartridge. Assess and manage as for any form of trauma – external haemorrhage control may necessitate firm pressure over a large wounded area. The risk of wound sepsis is particularly high.

Military Weapons

Assault rifles and automatic weapons are now readily available to criminals and terrorists. This need not unduly trouble prehospital personnel. Treat victims as described earlier. It would be sensible to presume anyone wounded by bullets from military weapons to have serious injury until proved otherwise.

FURTHER READING

Greaves I, Dyer P & Porter K, eds (1995) *A Handbook of Immediate Medical Care*. London: WB Saunders.
Knight B (1991) *Simpson's Forensic Medicine*, 10th edn. London: Edward Arnold.

chapter twenty-nine:

BURNS

Burns are the third highest cause of deaths due to accidents. In 1988 in England and Wales 900 people died from fire, and serious burns resulted in 15,000 admissions to hospital. Almost 150,000 patients present to accident and emergency departments in the UK with burns each year.

ANATOMY OF THE SKIN

The cells of the epidermis come from the germinal layer; they gradually migrate upwards, and the outer layer is shed continuously. The epidermis acts as a barrier against water, bacteria and external injurious substances, and protects against wear and tear. The dermis consists of strong connective tissue containing numerous nerve endings to provide sensation, and the skin adnexa which include sweat glands, hair follicles and sebaceous glands. The functions of the skin are:

- Protection from injury
- Temperature control
- Prevention of excess water loss
- Detection of the nature of the immediate environment

Depth of Burns

The anatomy of burn depth is shown in Figure 29.1.

Simple erythema
Simple erythema is a superficial burn with no skin loss, e.g. sunburn. The skin is red and tender; this heals in 5–10 days with no scarring.

Superficial partial-thickness burn
Blisters are thin-walled and the burn is extremely painful. The skin is red and moist with a granular appearance and the germinal layer is not penetrated; an example is a scald from boiling water. Healing takes 10–20 days and there is minimal scarring.

Deep partial-thickness burn
A deep partial-thickness burn can be produced, for example, by boiling fat; it is deeper than the superficial partial-thickness burn and the blisters are thick-walled. The underlying skin is granular, and white in appearance with pin-point red mottling; sensation may be dulled. Healing is by migration of epithelial cells from the edge of the wound or skin adnexa, which takes 25–60 days. This burn type causes severe scarring and contractures, and is treated with excision and early grafting.

Deep (full-thickness) burn
Full-thickness burns are caused by prolonged contact with the burning agent or dry heat. The appearance is white, leathery or charred, and there is no sensation. This burn affects the full thickness of the skin, and may extend further into fat, muscle or bone; it does not heal. Treatment includes tangential excision and either skin graft or free flap repair depending on the depth.

FACTORS AFFECTING THE DEPTH OF THE BURN

Type of Burning Agent

Wet heat
Wet heat is the most common burning agent, for example boiling water from a kettle; this produces a scald which is a superficial partial-thickness burn. Superheated steam produces a deep partial-thickness burn as the temperature is greater and large amounts of energy are released as the steam condenses.

Dry heat
Dry heat may be a flame burn or a contact burn, e.g. with hot tar. These are direct burns and are often deep. Flame burns are often associated with inhalation injuries and other injuries.

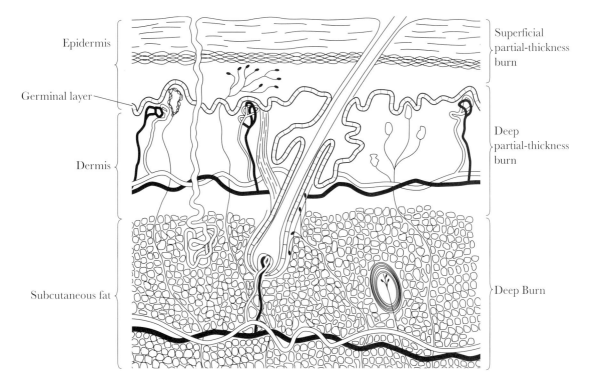

Fig. 29.1 *The skin in burns*

Flash burns

Flash burns are associated with explosions where the patient is subject to intense heat for a few seconds. These are usually partial-thickness burns and the patients commonly have other associated injuries.

Chemical burns

The severity of chemical burns depends upon the agent, the time of contact and the concentration. Some alkaline substances, e.g. wet cement, are highly corrosive and will continue to burn until completely removed. Acid burns usually produce less damage but will continue to burn if left on the skin. An exception to this is hydrofluoric acid which penetrates deeply and produces extensive tissue destruction and pain; these burns require treatment with calcium gluconate.

Electrical burns

See Chapter 41 on electrocution.

Radiation burns

The most common radiation burn is sunburn. See Chapter 43 on nuclear incidents.

Duration of Exposure to the Burning Agent

As the time of exposure to the burning agent is increased, the severity of the burn increases.

PATHOPHYSIOLOGY OF BURNS

In a burn wound there are three zones:

- The zone of coagulation
- The zone of stasis
- The zone of hyperaemia

The *zone of coagulation* is the central zone where cells have been destroyed by the thermal injury, producing an avascular area.

In the *zone of stasis* cells have been injured by the heat and should survive; however, they may die during the first 48 hours owing to associated vasoconstriction and microthrombus formation which reduce the blood supply.

In the *zone of hyperaemia* there is minimal thermal damage but marked vasodilatation and an acute inflammatory response. Owing to vasodilation and changes in the blood vessel walls, large amounts of fluid leak from the surface of the burn. The amount of fluid loss is dependent on the extent of the burn. This fluid loss tends to occur over the first 36 hours after the burn injury, and if the burn is large enough this can result in hypovolaemia. Thus fluid replacement is vital in burn management, and the type and the amount of fluid to be given are discussed below.

The pain from a burn is produced by the exposure of nerve endings in burnt skin as well as by inflammatory mediators.

Thermal damage to cells allows sodium to enter the injured cells producing a serum sodium deficit. Dead red blood cells release haemoglobin and damaged muscle releases myoglobin. This, combined with hypovolaemia, can lead to renal impairment. If the burn injury is severe, cardiac output can drop owing to the metabolic effects of the burn on the myocardium. Cardiac output also decreases if the burn injury is extensive and there is a large fluid loss with no replacement. This leads to an increase in heart rate and peripheral vascular resistance to maintain blood pressure and coronary and cerebral blood flow. As a result there is a reduction in blood flow to peripheral tissues and the gut, which leads to bacterial transfer from the gut into the blood stream, producing burn sepsis. The patient's immune system is depressed following a burn, leading to an increased susceptibility to infection. Bacterial infection delays healing and can convert a partial-thickness burn into a full-thickness burn. Thus it is important to wear gloves when treating or moving a burns patient. If a burn is extensive it is important to remember that the patient will lose heat rapidly and become hypothermic.

FACTORS AFFECTING THE OUTCOME OF BURNS

Factors affecting the outcome of burn injuries include the source and the depth of the burn – see above. Other factors are discussed below.

Extent of Burn

It is important to assess the extent of the burn accurately. In most accident and emergency departments the Lund and Browder chart is used for the estimation of percentage burn (Figure 29.2). This chart takes into account the differences in body surface area between adults and children when assessing the extent of the burn, so that the volume of fluid lost can be calculated correctly when estimating fluid replacement. For pre-hospital use a simpler method is the Wallace *rule of nines* for adults, and the *rule of fives* for children and infants (Figure 29.3). Another method uses the approximation that the patient's hand (flat with the fingers together) is equal to 1% of the patient's body surface area. This method is useful in assessing patchy burns present all over the body (Fig 29.4).

Burn Site

Burns in certain areas of the body have a worse prognosis than others. Burn sites with a poor prognosis are:

- Face
- Hands and feet
- Eyes
- Ears
- Perineum

Burns to the hands and feet, especially deep or deep partial-thickness burns, can produce extensive scarring and disability. Any facial burns can produce scarring and are often associated with an inhalation injury. Burns to the ears and eyes can produce long-term problems. A burn to an eye can cause blindness, eyelid deformities or corneal scarring. Ear burns can lead to deformity and infection. Burns to the perineum are difficult to dress and are susceptible to infection.

Circumferential burns

If there is a circumferential burn to the neck this can cause airway obstruction. Circumferential burns to the limbs produce constriction causing oedema and distal ischaemia. A circumferential burn to the chest can lead to respiratory failure.

Inhalation Injury

Inhalation injury is now the major cause of death in burns. It can be caused by three different mechanisms. The first is direct thermal injury by inhalation of flames, steam or hot gases. The second is inhalation of smoke containing water-soluble substances which react to form alkalis or acids, e.g. hydrogen chloride, ammonia or phosgene (produced by burning polyvinyl chloride), and lipid-soluble substances such as acrolein which can be attached to inhaled carbon particles. The third mechanism of injury is systemic poisoning (e.g. carbon monoxide, cyanide).

The upper airway is damaged by either direct thermal injury or smoke inhalation. This leads to oedema and sometimes obstruction of the upper airway which can have a rapid onset. The lower airway is damaged by smoke; in addition, superheated steam can produce thermal damage to the alveoli and this has a poor prognosis. Smoke inhalation can cause sloughing of the airway lining, producing obstruction and inflammation. The latter leads to the loss of protein-rich fluid into the lungs, causing pulmonary oedema and hypoxia.

Systemic toxicity is caused by the inhalation of chemicals, e.g. cyanide from burning polyurethane foam, which cause cell death. Another common inhaled gas is carbon monoxide, which binds to haemoglobin to produce carboxyhaemoglobin, making the haemoglobin unavailable for oxygen carriage. Inhalation injury should be rapidly assessed and treated promptly (see Chapters 4 and 5).

Electrical Injury

Electrical injuries are discussed in Chapter 41.

Age of the Patient

There is a greater mortality rate in children under 5 years old, as a child's surface area is greater in relation to their total body size and they will thus lose proportionally more fluid from the same percentage burn compared with an adult. In the elderly

NAME _____ WARD _____ NUMBER_____ DATE ____
AGE_____ ADMISSION WEIGHT_____

LUND AND BROWDER CHARTS

IGNORE
SIMPLE ERYTHEMA

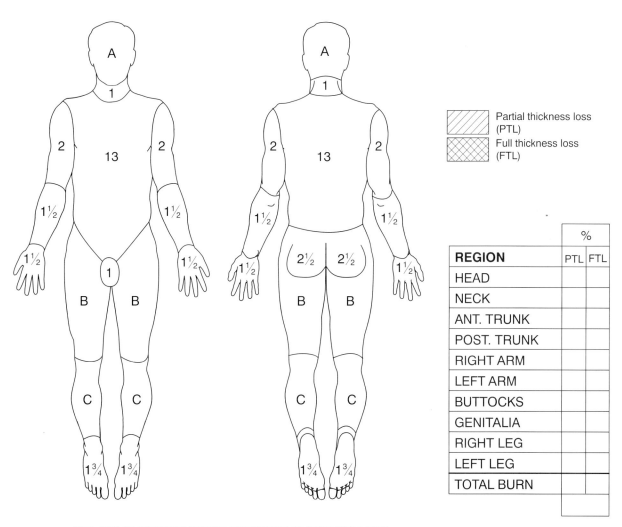

		%	
REGION		PTL	FTL
HEAD			
NECK			
ANT. TRUNK			
POST. TRUNK			
RIGHT ARM			
LEFT ARM			
BUTTOCKS			
GENITALIA			
RIGHT LEG			
LEFT LEG			
TOTAL BURN			

RELATIVE PERCENTAGE OF BODY SURFACE AREA
AFFECTED BY GROWTH

AREA	AGE 0	1	5	10	15	ADULT
A=½ OF HEAD	9½	8½	6½	5½	4½	3½
B=½ OF ONE THIGH	2¾	3¼	4	4½	4½	4¾
C=½ OF ONE LEG	2½	2½	2¾	3	3¼	3½

Fig. 29.2 Lund and Browder chart. From Settler, J (1986) Burns: The First Five Days, *with permission from Smith and Nephew*

WALLACE'S RULE OF NINES

RULE OF FIVES FOR CHILDREN AND INFANTS

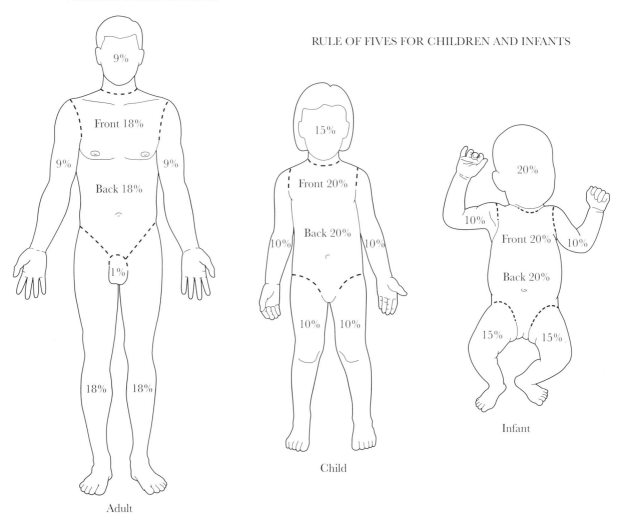

Adult

Child

Infant

Fig. 29.3 The 'rule of nines' (adults) and the 'rule of fives' (children and infants)

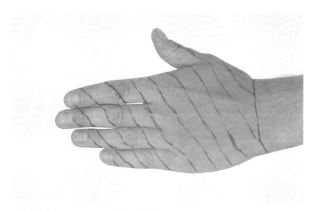

Fig. 29.4 One per cent of the body area

the mortality rate is also greater, firstly because ageing tissue does not heal as well as younger tissue, and secondly because patients often have associated medical conditions which affect morbidity and mortality, as well as a reduced physiological reserve.

Associated Injury

Associated injuries are common in patients suffering from burns who may have jumped to escape the fire, or have been involved in an explosion or a road traffic accident where petrol has ignited. In all these cases associated injuries should be looked for in the primary and secondary surveys.

Associated Medical Conditions

If a patient has a respiratory disorder the mortality from an inhalation injury will increase. A burn may cause further problems for patients with heart conditions through either emotional or physical stress. Patients with diabetes mellitus, on steroid therapy or with peripheral vascular disease will have delayed healing.

CRITICAL BURNS

The burns listed below should be regarded as critical and will normally require specialist management in a burns centre following assessment in the accident and emergency department. Consideration should be given to direct transfer from the scene of the accident to a regional burns centre.

Critical burns

- Simple erythema over more than 75% of the body surface area
- Partial-thickness burn exceeding 10% surface area in a child, 15% in an adult and 5% in an elderly patient
- Deep burn over more than 10% of the body surface area
- Inhalation injury
- Burns complicated by a fracture or major soft tissue injury
- Burns in patients with associated medical conditions
- Any chemical or electrical burns

ASSESSMENT AND MANAGEMENT

Safety at the Scene

The approach to the scene is described in Chapter 1. Ensure that the environment is safe for you and the patient; if necessary wait for the fire service to put the fire out or to rescue the burns patient. Remember that just opening a door or window increases the oxygen supply to the fire, increasing its intensity or possibly causing an explosion, thus endangering the lives of both you and the patient.

Stopping the Burn Process

Dry and wet heat
Once the patient is safe it is necessary to prevent further harm. If the patient's clothes are smouldering or in flames, place the patient on the floor and wrap them up in a blanket to put the flames out. If the clothes are smouldering or have hot liquid on them, they must be removed quickly; if the clothing is stuck or

burnt onto the skin the clothes must be cut around and soaked with clean cold water to minimize the burn process. If the burn area is extensive from either dry or wet heat (e.g. flame or scald) then it can be soaked with clean cold water, but do not leave the water on the burn, as this will increase heat loss from the body surface and the patient may become hypothermic. If the flame burn or scald area is small (less than 10%), cold water on a clean, sterile towel can be left on until the patient is in hospital as this reduces the burn process and alleviates pain.

Tar burns
Do not remove the tar but immerse in cold water to cool the area to stop the burning process.

Chemical burns
Continuously wash the burn with large quantities of water for 10 or more minutes at the scene, then transfer the patient to hospital.

Primary Survey

Assessing the airway
The airway should be assessed as explained in Chapters 2 to 5.

Assessment of breathing
The breathing should be assessed as explained in Chapters 2 to 5.

Specific signs and symptoms of inhalation must be looked for, including certain aspects of the history. These include:

- History of being confined with the fire in a closed space
- History of unconsciousness at the time of the incident
- Exposure to smoke or gas during the incident
- Evidence of burns to the face
- Singed nasal hair
- Cough or carbonaceous sputum
- Blistering or redness in the mouth
- Evidence of laryngeal oedema, e.g. hoarseness, stridor
- Wheezing
- Signs of airway obstruction or respiratory distress
- Full-thickness burns to the nasolabial area of the face or posterior pharyngeal swelling
- Signs of respiratory failure: the patient who is unable to speak owing to shortness of breath or exhaustion, or who is unconscious

If the patient is unconscious and unresponsive then oxygen should be given via a bag and mask, and only in extreme circumstances (respiratory or cardiac arrest) should intubation be considered in the field. This should be done using a smaller tube than normal because the airway will often be narrowed owing to oedema. It is best to transfer the patient to the nearest accident and emergency department for definitive airway management.

If there is marked wheezing, nebulized salbutamol at the scene may help.

> **If there is any evidence of an inhalation injury or a critical burn the patient should be given the highest concentration of oxygen available (100%)**

Assessment and treatment of carbon monoxide poisoning

Most burns patients from a fire in an enclosed environment will have inhaled carbon monoxide. Carbon monoxide is a by-product of incomplete combustion of carbon and has a higher affinity for haemoglobin than oxygen (approximately 200 times greater). If large amounts of carbon monoxide are present, oxygen is displaced from haemoglobin and large quantities of carboxyhaemoglobin are produced. Because the binding of carbon monoxide to haemoglobin is much stronger than that of oxygen it also makes it difficult for the haemoglobin to release oxygen at the tissues, which further aggravates tissue hypoxia. The half-life of carboxyhaemoglobin in room air is 320 minutes; on 100% oxygen it is 80 minutes, and on 100% oxygen at 3 atmospheres (hyperbaric oxygen) it is 23 minutes. The signs and symptoms of carbon monoxide poisoning include lethargy, muscle weakness, headache, nausea and vomiting. When carbon monoxide poisoning is more severe the patient will have dilated pupils, cyanosis and pulmonary oedema. However, the cherry-red mucosa which is classically described is rarely seen. The signs and symptoms of mild carbon monoxide poisoning are:

- Lethargy
- Muscle weakness
- Headache
- Nausea
- Vomiting

The signs and symptoms of severe carbon monoxide poisoning are:

- Cyanosis
- Coma
- Pulmonary oedema
- Dilated pupils

Any person with carbon monoxide poisoning should be given 100% oxygen and transferred to the accident and emergency department immediately. Pulse oximetry, which measures oxygen saturation, does not alter in carbon monoxide poisoning as it will not detect the difference between carboxyhaemoglobin

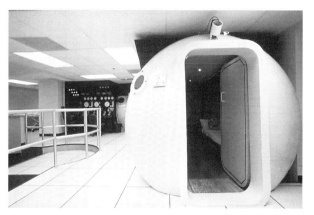

Fig. 29.5 A hyperbaric chamber

and oxyhaemoglobin. Pulse oximetry may therefore appear falsely reassuring in a patient with carbon monoxide poisoning. The levels of carboxyhaemoglobin can only be measured from an arterial blood sample. The patient is considered for hyperbaric oxygen (Figure 29.5) if:

- The patient is unconscious at any time
- The carboxyhaemoglobin concentration exceeds 20%
- Neurological signs and symptoms are present
- The patient is pregnant

Patients with carboxyhaemoglobin levels of 50–60% are comatose and require ventilatory support.

The diagnosis of carbon monoxide poisoning may be straightforward if the patient is found in a fume-filled car with the exhaust connected to the interior. However, the symptoms are unfortunately vague and non-specific, and a high index of suspicion must be maintained especially in chronic carbon monoxide poisoning, which may occur in poorly ventilated accommodation.

Assessment of circulation

It is important to assess pulse, blood pressure and capillary refill in any burn, but especially in a critical burn (>15% in an adult; >10% in a child). An intravenous infusion must be started in a patient with a critical burn if the transfer time is greater than 20 minutes, as vast quantities of plasma will be lost from the burn. However, it is important to realize that a patient suffering from burns alone is unlikely to be initially hypovolaemic at the scene. If the burns patient is in hypovolaemic shock immediately after the burn it is advisable to give the locally recommended fluid for hypovolaemic shock due to trauma, and the cause of the hypovolaemia should be assumed *not* to be the burn. Intravenous access requires two large-bore cannulae in the antecubital fossa. If this area is burnt it is preferable to site the intravenous line somewhere else in the upper limb; if this is not practicable the lower limb should be considered. In burns units, plasma protein fraction has been recommended as the ideal replacement fluid for burns as this closely resembles the fluid lost and maintains body functions as close to normal as possible. This is not practical outside hospital. It is also suggested that plasma substitutes are of value if there has been a delay of 1 hour or more in giving a patient fluid after a burn; this is because of their plasma expanding properties. There is still controversy over which fluid to give initially. There has been a trend away from using plasma or other colloids, and at present the recommended initial fluid is Hartmann's solution. This is partly on clinical grounds as well as for reasons of cost, and it has been shown in a number of centres that electrolyte and plasma infusions give comparable results. If Hartmann's solution is unavailable normal saline is a suitable alternative.

In pre-hospital care rapid transfer of a burns patient to appropriate definitive care must never be delayed while an intravenous infusion is set up; consider setting up an infusion in transit.

Fluid requirement formulae A number of formulae for fluid replacement following a burn are available. These formulae are not relevant to pre-hospital care, and are given here for information only.

The *Muir and Barclay formula* is commonly used in burns units and in accident and emergency departments in the UK. This gives the amount of colloid required in the first 4 hours:

Fluid (ml) = 0.5 × (weight in kg × percentage surface area burnt)

The Parkland formula is commonly used in North America and is used to calculate crystalloid requirements, which are greater than the volume of colloid which would be required. The amount of fluid (Hartmann's solution) required in the first 8 hours is:

Fluid (ml) = 2 × (weight in kg × percentage surface area burnt)

ANALGESIA

The ideal analgesic agent is morphine at 0.1 mg/kg body weight, given intravenously with an appropriate antiemetic. However, this is unavailable at the scene in the UK unless a doctor is present. Often the patient with a full-thickness burn will not request analgesia as there is no pain. Partial-thickness burns are extremely painful, and either nitrous oxide and oxygen inhalation (Entonox) can be self-administered by the patient or the patient can be given nalbuphine (Nubain) intravenously. Nalbuphine is now available on a number of paramedic ambulances and can be given as a 10 mg dose intravenously, repeated if the pain relief is not sufficient with the first dose. No analgesic drug should be given intramuscularly or subcutaneously in severe or moderate burns, as it will remain unabsorbed owing to poor circulation.

> It is essential that hospital medical staff are made aware that nalbuphine has been given

SECONDARY SURVEY

During the secondary survey a full history should be ascertained. This should include the following details:

- Time of the burn
- Burning agent
- Is the patient complaining of pain?
- Has the patient jumped or been involved in an explosion?
- Was the patient in a confined space?
- Has the patient lost consciousness at any time?
- A brief medical history, drug and allergy history
- Tetanus status of the patient

During the secondary survey a head-to-toe examination is performed to see if any other injuries have been sustained by the patient.

INITIAL DRESSINGS FOR BURNS

If the burn affects less than 10% of the skin surface area, then a clean dressing soaked in cold water or normal saline can be used to reduce the effect of the burn (both the pain and the burning process). If the burn is over 10% then a sterile clean cloth or cling film can be placed over the burn to reduce air currents which will reduce pain and prevent contamination of the burn. These emergency burn dressings allow the burn to be reassessed in the accident and emergency department so that a definitive burn dressing can be applied. If the patient is to be transferred to a burns unit, cling film should be placed on the burn so that it can be easily reassessed at the unit. It is important to know the local burns unit policy on dressings when transferring burns patients.

> Under no circumstances should any cream (antibiotic or otherwise) be applied to a burn before hospital assessment

DISPOSAL

All burn patients should be transferred to hospital and from there a decision can be taken as to whether the patient needs to be transferred to a burns unit, admitted to the hospital from the accident and emergency department, or treated as an outpatient. Critical burns should if possible go direct to the burns unit – these are:

- Partial-thickness burns over 10% in a child or the elderly and over 15% in an adult
- Full-thickness burn of over 5% at any age
- Extensive burns to the hands, feet, genitalia, perineum or face
- Severe electrical burn
- Severe chemical burn
- Inhalation injuries

FURTHER READING

Davis D (1985) *ABC of Plastic and Reconstructive Surgery.* London: BMJ Publications.

Eaton C J (1993) *Essentials of Immediate Medical Care.* Edinburgh: Churchill Livingstone.

Greaves I, Dyer P & Porter K (1995) *A Handbook of Immediate Care.* London: W B Saunders.

Pre-Hospital Trauma Life Support Committee of the National Association of Emergency Medicine Technicians (1990) *Pre-hospital Trauma Life Support*, 2nd edn. In cooperation with the Committee on Trauma of the American College of Surgeons.

Settle JAD (1986) *Burns: The First Five Days.* Smith and Nephew Pharmaceuticals.

Skinner D, Driscoll P & Irlam R (1991) *ABC of Major Trauma.* London: BMJ Publications.

Wardrope J & Smith JAR *Management of Wounds and Burns.* Oxford Handbooks in Emergency Medicine. Oxford University Press.

chapter thirty:

WOUND MANAGEMENT

According to the 1987 mortality statistics of the Office of Population Censuses and Surveys, 432 deaths (2.5% of deaths from accidents) in the UK were due to wounding. Throughout the country 3 million wounds are treated annually in accident and emergency departments. Thus there are a large number of wounds inflicted by accidents and it is vitally important to assess and manage a wound correctly to reduce the long-term problems this may cause the patient.

ANATOMY OF THE SKIN

See Chapter 29.

DEFINITIONS

Wound Any interruption by violence or surgery of the continuity of the external surface of the body or the surface of an internal organ. Legally this used to mean the whole thickness of the skin must be broken and an internal injury alone would not qualify as a 'wound'. However, this part of the definition is no longer used. Strictly, *a wound is a disruption of the continuity of tissue*.

Cut (incised wound) A breach of the skin caused by a sharp edge.

Laceration A breach of the skin caused by a blunt force; it is usually irregular in shape.

Contused wound Loss of continuity of the tissue with surrounding bruising.

Penetrating wound A wound produced by a pointed object which produces a fine path into the body.

Contusion An area of bruising due to the effect of blunt force which does not produce a break in the skin.

Haematoma A swelling composed of blood which is present underneath the skin. This is produced by a blunt direct force without breaking the skin.

Abrasion Removal of a portion of the surface of the skin. It is usually the outer layers of the skin that are damaged and there is often oozing from the capillaries on the surface of the dermis.

Puncture wound A wound with a narrow path made by, for example, a nail.

Avulsion The forced separation of two parts; with wounding, this is when a flap of skin has been partially or completely removed.

Amputation Removal of a portion of a limb or the complete limb, accompanied by profuse bleeding.

Closed wound An internal injury caused by a blunt direct force to the surface of the body. The skin itself is intact, but there is injury to the underlying tissues. This could be in the form of a simple contusion as defined above. Over the chest or abdomen this may lead to internal injury to the ribs and lungs or the rupture of hollow organs respectively. In the case of a crush injury to the limb or finger this may produce external bruising or contusion, and there may be extensive underlying damage with bony injury.

PATHOPHYSIOLOGY

Wound healing can be divided into two types. Healing by primary intention occurs when the wound is a simple cut with minimal tissue loss. Healing by secondary intention occurs when there is significant tissue loss from the wound. The phases of wound healing are the same in primary and secondary intention. However, in secondary intention healing there is more emphasis on wound contraction.

Phases of Healing

Inflammation

During wounding blood vessels are torn, and initially they contract, reducing the blood loss from the open end. Blood is released into the wound which triggers the activation of platelets and initiates the coagulation cascade, which ultimately leads to the production of fibrin from fibrinogen and produces a clot in the wound. A complex sequence of events gives rise to the activation of other biological compounds including vasodilators, which increase the capillary permeability in the area producing swelling and oedema; other compounds are released which attract cells to the wound. These cells include polymorphonuclear cells, granulocytes and macrophages which remove tissue debris and bacteria. The macrophages initiate the healing of the wound by stimulating the production of blood vessels and attracting fibroblasts, cells that produce the extracellular matrix which contains collagen. The inflammation process occurs over a period of up to 4 days, with a maximum response at 24 hours. The wound at this stage will have a clot on the surface and the surrounding tissue will be red and oedematous.

Cell proliferation and matrix deposition

During the next stage, which lasts up to 30 days, there is an increase in cell proliferation, especially in fibroblasts which produce collagen. Collagen is laid down haphazardly in the scar tissue. At the same time epithelial cells at the wound margins start to move in to cover the wound. New capillaries are formed, giving the base of the wound a granulated appearance *(granulation tissue)* and the epithelial cells grow over the granulation tissue beneath the clot. The epithelium over the granulation tissue is extremely delicate and can often be damaged with either removal of the clot or repeated dressings. At this stage the wound space becomes organized and it is very vascular. The scar and surrounding tissue are red owing to the increase in blood flow to the area. During this phase the contraction of the wound is initiated. This is caused by two components: firstly by the myofibroblasts, and secondly by the maturation of collagen which occurs in the third phase.

Matrix remodelling

This third phase overlaps with the first two phases and occurs between days 1 and 300. However, the wound is regarded as 'healed' at 30 days. During phase three the matrix of collagen is remodelled, there are changes in orientation of the collagen fibres, and the collagen becomes cross-linked biochemically producing an increase in its tensile strength. This, in combination with the contractility provided by the myofibroblasts, produces further contraction of the scar tissue. The scar becomes less vascular, less cellular and appears white.

With primary intention healing the two edges of the wound are opposed and there is healing with minimal scarring. With secondary intention healing there is a defect in the wound and the vascular granulation tissue matures in the base of the defect, initially producing a red, very vascular area which converts into a dense mass of fibrotic tissue which is white and avascular. With secondary intention healing wound contraction is more prominent and brings together the structures on either side of the wound. This can lead to significant deformity or contractures if the defect has been large.

Factors Affecting Wound Healing

Age

As tissue ages, the healing process slows.

Nutrition

Any decrease in protein intake causes a reduction in the essential amino acids available for tissue repair. A decrease in vitamin C intake causes poor tissue healing and produces the characteristic picture of scurvy. Zinc is also vitally important for the synthesis of collagen.

Diseases

Disease processes, specifically diabetes mellitus and haematological problems such as anaemia, will decrease the efficacy of wound healing.

Drugs

Steroids dampen the inflammatory response and over long periods can cause the skin to thin, making it more susceptible to damage.

Infection

If there are more than 100,000 bacteria per gram of tissue at the time the wound is repaired, infection is likely to occur.

Foreign body

Any foreign material in a wound which is not removed at the time of repair can give rise to further inflammation and infection, and prevent wound healing.

Poor blood supply

Pretibial wounds, especially in the elderly, have a reduced blood supply. This reduces the influx of inflammatory cells, and the supply of oxygen and nutrients required for healing.

Adhesions, movement and drying

All these affect the degree of wound healing. 'Adhesions' occur when dressings stick to a wound: every time the dressing is replaced the re-epithelialization is disrupted and the granulation tissue bleeds. This also occurs if there is movement of the dressing around the wound. Drying of a wound, although once thought to be ideal for healing, reduces the amount of re-epithelialization and thus reduces the rate of healing.

Ionizing radiation

Ionizing radiation causes a reduction in the rate of healing.

Hypoxia

Hypoxia is associated with poor blood supply. If a patient is severely wounded with a reduction in oxygenation of the tissue and a reduction in the blood supply due to hypovolaemia, both of these will be detrimental to the establishment of the initial phase of wound healing. Thus it is vitally important to maintain the airway, breathing and circulation during wound management.

IMMEDIATE MANAGEMENT OF WOUNDS

Firstly, it must be remembered that the primary survey comes before dealing with any soft tissue injury.

Airway

The airway must be secured using the procedure described in Chapters 4 and 5. Any severe facial injury can produce major bleeding. This may be external from obvious lacerations or internal from facial fractures (see Chapter 22).

Breathing

Ensure that the respiratory rate of the patient is adequate. In any penetrating wound to the chest the object must be left *in situ*, and if there is an open pneumothorax a dressing sealed on three sides must be placed over the wound thus preventing a sucking chest wound (see Chapter 23). A patient who has suffered a severe blunt injury to the chest may have massive internal bleeding producing a haemothorax. Unfortunately there is little that the paramedic can do except provide high-flow oxygen, maintain the upper airway, obtain intravenous access to provide large volumes of fluid and transport the patient to hospital as soon as possible.

Circulation

Circulation must be assessed (see Chapters 19 and 20). Intravenous access must be obtained, preferably two lines (16 or 18 gauge), and intravenous fluids commenced.

Control of external haemorrhage
There are three different kinds of bleeding:

- Arterial bleeding is bright red in colour and often under pressure, spurting from the wound. If a large artery has been severed, e.g. the femoral artery, a large volume of blood may be lost
- Venous bleeding is dark red in colour and tends to be slower than arterial. However, the veins are capacitance vessels, and if they are full, a large amount of blood can be lost
- Capillary bleeding or oozing from capillaries typically occurs with an abrasion. If capillary bleeding is caused by a blow to the skin with no break, this will produce damage to the capillaries beneath the skin and cause a contusion or bruise

It is important before treating a wound to ensure personal protection with gloves, glasses or face guard and apron or overalls. Firstly, cut or remove the clothing away from the wounded area thus exposing the wound. At this time it is useful to make a mental note of the size and depth of the wound and the sort of bleeding occurring. The majority of wounds show a mixture of both arterial and venous bleeding. It is important to note if it is a major arterial bleed.

Control of bleeding from an open wound Apply direct pressure to the wound with a clean, large gauze pad (dry or moist). The gauze pad can be moistened with sterile water or saline if it is available. The direct pressure must be constant. If a gauze pad is not available just use your gloved hand, provided that you have ascertained that there are no sharp objects in the base of the wound. Three layers of gauze can be placed on the wound and the bandage placed over these layers of gauze to secure them in position. The entire wound should be covered and the bandage secured. It is important to elevate the injured area above the heart if possible to reduce blood flow to the area. If direct pressure to the wound is not sufficient and the wound is still bleeding, do not remove the dressing but apply indirect pressure to specific pressure points. These are areas where the arteries providing blood to specific areas can be pressed against bone, thereby reducing the flow of blood to the wound. Five important pressure points are:

- The femoral artery in the groin, which can be compressed against the pelvis
- The brachial artery approximately 2 cm in from the medial epicondyle of the elbow, which can be compressed against the lower end of the humerus
- The superficial temporal artery, which can be palpated just anterior to the tragus of the ear and can be compressed against the temporal bone to reduce bleeding from scalp lacerations on that side
- The supraorbital and supratrochleal arteries supplying the forehead, which can be compressed against the supraorbital margin to reduce bleeding from lacerations of the forehead
- The facial artery, which can be compressed against the mandible approximately halfway from the angle of the mandible to the tip of the chin to reduce bleeding from the lower half of the face

Direct pressure should only be applied for 10 minutes at a time with release of the pressure and review to see if the bleeding has stopped. If it has not stopped then the pressure can be reapplied.

Splinting is also effective in reducing movement of the limb, thereby reducing the amount of bleeding. Splinting is also an advantage in patients who have an open fracture (see Chapter 25). The air splint is useful because it has the double advantage of splinting the appropriate limb and providing direct pressure to the wound.

Tourniquets are used as a last resort where the patient is exsanguinating, e.g. from a sudden traumatic amputation, or in a severe crush injury when the application may protect the patient from toxins arising from the crushed part. If a tourniquet is to be applied it should be tight enough to prevent both arterial and venous flow. If the tourniquet is too loose it allows arterial flow and leads to venous engorgement in the limb and further bleeding. It is important to use wide, flat material and apply a rolled pad to the artery underneath. The tourniquet must be tightened until no further bleeding occurs. The time of application of the tourniquet, the name of the person applying it and its position must be recorded. The tourniquet must never be covered. It should be released when an adequate external compression bandage has been applied to the area. It is advisable to mark on the patient that a tourniquet has been applied so that it is not forgotten once the patient has been transferred to hospital. Once applied, tourniquets are best removed in hospital.

Control of external haemorrhage of an open wound with a sharp object protruding When a sharp object is protruding from a wound it is important not to remove the object. The edges of the wound are pushed against the sharp object by placing pads on either side. The pads on either side of the protruding object should be high enough to allow a bandage around to provide compression.

SPECIFIC WOUND MANAGEMENT

Wound Assessment

During the history relevant details regarding the patient should be obtained (see Chapter 18).

Mechanism of injury
The mechanism of injury is how the wound came about. The broad categories used are blunt injury and penetrating injury.

Blunt injury Blunt injury may occur, for example, in a road traffic accident. The severity of the blunt injury depends on the speed and direction of impact; in road traffic accidents, the greater the speed of the vehicle the greater the severity of the injury to the occupant, and injury patterns can be predicted. For example, a frontal collision is more likely to result in injury to the front of the head, the neck, the front of the chest, abdomen, pelvis and the femur. However, a side impact will cause rotational injury to the head and neck, and injure the lateral side of the chest and abdomen as well as the hip (see Chapter 18).

Blunt injuries are also caused by being hit by a blunt object, e.g. a baseball bat. It is not always necessary for the skin to be broken; if a baseball bat hits the abdomen with severe force it will sink in and make no visible impression. However, there may be an abrasion or contusion left after the impact. The force with which the baseball bat hits the stomach causes indentation and can produce underlying bony or internal organ damage. This applies also to any significant blunt force on the chest causing fractured ribs and underlying pulmonary contusion.

Another type of blunt injury is the crush injury; this typically occurs when fingers are trapped, for instance in machinery, a car door, or underneath someone's foot in a contact sport. In this instance the skin may not be damaged, although there often is a split laceration due to pressure. There is marked contusion and eventually gross swelling of the part crushed, owing to the tissue damage which occurs underneath the skin. There may be no bony injury, but there is often long-term swelling and damage to the soft tissue which takes time to heal.

Penetrating wounds The damage produced by a *stab wound* depends on the area of the body involved, and the velocity and force with which the stab has been produced. It is important to remember in a stab wound that only structures lying in the path of the stabbing implement are damaged. Thus if there is a stab wound to the leg muscle, nerve or vessel damage may also occur. However, if there is a stab wound to the abdomen, any of the viscera underlying that area of the stab wound can be damaged.

The damage caused by a *bullet wound* depends on the shape of the bullet, the velocity, the angle at which it was fired and the distance of the person from the weapon. When a bullet penetrates the skin, the energy is dissipated from the bullet to the tissue and the cells of the tissue are moved directly away from the site of impact by the energy exchange. This causes damage to the tissue on either side of the pathway of the bullet as well as the tissue damaged by the bullet. The path of the bullet varies and it is not just tissues adjacent to the entrance site that are damaged. The bullet may take any path through the body, depending on the amount of kinetic energy it contains when it first hits the body. It is also important to note that there is a great deal of contamination from a bullet wound due to clothing and foreign material being drawn in with the bullet.

Bites can be produced by animals or humans, and there is a risk of wound infection. Providing they are cleaned and left open they usually heal. However, any dog bites or animal bites to the face are usually seen by a plastic surgeon as these wounds require debriding before suturing. The most common human bite wound is a laceration over the knuckle from a punch, and these wounds are likely to become infected; patients with this type of wound are always given antibiotics. Bites that produce lacerations can damage underlying tissue.

Puncture wounds can be caused by bites, dirty nails or sharp objects. Since these wounds are caused by a sharp point and the wound closes over, they are prone to infection especially with anaerobic bacteria. These patients need antibiotic cover. With a puncture wound, again only structures in the path of the puncturing object are damaged. This usually involves muscle and occasionally nerves and tendons.

Environment in which the injury occurred

It is important to observe where the wound occurred, i.e. indoors or outside, and also if the area outside was tetanus-prone. Tetanus-prone wounds are any wounds more than 6 hours old, those with a large amount of necrotic tissue present, and wounds that have been in contact with soil or manure. Other tetanus-prone wounds are puncture wounds or wounds that are infected (Table 30.1).

The temperature of the environment is also important; frost-bite will reduce wound healing.

Time of injury

If the wound is more than 6 hours old it is more likely to have been infected. An untreated wound more than 3 hours old will have more than one million bacteria per gram of tissue. In all traumatic wounds there is an infection rate of approximately 15%. One way to reduce wound infection is, if possible, to clear away any debris around the wound, apply a clean sterile dressing or gauze and transfer the patient to an emergency department so that the wound can be cleaned and treated. However, if the wound is more than 6 hours old it will be highly contaminated, and it is preferable for this wound to be cleaned in the accident and emergency department and to remain open with an appropriate dressing. It would not be sutured immediately and may be left open to heal or be sutured at a later stage.

Examination

Pre-hospital examination of the wound includes observation of the size, shape and depth of the wound, and of any underlying structures that have been exposed or are protruding from the wound, e.g. bone, tendons, vessels, nerves or subcutaneous tissue. At the scene it is important to note movement and sensation distal to the wound so the examining hospital doctor can assess if distal function has deteriorated.

Wounds at Specific Sites

Scalp wounds

For scalp wounds it is important to replace any skin flaps and provide direct pressure on the site of the wound with a sterile gauze and secure it with a bandage. If neck injury is not suspected, lie the patient down with the head raised.

Neck wounds

Neck wounds, either open or closed, can produce swelling around the larynx and trachea due to bleeding and haematoma formation which can compromise the airway. Thus the airway must be protected early to prevent any deterioration.

Wounds of the palm of the hand

It is important to place a sterile pad over a wound in the palm of the hand, with the patient's fingers placed over the gauze to apply pressure over the injury. Then bandage the fingers down. The same principles apply for wounds in joint creases, for example, at the elbow the pad can be placed in the crease of the elbow and the elbow flexed to exert pressure over the pad to reduce the bleeding. The pressure can be released every 10 minutes to see if the bleeding has stopped.

Bleeding from the ear, nose or facial injuries

See Chapter 22.

Table 30.1 Tetanus: treatment and prophylaxis

Immunization status of patient	Treatment
Tetanus-prone wounds	
Tetanus course or booster up-to-date (within the last 10 years)	No treatment unless a very high risk of infection
Completed course for tetanus > 10 years ago	One dose of tetanus booster plus human tetanus immunoglobin IM
Has not had a complete course of tetanus immunization	A complete course of tetanus immunization plus one dose of human tetanus immunoglobin IM
Unknown	Full tetanus course plus one dose of tetanus immunoglobin IM
Wounds not tetanus prone	
Covered for tetanus	No action required
Completed course for tetanus > 10 years ago	One dose of tetanus booster
Has not had a complete course of tetanus immunization	A complete course of tetanus immunization
Unknown	Full tetanus course

Chest wounds
See Chapter 23.

Abdominal injuries
See Chapter 24.

Eye wounds
Any contusion, laceration or penetrating wounds to the eye should be covered by a sterile dressing and the sterile dressing bandaged *in situ*. The bandage should really cover both eyes as this prevents any movement of the eye which could cause further damage. The patient should be kept as still as possible with the head slightly raised, provided there is no neck injury.

Varicose vein injuries in the lower leg
Apply direct pressure to the wound with gauze, lie the patient down and elevate the leg. The patient should be transferred to hospital with the leg elevated.

Management of Specific Types of Wounds

Flap wounds
It is important to make sure that the flaps are replaced and a sterile gauze dressing, dry or moist, is placed over the top.

Foreign body wounds
If there is a large impaled object then this should not be removed and a bandage should be applied around the area. If there is a small foreign body, either glass or grit, on the surface and not embedded it can be removed. If small particles of glass or grit are embedded these will be more difficult to remove, and a sterile dressing, dry or moist, should be placed over the wound and the personnel at the hospital notified on arrival.

Crush injuries
Crush injuries can range from a fingertip crushed in a car door to a major crushed chest in a road traffic accident. The crush of a fingertip is common and causes local tissue damage, possible fracture and marked swelling. This should be covered with either a dry dressing or a moist saline soak, elevated, and the patient taken to hospital. With extensive crush injuries to the limbs it must always be borne in mind that there is a possibility of a release of toxins once the crush has been released. This is more likely if the limb has been crushed for longer than 10 minutes. In these instances it is important to control the airway, breathing and circulation before the crush is released. Once the object crushing the limb has been released it is important to cover the external wound, splint the limb and transfer the patient to hospital as soon as possible.

High-pressure injection injuries
Injuries may occur from a high-pressure oil or grease gun, and initially very little injury may be evident. However, these type of injuries must be seen in hospital as in high-pressure injection there may be severe damage and necrosis to the tissue underlying the skin, despite it initially looking undamaged. These injuries can lead to extensive loss of soft tissue.

Puncture wounds
See above.

Bites
See above.

Amputation
When either a limb or a digit has been completely severed there can be massive bleeding, but bleeding is usually limited as the vessels have been torn and have retracted into the wound. The area should be covered with a sterile saline soak or sterile gauze, direct pressure applied and the stump elevated. The amputated part should be wrapped in cling film or a polythene bag. The bag can then be wrapped in gauze and placed in a plastic bag containing ice. It is important not to place the amputated part directly in contact with either cotton wool, gauze or ice as this will cause damage.

Abrasions
Abrasions are superficial wounds which are usually caused by shearing or friction and usually contain grit or debris. It is important not to try to clean them at the scene, as this can be extremely painful, and it is best to cover the abrasion with a sterile dressing, preferably moist, and transfer the patient to hospital so that the abrasion can be cleaned adequately under local anaesthesia to prevent tattooing.

Contusions
Where there are severe contusions to a limb, hand or digit, the injured part should be immobilized in a splint, elevated and, where possible, ice or a cold compress used to alleviate the pain and swelling.

Basic Dressings

It was originally thought that wounds should be kept dry to prevent infection and aid healing. However, it has been shown that it is important to keep the wound environment moist, and a specific level of moisture is required for ideal healing. Re-epithelialization of wounds occurs 40% faster in a moist environment; this is because a wound deprived completely of any exudate actually heals more slowly, as the exudate contains growth factors required to encourage new vessel formation and re-epithelialization.

The ideal wound dressing should promote gaseous exchange, maintaining the correct oxygen tension and pH of the wound surface. There should be high humidity in the wound and an equilibrium between exudate absorption and the amount of moisture at the wound surface. The temperature of the wound should be maintained near to core temperature which enables the cells to function maximally for regeneration and phagocytosis. The dressing should aid the removal of dead tissue, bacteria and any unwanted chemicals, and should provide a barrier to the outside environment, preventing bacteria entering the wound as well as protecting against environmental changes in temperature. It should preferably be non-adherent, non-allergenic and have good mechanical properties to protect the wound from external forces. Currently there is no one particular dressing that provides all of these features. However, there are numerous micro-environment dressings available which include thin films, hydrocolloids, hydrogels, foams and alginates. All of these may be used at different times with different wounds, and are all utilized in the long-term treatment of wounds.

In pre-hospital wound treatment where the wound needs to be covered quickly with the cleanest possible material, the most useful dressings should be sterile, usually gauze pads or larger bulky dressings if required to stop excessive bleeding. It is unlikely to be a clean environment at the scene, but any further contamination of the wound should be prevented. If sterile water or normal saline is available then some of the gauze may be moistened to provide a moist contact with the wound to prevent the sterile dressing becoming adherent to the wound. The dressing can be secured in place using a non-sterile bandage. Occlusive dressings can be used for wounds of the abdomen or chest, particularly of the abdomen where bowel has been exposed, as this prevents loss of moisture. Cling film has already been mentioned as a dressing for burns.

FURTHER READING

Falanga V (1988) Occlusive wound dressings: why, when, which? *Archives of Dermatology* 124: 872–877.

Haywood I & Skinner D (1991) Blast and gunshot. In: Skinner D, Driscoll P & Earlam R (eds) *ABC of Major Trauma*, pp 88–90. London: BMJ Publications.

Szycher M & Lee SJ (1992) Modern wound dressings: a systematic approach to wound healing. *Journal of Biomaterials Application* 7: 142–212.

Walton LR & Earle Matory Jr W (1993) Wound care. In: Saunders CE & Ho MT (eds). *Current Emergency Diagnosis and Treatment*, 4th edn, pp 377–403. Lang Medical.

Wardrope J & Smith JAR *The Management of Wounds and Burns*. Oxford University Press.

Wijetunge DB (1994) Management of acute and traumatic wounds. Main aspects of care in adults and children. *American Journal of Surgery* 167 (1a): 56s–60s.

Winter GD (1962) Formation of scab and rate of epithelialisation of superficial wounds in the skin of the young domestic pig. *Nature* 193: 293–294.

chapter thirty-one

OVERVIEW OF TRAUMA RESUSCITATION

SAFETY

The first priority at all times is to be safe: are you safe, is the scene safe, is the casualty safe?

> Safety – self, scene, casualty

Remember that the fire service have overall responsibility for the safety of an accident scene.

ASSESSMENT

The first role of the paramedic, particularly if the ambulance service is the first emergency responder to arrive, is a brief assessment of the scene. What is the nature of the incident? Are there any specific hazards? What emergency response is present and what will be required? Do you have the equipment you require? How many casualties are involved, and what are the mechanisms and nature of their injuries?

Assess

- Safety
- Hazards
- Casualties – numbers
- Mechanisms of injury
- Emergency services – present and required

On arriving at the scene of an accident, always identify yourself to the senior representatives of the other emergency services. An important early priority must be to assess the casualties for priority of treatment and evacuation: this is triage (see Chapter 56).

> On arrival at an accident, identify yourself to the other emergency services

PATIENT MANAGEMENT

The first and most important part of the management of any trauma victim is the *primary survey*. This must be performed rapidly, carefully and in a standard manner; it is the basis of all good trauma care. During the primary survey, life-threatening problems are identified and dealt with; other problems can wait.

> The role of the primary survey is to identify and treat life-threatening problems

The primary survey not only identifies but treats life-threatening problems.

> Primary survey = identification of problems + treatment

The Primary Survey

Obstruction of the airway causes death more rapidly than disruption of breathing, which in turn is more rapidly fatal than circulatory compromise. For this reason, the primary survey must rigidly follow the 'ABC' sequence – airway, breathing and circulation – to which are added control of the cervical spine to prevent progression of neurological deficit (potential or actual) due to neck injury, and control of overt haemorrhage as an adjunct to management of the circulation, thus:

airway with cervical spine control
breathing
circulation with control of overt haemorrhage

The primary survey is completed by 'disability' and 'exposure'. In the primary survey, the assessment of disability is 'AVPU' (see below) and pupillary response to light. The degree of exposure must be judged according to the patient's injuries (severity and location), environment, sex and age. Although due regard must always be made for the patient's modesty, exposure must be sufficient for the proper management of the patient's injuries.

The full primary survey

- Airway with cervical spine control
- Breathing with oxygen
- Circulation with control of overt haemorrhage
- Disability
- Exposure

Approaching the patient

On approaching the patient, introduce yourself, and explain what you are about to do. Remember that casualties can often hear what is said to them although they give no sign of this at the time. If the patient speaks to you, however incoherently, it means that the airway is clear and the patient is breathing; otherwise proceed to assess the airway.

Airway with cervical spine control

If the patient is breathing quietly and comfortably, no other action may be necessary than to apply oxygen at 12–15 litres per minute via a face mask with reservoir. If, however, you feel the airway is at risk, either the insertion of an airway (nasopharyngeal or oropharyngeal) or putting the patient in the recovery position should be considered. If the airway appears obstructed or partially obstructed, any obvious removable obstruction should be removed digitally or by suction, and simple airway manoeuvres applied (see Chapters 3–5). These are *chin lift* and *jaw thrust*.

All trauma victims require high-flow oxygen

Both the head tilt and chin lift, as well as the recovery position, are best avoided if there is any possibility of cervical spine injury, and immobilization of the cervical spine should be maintained manually at first, then by semirigid collar and tape throughout resuscitation. Remember, however, that the airway takes precedence over the cervical spine, and if it is absolutely necessary to compromise the cervical spine (for example, by performing a head tilt) to achieve a patent protected airway, then this must be done.

Airway takes precedence over cervical spine

The jaw thrust manoeuvre is safe in cervical spine injury.
If simple airway manoeuvres are successful in clearing the airway, an oral or nasopharyngeal airway can be inserted if tolerated, and oxygen applied. Otherwise it will be necessary to proceed with *stepped airway care* as follows.

1. Airway clearance – manual and aspiration
2. Manual airway opening manoeuvres:
   chin lift
   jaw thrust
3. Oropharyngeal airway
4. Nasopharyngeal airway
5. Oral tracheal intubation
6. Cricothyroid jet ventilation

Nasopharyngeal airways are often better tolerated than oral ones but are a last resort if there is any possibility of basal skull fracture (consider in the patient with a partial obstruction and clenched teeth).
When – and *only* when – the airway is patent and protected, it is possible to move on to the assessment of breathing. However complex the airway manoeuvre that is required, it must be completed before the breathing is considered.

Breathing

Assessment of breathing begins with the *neck*:

trachea
neck veins

Then examine the *chest*:

- LOOK for movement, instability, flail segments, wounds
- PALPATE for surgical emphysema, tenderness, wounds, paradoxical movement
- PERCUSSION for resonance or dullness
- LISTEN with a stethoscope for breath sounds

Hyperresonance with reduced breath sounds suggests a pneumothorax; dullness with reduced breath sounds is indicative of a haemothorax. Remember, the role of the primary survey is the identification and treatment of life-threatening injuries.

Life-threatening chest injuries

- Airway obstruction
- Tension pneumothorax
- Open pneumothorax
- Massive haemothorax
- Flail chest
- Cardiac tamponade

If the clinical signs suggest a tension pneumothorax, an intercostal needle thoracocentesis should be performed (Chapter 23). Penetrating chest wounds should be covered with a dressing and sealed on three sides.

Remember to examine the back of the chest

When – and *only* when – life-threatening breathing problems have been identified and treated where possible, is it appropriate to move on to the circulation.

Circulation with control of external haemorrhage

The patient must be assessed for signs of shock; at the same time, obvious external haemorrhage should be controlled by external pressure. In the trauma patient the causes of shock are:

- Hypovolaemic
- Cardiogenic
- Neurogenic

Septic shock is unlikely to be a problem in the trauma victim unless rescue is particularly prolonged (for example, following a natural disaster such as an earthquake).

Hypovolaemic shock is by far the most likely cause for shock in the trauma victim and may be classified as in Table 31.1. Haemorrhage may be divided into:

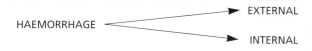

Significant external haemorrhage is likely to be obvious. The location of internal (concealed) haemorrhage may be:

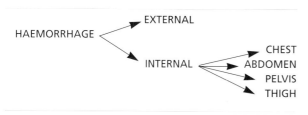

Brief palpation of the abdomen and pelvis will aid the location of bleeding. Significant haemorrhage into the chest should already have been identified during the assessment of breathing. Severe shock may result from bleeding into the thighs from femoral fractures, although this is uncommon.

Cardiogenic shock may result from tension pneumothorax or cardiac tamponade, usually secondary to penetrating injury.

Neurogenic shock is rare. Never assume that shock is neurogenic as any accident severe enough to cause spinal injury is also likely to be capable of producing haemorrhage from other associated injuries.

> **Isolated head injuries do not cause shock**

All patients with significant trauma should have an intravenous cannula inserted and should receive fluid replacement. Crystalloids are usually recommended for grade I and II shock and crystalloid followed by colloid for grade III and IV shock. Ideally, therefore, intravenous access should be obtained using the largest possible cannulae (usually 16 G or 14 G).

If transfer times are likely to be short, and particularly if on-scene conditions are likely to make intravenous access difficult, it is *far more appropriate* either to obtain intravenous access *en route* or to wait until arrival in a warm and well-lit accident and emergency department.

> **Intravenous access must never delay patient transfer**

Disability

Disability is assessed during the primary survey using the 'AVPU' system and pupillary assessment to light (PERL – 'pupils equal and reactive to light').

Pupillary reactions are examined and the patient's response classified as follows:

A > Alert
V > Patient responds to Voice
P > Patient responds to Pain
U > Patient Unresponsive

Table 31.1 Classification of hypovolaemic shock (adult)

	Class I	Class II	Class III	Class IV
Blood loss (mL)	Up to 750	750–1500	1500–2000	> 2000
Blood loss (%BV)	Up to 15%	15–30%	30–40%	> 40%
Pulse rate	< 100	> 100	> 120	> 140
Blood pressure	Normal	Normal	Decreased	Decreased
Pulse pressure (mmHg)	Normal or increased	Decreased	Decreased	Decreased
Respiratory rate	14–20	20–30	30–40	> 35
Urine output (ml/hr)	> 30	20–30	5–15	Negligible
CNS/mental status	Slightly anxious	Mildly anxious	Anxious and confused	Confused and lethargic
Fluid replacement (3:1 Rule)	Crystalloid	Crystalloid	Crystalloid and blood	Crystalloid and blood

Exposure

In the primary survey, 'E' is for exposure. The degree of exposure that is appropriate depends on the clinical situation. Exposure of the chest is always necessary for assessment of 'B' and other exposure must be performed as necessary to ensure that *no significant injury is missed*. For reasons of privacy, warmth and good lighting, this part of the primary survey is often best performed in the ambulance. Motor-cycle leather trousers should only be removed after careful consideration, as they may act to tamponade significant lower limb bleeding from pelvic or long-bone fractures by acting like a pneumatic anti-shock garment.

Once the primary survey is complete, it may be appropriate to move on to the secondary survey. Short transfer times and the identification of significant problems during the primary survey usually mean that the secondary survey is delayed until arrival at hospital.

> **Performing a secondary survey must never delay patient transfer to hospital**

If there is any suggestion of a change in the patient's condition during either the primary or secondary surveys, always follow the same routine: go back to airway (A). If the change in the patient's condition is an increase in respiratory rate do not be distracted into returning to breathing (B), or if bleeding into returning to circulation (C): always return (however briefly) to A. The same principle applies if you become distracted during your examination.

> **If in doubt, go back to 'A' (airway)**

The Secondary Survey

The secondary survey is a 'head to toe' assessment of the patient with assessment of vital signs (including the Glasgow Coma Scale), during which all the patient's injuries will be identified.

It is vital to remember that the secondary survey was originally described for use in the accident and emergency department and included appropriate X-rays. The clinical examination itself, if it is to be appropriately thorough, will take time. The following description of a detailed survey, therefore, will rarely be appropriate in the pre-hospital environment which is often cold, uncomfortable and poorly lit. Furthermore, there is no point in delaying transfer to definitive treatment to perform an examination which will be repeated in hospital: the life-threatening problems will have been identified during the primary survey.

> **Remember the 'golden hour'!**
> **The time from injury to definitive surgical treatment in hospital**

The secondary survey should follow a logical order, starting at the head and working towards the feet. In principle a 'log roll' examination of the cervical spine should be included, but practical considerations suggest that this is best performed in hospital.

Head

Remember at all times that your most important role is to prevent secondary brain injury. Head injuries are classified in Figure 31.1.

Examine the scalp for lacerations, paying particular attention to the possibility of compound skull fractures. Do not insert your fingers into deep scalp lacerations!

Check for bruising and swelling to the face, scalp and behind the ears, and identify and record any alteration in facial contour. Do not forget to record blood or possible cerebrospinal fluid leakage from the nose or ears.

Chest

Life-threatening problems should already have been identified during the primary survey. This sequence should be repeated in the secondary survey:

- Trachea
- Neck veins
- Visual inspection
- Auscultation
- Percussion
- Palpation

In addition, the presence of bony injury to the chest (ribs, clavicles, scapulae, sternum), bruising, pattern bruising, lacerations and abrasions should be noted and recorded (Figure 31.2). Pay particular attention to seat-belt bruising (or its absence) in road traffic accidents.

Upper limbs

The first clue to an upper limb injury may be an abnormal position of the arm: check carefully for this and for swelling, bruising, lacerations and abrasions. Compound fractures should be noted. Always record that a fracture was compound before it was reduced. Examine each joint in turn for swelling, deformity and range of movement (normal and abnormal). Evidence of vascular or neurological compromise must also be sought.

Abdomen

Observe the abdomen for swelling, bruising, abrasions or lacerations and record their presence. Examine the abdomen gently for tenderness or rebound (see Chapter 15). Intra-abdominal pathology may be associated with tenderness, rebound and swelling, but it is vital to remember that in the early stages

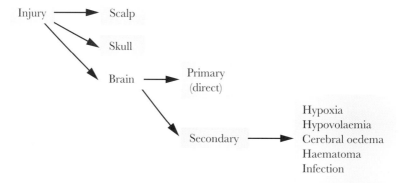

Fig. 31.1 *Classification of head injuries*

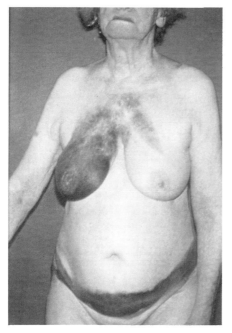

Fig. 31.2 *Secondary survey chest injuries*

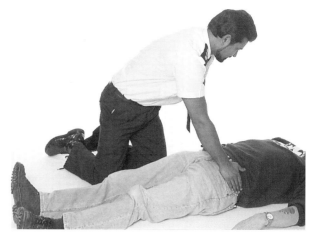

Fig. 31.3 *Springing the pelvis*

abdominal injuries may be concealed (silent). Patients who have blunt chest and leg injuries probably have abdominal injuries as well, as the mechanism of injury is unlikely to have missed the unprotected part of the body that lies between.

Chest injury + leg injury = abdominal injury

There is no role for the measurement of pelvic girth or for auscultation of the abdomen in the pre-hospital environment.

Pelvis

Bleeding into the pelvis is a common cause of concealed haemorrhage and should not be forgotten if there is shock without external bleeding or evidence of intrathoracic or intra-abdominal haemorrhage. Pain on springing the pelvis (Figure 31.3) may give some indication of pelvic injury, but is not particularly reliable. Suspicion of the possibility of pelvic injury should arise from a knowledge of the mechanism of injury.

Lower limb

The lower limbs are examined for abnormal position, deformity, swelling, bruising, lacerations and abrasions. Compound fractures may be noted. The knee and ankle should be examined for evidence of fracture, dislocation, deformity or swelling and movement (normal or abnormal) as well as the superficial injuries listed above. As with the arms, neurological and vascular damage must be confirmed or excluded (Table 31.2).

Having completed the secondary survey make sure all your findings have been recorded.

If it isn't written down, it wasn't done

Preparation for Transport

More often than not, transfer of the patient will begin before

Table 31.2 Limb examination

Superficial	Lacerations
	Bruises
	Abrasions
	Swelling
Bones	Simple fractures
	Compound fractures
Joints	Swelling
	Deformity
	Abnormal movements:
	fracture
	dislocation
Nerves	Neurological damage
Arteries	Vascular compromise

the secondary survey, at a time when only 'ABCDE' and other major injuries have been identified. Remember that major fractures, dislocations and soft tissue injuries should be identified during 'E' of the primary survey and not during the secondary survey. Whenever preparations for transport are made the principles remain the same.

Airway
Ensure that the patient's airway is safe and will remain protected during any handling. The patient should continue to receive high-concentration oxygen and should be moved in such a way that the risk of spinal injury is minimized.

Breathing
Confirm that the patient is breathing, or if not, that supported respiration is in progress and can be continued during transfer.

Make sure that any cannulae or chest drain inserted are fastened securely.

Circulation
Make sure that the patient's condition can be observed and that a central pulse is easily at hand. During short periods of transfer (for example *into* an ambulance) drips should be switched off and the fluid bags placed against the patient; alternatively, if enough pairs of hands are available, infusion bags may be carried at shoulder height and handed into the ambulance.

Disability
Assessment of 'AVPU' and pupillary reactions should be repeated as soon as the patient is in the back of the ambulance.

Exposure
The patient should be reasonably covered during transfer. It may be appropriate to remove clothes or blankets during transport to facilitate observations.

When positioning the patient in the ambulance, if the patient has severe unilateral injuries (or more significant injuries on one side), place the patient with the injured side against the gangway. This will aid access both for observation and practical intervention if required.

In Hospital

The role of the paramedic in the hospital management of trauma is vital. Only the paramedic can give details of the accident and, most importantly, of the mechanism of injury. The ambulance service report form should be given (ideally) to a doctor or to the senior nurse involved with the case. If a verbal hand-over is required, the system of 'ABCDE' with secondary survey can be used. Identified problems and appropriate therapeutic interventions can be listed, starting with those affecting the airway, followed in turn by breathing, circulation and disability problems. Injuries noticed during 'exposure' and the secondary survey are reported last.

5

PAEDIATRICS

chapter thirty-two

OBTAINING A PAEDIATRIC HISTORY

A paediatric history is made up of two elements:

- The account of what has happened
- Background information about the child which might affect the current or future situation

Even in the early stages of treating a patient, there are essential facts which provide vital help in deciding what to do. In addition, a considerable amount of information is available in the pre-hospital situation which is difficult or even impossible to obtain later. Conversely, the past medical records are usually obtainable by hospital staff whereas out of hospital only verbal information is available.

Immediate assessment: a few brief details are AMPLE

THE AMPLE FORMAT

Immediate assessment (see Chapter 33) and appropriate action take precedence over the history at all times. However, even in the first few seconds some relevant information can be vital. This should take the form of a few short, structured questions. The 'AMPLE' format is widely used and is easy to remember:

A > Allergies
M > Medicines
P > Past medical history
L > Last food and drink
E > Events leading up to the current problem

Allergies

It is especially important to know about allergies if any drugs may be given. Adrenaline is not a problem and is a major treatment for severe allergic reactions. Occasionally, an allergic reaction to medicines or foods is the *cause* of the illness.

Medicines

Any medicines that the child may have already taken will influence his treatment. Regular medication gives much information about known medical problems and the current state of health. For instance, a child with asthma who is taking regular steroids has an illness which has been difficult to control.

Past Medical History

The medical history has a major bearing on the current problem. At this stage just a list of important past illnesses is required. Even in young children the past history can be surprisingly complicated! Children with congenital problems frequently present with urgent problems such as fits and chest infections. Certain illnesses such as asthma also lead to recurrent problems.

Last Food and Drink

The presence of food and drink in the stomach is a major risk factor for regurgitation. This may lead to airway and breathing problems. To be forewarned is to be in a position to take action if necessary. This knowledge is particularly important in the child with a reduced level of consciousness or in whom narcotic analgesic drugs may be given. Children often vomit after minor injuries and during the course of many illnesses.

Events Leading up to the Current Problem

Brief details of the course of an illness or the mechanism of an injury together with the nature of the present complaints are extremely helpful.

THE STORY FROM THE SCENE

Every police officer knows how much information can be gathered from the scene of an incident. The pre-hospital worker has a unique insight into this source of information. At a child's home, the normal living environment reveals much about the child's daily life. The family's social circumstances and habits may give useful clues as to the current problems. The apparent health and well-being of the other children in the household is also important.

When attending an accident, the circumstances leading up to the event can be a valuable guide as to the nature and severity of any injuries. The environmental conditions, the position of casualties and the proximity of other objects such as vehicles all give useful clues as to the mechanism of injury.

THE CARER'S TALE

Children are unique in often having someone in close proximity who is looking after them. This person, who is usually a parent but may be a relative, friend or teacher, can usually give a good account of what has happened. Depending on their relationship to the child, they may also know about other parts of the history. Teachers, for instance, often know about illnesses and medication.

WHAT THE BYSTANDER SAW

People at the scene of an incident often give valuable information. Such people may include passers-by, neighbours or professionals such as police officers and firefighters. Sometimes the accounts may differ, but usually the essential details are consistent. After the incident, all these people disperse and this part of the history may be lost for ever.

THE CHILD'S OWN ACCOUNT

It goes without saying that children vary widely in their ability to communicate. A neonate may make signals that are only understood by its mother whereas teenagers use the same level of communication as adults. The type and level of language used is also influenced by the child's intelligence and environment. Consequently, communicating with a child is a difficult art which comes more naturally to some than to others.

The person trying to elicit a medical history from a child must pitch the questions at the right level and continually reassess the responses of the child. It is obviously a mistake to phrase a question in language that a small child cannot understand. However, it is equally ineffective to address older children with questions in 'baby language' that leave them feeling patronized.

Children often respond very well to appropriate questions. Their account of events can be extremely accurate. It should not be assumed that an adult's story of events is any more credible than an older child's.

WHAT OTHER HEALTH PROFESSIONALS ASK

Doctors and nurses all take histories; they use slightly different structures according to differing professional needs. The 'AMPLE' format described above is probably the best one in the immediate care situation, but it is important to understand other methods. Doctors divide the information into:

- Presenting complaint and history of presenting complaint – what has been happening to prompt the current need for help
- Past medical history – past illnesses and operations
- Social history – the environment that the child lives in and the people that they live with
- Family history – medical problems of other family members
- Drugs and allergies – the child's current and past medication and known allergies
- Review of systems – a checklist of the different body systems involving inquiry into possible problems with each

Nurses use a variety of structures which focus on the environment needed to care for the child during the illness.

RELEVANT IMMEDIATE QUESTIONS

The 'AMPLE' structure describes most relevant details; the depth of inquiry should vary with the immediacy of the situation. Once again it should be emphasized that immediate assessment and corrective interventions take precedence over almost all questioning. The questions below should be addressed to the most appropriate person, be that the carer or the child.

Breathing problems, fits, pain, injury and general symptoms of infection are responsible for the majority of paediatric emergencies. A systemic consideration of some useful urgent questions is helpful. These questions make up the 'E' (events) and some of the 'P' (past medical history) of 'AMPLE'. The list below is by no means exhaustive, but it serves to illustrate the technique of direct questioning to ascertain the need for urgent action. The form of the question must be tailored to the situation and the people.

Airway

Diagnosis of the problem:

- When did the problem start?
- Is there reason to suspect an inhaled foreign body?

Severity of the problem:
- Has the child been distressed?
- Has the child been drooling?
- Can the child eat and drink?

Breathing

Diagnosis of the problem:

- When did it start?
- Has it ever happened before?

Severity of the problem:
- Has the child been responding normally?
- Has the child been distressed?
- Has the child ever needed steroids?
- Has the child ever been admitted to hospital with breathing problems before?
- If admitted, has the child ever been on an intensive care unit?

Circulation

Diagnosis of the problem:

- When did it start?
- Has the child any heart problems?
- Does the child have a rash? – meningoccocal septicaemia causes purpura (bruises)
- Has the child had any diarrhoea or vomiting?

Severity of the problem:
- Has the child been responding normally?

Disability

- When did it start?
- Has the child been responding normally?
- Does the child have a rash?
- Has the mother (or other carer) noticed any agitation, or an odd cry or affect?

Environment

- In what position is the child most comfortable?
- Is the child too hot or too cold?

Fits

Diagnosis of the problem:

- Has the child ever had fits before?
- Has the child been generally unwell in any way before the fit?
- Has the child had a raised temperature?
- Have the child's eyes rolled up at the time of the attack? (Mothers often notice this)
- Was the child playing when it suddenly it went limp and collapsed? Febrile convulsions often occur with minimal tonic/clonic activity

Severity of the problem:
- How long did the fit last?

Glucose

Diagnosis of the problem:

- Does the child have diabetes?
- Has the child had his or her normal insulin dose?
- Has the child been eating and drinking normally?

Severity of the problem:
- Has the child been behaving and responding normally?

Immediate Needs

- Where does it hurt?
- How bad is it?

Summary

This system is summarized below:

- Airway
- Breathing
- Circulation
- Disability
- Environment
- Fits
- Glucose
- Immediate needs

It is important to note the differences (and similarities) between this system and the 'ABCDE' of trauma resuscitation.

FURTHER BACKGROUND QUESTIONS

In the situation of immediate care, extensive consideration of the child's background is often irrelevant and may be counter-productive. However, it is useful to have some appreciation of the special features of a child's history.

Maternal Health and Pregnancy

The health of the mother may affect the development of the fetus. Maternal infections such as rubella may lead to a damaged baby.

Birth Problems

A difficult birth (caesarean section or forceps delivery) may later manifest itself as developmental problems or fits. Was the child on the special care baby unit (SCBU)? If so, then the perinatal period was not as smooth as it might have been.

Development

The continuing rapid development of a child distinguishes it from the adult. Questions should be asked about relationships, behaviour, play, school, sports and activities.

Immunizations

Children in the UK benefit from a planned programme of immunizations. The immunizations received by the child should be ascertained.

Siblings

The health of brothers and sisters may give useful information concerning a child's illness.

Exploration of the Current Problem

It is important to listen to the story told by the child or the carer. Direct questions will involve expanding on the 'AMPLE' format and the systematic 'A–I' approach above. The particular complaints that are common in children may also involve:

- Raised temperature or shivering
- Lethargy or drowsiness
- Headache and neck stiffness
- Aches and pains
- Cough, cold, sore throat and earache
- Feeding problems
- Diarrhoea and vomiting
- Reduced or increased urine output (? normal wet nappies in a small child)
- Difficulty sleeping

Sometimes the worries of the parents and other carers pre-dominate over the symptoms of the child, and these problems must be explored also.

LANGUAGE PROBLEMS

The UK is a multicultural society and children reflect this in the languages that they speak. Most children speak excellent English, but in a crisis they may revert to the language that they speak at home. Gentle rephrasing of the questions may be suc-cessful, but sometimes another person is needed to act as a translator.

EARLY SUSPICIONS OF CHILD ABUSE

Several different types of child abuse are now recognized. These are:

- Physical abuse (non-accidental injury)
- Emotional abuse
- Neglect
- Sexual abuse
- Organized or ritual abuse

There are patterns of physical signs for some types of abuse, but the history and the context in which the events occurred are the most important first indicators to alert the health worker. The following features of a history of injury might point to abuse:

- Inappropriate delay in seeking help and advice after a significant injury
- Previous history of frequent accidents
- The history of the accident is not a likely mechanism for that injury
- Vague or absent history of an accident
- Different carers give different explanations for the same injury
- The child gives a different history

- The injury is supposed to have been sustained in a way that is inconsistent with the child's development, e.g. a fall before the child has started walking
- The adults with the child are either unconcerned or hostile during questioning

The pre-hospital worker is in a unique position to note two particular factors:

1. The *home* – the environment from which a child comes is often seen by pre-hospital workers. This environment may have changed by the time others (such as social workers) can visit it.
2. The *initial story* – one of the best pointers to physical abuse is inconsistency in the history, both between those telling it and in respect of the likely mechanism of injury. Such inconsistencies may well have been 'ironed out' by the time the tale is told to hospital staff.

RECORD-KEEPING

Good, legible records are of vital importance, although 'good' should not be taken as meaning 'long'. Accurate details help medical and nursing staff to deliver appropriate care while giving due consideration to the pre-hospital situation and treatment. The history given (and recorded) often makes sense of what later seem to be inexplicable events and actions. In addition, paramedics are often judged by the quality of their written information.

Sometimes, many months or years later, the pre-hospital records provide important information. Cases involving children may be the subject of social investigation and legal actions may be delayed until the child reaches maturity. At such a time, the paramedic may be called to give evidence in court. Failure to make sense of one's own records is acutely embarrassing, to say the least! In cases of litigation where a health worker is involved, the court may sometimes take the view that the quality of the records may reflect the quality of the care given. In any case, actions omitted from the records will be taken as omissions from the actions of the worker involved.

Derogatory comments or criticisms are best not recorded in the notes. Children can be very difficult to manage – but they learn their strange behaviour from adults! However, a record of the paramedic's opinion on such episodes is often hard to justify at a later date. Any concerns are best communicated directly to hospital staff.

Pre-hospital record-keeping is a rapidly evolving field. Dictating machines and small computers may be the record-keeping devices of the future.

How to Hand Over the History to the Hospital

Good communication is vital at the point where the care of the patient is transferred from the pre-hospital workers to the hospital. It should include both handing over the written records of the history and some direct discussion. What happened when the ambulance arrived and on the way to the hospital is now part of the history!

FURTHER READING

Advanced Life Support Group (1993) *Advanced Paediatric Life Support*. London: BMJ Publications.

American Heart Association & American Academy of Pediatrics (1990) *Pediatric Advanced Life Support*. Dallas: American Heart Association.

Morton RJ & Phillips BM (1992) *Accidents and Emergencies in Children*. Oxford University Press.

chapter thirty-three:

ASSESSMENT OF THE ILL OR INJURED CHILD

Assessment should be carried out in a structured fashion, correcting problems as they are identified. The aim of the pre-hospital assessment is management of the child's condition rather than specific diagnosis.

DIFFERENCES BETWEEN ASSESSING ADULTS AND CHILDREN

The principles of paediatric assessment are identical to those applicable for an adult. Problems arise because the range of ages – and hence sizes – of children affects physiological measurements, drug doses and equipment sizes. An expected adult weight range is 45–90 kg; that is a two-fold difference. Children's weights may easily vary from 3 kg to 60 kg: a twenty-fold range. A factor of two is often disregarded – most adults are given a standard dose of drugs and assumed to have similar physiological parameters. A twenty-fold difference is impossible to ignore; treatment must be tailored to the size of the child.

The age of a child is usually known but the weight is more difficult to ascertain. Because of this it is important to be able to estimate a child's weight from a knowledge of the age. A method of doing this is shown in Table 33.1

The weight of a child in kilograms can be approximately calculated by the formula:

Weight in kg = (age in years + 4) × 2

This works well between the ages of 1 year and 10 years.

The average birthweight of a full-term infant is 3.5 kg; this has usually doubled by 5 months of age and tripled by 12 months. Surface area is needed to assess the area of a burn. It is best to use a Lund and Browder chart, but a quick estimate can be made on the basis that the palm of the patient's hand and adducted fingers are approximately equivalent to 1% of the body surface area (see Chapter 29).

The conditions with which children present are different. They do not generally suffer from the degenerative diseases of adult life, but have problems with infective conditions. Their fast metabolism and low reserves mean that they become ill (and cold) very quickly, but their general health and high capacity for repair make for a speedy recovery.

Children usually die from *hypoxia* (secondary to respiratory distress or depression) or from *hypovolaemia* (fluid loss or maldistribution). These lead to cardiac asystole which has a very poor prognosis. Therefore, it is vital to recognize and reverse these conditions before terminal bradycardia supervenes. Coronary artery disease and thus ventricular fibrillation is uncommon in children.

Children differ in their body proportions from adults. They also have a more elastic skeleton. These facts make for a different pattern of injury and for an airway that can be more difficult to manage.

The interaction with the assessor is as variable as the age of the child. Only practice can teach the subtle parts of this relationship, but those with children of their own have a distinct advantage.

Table 33.1 Estimating a child's weight

Age	Weight (kg)
2 months	5
6 months	7.5
1 year	10
3.5 years	15
6 years	20
10 years	30
13 years	40
14 years	50

IMMEDIATE ASSESSMENT

The 'SAFE' approach should be used. Children are usually easy to move to a safer place.

For paediatric cardiac arrest protocols see Chapter 35.

Airway

First, *check for responsiveness*. A response is usually immediately obvious. If it is not, then gentle shaking may establish verbal communication with an older child. The young child will respond by eye movement, cry or body posture – the mother will know. Failure to respond indicates a significantly lowered level of consciousness and therefore an airway at risk. There may be a need for airway opening manoeuvres and action to protect the airway.

Partial upper airway obstruction is suggested by:

- Snoring – the familiar sound of obstruction caused by the soft tissues of the mouth and pharynx ('the tongue falling back' is the usual oversimplified but easily understood explanation); it often accompanies the reduced muscle tone of a lowered level of consciousness
- Rattling or gurgling – the sound of fluids in the upper airway

For airway opening manoeuvres, recovery position and suction clearance of the airway, see Chapter 4.

Stridor is a harsh, 'crowing' noise which is heard best in inspiration – this differentiates it from wheezing, which is usually loudest in expiration. Stridor suggests obstruction at the level of the larynx and upper trachea. General illness and raised temperature usually indicate an infection causing swelling. Obstruction by a foreign body is the other main cause.

> Do not examine the throat with any instrument in children with stridor or suspected partial airway obstruction – doing so may convert the problem to complete obstruction

Drooling, the inability to swallow saliva, suggests blockage at the back of the throat.

> Cyanosis and reduced haemoglobin saturation readings on a pulse oximeter are very late signs of airway obstruction

For management of laryngotracheal obstruction see Chapter 3. For choking protocols see Chapter 4.

Ask yourself if this child needs

- The recovery position?
- A sitting-up position?
- Suctioning?
- Manual maintenance of the airway?
- An airway adjunct?
- Intubation?
- Oxygen?
- Nebulized adrenaline (used to temporarily reduce swelling of the upper airway) in a dose of 0.5–1 mg nebulized with oxygen?

All children with the problems identified below will benefit from high-concentration oxygen therapy. There is no need to assess 'risk' as in adults with chronic lung disease. Only a small group of infants with congenital heart disease need controlled oxygen therapy.

> It is not worth struggling to make an unwilling child wear an oxygen mask

The need for aids to maintain the airway is assessed on the same criteria in the child as in the adult. However, if a child's airway can be maintained by simple manoeuvres, an oropharyngeal (Guedel) airway is best avoided. This is because retching is easily induced in children and may be followed by laryngospasm or aspiration. For assessment of artificial airway and endotracheal tube sizes, see Table 33.2.

> Assess the need for cervical spine protection before any airway intervention

The presence or absence of the gag reflex gives no useful information. Testing for it in children may easily induce retching or laryngospasm and create an airway problem.

Table 33.2 Airway and endotracheal tube sizes

Oropharyngeal airway size	= approximately the distance from the centre of the lips to the angle of the jaw
Nasopharyngeal airway size	= approximately the distance from the tip of the nose to the tragus of the ear
Endotracheal tube size:	
Internal diameter (mm)	$= \dfrac{\text{age in years}}{4} + 4$ (neonate 3–3.5 mm tube)
Oral tube length (cm)	$= \dfrac{\text{age in years}}{2} + 12$
Nasal tube length (cm)	$= \dfrac{\text{age in years}}{2} + 15$

Breathing

Look, listen and feel for breathing. The absence of breath sounds indicates the need to follow procedures for cardiorespiratory arrest (Chapter 35).

Look for:

1. Difficulty in talking – a child who is unable to speak because of laboured breathing is very unwell.
2. An abnormal respiratory rate – usually fast, laboured breathing (Table 33.3). Very slow respiratory rates may occur just before respiratory arrest or in children poisoned with narcotic drugs, e.g. methadone.
3. Recession of the chest wall – the indrawing of the elastic tissues of a child caused by increased respiratory effort.
4. Wheezing and rattling, grunting and panting.
5. Nasal flaring and use of the shoulder and neck muscles during breathing.
6. Unequal or diminished breath sounds.

Absence of breath sounds means that the movement of air in the lungs is so diminished that it cannot be heard

All the above suggest that the child is struggling to achieve normal respiration. Failure to adequately oxygenate the blood and hence the tissues is shown by:

tachycardia – the hypoxic nervous system is stimulating the heart (for normal values see Table 33.3)

cyanosis – a late sign

irritability, confusion or reduced responsiveness mean that the brain is short of oxygen – this is an extremely worrying sign

The oxygen saturation shown by the pulse oximeter should be close to 100% in a normal, healthy child

Ask yourself if this child needs

- Oxygen?
- A bronchodilator, e.g. salbutamol?
- Intubation and ventilation?

All wheezy children will benefit from nebulized bronchodilators, whether they are known to be asthmatic or not. Ask the parents how much of this type of drug the child has already had, and look for agitation, tachycardia and tremor – the signs of overdosage. Remember, however, that these may also be signs of hypoxia.

Ventilation is indicated as an emergency procedure for respiratory insufficiency in a child in the same way as in an adult. Suggested ventilator settings for children are:

tidal volume 10 ml per kg

minute volume 100 ml per kg

The assessment of chest injury uses the same techniques in children as in adults. Because of the elastic chest wall, children are far less likely to have rib fractures than adults, although they may have severe underlying lung damage (see Chapter 23).

Breathing: what to look for

- Difficulty talking
- Abnormal respiratory rate
- Chest wall recession
- Wheezing and rattling, grunting and panting
- Nasal flaring and accessory muscles
- Unequal or diminished breath sounds
- Tachycardia
- Cyanosis
- Irritability, confusion, drowsiness

Circulation

Check for a central pulse (over 5 seconds). The brachial or femoral pulses should be used in infants rather than the carotid pulse, as their necks make carotid palpation difficult. The absence of a central pulse (or a rate of less than 60 beats per minute in infants) indicates the need to follow procedures for cardiorespiratory arrest (see Chapter 35).

In a child with ventricular fibrillation and no obvious precipitating factors, the cause could be poisoning with tricyclic antidepressants

Look for:

1. A fast or slow heart rate (for normal values see Table 33.3). Fast heart rates usually mean that either (a) there is a cardiac arrhythmia, or more commonly (b) the nervous system has detected a problem with the body (such as hypoxia, hypoglycaemia, pain or fear) and is 'instructing' the heart to beat faster. A slow heart rate usually means that something is wrong with the heart itself. The worst cause of this is severe hypoxia (or hypovolaemia) and, in this case, terminal bradycardia and asystole are only seconds away. This is the mechanism of most cardiac arrests in children. Occasionally, bradycardia is seen with poisoning and severe head injury; it may also occur in syncopal attacks.

Table 33.3 Respiratory and pulse rates in children

Age (years)	Respiratory rate (breaths/minute)	Pulse rate (beats/minute)
Under 1	30–40	110–160
1–5	25–30	95–140
6–12	20–25	80–120

2. Abnormal systolic blood pressure – this varies with age. A useful formula to calculate the expected systolic blood pressure is:

systolic blood pressure (mmHg) = 80 + (age in years × 2)

Blood pressure can be difficult to measure in young, restless children. It will not fall until very late in shock. It may be raised with intracerebral and renal problems.
3. A raised capillary refill time – it should be less than 2 seconds if the circulation is satisfactory. However, peripheral shutdown in a cold, wet child can easily produce a prolonged refill time.
4. Pallor and coolness of the skin – the body diverts blood away from the skin when there are circulatory problems and these signs are thus very useful.
5. Active bleeding

Blood volume is approximately 80 ml/kg

Inadequate circulation will reduce tissue oxygenation and thus may also cause:

a raised respiratory rate
altered mental status as detailed above

Circulation: what to look for

- Fast or slow heart rate
- Abnormal systolic blood pressure
- Increased capillary refill time
- Pallor and coolness of the skin
- Active bleeding
- Raised respiratory rate
- Instability, confusion, drowsiness

The ECG is rarely as helpful in making a diagnosis in children as it is in adults, except for arrhythmias. A cardiac monitor does, however, provide constant information about the heart rate.

Ask yourself if this child needs

- Oxygen?
- Pressure haemostasis?
- Intravenous fluids?
- Vagal manoeuvres (tachyarrhythmia)?
- Sitting up (pulmonary oedema)?
- Urgent penicillin therapy (meningococcal septicaemia)?

The need for venous access and the site should be assessed carefully. There is nothing worse than looking for veins on a screaming child who is covered with bruises from previous attempts by someone else. Remember the possibility of intraosseous infusion.

Bolus fluid therapy should be calculated at 20 ml/kg and after further assessment repeated as necessary

Disability

Look for:

1. A reduced level of consciousness. This is the most important sign of any problem which is affecting the brain. Even sleepy children should be fairly easy to rouse. The 'AVPU' scoring system is as useful for children as for adults:

A > Alert
V > Voice elicits a response
P > Pain elicits a response
U > Unresponsive

Note: the parents of an ill child are usually in a highly distressed state, so be careful how you elicit the pain response; pressure on a fingernail is probably the most subtle way.

Consider hypoglycaemia as a cause for a reduced level of consciousness

2. Abnormal pupils – look for size, equality and reactivity. These features can be affected by both drugs and brain disease. Dilated, fixed or unequal pupils are worrying signs in children as they are in adults.
3. Abnormal posture and limb movements – children may be flaccid or show abnormal posturing. Limb movements may be unequal; sometimes this is congenital but it is best never to assume so.

Severe intracerebral problems may also cause:
airway obstruction
respiratory depression (respiration, unlike the heart-beat, requires an intact brain stem)
bradycardia and hypertension

Signs of an intracerebral problem

- Reduced level of consciousness
- Abnormal pupils
- Abnormal posture and limbs movement
- Airway obstruction
- Respiratory depression
- Bradycardia and hypertension

Ask yourself if this child needs

- The recovery position?
- Other airway care?
- Oxygen?
- Ventilation?
- Intravenous access?
- Glucose?
- Urgent penicillin therapy?

Exposure and Environment

Look for:

1. Cold extremities.
2. Shivering.
3. Wet clothing.
4. Pyrexia and clamminess.
5. The position in which the child is most comfortable.
6. The proximity of the mother or other carer.

> In a child, cold limbs usually indicate a
> cold trunk and head

Attention to these details early on can radically change the well-being (and demeanour) of a child.

A child may well need clothing removed to facilitate assessment. However, children easily become cold and embarrassed.

Ask yourself if this child needs

- Wet clothing removed?
- Warmth?
- Cooling measures?
- Repositioning or support of a limb?
- His or her mother?
- Covering up (embarrassment)?

Fits

Look for:

1. Frank tonic or clonic activity.
2. Spasmodic twitching.
3. Post-ictal drowsiness.
4. Gurgling, rattling or other signs of airway obstruction.
5. Cyanosis – during a fit there is a very high demand for oxygen, coupled with respiratory inadequacy.
6. Signs of head injury.
7. Signs of other injury caused by a convulsion (e.g. a bitten tongue and intraoral bleeding).
8. Reasons to consider hypoglycaemia.

It is very difficult to assess or manage a fitting child. Hence termination of the convulsion must be an immediate aim.

Ask yourself if this child needs

- The recovery position?
- Other airway care?
- Oxygen?
- Intravenous access?
- Anticonvulsant therapy, for example rectal diazepam?
- Cooling measures?

- Glucose?
- Urgent penicillin therapy?

Glucose

Children are like fast-burning little engines and become short of oxygen and fuel very quickly. Their fuel is glucose and they have relatively low glycogen reserves. Glucagon will therefore be less consistently effective than in adults.

Look for:

1. Restlessness, agitation or other mental change ('jitteriness' in a neonate).
2. A reduced level of consciousness.
3. Signs of insulin usage. (All diabetic children will be on insulin – oral hypoglycaemic drugs are generally only used in adults. This does not mean, of course, that a child cannot take someone else's drugs and become hypoglycaemic!)
4. A low blood glucose level on testing with a reagent strip (if available).
5. Convulsions – can be caused by hypoglycaemia.

Ask yourself if this child needs

- The recovery position?
- Other airway care?
- Oxygen?
- Intravenous access?
- Glucose or glucagon therapy?

History

After immediate problems have been assessed and appropriate action has been initiated, further information may be sought. The 'AMPLE' structure is recommended as providing adequate historical detail in the pre-hospital situation. Appropriate immediate questions are discussed in Chapter 32. Some of the answers will give enormous help in the assessment of both the type of problem and the likely severity.

Ask yourself

- Are the answers to these questions going to affect the immediate management of this child?

Immediate Needs of the Child

Some immediate needs will have been assessed, under 'environment'. These needs include the provision of warmth, the removal of wet clothing and the need to ensure psychological support from the mother or other carer. A position of comfort is also mandatory; it may be life-saving in conditions such as epiglottitis.

The relief of suffering is as usual of paramount importance. This may entail assessing:

1. *The need for analgesia* – this can be very difficult to assess in a distressed child. Exact localization of pain is difficult in very young children, but careful observation and discussion with the mother often helps. If analgesic drugs are available, they can turn an unmanageable situation into a calm one. They also reassure the carers. It is far better to give analgesia freely to children who may be in pain than to withhold it on the spurious grounds that it alters conscious level or masks pupillary or abdominal signs. Gaseous analgesia (Entonox) may be inappropriate for younger children as they find it frightening and do not have enough inspiratory force to open the demand valve.

2. *The need for limb splintage* – simple limb support with troughs and pillows can be very helpful in children with limb injuries. Distal circulation should be assessed before and after positioning limbs in the same way in children as in adults.

3. *The tolerance of cervical and spine splintage* – conscious children often do not tolerate this sort of device very well. If a collar is distressing a child significantly, it is better to remove it. The mother's hands and pillows can be more acceptable substitutes. A child who is struggling to remove a collar is actually moving the neck more than a child with no splint who is lying still. The indications for spinal immobilization are the same in children as in adults, although young children are less accurate in localizing the pain of spinal injury.

Ask yourself if this child needs

- Drugs to relieve pain
- Splintage
- Freedom from splintage

FURTHER ASSESSMENT

For further information concerning the recognition of the seriously ill child, see Chapter 34.

For further assessment of injuries see Chapter 36.

The Needs of the Parents

The needs of the carers cannot be ignored. These may vary from simple reassurance to medical treatment. The satisfactory treatment of children depends on the support of those closest to them. The mental state of a child may be inseparable from that of the mother. Parental anxiety or difficulty coping is a good reason for admitting a child to hospital.

Fluid Loss and Dehydration

Look for:

1. Purpura – these small bruises may be the first sign of meningococcal septicaemia.
2. Abdominal pain, tenderness or rigidity following trauma or illness. Large amounts of fluid or blood can be 'lost' into the abdomen. The elastic ribs and low liver and spleen increase the possibility of intra-abdominal damage.
3. Dehydration, shown by a dry, non-elastic skin or sunken eyes. In infants a floppy anterior fontanelle is a useful, if late, sign of severe fluid loss. Diarrhoea and vomiting can quickly dehydrate a small child.
4. Wet nappies confirm urine output in young children. The child's carer will know their normal state.

Level of Consciousness

Although the 'AVPU' method is quick and convenient, the Glasgow coma scale (GCS) is the standard method of scoring a reduced level of consciousness from any cause. The standard (adult) GCS is suitable for children of school age, but a special variant of the GCS is more appropriate in children under 4 years old. Table 33.4 gives an example of the children's coma scale.

Even in experienced hands, the children's coma scale is difficult to apply, and even more difficult to remember. Do not delay a transfer to perform a coma scale assessment; use 'AVPU and pupils'.

Table 33.4 The Glasgow Coma Scale in children

Response elicited	Score
BEST EYE OPENING RESPONSE	
Open spontaneously	4
React to speech	3
React to pain	2
No response	1
BEST MOTOR RESPONSE	
Moves normally and spontaneously or obeys commands	6
Localizes pain	5
Withdraws in response to pain	4
Flexes abnormally to pain (decorticate movements)	3
Extends abnormally to pain (decerebrate movements)	2
No response	1
BEST 'VERBAL' RESPONSE	
Smiles, follows sounds and objects, interacts	5
Cries consolably or interacts inappropriately	4
Cries with inconsistent relief or moans	3
Cries inconsolably or is irritable	2
No response	1

Poisoning

Bizarre symptoms and signs and unexplained combinations of findings suggest poisoning. Younger children may ingest substances accidentally; older children may experiment with drugs. Look for the most common signs:

confusion, agitation and drowsiness
tachycardia
dilated pupils
evidence at the scene (which is of enormous help to hospital staff)

Other Important Findings

1. Raised temperature – a hand on the abdomen may reveal an obvious pyrexia. This often accompanies a fit: febrile convulsions are common between 5 months and 5 years of age. Children with epilepsy are more likely to have a fit during a pyrexia.
2. Neck stiffness indicates inflammation of the meninges, i.e. meningitis. This is often accompanied by pyrexia, headache and drowsiness; however, the diagnosis can be difficult.
3. Rashes usually indicate systemic infection, allergy or specific skin disease. Purpura is the most worrying skin sign (suggesting possible meningococcal septicaemia, or other cause of vasculitis).
4. Drawing up the knees suggests pain in the abdomen.
5. Signs of congenital abnormality – children with congenital problems are often prone to fits and chest infections.
6. The relationship and interaction with the parents and the other family members is always important to note.

Upper Respiratory Tract Infection

Young children may have upper respiratory problems up to ten times a year. Such infections may precipitate asthma attacks or lead to more serious chest infections.

Look for:

1. A cough and/or a runny nose – the most common signs of infection. The barking cough of croup is important to recognize as it may accompany stridor. Whooping cough is very distressing. Severe coughing empties the lungs and is followed by an inspiratory 'whoop'. Children with upper respiratory infections often have a sore throat. There may be enlarged lymph nodes in the neck or even in the abdomen (adenitis) which can mimic appendicitis. Asthma may cause nocturnal coughing.
2. Pulling at the ears – young children may pull at their ears if they have earache. Otitis media (infection of the middle ear) is a frequent accompaniment of upper respiratory infection in children.

Signs of Child Abuse

See Chapter 32 for elements of a history which lead to suspicions of abuse.

Signs suggestive of non-accidental injury

- Unexplained head, facial, chest or limb injuries – especially in children who are not able to walk, and thus fall (few children walk before the age of 11 months)
- Multiple bruising
- Injuries of different ages
- Unusual burns (e.g. those of a 'glove' or 'stocking' distribution)
- Unusual cuts and bruises – imprints of hands, sticks, cords, shoes, belts and teeth may be present

Continuing Assessment

Assessment should continue during initial treatment and transportation. Children may change their physiological status very rapidly. It is particularly important to assess the effect of any interventions.

Monitoring needs to be appropriate to the child's condition and should not replace careful observation. It needs to be considered in terms of usefulness of information obtained and acceptability to the child. In a conscious child, this probably means *pulse oximetry* is better than *ECG monitoring* which is better than *blood pressure monitoring*.

Consideration of Other Children in the Vicinity

In many situations, such as severe infections, fires, poisoning and abuse, other children may have been exposed to the same agents as the patient. In such cases it is appropriate to assess the risk to these children also. Sometimes, full assessment (and the need for speed) may necessitate bringing other children into hospital along with the primary patient.

FURTHER READING

Advanced Life Support Group (1993) *Advanced Paediatric Life Support*. London: BMJ Publications.

American Heart Association and the American Academy of Pediatrics (1990) *Pediatric Advanced Life Support*. Dallas: American Heart Association.

Morton RJ & Phillips BM (1992) *Accidents and Emergencies in Children*. Oxford University Press.

chapter thirty-four

THE SICK CHILD

Children tend to be treated with a greater sense of urgency than adults. This reflects both the instinct that most adults have to protect the young and the generally held view that children can 'go off' quickly. This sense of urgency is useful in that it focuses care on the child. It must not, however, be allowed to deteriorate into a sense of panic. If carers are happy about their diagnostic and treatment abilities then they will be able to care for children with confidence. Gaining this confidence requires both training and practice.

It may seem obvious to state that recognizing that a child is ill is the key to ensuring that the best outcome is obtained. In fact there is a definite skill to this, and this skill has to be studied and practised like any other. The importance of the ability to recognize the severity of childhood illness cannot be overemphasized – a decision to rapidly transport a child to hospital may mean the difference between life and death. A considerable proportion of this chapter is devoted to this skill.

Once the seriousness of their condition has been established some children may need interventions prior to and during transport. Some appropriate treatments are discussed at the end of this chapter. Specific conditions are not dealt with in detail since the priority for seriously ill children is rapid, safe transportation to an advanced facility, rather than diagnosis and treatment at the scene.

RECOGNITION OF SERIOUS ILLNESS

Health workers with a great deal of paediatric experience will intuitively recognize a very sick child. Those with less experience should approach the assessment of each child systematically to try to decide whether serious illness is present or not. This systematic approach should follow the familiar 'ABC' pattern.

Airway

The airway may be patent or obstructed, protected or unpro-

tected. Obstruction may be partial or complete and protection may be secure or insecure. Any child who has anything other than an open and securely protected airway is seriously ill.

Airway patency

If the child is conscious then a simple question such as, 'How are you?' or 'What's wrong?' should start the assessment. If the child answers then this confirms that the airway is patent, and implies that pharyngeal and laryngeal function are such that it is protected. Remember there are many reasons why a child fails to answer such questions (fear of strangers and inability to talk being two obvious ones), and silence does not therefore imply that the airway is obstructed.

In an unconscious child an appropriate airway opening manoeuvre should be performed, and breathing should be assessed as described below.

Airway protection

An airway may be insecure either because the protective pharyngeal and laryngeal reflexes are absent (usually because conscious level is decreased for whatever reason) or because there is a developing pathological condition which places the airway at risk. A child with a significantly reduced conscious level (responds to pain or verbal stimuli only, or is unresponsive) should be considered to be seriously ill since the airway is at risk.

Breathing

An apnoeic child is fairly easy to spot and is clearly seriously ill. It is much more difficult to recognize children with inadequate breathing; these children are potentially as ill as those who are apnoeic, and the earlier they are picked out the better their prognosis. Adequacy of breathing should be examined as follows.

Work of breathing

As breathing becomes more difficult more effort is required to

Table 34.1 Normal respiratory rates in children

Age (years)	Respiratory rate (breaths/min)
< 1	30–40
1–5	25–30
6–12	20–25

Table 34.2 Normal pulse rate and systolic blood pressure in children

Age (years)	Pulse rate (beats/min)	Systolic blood pressure (mmHg)
Newborn	160	60–80
< 1	110–160	70–90
2–5	95–140	80–100
6–12	80–120	90–110
13 +	60–100	100–120

maintain it. This fact can be used to try and spot children with breathing difficulty. Respiratory rate will increase from normal. Normal ranges vary depending on the age of the child (Table 34.1).

Respiratory rate should be counted by exposing the chest. Exposure will also enable another major sign of increased respiratory rate to be seen – *recession*. Recession is the appearance of indrawing that occurs while the chest is expanding during inspiration. It can be seen in a number of areas: intercostal (between the ribs), subcostal (below the ribs) and sternal. The last is usually only apparent in younger children (< 2 years old) who have very elastic chests. Extra noises may be heard during the breathing cycle. Wheezes (both during inspiration and during expiration) indicate that respiratory work is raised because of the increased pressure associated with narrowing of the airways. Severe upper airway obstruction (such as that caused by a foreign body) can result in stridor. It is important to note that the loudness does not correspond to the severity of the problem. In fact, silence in a previously noisy chest can be one of the most worrying signs of all, in that it may indicate either exhaustion or total obstruction.

Effectiveness of efforts to breathe

Initially, as the work of breathing increases, effectiveness will be maintained, but eventually the body will not be able to keep up the effort and signs of inadequate breathing will appear. Depth of breathing (or in infants abdominal movement) can be a useful indicator, as can a falling respiratory rate.

If breathing is inadequate the effects do not manifest themselves only in the chest. Hypoxia (reduction in oxygenation) initially causes the heart rate to rise as the body attempts to deliver more blood to the tissues to make up for the lower concentration of oxygen. Eventually, however, the heart rate falls to below normal levels: this is a very serious sign and usually indicates imminent death. Hypoxia will also affect conscious level. First of all the child becomes agitated, but, as the low oxygen delivery continues, drowsiness and then unconsciousness will ensue.

The advent of pulse oximetry has been a great advance in non-invasive monitoring. It allows oxygen saturation to be measured in any situation and is an invaluable tool in assessing the adequacy of breathing. Saturation may be normal if breathing is adequate, may be low (less than 95% on air) if there is some impairment, or very low (less than 90% on air or less than 95% on oxygen) if breathing is seriously impaired. The great advantage of using pulse oximetry is that continuous objective assessment of breathing can be undertaken.

Circulation

Circulation may be present or absent and, if present, may be adequate or inadequate. It is fairly easy to decide that circulation is absent by palpating a large artery (carotid or femoral in a child, or brachial in an infant) for 5 seconds to see whether any pulse is present. As with breathing, however, it is not the ability to spot the child that has already died that is important, but rather the recognition of the child in a life-threatening condition. To achieve this aim the state of the child's circulation must be systematically examined.

Decreased capillary refill time and increasing peripheral pallor and coolness are early signs of a failing circulation in children. The capillary refill is measured by applying gentle pressure (enough to squeeze out the blood) over a nail bed for 5 seconds, then releasing the pressure and counting the time in seconds that it takes for the blood to return. The normal time is less than 2 seconds.

Both pulse rate and blood pressure can be measured, but the assessment and interpretation of these figures is fraught with difficulty, especially in the very young. The normal values vary with age and, in the case of blood pressure, the equipment needed for accurate measurement is also age-specific. Furthermore, significant interpretable changes occur later rather than earlier. For those who do manage to measure these parameters accurately, normal values are shown in Table 34.2. A raised respiratory rate and a decreased level of consciousness may both result from circulatory inadequacy.

Disability

Disability assessment involves a rapid evaluation of conscious level. Children with reduced conscious level for whatever cause should be classed as seriously ill and treated accordingly. The simple 'AVPU' system shown below is recommended:

A > Alert
V > Responds to Voice
P > Responds to Pain
U > Unresponsive

Any voice prompt can be used – calling the child's name is recommended. Remember very young children may not recognize

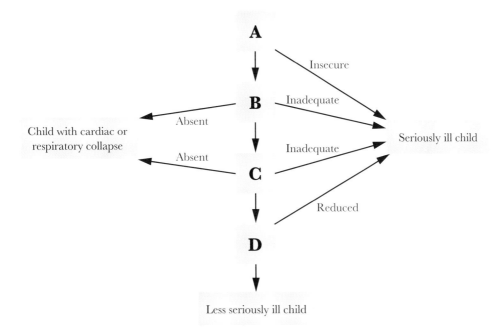

Fig. 34.1 *Summary of recognition pathways; A, airway; B, breathing; C, circulation; D, disability*

words – but all should recognize the sound of a voice. The painful stimulus should only be applied if there is no response to voice. Initially a peripheral stimulus such as fingernail bed pressure should be used; if there is no reaction this should be followed by a central stimulus such as supraorbital ridge pressure. While an examination of the pupils for size and reactivity is often recommended at this stage, there are no pupillary signs of serious illness that are present when conscious level is normal.

Assessment Summary

The recommended approach to assessing whether a child is seriously ill is summarized in Figure 34.1. Note that there are three possible outcomes to this. First, the child may be found to be in respiratory or cardiorespiratory arrest; in such a case the appropriate resuscitation should be started and rapid transport to an advanced facility should be arranged. Secondly, the child may be assessed as seriously ill; in these cases appropriate levels of resuscitation should be commenced (see below) and again rapid transport should be arranged. Finally, the child may be found to be less seriously ill. In such cases transport to another facility where further evaluation can be carried out will usually be appropriate; speed is less important in these latter cases – but this does not imply that time should be spent attempting procedures at the scene that could be done as well or better in hospital.

APPROPRIATE TREATMENT

Even in the best of circumstances performing procedures on children can be practically difficult and emotionally draining for the professional involved. The difficulties encountered are worsened by adverse conditions and inexperience of the operator. Since the circumstances of most pre-hospital care are not ideal, and because very few paramedics will attend seriously ill children often enough to keep a high level of proficiency in practical procedures, resuscitative procedures should be limited to those necessary for safe transportation.

Airway

Both opening and maintenance of the airway are essential. Simple opening manoeuvres should be performed first – head tilt, chin lift and jaw thrust can be used in children. The head should be kept in the neutral position in infants (< 1 year old), as overextension may cause deformation of the soft trachea with consequent airway obstruction.

Oropharyngeal airways can be used as simple adjuncts to airway opening. The appropriate size should be found by placing the airway vertically at the side of the face and selecting the one that reaches from the angle of the jaw to the level of the incisor teeth. The selected airway should be inserted the 'right way up' by depressing the tongue (using a tongue depressor or a laryngoscope blade) and slipping the airway into the mouth until the flange lies at the lips. Attempts to insert an airway using the adult twisting technique may cause considerable damage to the soft palate, and may compromise the airway as bleeding occurs. Nasopharyngeal airways are not routinely used in children.

Beware of interfering with a child who has severe stridor and is managing to maintain a critical airway. These children often wish to sit up during transport and should be allowed to do so. Attempts to make things better by lying the child down and opening the airway may prove to be the last straw, and can precipitate respiratory arrest. Once this has occurred it can be extremely difficult to re-establish ventilation. The sensible approach to such a situation is to provide high-flow oxygen, and to transport the child calmly to an advanced facility (preferably warning that facility of your imminent arrival so that appropriate preparations can be made).

Breathing

All children with inadequate breathing should be given oxygen in the highest possible concentration. Worries about potential oxygen toxicity are totally misplaced in such situations. Paediatric oxygen masks with rebreathing bags are available and can achieve an inspired concentration of 85% with high gas flow rates.

If respiratory support is required it can be given either by using a bag–valve–mask system, or by intubating the child and using a self-inflating bag or mechanical ventilator for ventilation.

The bag–valve–mask option is technically simple and can be initiated quickly when necessary. A child need not be apnoeic or unresponsive before support is given in this way. An appropriately sized mask can be quickly selected by considering the size of the child's face – the mask should cover both the mouth and nose; the choice between round and shaped masks is largely to do with operator preference. Three sizes of self-inflating bag are available – infant, child and adult. If in doubt use an adult bag since it is always worse to underventilate than to overventilate. Adequacy of ventilation can be judged by looking for chest excursion.

Attempts at intubation are only indicated in apnoeic children, and then only once other avenues have been exhausted. Paramedics are unlikely to be skilled or practised in these techniques in children, and critical time should not be lost to failed attempts. However, if the decision to intubate has been made then the correct equipment must be selected and the correct technique used; these will depend on the age of the child.

A correctly sized tube can be selected by looking at the size of the child's little finger, or by using the formula below:

$$\text{internal diameter (mm)} = \frac{\text{age in years}}{4} + 4$$

Infants and very young children (below the age of 2 years) have a long, floppy epiglottis, and this cannot be elevated sufficiently to allow the cords to be seen if the standard intubation technique is used. Consequently it is necessary to directly lift the epiglottis with the laryngoscope. This is achieved by passing the laryngoscope almost to the oesophagus and slowly withdrawing it in the midline. As the laryngoscope is withdrawn the epiglottis will remain elevated and the cords will come into view. A tube can then be passed through the cords and ventilation commenced. It is said that a straight paediatric blade is necessary to allow this technique to be performed, and it is certainly true that having one can make things easier. However, a standard or even a long adult blade can be used with success, since in a small mouth the curve of the adult blades is almost indiscernible. In children over 2 years old the standard technique can be used of passing the laryngoscope blade into the vallecula and lifting the epiglottis upwards and forwards to reveal the cords. As discussed above, adult-sized blades can be used if necessary.

Once the child is intubated, ventilation should be started and the position of the tube checked by listening with a stethoscope. Adequacy of ventilation is judged by looking for a reasonable rise and fall of the chest.

Circulation

If circulation is present then circulatory resuscitation is rarely necessary in the pre-hospital phase of care. Gaining intravenous access can be extremely difficult in children, and time should not be wasted unless access is essential.

If vascular access is required (usually because of progression to cardiorespiratory arrest) then strict time-limiting protocols should be adopted. A vein should be identified and the area prepared as usual; if standard techniques do not work within *90 seconds* then the procedure should be abandoned and an intraosseous line should be inserted. This is usually achieved in the medial surface of the upper tibia using a specially designed intraosseous needle. Both drugs and fluid can be introduced through this route.

Treatment Summary

Once the seriousness of a child's condition has been recognized it is important that treatment is limited to that necessary for rapid, safe transportation. This will include attention to the airway and to breathing, but will rarely involve circulatory management. Sticking to these appropriate levels of paramedical intervention is essential if the benefits of pre-hospital care are to be maximized. Diagnosis can be made and specific treatments administered in the receiving unit on arrival.

chapter thirty-five:

PAEDIATRIC CARDIAC ARREST

Cardiorespiratory arrest occurring in children is a far rarer clinical event than in adult practice. Unfortunately, the outcome for children is much poorer than for adults, particularly when the arrest occurs out of hospital.

PAEDIATRIC LIFE SUPPORT

In adults cardiac arrest is usually secondary to a primary cardiac event such as myocardial infarction:

primary cardiac event (e.g. myocardial infarction)
↓
cardiac arrest (ventricular fibrillation, asystole, electromechanical dissociation)
↓
respiratory arrest

This is not true, however, for children, in whom the underlying event is hypoxia followed by respiratory arrest:

primary respiratory event
↓
progressive bradycardia
↓
asystolic arrest

The outcome of paediatric cardiac arrest is therefore worse than adult cardiac arrest, not only because the arresting rhythm is asystole but also because the arrest takes place late in a sequence of rapidly worsening illness. It is easier to prevent paediatric respiratory arrest than to treat it.

For the youngest children (i.e. infants) the usual clinical cause is sudden infant death syndrome. For older children, the underlying cause is hypoxia secondary to clinical situations of severe sepsis, drownings, poisonings, aspirations and inhalations to the respiratory tract and trauma.

In 1992 the European Resuscitation Council issued a set of guidelines (see Further Reading) aimed at improving the quality of basic life support and advanced life support for paediatric cardiac arrests. Paramedics have a clear role to play in the institution of both basic and advanced life support for paediatric cardiac arrests occurring out of hospital.

A second obvious difference in the management of paediatric cardiac arrest is that a wide range of sizes of equipment will be required, and that a great variation in drug dosage will be required for babies and children from birth to age 15 years.

Normal Values

Before discussing methods of resuscitation it is important to be aware of some of the normal physiological parameters for children (Table 35.1).

BASIC LIFE SUPPORT

Because paediatric care includes children ranging in age from 1 day old to 15 years old and thus covers considerable variations

Table 35.1 Normal physiological values in children

Age (years)	Heart rate (beats/min)	Respiratory rate (breaths/min)	Systolic blood pressure (mmHg)
< 1	110–160	30–40	70–90
2–5	95–140	25–30	80–100
6–12	80–120	20–25	90–110
> 12	60–100	12–16	100–120

in size, the basic life support procedures are different for infants (aged under 1 year) and children (aged 1 year to 15 years).

Infants

For infants, basic life support starts with checking for responsiveness by shaking and gently pinching the infant while shouting for help. The next step is to open the airway by the head tilt or chin lift manoeuvre. When this is achieved, check the breathing by looking, listening and feeling for any signs of respiration. If breathing is found to be absent it is necessary to deliver five breaths, taking no more than 10 seconds to achieve this. When this has been performed, check for a brachial pulse – it is very difficult to feel a carotid pulse in infants because of their short necks.

In infants check the brachial pulse

If the pulse is absent or the infant is found to be profoundly bradycardic (i.e. the pulse rate is less than 60 per minute) then chest compression should begin. To achieve this two fingers are placed on the lower sternum, a finger's breadth beneath the nipple line (Figure 35.1). The chest is compressed to a depth of

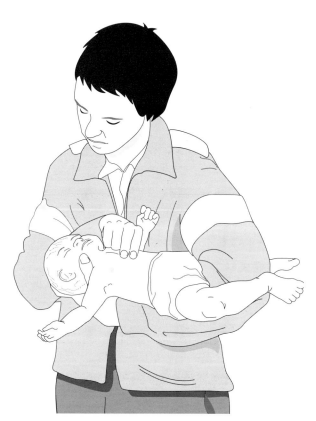

Fig. 35.1 *Correct hand position for cardiopulmonary resuscitation in infants*

2 cm and five rapid compressions are administered. This should be followed by a cycle of five compressions to one breath.

If the pulse is below 60/min commence basic life support

The paramedical crew attending such a call should in the first instance continue basic life support measures while efforts to commence more advanced life support are considered. The crew will have adjuncts to aid this cardiopulmonary resuscitation (CPR). The American Heart Association in its *Paediatric Advanced Life Support Manual* lists some of the equipment required for pre-hospital basic life support units, which includes:

- Rigid cervical collar
- Oropharyngeal airways
- Self-inflating bags
- Face masks
- Oxygen delivery devices
- Portable suction catheters
- Blood pressure cuffs
- Backboard
- Extremity splints
- Burn dressings

Children

For children over 1 year old the following sequence is used:

- Check responsiveness
- Open airway
- Check breathing
- Check (carotid) pulse
- Commence respiratory support or CPR as appropriate

Chest compressions are given using the heel of one hand for children aged 1–10 years, and a two-handed technique for children aged 10–15 years. In both instances the heel of one hand is placed on the lower sternum, one finger's breadth above the xiphisternum, and the chest compressed to a depth of 3 cm (Figure 35.2). Five chest compressions are given and then a cycle of one breath to each five compressions is maintained.
The approach to paediatric cardiac arrest is summarized in Figure 35.3.

ADVANCED LIFE SUPPORT

The trained paramedic should be able to institute more advanced life support measures to augment cerebral and cor-

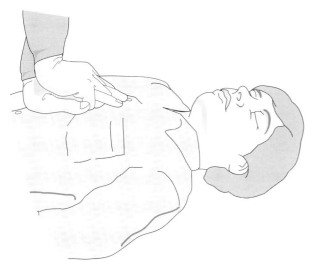

Fig. 35.2 *Correct hand position for CPR in children over 10 years of age*

onary circulation during basic life support and to attempt to terminate the cardiac arrest and restart the cardiovascular and respiratory systems.

The *Paediatric Advanced Life Support Manual* lists suitable equipment for pre-hospital advanced life support units. The list includes:

- Monitor defibrillator
- Laryngoscope with straight and curved blades
- Paediatric stylets
- Paediatric Magill forceps
- Endotracheal tubes, size range 2.5–8.0
- Intravenous catheters
- Intraosseous needles
- Intravenous fluids
- Resuscitation drugs

The paramedic needs training in the use of all the above equipment. Training will be required to connect the child to a cardiac monitor and to determine correctly what cardiac rhythm underlies the cardiorespiratory arrest. Training is also required in intubation and securing an airway. The paramedic needs to be familiar with the methods of intravenous or intraosseous access to the circulatory system (see Chapter 6). Finally, the paramedic needs training in the use of drugs useful in treating cardiac arrest.

The size of the endotracheal tube used for intubation and the dosage of the drugs used in arrest depend on the age and size of the child. Two important formulae will assist the paramedic to choose correctly. To estimate the weight of the child, add 4 to the child's age in years and double it. For instance, a 4-year-old child will weigh approximately 16 kg.

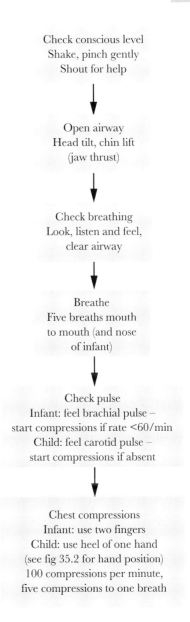

Check conscious level
Shake, pinch gently
Shout for help

↓

Open airway
Head tilt, chin lift
(jaw thrust)

↓

Check breathing
Look, listen and feel,
clear airway

↓

Breathe
Five breaths mouth
to mouth (and nose
of infant)

↓

Check pulse
Infant: feel brachial pulse –
start compressions if rate <60/min
Child: feel carotid pulse –
start compressions if absent

↓

Chest compressions
Infant: use two fingers
Child: use heel of one hand
(see fig 35.2 for hand position)
100 compressions per minute,
five compressions to one breath

Fig. 35.3 *An approach to cardiac arrest in infants (less than 1 year old) and children (over 1 year old)*

Weight in kg = (age in years + 4) × 2

To estimate the endotracheal tube size (internal diameter in mm), the age is divided by 4 and 4 added:

$$\text{Endotracheal tube size} = \frac{\text{age in years}}{4} + 4$$

For example, a 6-year-old child would require an endotracheal tube of 5.5 mm.

Arrest Algorithms

When the child is placed upon a cardiac monitor the first decision, as in adult practice, is to determine which arrest rhythm the child is suffering from.

Asystole

The algorithm for the management of paediatric asystole is given in Figure 35.4. Asystole is by far the most common rhythm found in paediatric cardiac arrest, particularly arrest occurring outside hospital. Treatment is intubation and ventilation with supplemental oxygen to try to give an inspired oxygen content of 100%. Circulatory access should then be gained as rapidly as possible.

With skill it is possible in some cases to gain intravenous access. For younger children this may involve using a vein on the back of the hand or the dorsum of the foot, as large antecubital veins are not as readily found as in adults. If intravenous access is not successful, intraosseous access should be obtained (Chapter 6). Research shows that with a minimum of training it is easy to gain intraosseous access. Fluids or drugs given by this route are rapidly diffused into the venous system and therefore gain access to the central circulation as effectively as by peripheral cannulation.

Once access is achieved, adrenaline in a dose of 10 μg/kg (0.01 ml of 1: 10,000 solution) is administered. Thus, for a child aged 1 year the weight will be 10 kg and the first dose of adrenaline will be 100 μg, or 0.1 mg, and the paramedic would give 1 ml of adrenaline 1 in 10,000 solution as the first dose.

The initial dose of adrenaline is 10 μg/kg

Cardiopulmonary resuscitation is then continued for 3 minutes, by which time there is a need for a further dose of adrenaline. The dose of adrenaline for the second and successive doses is not 10 μg/kg but 100 μg/kg. Therefore, the second dose for a 10 kg child would be a total of 1000 μg, which is 1 mg or 10 ml of 1 in 10,000 adrenaline. Cardiopulmonary resuscitation is then continued for a further 3 minutes, after which a further dose of adrenaline 100 μg/kg is necessary.

The subsequent doses of adrenaline are 100 μg/kg

While this cycle continues, consider whether to augment the resuscitation by giving the child a fluid bolus, normally 20 ml/kg of normal saline, particularly if the history suggests hypovolaemia.

If intravenous or intraosseous access is not possible, adrenaline may be delivered at a dose of 100 μg/kg via the endotracheal tube. However, if 1 in 10,000 adrenaline is used for this, large volumes would be required, so for this method of administration more concentrated adrenaline (typically 1 in 1000) is recommended.

The use of vagolytic drugs such as atropine is controversial and is not included in the European Resuscitation Council guidelines for asystole. However, the drugs do have a role in treating bradycardia before asystole ensues.

Electromechanical dissociation

Electromechanical dissociation (EMD) can be found in paediatric practice. The treatment is as follows (Figure 35.5):

- Intubation
- Ventilation with 100% oxygen
- Intravenous or intraosseous access
- Adrenaline 10 μg/kg
- CPR for 3 minutes
- Consideration of underlying cause of EMD
- High-dose adrenaline 100 μg/kg
- Continue CPR

Electromechanical dissociation is usually secondary to some known cause, such as profound hypovolaemia, tension pneumothorax, cardiac tamponade, drug overdose or hypothermia. It is therefore necessary for the paramedic to consider whether any of these problems are present. It is strongly recommended that the child is given a fluid challenge of 20 ml/kg of fluid such as normal saline for this particular arrest rhythm.

Ventricular fibrillation

Ventricular fibrillation in cardiac arrest occurring out of hospi-

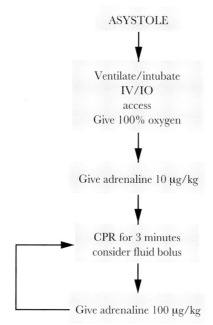

Fig. 35.4 *Management of asystole in children*

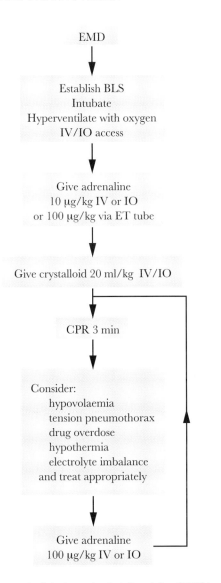

Fig. 35.5 *Management of electromechanical dissociation (EMD) in children. BLS, basic life support; CPR, cardiopulmonary resuscitation; ET, endotracheal; IO, intraosseous; IV, intravenous*

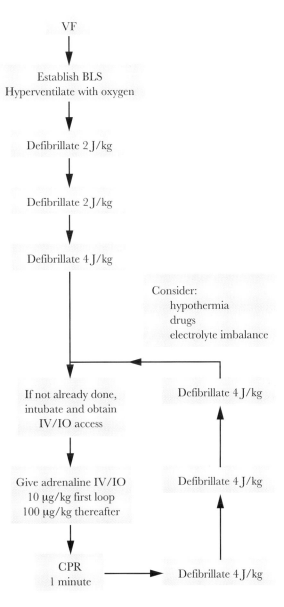

Fig. 35.6 *Management of ventricular fibrillation (VF) in children. BLS, basic life support; CPR, cardiopulmonary resuscitation; IO, intraosseous; IV, intravenous*

tal is rare, but may occur typically with some poisons, such as with tricyclic antidepressant drugs, and also with drowning in cold water and hypothermia.

If ventricular fibrillation is diagnosed when the child is placed on a cardiac monitor, it is important that the child is defibrillated. This can be achieved by a precordial thump, although great care should be taken not to traumatize the chest and cause further problems. Thereafter the child can be defibrillated with a shock of 2 joules per kg. If there is no response a further shock of 2 J/kg is delivered and if again there is no response the shock is increased to 4 J/kg.

If after these three shocks the child is still in ventricular fibrillation, the next step is intubation and ventilation with supplemental oxygen. This is followed by gaining circulatory access through an intravenous or intraosseous route and giving a dose of adrenaline (10 µg/kg). Cardiopulmonary resuscitation is continued for 1 minute only before the rhythm is checked on the monitor, and if the child remains in ventricular fibrillation three further shocks all at 4 J/kg are delivered, with pauses in between to check for any return of pulse. If this second set of shocks is unsuccessful then high-dose adrenaline (100 μg/kg) is used and cardiopulmonary resuscitation continued again in a cycle for 1 minute.

Thereafter treatment consists of a cycle of CPR resuscitation for 1 minute followed by three shocks of 4 J/kg, followed by high-dose adrenaline with continuation of CPR, and so on. If the cause of the ventricular fibrillation is known to be secondary to imbalance of electrolytes (particularly potassium) or hypothermia, then measures to correct the underlying situation should be taken. If these measures are unsuccessful after three cycles, it is possible to consider an alkalizing agent, such as sodium bicarbonate. The use of specific antiarrhythmic drugs such as lignocaine, in a dose of 1 mg/kg, can also be considered. The management is summarized in Figure 35.6.

In order to give a safe defibrillatory shock to a young child or infant, it may be necessary to use special paediatric paddles which are smaller than adult paddles. In addition, it is also necessary to use some form of electrogel or electrode pad between the child's skin and the defibrillator paddles.

CONTINUATION OF CARE

The paramedical team having instituted or continued basic life support, and started the advanced life support appropriate to the child's clinical situation, next need to consider transporting the child to hospital. This should be achieved without any break in cardiopulmonary resuscitation or any of the cycles.

In addition, adequate warning should be given to the receiving hospital who may have a specific team for paediatric cardiac arrests that can be there to receive the child on arrival to the accident and emergency department.

It is hoped that the improvement in first-aid skills by members of the public, the use of skilled paramedics to take over resuscitation in pre-hospital care, and the establishment of specialized paediatric arrest teams, will improve the outcome for children who should suffer such an unfortunate event.

FURTHER READING

Advanced Life Support Group (1993) *Advanced Paediatric Life Support*. London: BMJ Publications.

American Heart Association & American Academy of Paediatrics (1990) *Paediatric Advanced Life Support Manual*, American Heart Association.

Greaves I, Dyer P & Porter K, eds (1995) *Handbook of Immediate Care*. London: WB Saunders.

Guidelines for Paediatric Life Support. Paediatric Life Support Working Party of the European Resuscitation Council (1994) *Resuscitation* 27(2): 91–105.

chapter thirty-six:

THE INJURED CHILD

Major injury in childhood poses special difficulties to health-care professionals. One of the principal difficulties is that although injury in childhood is very common (one in three children are injured each year), true multisystem trauma occurs relatively infrequently and any one practitioner is likely to have only limited experience of the condition. It is therefore of vital importance that certain rules are firmly held so that assessment and resuscitation can be approached methodically, efficiently and thoroughly. These rules are:

- The 'ABC' priorities are the same as for adults
- The practicalities are different

DIFFERENCES BETWEEN CHILDREN AND ADULTS

Children differ from adults in the following ways.

Size

Smaller size means that a child sustains more injuries than an adult would sustain from the same force. Multiple system injury is more likely in children than adults given a similar force.

Shape

The child's relatively large head means more forces may be applied through the neck during deceleration. A falling child tends to land head first.
Formulae for calculating the area of a burn are also different.

Skeleton

The skeleton in children is very elastic. The child may sustain internal organ damage without overlying fracture, e.g. spinal cord damage may occur without radiological evidence of any fracture or dislocation of the spine. More importantly, lung contusion may occur without overlying rib fracture. Fracture of one or more ribs in childhood is extremely uncommon, and is very serious. It indicates that enormous force has been applied and internal damage is likely to be severe.

Surface Area

The larger surface area relative to body size in children means more rapid heat loss.

Sequelae

The physical and psychological results of the injury will remain with the child for a long time.

Psychology

Assessment and treatment of a frightened child who is in pain need a careful and gentle approach. The psychological impact on the carer of having to deal with a distressed child may also significantly alter performance.

Equipment

Appropriately sized and designed equipment must be available to allow appropriate treatment.

Specific Differences in Treatment

Specific differences exist between the anatomy and physiology of the child which have an immediate practical bearing on what injuries may have been sustained and on how the child is treated. These differences are listed below under the 'ABCD' headings:

A > Airway with cervical spine control
B > Breathing with oxygen
C > Circulation with haemorrhage control
D > Disability

Airway

The differences in a child's airway when compared with an adult are:

- Relatively large tongue
- Relatively large epiglottis
- Relatively short trachea
- The narrowest part of upper airway is below the level of the cords
- The larynx is more difficult to visualize

The practical consequences of these differences are as follows.

1. The best way to insert an oral airway is by depressing the tongue with a tongue depressor or the blade of a laryngoscope. The oral airway is then inserted directly rather than rotated through 180 degrees as with an adult.
2. Nasopharyngeal airways are more difficult to insert in the very small child.
3. Orotracheal intubation requires a different technique. The large, floppy epiglottis may be incorporated by the laryngoscope blade and lifted out of the way to allow better visualization of the cords.
4. In children under 6 years old an uncuffed tube should be used. A useful way of remembering the right size of tube is that it should be the size of the child's small finger. Alternatively, use the formula:

$$\text{internal diameter (mm)} = \frac{\text{age in years}}{4} + 4$$

5. When inserted, the black vocal cord marker near the tip of the endotracheal tube should be placed at the level of the cords.
6. After placement be sure to listen for air entry high in the axillae, as noises can be easily transferred from one side to another.
7. Surgical cricothyroidotomy should not be performed in children; only needle cricothyroidotomy is appropriate.

Breathing

Children breathe rapidly. They have a low reserve of oxygen and their metabolism uses oxygen very quickly; if ventilation is impaired cyanosis ensues rapidly. If ventilatory support is needed then the rate of ventilation should be around 20 breaths per minute for a child and 40 breaths per minute for an infant. The volume of the ventilation is best judged by watching the child's chest move.

Children do not tolerate tension pneumothorax well. This is because the mediastinum is very mobile and it can be pushed across to compress the other lung by the increased pressure within the injured hemithorax. Repeated assessment of air entry in the ventilated child is therefore of paramount importance.

Circulation

The heart rate in children is faster than in adults (Table 36.1). The blood pressure also varies with age. In children under 1 year old the minimal acceptable normal systolic pressure is 70 mmHg. In children older than 1 year the expected systolic pressure can be worked out by the formula:

$$\text{systolic pressure (mmHg)} = 80 + (\text{age in years} \times 2)$$

The circulating blood volume of a child is roughly 80 ml per kilogram, which means that the total blood volume of a neonate is likely to be around 240 ml.

Children respond to a decrease in blood volume by tachycardia. The first response to blood loss is therefore tachycardia. The next response is usually cool skin at the peripheries, with a drop in blood pressure as a late sign.

The practical implications of these features are that assessment of a child's circulatory status is very difficult:

- Heart rate, which is the first sign of blood loss, is likely to be affected by fear and pain
- Peripheral skin temperature will be affected by ambient conditions
- Low blood pressure is a late feature

Repeated and frequent assessments are therefore necessary so that changes can be detected early. The period of 'compensated' shock lasts for a long time.

If there is a suspicion of circulatory compromise or if injuries are apparent which would indicate significant blood loss then a fluid bolus should be administered. The best route of access to the circulation is through the antecubital fossa as in an adult, or in the dorsum of the hand in a child under 1 year old. Venous access can be extremely difficult. Techniques of intraosseous infusion and venous cutdown can be performed in the emer-

Table 36.1 Mean heart rate in children

Age	Mean heart rate (beats/min)
Newborn – 3 months	140
3 months – 2 years	130
2 years – 10 years	80
More than 10 years	75

Table 36.2 Cannula sizes

Age (years)	Cannula size (gauge)
Under 1	23
1–2	21
3–12	20
More than 12	18

Table 36.3 Glasgow Coma Scale for children under 4 years old

Verbal Response	Score
Smiles, follows sound and objects, interacts	5
Cries consolably or interacts inappropriately	4
Cries with inconsistent relief or moans	3
Cries inconsolably or is irritable	2
No response	1

gency room. If no point of access can be seen, taking a patient to a hospital that is within 10 minutes transfer time may be more appropriate than attempting the difficult process of cannulation. If cannulation can be achieved, however, the bolus that should be administered is 20 ml/kg of crystalloid solution (preferably warmed).

Cannula sizes are given in Table 36.2.

Disability (neurological status)

Children frequently sustain head injury because of the relatively large size of the head. Vomiting after head injury is common and does not necessarily imply increased intracranial pressure. Persistent vomiting is more worrying, however. Children sustain fewer intracranial haematomas after head injury but are more liable to develop cerebral oedema than adults. It is therefore especially important that episodes of hypotension or of hypoxia are avoided wherever possible. Adequate ventilation with a high concentration of oxygen is therefore mandatory and attempts to correct any hypotension due to volume loss should be made if this is technically possible.

Seizures after head injury are more common than in adults but are usually self-limiting. Infants can lose a large proportion of their circulating volume from scalp lacerations or into haematomas within the scalp. Head injuries do not otherwise cause shock.

Assessment using the Glasgow Coma Scale is likely to be more difficult than in an adult because of the child's inability to cooperate.

The practical implications of these changes are that attention to the airway, breathing and circulation will protect the child from secondary brain injury. The Glasgow Coma Scale has to be modified for children younger than 4 years of age. The assessment of the verbal component of the score is as outlined in Table 36.3.

NON-ACCIDENTAL INJURY

Health-care professionals have a responsibility for the protection of children. It is important that a child who is being deliberately abused is identified and protected from further injury. All health-care professionals need to be aware of the features of non-accidental injury. Suspicion should be aroused by:

- A history that does not fit the apparent injuries
- A delay in seeking help
- An inappropriate response from the child or carers
- Inconsistent history of the injury

Injuries that are especially associated with a non-accidental cause include:

- Injuries around the mouth
- Injuries around the genital area
- Long-bone fractures in children under 3 years old
- Bizarre injuries such as cigarette burns or rope burns

It is important the pre-hospital personnel pass on any suspicions to the health-care professionals to whom the case is handed on at the hospital.

SUMMARY

Multiple system injury in childhood is relatively uncommon and is distressing for health-care professionals. The principles and priorities of assessment and management are the same as for the adult population. Some differences in the techniques of resuscitation must be practised.

FURTHER READING

American Heart Association and American Academy of Paediatrics (1990) *Pediatric Advanced Life Support*. Dallas: American Heart Association.

American College of Surgeons (1993) *Advanced Trauma Life Support Programme for Physicians*.

Morton RJ & Phillips BM (1992) *Accidents and Emergencies in Children*. Oxford University Press.

6

CARE OF THE ELDERLY

chapter thirty-seven

THE ELDERLY PATIENT

Throughout the twentieth century in the UK there have been improvements in public health, nutrition and housing, and medical advances, especially the discovery of antibiotics. These have led to a steady increase in the numbers of people reaching not only the statutory retirement age, but their 80s and 90s, and older; for example, the number of centenarians in the UK rose from around 200 in 1951 to 4000 in 1989. In the second half of the twentieth century the number of pensioners will have increased from 5.25 million in 1951 to a projected 10 million by the millennium. Furthermore, the greatest increase is in the numbers of the very old, with a rise in those aged over 80 years from 0.75 million to 2.5 million, accompanied by no change in the overall population. We see therefore a relative reduction in numbers of younger people who may be called upon to support their elders both financially and physically. The burgeoning cost of caring for our oldest citizens is the subject of vigorous political debate as we look to the year 2020, with a further projected increase in people aged over 75 years of over 30%. The decrease in the proportion of those able and willing to care for the old highlights the ever more precarious support systems for our most frail citizens.

Why do old women outnumber men by 2 or 3 to 1? The ravages of two world wars, and other factors (such as the capacity for young and middle aged men to 'self-destruct' with industrial accidents, smoking and excess alcohol consumption), have left many widows now in their 80s and 90s. Thus, nearly half of women over 75 will live alone. Old age may also bring with it an accumulation of illnesses which result in a reduced capacity to function independently: half of those old people over 85 will be housebound or unable to leave their homes without assistance. In summary, old age may bring a combination of factors rendering the old person especially vulnerable to an acute breakdown in their capacity to cope:

- Social isolation
- Poor housing
- Low income
- Precarious functional capacity
- Dependency on others

Moreover, many old people are fiercely proud and independent, and may fail to recognize or acknowledge their increasing vulnerability. This is the backdrop to emergencies occurring in vulnerable old people, and the factors described here are essential for an understanding of the emergency situations involving old people to which the paramedical workers may be called.

THE AGEING PROCESS

Physical Ageing

Scientists have great difficulty in distinguishing the 'pure' effects of ageing from abnormal or pathological ageing. Strictly speaking, for a process to be due entirely to ageing, it should be present in everyone and should be progressive and deleterious. In practical terms, most clinicians will include conditions which have a strong association with growing older. Table 37.1 describes some important physiological changes associated with growing older and the common clinical consequences of these changes. What is remarkable is the extraordinary variability in individuals' susceptibility to the ravages of ageing. Thus, while the changes described in muscle are true for most old people, a marathon runner aged 80 will have muscle which is virtually indistinguishable structurally and physiologically from that of a fit 20-year-old. Inspection of the major clinical consequences of ageing highlights some of the major problems of old age which will be described later.

Ageing of the Psyche

Popular stereotypes need to be judged with caution. Many

Table 37.1 Physiological changes in the elderly

Change	Clinical consequences
Brain	
Shrinkage and loss of neurones (cerebral atrophy)	Increasing forgetfulness. Dementia. Vulnerability to toxic confusional states
Peripheral and autonomic nervous system	
Reduced awareness of touch, temperature, pain. Impaired proprioception. Impaired control of posture and balance	Hypothermia. Postural hypotension. Falls, urine incontinence, constipation
Eye	
Cataracts. Macular degeneration. Stiffening of lens	Impaired eyesight. Presbyopia (failure to accommodate to near and distant vision)
Ear	Deafness
Bones, joints and muscles	
Thinning of bones (osteoporosis)	Fractures of femoral neck, wrist and vertebrae. Increased curvature of spine (kyphosis)
Osteoarthritis	Stiffening of knees, hips and fingers
Loss of muscle, strength and bulk capacity to respond to displacement	Immobility, falls

behaviours described as being associated with ageing may well be the habits of middle age carried into late life:

- Rigidity of personality
- Reduced sexual drive
- Decreased repertoire of activities
- Hypochondriasis
- Bowel obsession

Successful ageing embodies maintenance of interests, hobbies and work, adapting to changing capability, maximizing current abilities and avoiding negative attitudes to old age (ageism).

THE NATURE OF ACUTE ILLNESS IN OLD AGE

Some generalizations can be made. Firstly, acute illnesses in old people often fail to present with convenient and characteristic symptoms or physical signs:

- A myocardial infarct may present without crushing central chest pain and rather with a fall, acute onset of mental confusion or simply breathlessness
- Acute infections may fail to mount the response of an immune reaction (raised white cell count) or a raised body temperature

Acute illnesses in old people arise in the context of a general background of failing health such as:

- Memory loss and impairment of intellect. The elderly brain is especially susceptible to the toxic effects of any acute illness, so that acute onset of mental confusion may be a presenting symptom which resolves provided that the underlying cause is treated
- Failing eyesight or hearing
- Increase in postural sway so that acute illnesses may present as falls
- Impaired central control of bladder function so that acute illnesses may present with urinary incontinence
- Perhaps most importantly, an accumulation of other diseases; for example, a fairly trivial acute illness may arise in a person already compromised by heart failure and further limited by impaired mobility following an operation for a fractured neck of femur

Acute illnesses in old people often arise in a situation of precarious social circumstances in which the support network for the individual is already stretched. Such illnesses are often partly or wholly related to drug therapy.

The paramedic called to an emergency must be aware that an apparently minor illness in an old person can have very different consequences from the same illness in a young person. Consider two patients, one young and one old (Figure 37.1).

Case 1

A young man of 25 years old, previously fit, develops a runny nose which progresses to laryngitis and acute bronchitis with a painful hacking cough. The course of his illness is illustrated in Figure 37.1 (lower line) which plots his illness in terms of 'disability'. Because he feels unwell, has a fever and is in some pain from his coughing, he takes to his bed. However, being otherwise fit, he is able to get up to the toilet and to move around in bed. His

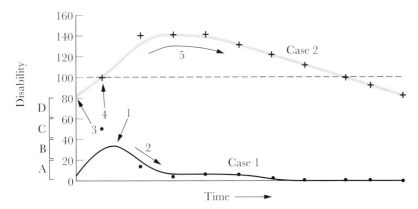

Fig. 37.1 The effects of acute illness in a young person (lower plot) and an elderly person (upper plot). Disability is on an arbitrary scale; 100 is the threshold for hospital admission. The elderly person's starting disability of 80 is due to arthritis of the knees (A), poor eyesight (B), cardiac failure (C) and carer stress (D)

wife is able to go to the pharmacist and gets some aspirin to relieve his symptoms. She is able to provide him with food and drinks and over a period of 48 hours he improves and is soon up and about. The maximal level of his disability (1 in Figure 37.1) is reduced by the lack of other illnesses (co-morbidity) and the presence of his wife to look after him. His quick recovery (2) is due to his general good health and a responsive immune system. He may never reach his doctor's attention and will not reach the 'disability threshold' for admission to hospital.

Case 2

An 85-year-old widow lives alone in a warden-controlled flat because of previous falls due to a combination of poor eyesight, osteoarthritis of her knees and cardiac failure. Her daughter has felt obliged to visit every day, and especially in the evenings and at weekends when there is no warden on duty. The background problems impose a level of disability illustrated by A–D in Figure 37.1. Thus even at her best she has a precarious existence close to the threshold for hospital admission (3 in Figure 37.1). Now follow her illness in Figure 37.1 (upper line). She develops a similar illness to Case 1 on Saturday afternoon and takes to her bed. Her legs, already stiff, seize up and she is unable to go to the toilet, gain access to food or fluids, or contact the warden who is off duty. Her daughter arrives to find her lying in a wet bed, acutely embarrassed and with a hacking cough. She is complaining bitterly of pain in her knees and her daughter is unable to move her, thus her level of disability rises further (4) to the point at which she requires emergency admission to hospital. Thereafter, the slower recovery (5) is due to the secondary effects of the respiratory infection on her mobility and her cardiac failure.

MAJOR MEDICAL PROBLEMS IN OLD AGE

The effects of ageing and acute or chronic illnesses often manifest as conditions best described as 'functional failure', as described above. Professor Bernard Isaacs, one of the first generation of academic geriatricians, characterized these common manifestations of illness in old age as the 'giants of geriatric medicine':

- Intellectual disorder (dementias and acute confusional states)
- Immobility, incontinence and instability (a tendency to fall)
- Visual and hearing impairment
- Depression
- Adverse drug reactions (approximately 10% of acute admissions to geriatric wards are as a result of adverse drug reactions)

Multiple ailments – so common in old people – often result in multiple drug therapy, thus increasing the risk not only of adverse drug reactions, but also of potentially serious drug interactions.

Intellectual Disorder

Some impairment of memory and concentration is so common in later life as to be considered normal and not indicative or predictive of dementia. This thought is a great relief to its victims, but occasionally is responsible for a delay in diagnosis of genuine dementia. This type is seldom in any way disabling. In simple terms, intellectual disorder is of two types: due to disease outside the brain (extrinsic), and due to intrinsic brain disease (dementia).

Extrinsic causes

Mental impairment may be caused by drugs, infections, hypoxia, dehydration, electrolyte disorders, disturbances of carbohydrate metabolism and renal and hepatic failure. Hypothyroidism and vitamin B$_{12}$ and folate deficiency very rarely cause intellectual impairment, although they may be found in association. Head injury with or without intracranial haemorrhage may be included in this category. The intellectual dysfunction associated with these extrinsic causes is usually short-lived, unless there is coexisting intrinsic brain disease.

Two cardinal features distinguish this type of mental disorder from dementia:

- Acute onset (and usually rapid resolution)
- Disturbed or fluctuating conscious level

Extrinsic causes of mental impairment
- Drugs
- Infections
- Hypoxia
- Dehydration
- Electrolyte disturbances
- Carbohydrate metabolism disturbances
- Renal and hepatic failure
- Hypothyroidism
- Vitamin B$_{12}$ and folate deficiency
- Head injury

Intrinsic causes

Dementia is a pathological state characterized by diffuse loss of brain tissue. When brain tumour and other focal conditions have been excluded, the usual causes are Alzheimer's disease, multifocal vascular disease, and a mixture of the two. Dementia also occurs in Parkinson's disease, Huntington's chorea and other rarer brain diseases.

Alzheimer's disease is a slowly progressive disease with a 10-year course on average. While some cases can present in the fifth and sixth decades, most appear in the eighth and ninth decades.

Vascular brain disease, also called multi-infarct dementia, occurs in hypertensive patients who suffer progressive loss of brain tissue, with or without focal neurological signs. The course of this disease is more rapid than that of Alzheimer's disease, and many patients die from cardiac disease or stroke.

The history

Patient's may give a very misleading history of the illness as they are unable to assess their current state, but may be able to talk convincingly and positively of their past life. Patients have considerable skills of deception. Be very wary of patients who make even the slightest lapse from consistency of accuracy in answering questions, and seek information from relatives who have watched them over a period of time. Tell-tale signs are:

- An increased use of the telephone, especially in the middle of the night
- Frequent losses of key, pension books, money, jewellery
- Accusations that others have stolen these
- Burning out kettles
- Leaving the gas on unlit
- Resistance to bathing and changing clothes
- Changes in sleep-wake patterns
- Soiling of clothes and neglect of personal appearance
- Leaving the house and getting lost
- Repeatedly asking the same question
- Misidentifying or failing to identify near relatives
- Speaking of the past as if it were the present, and of dead people, e.g. parents, as if they were still alive

Eventually a crisis occurs which carers can no longer accept, and this fracture of sound support may masquerade as a medical emergency.

Immobility

Immobility can be defined as an inability to occupy space (the life-space, ranging from anywhere in the world to the confines of an upstairs bedroom). From a clinical point of view, however, it can be considered as a restriction of everyday activities.

How commonly does restricted mobility occur?

An investigation in the UK by Age Concern in 1978 of people past retirement age revealed that about 40% had no difficulties getting about. In the remaining 60%, difficulties with hills and ramps were the most commonly reported (31%), while others were traffic and road crossing (23%), uneven pavements (16%), and steps and kerbs (4%).

What are the barriers to maintaining mobility in old age?

Physical barriers (often more than one):

- Joint problems, especially osteoarthritis of knees and hips
- Neurological deficit: impaired balance, stroke, Parkinson's disease
- Previous falls
- Sensory deprivation: deafness, impaired vision
- Cardiovascular and respiratory diseases

Mental barriers:

- Reduced expectations of an active life
- Loss of adaptability and creativity
- Introversion with reduced social contact
- Anxiety and fear of going out (or of allowing others to)

Social barriers:

- Retirement brings with it dangers of reduced social contact, and a drop in income. The retired person may regard a motor car as an unnecessary expense. Many regret having got rid of their car
- Living alone: an epidemic problem in ageing women
- Nowhere to go – insufficient outside interests or activities

What are the consequences of immobility?

Loss of choice. Any of the following choices may be lost:

- Being able to go where we want to be and thus be able to do what we want to do
- Being alone or with others
- Having the TV on or off (look around any hospital ward or old people's home)

Loss of capability:

- Getting to the toilet in time, answering the door or getting upstairs
- Social responsiveness
- Worsening physical dependency

An old person's world may thus contract and after becoming housebound he (or more often she) then becomes restricted to the lower half of the house and eventually perhaps to one room.

Incontinence

Anyone can become incontinent if not able or not allowed to have access to proper toilet facilities. The elderly are more vulnerable because of poor mobility, and frequency and urgency of micturition. Any acute illness is likely to be associated with deterioration in continence, but usually this is transient. Likewise, any change of environment such as admission to hospital may also lead to a temporary period of incontinence.

Extrinsic causes

One common cause for incontinence in old people is faecal impaction. It is easily diagnosed by rectal examination and quickly cured by enemas. Those suffering from chronic brain failure are more likely to develop difficulties with incontinence, which is partly due to a diminished response to sensation of bladder filling. Similar difficulties arise following the removal of indwelling catheters and continence may not be regained for several weeks in some cases. Finally, urinary tract infection may occasionally cause incontinence.

Drugs such as diuretics may exert adverse effects on an older person's bladder by their mode of action. Hypnotics and sedatives may lead to incontinence, especially at night. Anticholinergic drugs such as antidepressants, antiparkinsonian drugs and verapamil can lead to urinary retention with overflow.

Intrinsic causes

Intrinsic causes include disorders of the bladder, sphincter or their nerve supply.
Incontinence may be caused directly because of over- or under-activity of the bladder itself or the sphincter.

Instability

Balance

Balance is a set of biological strategies designed to maintain the body in the erect posture. Mechanisms involved include ocular, vestibular and proprioceptive (position sense) receptors found in the neck and elsewhere, especially in the weight-bearing joints and in the tendons and ligaments of the trunk. Under normal circumstances, the body undergoes oscillations around a fixed point known as the 'sway path'. As these balance mechanisms deteriorate with increasing age, sway increases.

Ocular mechanisms   Under normal circumstances, visual cues are constantly used to correct minor deviation from the fixed point. In old people visual acuity is frequently reduced, as is the threshold for light stimulation.

Vestibular mechanisms   The vestibule is mainly involved with rotatory movements of the head and neck, whereas the otolith organ is involved with acceleration and deceleration. With advancing age, these mechanisms are relatively inefficient. Vestibular mechanisms may be implicated in walking over uneven ground, or have some part to play in instability during rising from a chair.

Proprioceptive mechanisms   Position sense is important for maintaining balance. Sensory information from proprioceptors in the central spine and major weight-bearing joints may be impaired with ageing and arthritis. Failure of these mechanisms leads to an increased likelihood of falls.

Falls

How common? Very common!

About 20% of elderly men and 40% of elderly women will give a history of a recent fall, and the liability to fall rises with age: the probability going up from 30% chance of falling at the age of 65 years to 50% at the age of 85 years. The majority of falls are not reported and *only about 3% of elderly people who fall sustain an injury that requires medical attention.* Nevertheless, in an average-size health district of 250,000 people, with about 37,000 people over 65 years old, between 16 and 20 beds will be occupied by patients admitted as a direct result of a fall. It is one of the most common causes of emergency admission to an acute geriatric ward, often after a prolonged period lying on the floor unable to get up.

Where and when do falls occur?
Most falls occur indoors or very close to the house, in daytime. Falls on stairs are more likely to occur when the person is descending.

What are the clinical features?
Falls may be divided into two broad categories: extrinsic and intrinsic.

Extrinsic falls are those in which an external factor is responsible, e.g. tripping or accident. This type of fall occurs in a younger, fitter person, and the vast majority are unreported and cause no serious injury. The consequences are slight with no restriction in activities or loss of confidence. In *intrinsic* falls the dominant cause is failure of balance for the reasons described above and in which one or more precipitating factors (described below) may play a part. In this case the patient is older and more frail, and typically the consequences are much more serious regardless of physical injury: loss of confidence, restriction of activity and a loss of mobility may all result in fear of going out of doors unaccompanied.

Precipitating causes
Change of posture Getting out of a chair, an unstable situation requiring strength and coordination in antigravity muscles, is a typical precipitating cause. The reason is rarely postural hypotension, an uncommon cause of falls although much loved by medical students and doctors!

Extended movement In falls due to extended movement the person reaches out or up, which puts the centre of gravity outside the ground base, but owing to a slowing of postural reflex movements is unable to compensate by moving the feet quickly enough to prevent a fall.

Illnesses Any acute illness such as cardiac disease or arrhythmias, may lead to a fall, as may poor vision.

Drugs Diuretics, hypnotics and drugs for hypertension are particularly implicated in falls in the elderly.

What is the prognosis?
Falls in the very old often indicate serious underlying disease and have a gloomy outlook. About a quarter will die within a year of their index fall. If they have lain for more than an hour, half will be dead in 6 months.

Visual Impairment

A few generalizations can be made about the special problems old people with failing vision may encounter:

- The additional burden of other handicaps
- Less opportunity to manipulate their physical and social environment to their needs
- Less advantages than younger people in seeking registration as either blind (acuity worse than 6/60 – unable to read top line of Snellen chart) or partially sighted (no better than 6/60 – able to read the top line)

Thus, visual handicap remains grossly underreported both to doctors and registering authorities.

The ageing eye
The following changes are seen in the ageing eye.

Cornea The cornea becomes slightly more opaque with slight scattering of light and reduction in light transmission, especially at the ultraviolet end of the spectrum. Specific diseases rather than age itself are responsible for any visual handicap.

Lens The largest contribution to the visual consequences of the ageing process is made by changes in the lens: it becomes thicker, stiffer, denser and more yellow (filtering out blue and violet). The main consequence is presbyopia or reduced ability to accommodate.

Ciliary apparatus Thickening of the ciliary apparatus may lead to closed angle glaucoma (see below).

Retina The blood vessels of the retina become narrower. Macular deterioration reduces spatial discrimination, black and white contrast and colour perception.

Eye diseases
Most people enter retirement with some form of corrected optical problem (usually presbyopia and astigmatism). All elderly people with visual disability (worse than 6/36) have a disease, *not* simply the effects of normal ageing.

Most of the major eye diseases encountered are progressive but amenable to treatment, so accurate diagnosis is essential. The four major diseases of the eye in old age are:

- Cataract (clouding of the lens of the eye)
- Macular degeneration (deterioration in central vision)
- Glaucoma (increase in pressure of fluid within the eye)
- Diabetic retinopathy (visual failure due to small vessel disease of the retina)

Hearing Impairment

Deafness is a common problem in the elderly, which increases in prevalence with age, 30–40% of people over 75 years having some degree of hearing loss.

Pathology

Acquired causes are either conductive or sensorineural deafness, and are superimposed upon an age-related sensorineural hearing loss termed *presbyacusis*. Presbyacusis is characterized by a predominantly high tone hearing loss caused by degeneration and atrophy of the sensory cells and neuronal connections within the cochlea.

Symptoms

Difficulty understanding speech is the most distressing and common consequence of hearing impairment. High tone hearing loss particularly affects consonant as opposed to vowel sounds. Since much of the information in speech is encoded in consonant sounds, when these are imperfectly heard, speech is almost unintelligible. Frequency discrimination, sound localization and reaction time are also impaired. In some patients distressing tinnitus (whistling or ringing) and abnormal loudness perception may add to their problems.

Social consequences

In most elderly patients difficulty in hearing speech is first noticed during group conversation. As with many other disorders in old age, this inability to communicate effectively often leads to loss of independence and social isolation. In some individuals irritation and unhappiness caused by deafness may progress to clinical depression. Alternatively, others may feel 'left out' and if unable to lip-read in group discussions, may become suspicious and harbour paranoid ideas.

Hearing aids

Hearing trumpets are still available and, although they may appear outdated, are still effective. Postaural and body-worn aids are readily available; these aids have a volume control and settings marked 'O' for off, 'M' for on (microphone), and 'T' for use with telephones fitted with an induction coupler (telecoil) loop, which cuts out background noise. Some public buildings and phones are also fitted with coupler loop systems. Bone conductor aids are available to patients with severe middle ear disease causing profound conductive deafness.

A hearing aid is most useful in face-to-face conversation when lip-reading augments the comprehension of speech. Group discussions are still difficult owing to amplification of ambient noise and reverberant sound which interferes with what the patient wishes to hear.

Depression

Depression is both a subjective mood state and an objective psychiatric illness. It is important to distinguish one from the other.

The psychiatric illness of depression is characterized by low mood, unaffected by external circumstances, feelings of unworthiness and helplessness. Suicidal ideas may be present. The future looks bleak. There is appetite disturbance, usually leading to weight loss. Sleep disturbance, characteristically early morning wakening, occurs. Concentration is poor, there is a decrease in normal interests, even in family and friends. In a severe illness, psychotic phenomena may be present, i.e. delusions and hallucinations. Delusions are usually of poverty or are nihilistic (thinking things have disappeared, never to exist again). Hallucinations are usually of a second person who makes derogatory statements, e.g. 'You are dirty', 'You should be dead'. In elderly patients with depression hypochondriacal ideas are more often present, e.g. worries about heart disease or cancer. This is often in the setting of real illness which is then exaggerated by fears and worries.

In summary, depression in the elderly is characterized by:

- Appetite disturbance
- Weight loss
- Sleep disturbance (early wakening)
- Poor concentration
- Decrease in normal interests
- Delusions and hallucinations
- Hypochondriasis

Masked depression

Hypochondria or anxiety symptoms predominate and there is no complaint of depression, although symptoms are present and can be revealed by questioning.

Pseudodementia

Pseudodementia is the term given to a syndrome that presents with *poor self-care* and *poor cognitive ability*. This change in function is brought about by a retarded depression. All the features mentioned above will be present; lack of interest will result in poor self-care and cognitive function. These patients will often answer 'don't know' to questions rather than confabulate. The history of onset of the illness is weeks or months rather than years as in a true dementia. There may be a family or previous history of affective disorder.

Prevalence of depression

A study of prevalence of depression in a community survey amongst elderly people conducted in the UK and USA in 1976 showed that 22% were possibly depressed, 13% had a minor depressive disorder and 1.6% had a major depressive disorder.

> Depression is a major health issue in people over the age of 65 years

Adverse Drug Reactions

Table 37.2 indicates the common culprits that cause problems

Table 37.2 Drugs that may cause problems in elderly patients

Drug group	Symptoms and signs
Diuretics	Falls, confusion, dry mouth, dehydration, postural fall in blood pressure, urinary incontinence
Compound analgesics	Drowsiness, confusion, falls, constipation
Tricyclic antidepressants	Greater risk of anticholinergic effects: urine retention, constipation, dry mouth, postural hypotension and confusion
Digoxin	Reduced renal excretion. Increased risk of side-effects such as sickness, diarrhoea, slow pulse rate and other heart rhythm disorders causing dizziness, fainting or falls
Beta-blockers	Falls, confusion, heart failure, slow pulse, postural hypotension, asthma attacks, cold limbs
Hypnotics	Increased and prolonged effects. Confusion, drowsiness, staggering and falls (especially at night)

in old people. The paramedic called to see an old person should (with permission) search for all medications (both prescribed and 'over the counter') and bring them with the patient to hospital. They may be crucial in assisting diagnosis, especially when the patient is unable to give an accurate history.

COMMUNICATING WITH OLD PEOPLE

Problems such as impaired hearing, anxiety, neurological problems (stroke, dementia, depression) and the effects of social isolation may cause problems in communicating with old people. Simple measures such as ensuring that a hearing aid is switched on and that dentures are worn may make a huge difference. In people with impaired hearing, ensuring good

lighting and that the patient can see your face clearly may assist with lip-reading, at which many old people are extremely adept. Further tips to assist with communication and obtaining a reliable history are given below.

1. *Introduce yourself.* Patients do not know who you are and it is a simple courtesy to tell them.
2. *Shake hands.* This friendly action provides information on the patient's vision (does the patient see and attend to the hand? Does he miss it when he reaches out his own hand?) and on the strength of grip, the temperature and moisture of the palm, and the general feeling of eagerness or apathy.
3. *Sit down close to the patient.* It is off-putting to be asked questions by someone who is towering over you. Get down to the patient's level both physically and psychologically. Speak clearly, have your face in a good light and never put your hand over your mouth.
4. *Don't waste questions.* Have a clear purpose in mind with every one you ask.
5. *How well does the patient hear you?* Watch the movement of the head, the facial expression and the response to questions, rather than directly asking if the patient hears you. Further guidance is given in the section on impaired hearing.
6. *How credible is the patient as a witness?* Begin by asking name, address, date of birth and current age. Check these against your own information. Discrepancies are very significant.
7. *How good is the patient's memory?* Avoid or postpone 'formal' tests of cognitive function. You will obtain just as much information, without risking upsetting the patient, by asking about family: the name of spouse (including wife's maiden name where appropriate), the names of sons, daughters, sons-in-law, daughters-in-law and grandchildren.
8. *How well is the patient oriented?* Establish first orientation by saying, 'You know who I am, of course, don't you?' and following with, 'Well, who am I?' and 'What is my job?'. If you are still in doubt about orientation continue with, 'You know what place this is, don't you?'. Orientation for time is best tested by asking about the month or the time of year, rather than the day of the week. Knowledge of the time of day is also a good guide; but do not ask more questions than you need.

THE HOME ENVIRONMENT: CLUES TO AID DIAGNOSIS AND MANAGEMENT

The paramedic may be in a unique position as 'Sherlock Holmes' when called to attend an old person at home. The major illnesses of old age often leave environmental clues to give assistance to the hospital or primary care team. This investigative role of the paramedic is especially crucial when the patient is a recluse, perhaps not well known to neighbours or to the primary care team, or is reluctant to go to hospital and may deny that problems exist.

A useful starting point is to consider who initiated the emergency call; was it:

- The patient? (probably wants help – consider fear and loneliness as well as genuine illness)
- A neighbour? (consider antisocial behaviour or genuine concern about failure of the patient to cope)
- Relatives or carers? (consider severe dependency and carer stress. Has the general practitioner been involved? If not, why not?)

Once the paramedic has arrived at the patient's home, careful observation of the following can help in assessing the patient.

1. *The garden and outside of the house* – is it well maintained? If so, by whom? If not, is this because of low income, lack of interest or lack of ability?

2. *Access to the house* – if this is difficult, is the patient a voluntary recluse or socially isolated, or is it because of neglect of maintenance, fear of assault or burglary? Check with neighbours.

3. The patient who is *slow or unable to answer the door* may be deaf, immobile or ill. Alternatively, the doorbell may not work.

4. *The letter-box test* – lift the flap and sniff! If the smell is unpleasant, consider severe neglect, urine or faecal incontinence of cats as well as humans.

5. *The general state of repair, maintenance and cleanliness* inside will give clues to the person's general level of household competence. Is the house well heated? If there is central heating, is it used? If the house is clean and tidy, who does it? At the other extreme, the visitor's feet may stick to the carpet and there may be extreme neglect and squalor. An interesting and not uncommon condition is what geriatricians call the 'senile squalor' (or Diogenes) syndrome. An elderly person (or occasionally a young person) lives in utter squalor, often surrounded by piles of junk or magazines to the extent that movement within the house is almost impossible. Surprisingly the person is not demented or ill, and may often have a middle-class background and have lived alone for many years. Usually they function reasonably well. People with long-standing psychiatric problems or alcoholism may also live in such squalor.

6. The *life-space* (see section on immobility): how much of the house does the person occupy? Are there walking aids or grab rails? Does the person go upstairs? Where are the toilet and bathroom? Are they used? Is there a commode? Does the person sleep in a chair? Can they get up and walk safely? Problems in these areas point to difficulties with mobility, recent or previous falls.

7. The *kitchen* – is there food around? Is there a refrigerator? If so, is there fresh food in it? Has the person been eating? Who prepares the food? Is the person capable of using the kitchen?

ABUSE OF OLDER PEOPLE

There has been increasing interest and concern about this important topic. Abuse may be physical, sexual or financial; it may be due to neglect by relatives, carers, or (it could be argued) by the Welfare State which leaves many old people on very low incomes or insufficiently supported in their own homes. Paramedics should be trained in the signs of non-accidental injuries. Much attention has been paid to this topic in children and adults in violent households, but only recently in elderly people. Injuries such as finger-mark bruising (especially on the upper arms), cigarette burns (which may not be self-inflicted), bruising around the head and neck and on non-extensor surfaces may be due to assaults and should be carefully documented. Usually they are blamed on falls, and in direct confrontation the old person will often deny abuse, which is often from a stressed carer on whom the old person depends. Physical abuse most often occurs within a caring relationship in which the carer, often inadequately supported, is dealing day and night with a person who is mentally or physically very dependent. Management of the situation demands care and treatment not only for the abused person, but also for the carer.

CONCLUSION

An understanding of the nature of illness in old age and especially the ways in which acute illness has to be considered in the context of social, physical and mental frailty is essential to the paramedic faced with the difficult task of dealing with the emergency in an old person's home. This important and fascinating area forms an ever-increasing proportion of emergency work.

FURTHER READING

Bennett GJ & Ebrahim S (1992) *Health Care of the Elderly*. London: Edward Arnold.

Pathy MSJ, ed. (1992) *Principles and Practice of Geriatric Medicine*. Chichester: John Wiley.

Pitt & Brice (1982) *An Introduction to the Psychiatry of Old Age*, 2nd edn. Edinburgh: Churchill Livingstone.

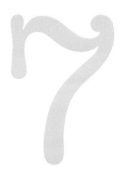

THE
HOSTILE
ENVIRONMENT

chapter thirty-eight:

HYPOTHERMIA

Hypothermia is a more complicated topic than is frequently appreciated, and its potential deleterious effects on people suffering trauma are not well researched. Hypothermia is defined as having a core temperature below 35 °C. Clinically, hypothermia can be divided into three categories:

- Mild: 32–35 °C
- Moderate: 30–32 °C
- Severe: below 30 °C

and into four groups according to circumstances:

- Immersion
- Dry
- Urban
- Diving

These categories are not strictly defined, but are descriptive. The underlying condition is broadly the same for each group but there are differences in terms of their treatment.

TYPES OF HEAT LOSS

There are four ways in which heat loss occurs from the body:

- Conduction
- Convection
- Radiation
- Evaporation

Conduction

Conduction is heat loss due to direct contact with the sur-roundings, e.g. the ground, air or water. The speed with which heat is lost to the surroundings depends on three factors:

1. The temperature difference between the body and the surrounding environment: the greater the temperature difference, the greater and quicker the heat loss.
2. The specific heat capacity of the substance in contact with the body. Denser substances take more energy to heat them up, e.g. water takes about 240 times more energy to heat than air. Thus, when a body falls into water it cools very quickly. Similarly, dense materials such as stone and metal conduct heat well, which is why they feel cold to the touch.
3. The surface area over which heat is lost. Children have a larger surface area for their weight than do adults and hence tend to cool more quickly.

The low conductance of air as compared with water is why low (still) air temperatures are tolerated much better than immersion in cold water.

Convection

Convection is in essence a form of conduction in which air (or water) that is cooler than the body comes into contact with skin and then moves away. While in contact with the skin it is warmed, and as it moves away new air comes in which is warmed in turn. As the rate of heat loss is greatest when the temperature difference is at its greatest, this causes a more rapid heat loss than simple conductive heat loss. It is this mechanism which explains why coffee is cooled by blowing on it (remember that the expired air will be warmer than the surrounding air and would therefore cool *less* quickly if conduction only was in progress).

The importance of convective heat loss is not great when a casualty is removed to a sheltered environment, but is highly significant when the person is exposed to wind. This is the 'wind chill' factor. The heat loss increases in relation to the square of the wind speed, thus a wind speed of 8 mph will remove four times as much heat as a wind speed of 4 mph. This relationship holds until the wind speed reaches 30 mph (13.5 m/s), at which stage the air is moving so rapidly that it is not in contact with the skin for long enough to be warmed to skin temperature and so heat loss increases little at winds over this speed.

Radiation

Radiation heat loss is generally the largest form of heat loss in the outdoor environment. All solid objects radiate heat to the sky when not absorbing heat from the sun. The human body radiates heat to surrounding solid objects. The degree of radiant heat loss depends on the difference in temperature between the two bodies (proportional to the fourth power of the difference between the two temperatures) and the emissivity of the surface (a black surface causes greater loss than white). The majority of this radiant heat loss is in the form of infrared radiation – hence the use of infrared detectors in searching for bodies.

Radiant heat loss is much more significant in the outdoor environment than in hospital, as in the latter the surrounding solid objects are at a much higher temperature (namely room temperature). Radiant heat loss to a mountainside with a temperature of 0 °C is highly significant, as the loss is proportional to the fourth power of the temperature difference.

Evaporation

Under normal conditions, evaporation is responsible for 20–30% of heat loss from the body. Approximately two-thirds of this occurs as 'insensible sweating' and one-third occurs through the air passages (inspired air requires to be both warmed and humidified prior to reaching the small airways). Evaporation of 1 g of water takes 0.6 kcal, and it is this high energy usage which explains why sweating is such an efficient means of cooling the body.

Evaporative heat loss is increased in the cold environment as cold air is dry. Thus heat loss from insensible sweating and from humidifying inspired air is increased. At high altitudes, where the air is thin, respiration increases in frequency and depth. As a result up to 4 litres of water a day is required to humidify the inspired air. This results in a heat energy loss of 2400 kcal.

Evaporative heat loss due to evaporation from wet clothing can also be significant.

Other Factors Affecting Heat Loss

In addition to the above-mentioned problems there are several other factors that will also affect heat loss. These include immobility (often secondary to injury or collapse) and hypothyroidism.

CONTROL OF HEAT LOSS

Physiological

The temperature of the human body is normally regulated within strict limits around an average core temperature of 37 °C, not usually altering by more than half a degree. The regulatory centre for this control lies within the hypothalamus at the base of the brain. On detecting a drop in the temperature of the blood reaching the brain, or on input from other sensory areas such as the skin, mechanisms to reduce heat loss and increase heat production are activated.

Reduced heat loss
Heat loss is reduced by:

- Stimulation of the sympathetic nervous system, causing constriction of blood vessels to the skin
- Curling into a ball, thus reducing the surface area of the body
- Abolition of sweating (although insensible evaporation will continue to occur)

Increased heat production
Heat production is increased by:

- Shivering – it should be appreciated that this results in an increase in energy and oxygen consumption by the body
- An increase in activity, e.g. running on the spot, foot stamping
- Metabolic heat production secondary to release of adrenaline and noradrenaline

Non-Physiological

Non-physiological methods of reducing heat loss include seeking shelter (possibly with a heating source) and the application of clothing. Protective clothing is a topic in its own right, but a few important principles are considered below.

Materials protective against heat loss
Many materials are used in cold-weather clothing. A problem with many is that their insulation abilities are dramatically reduced when wet (e.g. down has only about 10% of its dry thermal insulation value when it is wet). Wool remains one of the best materials in that it retains about 80% of its dry protective value when wet. Synthetic fibre-pile materials are nearly as good.

Other materials are now available which transmit water and sweat away from the skin to the outside, thus stopping evaporative heat loss from the skin. These are usually worn as a combination 'thermal' undergarment and a breathable outer garment. Most heat loss protection from clothes comes from their ability to reduce conductive and convective heat loss. Little protection from radiant heat loss is available, although microfibre materials are claimed to be effective.

The fingers are especially susceptible to heat loss because of their thin, cylindrical shape. Wearing mittens significantly reduces heat loss by effectively reducing the surface area of the fingers by combining them into a single unit. Blood flow to the brain is large and the skull is a good conductor. The scalp has little fat for insulation and its blood supply is not reduced in response to cold in the same way as other areas of the skin. Covering the head is therefore essential to reduce heat loss and a material such as wool is ideal.

The thermal or 'space' blanket is designed to protect against radiant loss and will also give some convective heat loss protection; it is therefore probably of more use in the pre-hospital setting as radiant heat loss is less in a warm room (although it is still present). The space blanket must not be used in isolation, however, as its conductive heat loss protection is very limited. There is no evidence to show whether the space blanket should be on the outside or inside of an ordinary blanket. It should also be remembered that use of the blanket will reduce radiant heat absorption from the sun, which can be significant even in a cold environment.

TYPES OF HYPOTHERMIA

Immersion Hypothermia

A person who falls into water rapidly becomes hypothermic owing to the high heat capacity of water (see above). Numerous other effects occur which are discussed in more detail in Chapter 39. It is important to realize that the person will continue to cool when removed from the water owing to evaporative and convective heat loss (Figure 38.1).

Dry Hypothermia

Dry hypothermia is in fact rarely dry; the term is used to distinguish it from immersion. This is the type of hypothermia found in people who are exposed on hillsides. The heat loss is usually slow and occurs as a result of all four forms of heat dissipation. There is usually a degree of exhaustion in addition to the heat loss.

Urban Hypothermia

Urban hypothermia is similar to dry hypothermia, but results from an injury or other medical problem. It is frequently seen in the elderly who fall and sustain a fractured hip and lie on the floor overnight; it also occurs, for example, following a stroke or

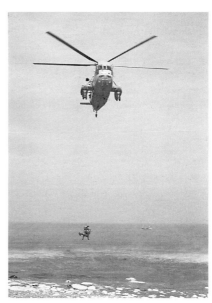

Fig. 38.1 *Immersion hypothermia*

in a drunk who falls down and lies in the gutter overnight. In this case the underlying medical problem is as important as the hypothermia.

This form of hypothermia also occurs in the victims of road traffic accidents, where the immobility enhances the other heat-losing processes. This is an underrecognized problem, and compounds the effects of hypovolaemic shock in that it increases oxygen requirements.

Remember that severe hypothermia can be protective to the brain (see Chapter 39), but mild to moderate hypothermia is not.

Diving Hypothermia

Diving hypothermia is similar to immersion hypothermia, but relates to deep diving. At depth, the type of gases breathed and their density mean a tremendous amount of heat is lost through the respiratory system.

CLINICAL EFFECTS OF HYPOTHERMIA

Hypothermia has a number of effects on the body, irrespective of its cause (Figure 38.2).

Some effects of the cold start as soon as the core temperature begins to drop, before true hypothermia has developed (Table 38.1).

Muscles

As cooling occurs the muscles become stiffer and uncoordinated

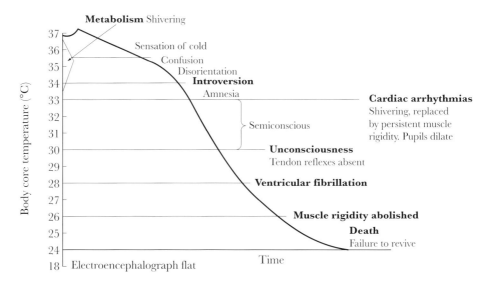

Fig. 38.2 *Effects of hypothermia. Reproduced from Eaton (1992)* Essentials of Immediate Care, *by permission of Churchill Livingstone*

and there is involuntary shivering. As the temperature drops further there is a reduction in the speed of nerve impulses to muscles. This results in increasing weakness and incoordination of movement. Shivering also depletes the muscle stores of glycogen and causes the accumulation of lactic acid and other metabolites. It also results in a marked increase in oxygen consumption by the body.

Table 38.1 Clinical freatures of hypothermia

Core temperature* (°C)	Clinical feature
36	Sensation of cold, stumbling, personality changes, mild confusion
35	Slurred speech, incoordination. Amnesia of events (on recovery)
34	Development of arrhythmias – typically atrial fibrillation
33	Shivering lost – replaced by muscular rigidity
31	Pupils become dilated. Loss of consciousness
30	Insulin ineffective. Risk of spontaneous ventricular fibrillation – often unable to defibrillate
26	Major acid–base disturbance
24	Significant hypotension
23	Apnoea
18	Asystole

* These temperatures are a guide and will vary between individuals.

As the core temperature reaches 33 °C, the shivering response is lost and replaced by persistent muscular contraction. This is less efficient than shivering as a means of heat production and results in the individual becoming literally 'stiff with cold'.

Cardiovascular System

As cooling sets in there is an increase in heart rate which directly relates to the increase in muscular activity (shivering). It is only as the core temperature drops significantly (below 32 °C) that the heart rate starts to drop. The heart, being a muscle, suffers in the same way as other muscles as the temperature drops, i.e. it becomes stiffer and less efficient. As the heart cools it also becomes 'irritable' and is prone to develop arrhythmias. Blood as it cools becomes thicker and more viscous, and is more difficult to pump around the body. The oxygen dissociation curve is shifted to the left, causing oxygen to be held more avidly by haemoglobin and therefore not given up in the tissues (it becomes a less efficient transporter).

Hypothermic patients develop a degree of dehydration. This is a complicated phenomenon, due in part to increased urine production (cold-induced diuresis) and complicated by fluid loss prior to hypothermia developing and reduced intake once developed. A redistribution of fluid also occurs, with intravascular fluid leaving the circulation for the extravascular compartment. This potentiates the increased viscosity of the blood.

Blood chemistry

Sodium With hypothermia and rewarming changes occur in the cell membrane permeability and in the sodium pump mechanism. The effects on serum sodium are not consistent and depend on the type and duration of hypothermia and on the method of rewarming.

Potassium Hypokalaemia is frequently seen in prolonged hypothermia and is due to potassium movement into cells. Hyperkalaemia may occur in association with the metabolic acidosis that is usually present.

Glucose Acute hypothermia is usually associated with raised glucose levels due to catecholamine-induced glycogenolysis. Prolonged hypothermia results in glycogen depletion leading to hypoglycaemia. The signs of hypoglycaemia will be masked by the hypothermia.

Amylase A rise in serum amylase levels is frequently seen in severe hypothermia and is associated with an ischaemic pancreatitis. Amylase is an enzyme produced by the pancreas and elevated levels in the blood are used as a marker of injury or inflammation of the pancreas.

Brain

With mild hypothermia the brain function becomes slower. An early change in personality can occur, e.g. a quiet person becomes noisy or an extrovert becomes withdrawn. As the temperature falls, confusion and disorientation set in. On further temperature reduction these symptoms become worse with increasing lethargy, leading to eventual unconsciousness. This train of deterioration is almost identical to that seen in other conditions where brain function is decreased, e.g. hypovolaemic shock.

The pattern of deteriorating brain function with falling temperature is therefore:

- Personality change
- Confusion
- Disorientation
- Lethargy
- Unconsciousness

CLINICAL RECOGNITION OF HYPOTHERMIA

The diagnosis of hypothermia in the field is frequently difficult, and often missed as attention is paid to the more obvious injuries.

History

The history frequently gives an indication of the likely presence of hypothermia and may well be the only indicator. Ask yourself the following questions:

- Has the patient been immobile for a prolonged period (after a fall, or trapped)?
- Is the patient wet (rain or immersion)?
- Has the patient been exposed to the wind?
- Has the patient open wounds, increasing heat loss?

Remember that temperatures do not have to be freezing to cause hypothermia.

Examination

There are few consistent signs other than the patient's skin feeling cold. Taking the temperature of the patient is the only conclusive guide, but this can be difficult and unreliable in the field. If a temperature is taken it should be performed with a low-reading thermometer. Oral temperatures can be difficult and dangerous to take in an unconscious or confused patient. Axillary temperatures are unreliable, but will at least give an indication of the degree of hypothermia. The best guide is a rectal temperature, which is usually not practical. If a mercury thermometer is used, it must be kept in position for 3 minutes. The answer to this problem may lie with the infrared tympanic thermometer which can give accurate readings within 1–2 seconds, unfortunately, they are expensive and not widely used in pre-hospital care.

Other signs include:

- Shivering – disappears around 33 °C.
- Pulse – initially raised, then falls (but other factors interfere, e.g. hypovolaemia and raised intracranial pressure). The pulse is difficult to feel and weak. It may be irregular owing to cold-induced arrhythmias
- Breathing – slow and shallow (although initially the rate may be raised)
- Breath – fruity, acetone smell due to incomplete metabolism
- Mental state – confusion through to unconsciousness (but other factors interfere, e.g. hypovolaemia and raised intracranial pressure)

Remember that the patient who is thought to be hypothermic must be examined for signs of injury or medical illness which may be masked by the effects of the hypothermia.

TREATMENT

Pre-hospital

The initial management of the patient is aimed at reducing

further heat loss. The patient must therefore be provided with protection against the elements. This involves replacing wet clothes, applying blankets (including a 'space' blanket) and providing shelter (e.g. tarpaulin rigged over a vehicle by the fire service at the scene of a road traffic accident).

The patient should be handled carefully, as sudden manoeuvres can precipitate cardiac arrhythmias. Insertion of an oral airway should be performed with care as the vagus nerve tends to be sensitive and stimulation can result in a severe bradycardia or asystolic arrest.

> **Careless handling of hypothermia victims may precipitate fatal arrhythmias**

Oxygen should be administered wherever possible, especially if injuries are present, and ideally it should be warmed and humidified (there are soda lime and water trapping devices which can be used to some effect in the field).

Warmed intravenous fluid should be administered, as this not only aids rewarming but replaces some of the fluid loss (warming devices are available).

The main pre-hospital danger is that the patient may suffer a cardiac arrest. This is most likely to be ventricular fibrillation. The protocols for treating arrests should be followed, but it must be appreciated that it may be impossible to defibrillate if the core temperature is below 30 °C. The relative protective effect of severe hypothermia on the brain gives rise to the edict that 'no body is presumed dead until it is warm and dead'. Thus resuscitation should be continued until the patient is adequately rewarmed.

> **No body is dead unless warm and dead**

No attempt should be made to actively warm the hypothermic patient pre-hospital by other means, such as hot-water bottles or heaters. This would result in peripheral heating, with opening of the skin and splanchnic blood vessels, resulting in the washing out of metabolites that have built up in the hypoxic tissue. When these arrive at the cold and 'sensitive' heart they can induce fatal arrhythmias.

In Hospital

Hospital care is only briefly covered as it falls outside the remit of this chapter, although some of these techniques can be used in pre-hospital care, especially if long transit times are anticipated.

The pre-hospital measures are continued, with regard being paid to injuries or medical problems. Further evaluation of the patient is undertaken, including ECG, chest X-ray, serum electrolytes, serum glucose, amylase, blood gases and a full blood count. The patient can then be managed by either active rewarming or passive rewarming.

Passive rewarming

In passive rewarming the patients are allowed to warm up on their own. Bringing a patient into a warm room does not actually warm the patient, it simply reduces heat loss and allows the patient to recover and warm up by their own metabolic efforts. This process is safe, although monitoring of electrolytes needs to be continued.

Active rewarming

Active rewarming involves actively reheating the patient. There are a number of methods that can be used.

Warm humidified oxygen It is the humidification that is primarily beneficial as it reduces evaporative heat loss (air transfers little heat).

Warmed intravenous fluids These fluids should be administered at a temperature of 37–39 °C if benefit is to be obtained.

Thoracic cradle heating Heat is applied to the thoracic region to achieve central warming. This can be done with a cradle of lights, although this method is being superseded by a warm air blanket system.

Peritoneal lavage A peritoneal dialysis catheter can be inserted and warmed fluids instilled into the abdominal cavity to cause central warming.

Oesophageal warming A closed circuit tube is inserted into the oesophagus and a warm fluid circulated through it. This causes central warming in a similar way to peritoneal lavage.

Extracorporeal rewarming A cardiopulmonary bypass machine can be used to reheat the blood.

Immersion Hypothermia

Patients who have undergone immersion hypothermia can be rapidly rewarmed by placing them in a bath at 40 °C with their legs and arms dangling out. This is permissible as the patient has been rapidly cooled and does not run into the same physiological problems as other hypothermic patients. This is discussed further in Chapter 39.

chapter thirty-nine:

NEAR-DROWNING

Drowning is a common cause of death in the UK, being the fourth leading cause of death in men under the age of 35 years and is the second leading cause of death in children, with 40% of all drowning deaths occurring in children under the age of 5 years. Alcohol and drugs are a significant predisposing factor. 'Near-drowning' is the term applied to a survivable drowning episode.

Death by drowning can be 'wet' or 'dry'. In 'wet' drowning, the individual aspirates water into the lungs, after an episode of breath-holding until the victim cannot hold the breath any longer. On inspiration much of the water is probably swallowed, but a proportion is inhaled. This inhaled water blocks the airways, only a proportion of it getting as far as the alveoli. The result is hypoxia which after a short period results in hypoxic cardiac arrest and hence death. It only requires 10 ml of inhaled water per kilogram of body weight to be fatal (Figure 39.1).

Fresh water in the alveoli is absorbed, resulting in haemolysis of red blood cells and haemodilution. Sea water, being hypertonic, causes withdrawal of water from the blood and no haemolysis. The changes that occur are of interest to the pathologist but not to the paramedic.

In 'dry' drowning no (or very little) water actually enters the lungs. This may be because of laryngeal spasm but is more likely to be because of primary cardiac arrest due to stimulation of the vagus nerve by cold water. It is this mechanism that causes the death of people who drop into cold-water. It is likely that this is the cause of death in 'spray drowning', deaths that occur in people on the surface of rough water. Vagal sensitivity is increased by hypothermia which occurs rapidly in cold-water immersion.

'Dry' drowning accounts for between 10% and 25% of drowning deaths, depending on the source of the information. It would seem to be higher in cold water drowning and this would fit the proposed mechanism.

PATHOPHYSIOLOGY

Immersion in Cold Water

When a body is immersed in cold water a number of effects occur, as described below.

Body temperature

When a person falls into cold water the body temperature rapidly starts to fall unless they are adequately protected (see Chapter 38). If the water temperature is much below 10 °C it is very difficult for the body to generate sufficient heat even if actively exercising, to prevent this temperature fall. The symptoms and problems related to hypothermia thus develop.

Respiratory system

Cold water has several effects: there tends to be a large intake of breath and breathing tends to occur at the maximum lung capacity, the breaths being rapid and shallow. This has the advantage of increasing the buoyancy of the individual; but this form of respiration is both inefficient and hard work, causing the subject to tire rapidly.

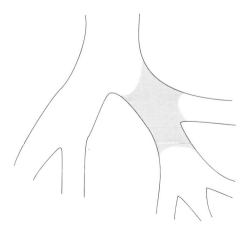

Fig. 39.1 Water blocking a small airway

When water temperatures are very low (5 °C or less) the ability to hold the breath dramatically reduces, maximal times being of the order of 5 seconds.

Cardiovascular system

Water exerts a pressure on the body and in the upright position gives an effect similar to applying a pneumatic anti-shock garment (PASG). This principle is easily understood if one appreciates that there may be a difference of 1.5 m between the neck at the surface and the soles of the feet. A height of 1.3 m is equal to 130 cm of water pressure, which equates to approximately 100 mmHg (mercury is 13 times as dense as water). This hydrostatic pressure effect is very important when removing patients from the water; if they are removed in the upright position there will be a sudden drop in blood pressure similar to that occurring on removal of a MAST (PASG) suit (Figure 39.2). Immersion in cold water also results in peripheral vasoconstriction due to the cold and the other changes that occur with hypothermia (e.g. reduction in circulating volume and fluid shifts between compartments).

The diving reflex

The diving reflex occurs in many mammals but its significance in adults is doubtful. It does seem to be more developed in children and probably explains why young children can survive prolonged cold-water immersion.

A reflex bradycardia occurs when cold water stimulates areas of the face and neck. This bradycardia, associated with the rapid cooling caused by cold-water immersion, can be protective of the victim by rapidly reducing the oxygen requirements of the brain and other tissues with a high metabolic requirement.

Other effects

The cold water, partly by producing hypothermia, and partly by a direct cold effect on the pharynx, causes intense vagal stimulation which results in a severe bradycardia or asystole. For this reason manipulation of the airway in a near-drowned person can cause cardiac arrest.

Effects of Near-Drowning

The effects of near-drowning are variable and depend on a number of factors: the temperature of the water, the length of time immersed and the amount of inhaled water. There is little difference between salt and fresh water.

Initial (primary) effects

The initial problem that occurs is hypoxia; the victim becomes confused, then lethargic and eventually unconscious, although patients frequently report that they experience a 'high'. Several divers have described this phase as being 'pleasant', in that they no longer cared what would happen to them. If the hypoxia continues then cardiac arrest will occur as a result of hypoxic myocardium. The victim will also suffer the associated prob-

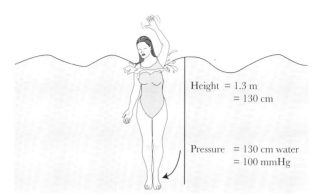

Fig. 39.2 *MAST effect. Pressure of water at feet in approximately 100 mmHg. This reduces to zero at the surface*

lems of hypothermia and the loss of hydrostatic pressure (as described above). In very cold water an asystolic arrest can occur owing to intense vagal stimulation.

Delayed (secondary) effects

Water inhaled into the lungs causes damage; this is multifactorial and includes the development of pulmonary oedema and a reduction in the amount of surfactant. As a result the subject may initially have few symptoms but may develop marked respiratory problems over several hours (usually 4–8). This problem is known as *secondary drowning*.

The other secondary problem is infection. Victims will have swallowed and inhaled water that may well contain microorganisms from sewage effluent or rat urine contamination (common in canals). Thus consideration should be given to the development of illness such as Weil's disease. Prophylactic antibiotics have not been shown to be of use.

DIAGNOSIS

The diagnosis would seem to be easily deduced from the circumstances; however, the picture is more complex, as the patient is likely to be hypothermic and may have other injuries associated with a fall or dive into water, or injuries sustained while in the water. The classic injury to the cervical spine occurs in the person who dives into shallow water thinking that it is deeper than it actually is.

The clinical picture may vary from a cardiac arrest (which may be ventricular fibrillation or asystolic) to a conscious patient with few signs or symptoms but who is at risk of secondary drowning.

Airway

Airway findings are variable: it may be totally patent, it can be obstructed by the tongue owing to unconsciousness, or it may be obstructed by water in the oropharynx.

Breathing

Breathing may be normal, but the chest should be auscultated as the presence of crepitations may indicate that secondary drowning is likely to occur. Breathing may be absent, either with or without cardiac arrest.

Circulation

The pulse is highly variable; many of the changes will be cold-related. A profound bradycardia may occur in relation to vagal stimulation.

TREATMENT

Removal from the Water

It is very important that the patient should be kept as horizontal as possible when removed from the water because of the loss of hydrostatic pressure to the body (Figure 39.3). This is especially important if the patient is hypothermic, and it is this combination that frequently led to deaths in the past — in World War II it was found that many shipwrecked sailors who were alive in the water had died by the time they were brought on deck.

Airway and Breathing

The airway should be checked and cleared with care being taken to maintain the neck in midline immobilization, as a cervical spine injury may have occurred on the fall or dive into the water. A cervical collar should therefore be applied unless cervical spine injury can be definitely excluded (e.g. in a swimmer who has got into difficulties). In the absence of a history of events it is safer to assume cervical spine injury. Protecting the neck is difficult while in the water but an inflated life-jacket (not a buoyancy aid) gives some neck protection.

On attempting to clear the airway, suction of the oropharynx should be used, although it must be remembered that in the hypothermic patient, any airway manipulation could cause vagal stimulation or laryngeal spasm. It is impossible to remove water from the smaller airways because of the capillary attraction between the wall and the water. This water will be absorbed if the patient survives. The patient should not be put in the head-down position as this does not help remove water from the lungs and will raise the intracranial pressure, which may already be elevated from the preceding cerebral hypoxia. Chin lift and jaw thrust should be used but head tilt avoided, in view of the risk of neck injury. Guedel or nasal airways can be used, but care is needed as vagal stimulation can occur.

In the apnoeic patient ventilation should be commenced. This is best undertaken via an endotracheal tube or laryngeal mask, as bagging via a mask tends to blow air into the stomach, which usually contains water, and thus increases the risk of regurgitation of stomach contents.

The breathing patient may be placed in the recovery position if spinal injury is excluded, the combination of hypoxia and swallowed water being a good stimulus for vomiting.

Circulation

In the absence of a palpable central pulse, cardiopulmonary resuscitation should be commenced and the appropriate cardiac arrest protocol followed. It should be appreciated that ventricular fibrillation may not be 'shockable' if the core temperature is below 30 °C. Cardiopulmonary resuscitation on its own can occasionally cure the patient by correcting the hypoxia (this has been recorded a number of times in children).

Bradycardias should be treated with caution; if caused by vagal stimulation their treatment improves the situation, but in the severely hypothermic patient it is frequently detrimental. A variety of other arrhythmias may be present due to hypothermia. Hypothermia, the loss of hydrostatic pressure and the presence of other injuries all contribute to a relative hypovolaemia. Intravenous access and warmed fluids are therefore required.

Hypothermia

It is clear from the preceding text that the near-drowned patient is frequently hypothermic. Once the patient is out of the water, wet clothes should be taken off as early as possible, otherwise continued heat loss will result from evaporation. First-aid measures must be aimed at preventing further heat loss.

Associated Injuries

The possibility of injuries must be considered and appropriate measures taken. The presence of hypovolaemia from a significant haemorrhage considerably complicates the clinical picture.

Further Treatment in Hospital

In the patient with cardiac arrest, continued resuscitation will

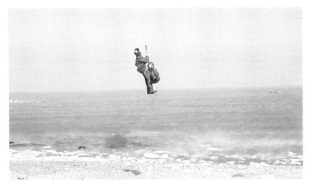

Fig. 39.3 Removal from the water

take place until the patient is warm but still not responding. Immersion hypothermia can be treated by rapid rewarming, in which the patient is placed in a bath at 40 °C with legs and arms dangling out. This should only be done where the cooling has been rapid (see Chapter 38). This treatment is only practicable and safe if the patient is conscious and sufficiently alert to cooperate. It should not be used for the unconscious patient. If a bath is unavailable a shower is an alternative, but is less efficient and requires even greater cooperation from the patient. The successfully treated patient will require the following investigations:

- Chest X-ray
- Blood gas analysis
- Full blood count, urea and electrolytes

The patient should be kept under observation owing to the risks of secondary drowning, and should not be discharged home unless the blood gases and chest X-ray are normal, and the patient is free from any symptoms, with a clear chest on auscultation.

chapter forty:

HEAT ILLNESS

In the UK heat illness is not a significant problem in civilian practice; it does, however, occur in the summer months and is frequently associated with strenuous activities such as sport or military exercises. Cases of heat illness do occur in other individuals such as labourers working outside in hot, humid conditions, or workers in industries such as steel manufacturing, where the working environment is hot.

As with other environmentally produced disorders there is a range of problems progressing through minor conditions (e.g. muscle cramps) to the life-threatening illness of heat stroke.

PHYSIOLOGY

In humans the core temperature is regulated to remain constant at around 37 °C. The centre for this regulation is sited in the hypothalamic region of the brain. Heat is produced through metabolism, either as a byproduct (for example of muscle contraction) or directly as a heat-producing mechanism. Heat loss occurs via a number of mechanisms and a fuller account is given in Chapter 38.

When excessive heat production occurs or the environmental temperature is raised, the hypothalamus detects a rise in the temperature of the blood passing through it and initiates heat-losing mechanisms. The vascular beds in the skin are opened in an attempt to lose heat by convection and conduction. Sweating is stimulated and the evaporation of this water causes significant heat loss via the energy required to cause the change of water from liquid to vapour – the latent heat of evaporation (0.6 Kcal/g). In extreme conditions 1.5 litres of sweat may be produced in an hour.

In the exercising individual the respiratory rate is increased, resulting in further heat loss through the evaporation associated with respiration.

There are two types of sweat glands in humans: the apocrine glands which are concentrated in the axilla, and the eccrine glands, which are the primary sweat-producing organs. Eccrine sweat is colourless and odourless (unlike that produced by the apocrine glands), the salt content can be varied depending on the amount of aldosterone production.

The redistribution that occurs in attempts to lose heat results in a marked increase in the blood flow to the skin and a reduction in the splanchnic and renal beds. This increased skin flow with the increased supply to muscles, in the exercising subject, results in a marked increase in cardiac output and produces a tachycardia. If the situation is prolonged then fluid loss from sweating and respiration results in a reduction in circulating volume. The physiological effects are summarized in Table 40.1.

Table 40.1 Physiological effects of heat illness

Respiratory	Increased respiratory rate – with increased fluid loss*
Cardiovascular	Dilated skin capillary beds Increased heart rate* Increased cardiac output* Relative or actual hypo-volaemia Reduced renal blood flow
Fluid and electrolytes	Dehydration Hyponatraemia (especially if fluid loss replaced by water only)
Skin	Warm and red – increased blood flow Increased sweating
Other	Decreased liver function Impairment of coagulation

* Exercise-related condition.

Acclimatization

Prolonged exposure to a hot environment results in acclimatization. Many of the changes that occur with this process are an attempt to reduce salt loss. The concentration of sodium in sweat is considerably reduced and the kidneys increase reabsorption of sodium. This process is the result of aldosterone secretion and possibly growth hormone release.

TYPES OF HEAT ILLNESS

Heat Cramps

Heat cramps usually occur in the muscles of the lower limbs, and are related to exercise. They occur in people in whom significant fluid losses due to sweating have been replaced with fluid with an insufficient salt content. As a result the individual becomes hyponatraemic and it is this electrolyte disturbance that is thought to cause the muscle cramps.

In the UK this has been a recognized problem in certain industries such as mining and steelworks. Experience has shown that adequate salt replacement relieves the problem.

Heat Syncope

Fainting related to the heat is not infrequently seen in accident and emergency departments during hot weather. Elderly people seem particularly prone to this condition. The likely mechanism is a degree of dehydration from sweating, combined with peripheral vasodilatation. If the person then stands for a long period, there is pooling of blood in the lower limbs (loss of the calf muscle pump) resulting in a drop in blood pressure and a subsequent syncope. Injuries can occur as a result of the fall. The condition is self-limiting as the supine position restores the circulating blood volume, but the patient should be rested and provided with an oral fluid intake. In the elderly patient this diagnosis should only be made after other, more serious diagnoses have been excluded.

Heat Exhaustion

Heat exhaustion is a condition caused by water or salt depletion. It typically occurs in subjects who are not acclimatized and who undertake vigorous exertion, for example in military training.

Diagnosis

The patient frequently develops the following symptoms and signs:

- Headache
- Dizziness
- General weakness
- Fainting
- Normal or mildly elevated core temperature (less than 40 °C)
- Tachycardia
- Orthostatic hypotension

It is very important the patient is treated at this stage, as if left untreated or allowed to progress, heat stroke (see below) will occur.

Treatment

The patient should be placed in a cool environment and an oral electrolyte solution provided. Care needs to be taken when cooling the patient as the traditional tepid sponging and fanning can increase core temperature by causing capillary shutdown in the skin and even stimulating a shivering response. This is a particular problem with younger children. Cautious cooling with a fan is appropriate.

In patients who have significant symptoms, intravenous fluid and electrolyte replacement is required.

Heat Stroke

Heat stroke is a serious life-threatening condition and requires rapid treatment. The condition normally occurs in hot, humid conditions where there is little wind, and it can occur in the absence of exercise. It has been seen in the UK under unusual circumstances such as people exerting themselves while wearing dry (diving) suits.

The condition occurs when the heat regulating systems fail to keep up with heat production, are unable to function effectively or fail (e.g. loss of sweating).

It is recognized that there are two clinical forms of heat stroke: *classic* and *exertional*. Classic heat stroke occurs during a period of sustained high environmental temperature and humidity. It tends to occur in older or debilitated people. Exertional heat stroke is caused by overproduction of heat as a result of exertion, and occurs primarily in young, fit subjects. Some individuals seem to be more prone to this condition than others, and the identification of these individuals is currently an area of interest to the military. Exertional heat stroke differs from classic heat stroke in that rhabdomyolysis and hypoglycaemia are a frequent problem. From the pre-hospital perspective the conditions are very similar.

Diagnosis

The diagnosis is primarily clinical. The symptoms and signs are:

- Temperature usually 41 °C or greater
- Skin is hot and dry, although sweating may still be present
- Weakness

- Nausea and vomiting
- Confusion progressing to lethargy and eventual coma
- Tachycardia and hypovolaemia
- Clotting abnormalities, including disseminated intravascular coagulation
- Hepatic damage – jaundice seen after 24 hours

Treatment

Early initiation of treatment in the pre-hospital phase is very important, as heat stroke if not corrected will result in rapid death due to damage to the central nervous system. This has been likened to frying eggs – the heat causes the protein to be denatured and irreversibly changed.

Cooling The patient should be cooled with care. Clothes should be removed. If there is likely to be a delay in transfer of the patient to hospital, then immersion in cool water should be considered. This rapidly cools the individual owing to the high specific heat capacity of water (i.e. its ability to remove heat rapidly). Care needs to be taken if the conscious level of the patient is altered, and in the unconscious patient protection of the airway is mandatory while performing this procedure. It is important to avoid the production of hypothermia.

Airway Oxygen is required at high concentration, and if the conscious level is altered, airway protection is necessary.

Cardiovascular system There is usually a degree of dehydration and therefore intravenous fluid is required.

Other Blood glucose levels should be checked using a reagent strip (for example BM stix®) and hypoglycaemia corrected. Fits can occur, and treatment is primarily aimed at airway control and maintaining oxygenation.

Further management in hospital

Hospital management is usually undertaken on an intensive care unit. Cooling needs to be continued, and electrolyte levels and the clotting status monitored.

chapter forty-one:

ELECTROCUTION

The frequency of accidental death by electrocution is about 0.54 per 100,000 population per year in the USA. Generated electricity accounts for over 90% of the deaths, the rest being due to lightning strike. Low-voltage electrical injuries (< 1000 volts) are common in the home and the workplace and are responsible for half of the deaths; high-voltage injuries occur in industrial settings. Lightning strike kills approximately 200 people annually in the USA, more than most other natural disasters combined.

PATHOPHYSIOLOGY

Electricity flows from the point of contact to the ground, producing heat directly proportional to the distance between these two points and the resistance of the tissues in between. The effects of electrical passage are generally worse with alternating current (AC) than with direct current (DC). The current follows the line of least resistance within the body. Skin has a high resistance when dry, followed by bone, muscle, blood vessel and nerve. The higher the resistance, the greater the damage produced.

Alternating current is generally more dangerous than direct current at any given voltage because it is more likely to induce ventricular fibrillation.

The points at which the electrical energy actually enters and leaves the body are marked by burns, the *entrance* and *exit wounds*. These are local lesions with a central charred region, an intermediate zone of whitish coagulation necrosis, and an outer area of brighter red, oedematous damaged tissue.

Alternating current in the domestic setting produces entrance and exit wounds of approximately the same size. In the industrial environment direct current is the most common cause of injury, and produces a small entrance wound and a much larger exit wound.

The greatest threats to life following electrical injury are a consequence of tissue damage, resulting in the release into the circulation of potassium and a product of muscle breakdown, myoglobin. These may cause cardiac arrhythmias and renal failure respectively.

When attending a patient who has suffered electrical injury, it is vital to remember the possibility of secondary blunt injury which may have resulted from the victim being thrown by the electrical contact. In any unconscious patient, therefore, cervical spine injury must be assumed and closed head injury suspected.

> **Suspect cervical spine injury in electrocution incidents**

AT THE SCENE

The scene of an electrocution is a hazardous environment for the rescuer: *are you safe to save?*

When dealing with electrical injury, the first consideration in the rescuer's mind must be personal safety. A rescuer unaware of the potential risks is in considerable danger, and if injured will become a liability, and worsen the situation.

> **Safety first!**

Ensure that the current is switched off before attempting to touch the victim or remove the victim from the electrical source. If possible, the current should be switched off at its source. The rescuer may have to separate the victim from the current using a non-conductive object, such as a dry broom handle. A victim may be unable to release an electrical source because currents in excess of 10 milliamperes will cause tetanic muscular contractions to occur. The only course of action will be to interrupt or discontinue the source of electricity, since separation of the victim from the source will be impossible.

In electricity pylon accidents it will be necessary to telephone the electricity board to prevent them reconnecting an interrupted source, which they will do as a matter of routine after 20 minutes – since the cause of most temporary interruptions is bird strike, which is generally not investigated.

When a worker on a utility pole is electrocuted, expired air ventilation can often be initiated by rescuers on the pole, with chest compressions if needed as soon as the victim can be lowered to the ground; in this situation, even if there is no loss of consciousness, a victim of high-voltage electrical shock should receive cardiac monitoring and transport to hospital because of the danger of delayed cardiac arrest from life-threatening arrhythmias.

Railway Accidents

Many electrical injuries occur on railways, a significant proportion of which are suicide attempts. Railway-related electrocution may be AC or DC; many lines are electrified on the 25,000 volt AC overhead system, whereas others are electrified on a 750 volt DC third rail system or the 630 volt DC fourth rail system which is used by the London Underground.

The railway is a hazardous environment; do not go onto a rail track unless you have to. Be aware of warning signs which indicate 'Reduced Lineside Clearance' or 'No Refuge'. Face oncoming traffic, and always wear a high-visibility tabard.

Telephones are clearly marked at crossings and signals and provide direct communication with British Rail (BR) Control. Obtain permission from BR before going on to the track and request an official railway lookout using these phones, or through your ambulance control. Use overhead line structure numbers, signal numbers or mile-post numbers to identify your exact location.

Using the lineside phones, the current isolation procedure and procedure for stopping trains is as follows. You should state:

1. 'Emergency call'
2. Your name
3. Where you are
4. Why you need the current switched off

Then wait for assistance!

Assume the electricity supply (whether overhead or a third or fourth rail system) is live until you have definite assurance that it has been switched off by BR. It is said that if the victim and the rescuer can remain more than 1 metre below the overhead wire at all times, it is not essential for the current to be switched off!

If a major incident occurs a BR incident officer will be appointed.

Remember: be seen, be alert, be safe to save

MANAGEMENT

After the safe extrication of the patient at the scene of an injury, immediate management follows basic principles with an evaluation of:

- Airway with cervical spine control
- Breathing
- Circulation

Emergency intervention and resuscitation will occur as for any victim of trauma, to achieve and secure an airway, establish adequate ventilation and provide fluid resuscitation. Accepted conventional algorithms for cardiac resuscitation should be followed in the case of cardiac arrest following electrocution.

The possibility of blunt trauma should be considered, and must be assumed to be present in any unconscious patient who has been electrocuted; the cervical spine should accordingly be immobilized, and the patient placed on a spine board until spinal injury can be excluded.

Oxygen should be administered and intravenous access obtained using two large-bore (14 or 16 G) cannulae in the antecubital fossae. Fluid infusion should be started, following accepted protocols for volume resuscitation; intravenous fluids are essential to treat or prevent shock (from the burn, or an associated secondary injury), and to optimize renal perfusion in the face of subsequent renal insult from myoglobin released from damaged muscle.

Cardiac monitoring is essential as there is a significant incidence of delayed arrhythmias following electrocution. Cardiac monitoring is generally continued in hospital for 24 hours in serious incidents.

A brief search should be made for any entrance or exit wounds, which should be covered with a clean, simple dressing during transfer to hospital.

LIGHTNING STRIKE

Unlike other forms of electrical injury, lightning strike rarely produces exposure long enough to cause breakdown of the skin, the primary insulator of the body to current flow. The current instead passes over the outside of the body, the 'flashover' phenomenon. The majority of the current thus passes outside the body. If the victim is wet, the flow of current may cause secondary burns as the fluid is turned into steam. Because of the flashover phenomenon, true entrance and exit wounds are uncommon.

The almost universal cause of death is respiratory arrest.

Lightning acts as a massive DC countershock, sending the heart into asystole that is normally temporary in the otherwise healthy young adults that are most often its victims. Unfortunately, the respiratory arrest that often accompanies cardiac arrest may last significantly longer than the cardiac event, and ventilatory support will be required in these patients. Patients who do not arrest immediately have an excellent chance of recovery: the victim who is moaning and groaning has a degree of stability of the vital signs, and recovery is the rule.

chapter forty-two:

CHEMICAL INCIDENTS

'Then all over the underground system people began collapsing. The commuters suffered bleeding from the nose, choking, loss of vision, burning in the throat. Several victims reported seeing brown plastic containers, like lunch boxes, wrapped in newspaper on the train floor, leaking a transparent liquid.'

The Tokyo underground gas attack
(*Daily Express*, 22 March 1995)

The above newspaper description of the chemical gas attack on a Japanese underground train in Tokyo in March 1995, which killed 7 people initially and put more than 4000 in hospital, graphically illustrates the hazards of chemical poisoning, irrespective of whether it is a deliberate terrorist attack or an accidental release. Many chemicals are unseen and the risks are not perceived until disaster strikes. Even then, the symptoms caused by chemicals may not be immediately recognized in the victims until the rescuers develop similar symptoms as a result of contamination.

When they occur, chemical disasters generate very high levels of media interest. On 3 December 1984 methylisocyanate leaked from a chemical plant in Bhopal in India. Precise figures are difficult to establish but between 150,000 and 200,000 people were affected and some 2500 died. The effects of this event are still being seen by health-care workers in the area.

The worst chemical incident in the UK was the explosion at the Nypro plant in Flixborough on 1 June 1974. This killed 29 people and injured over 100. Several thousand people needed to be evacuated from their homes while the incident was contained: it is another feature of chemical accidents that even if casualties are few, the social effects on the surrounding population can be enormous.

MANAGEMENT

Two aspects of the management of any chemical incident scene need to be considered:

organizational
clinical

The former is largely related to personal safety, protective clothing and decontamination, whereas the latter involves clear identification of the substance involved and its immediate and longer-term effects on those affected, along with the problems of decontamination of the seriously injured casualty. Common to both areas is the subject of information-gathering regarding the nature of the incident and the chemicals involved.

Safety at the Scene

The key to management of a chemical incident is to have a high index of suspicion, to protect oneself and to take advice from the experts. Remember that while a liquid chemical spill will be easy to see and hopefully contain, a toxic chemical gas cloud is no respecter of a police cordon tape.

Information-gathering

At the scene of any incident involving chemicals it is important to gather intelligence about the chemicals involved, their quantities, toxicity and the countermeasures that may be necessary. This information is needed quickly and it must be authoritative and accurate.

In the industrial setting there are a variety of regulations in the UK that govern the operation of sites handling dangerous substances. The most important of these are the Notification of Installations Handling Hazardous Substances Regulations 1982 (NIHHS) and the Control of Industrial Major Accident Hazard Regulations 1984 (CIMAH). Applications of these regulations to an industrial site will ensure that in the event of an accident, chemical spill or toxic release, the agents involved and all necessary arrangements for the management of the incident will have been the subject of pre-planning. The emergency services should therefore be aware of the chemicals involved and any special hazards or action necessary to combat the incident.

It is in the realm of transport accidents that uncertainty arises. Many thousands of potentially toxic and hazardous loads are carried on the roads of the UK every day. When one such load is involved in an incident it is essential that the attending emergency services can obtain information as to the load involved. There are a number of systems of hazard warnings that are of assistance to attending emergency services.

Hazard warning symbols

The standard diamond-shaped hazard warning symbols indicate to both the emergency services and the public the primary hazard present. Symbols represent hazards such as flammable solids or liquids, flammable or toxic gases, compressed gases, oxidizing agents and corrosive substances, amongst others. On multiloads the hazard warning diamond simply contains an exclamation mark.

The HAZCHEM action code system

The HAZCHEM code system is a set of code numbers and letters which when displayed on a vehicle carrying hazardous substances gives information about the appropriate firefighting methods and personal protection needed to deal with a spill (Figure 42.1). It also gives guidance as to whether or not the substance can be safely washed into drains, and whether evacuation of surrounding areas should be considered (Figure 42.2). The HAZCHEM plate displayed on vehicles (Figure 42.3) will also show the diamond warning sign, the United Nations (UN) number for the chemical carried and a contact number for specialist advice from the manufacturer.

ADR Kemler code

The ADR system is the European Road Transport system of hazardous load markings. Vehicles must bear a 40 cm × 30 cm label on both front and rear. The label is in two parts: the upper bears the Kemler code and the lower the UN substance number (Figure 42.4).

The Kemler code comprises two or three digits which indicate the properties of the load carried. The first digit describes the primary hazard, and the second and third digits the secondary hazards (Table 42.1). If the same number is repeated this indicates an intensified hazard. An 'X' in front of the UN substance number indicates that it must not be brought into contact with water. There is no provision in the ADR system for any words to be placed on the warning plate.

Hazchem Scale

FOR FIRE OR SPILLAGE

Hazchem	
UN No	

Issue No 1

1 JETS

2 FOG

3 FOAM

4 DRY AGENT

P	V	FULL	DILUTE
R			
S	V	BA	
S		BA for FIRE only	
T		BA	
T		BA for FIRE only	
W	V	FULL	CONTAIN
X			
Y	V	BA	
Y		BA for FIRE only	
Z		BA	
Z		BA for FIRE only	

E CONSIDER EVACUATION

Fig. 42.1 The HAZCHEM code system aide-mémoire *card (front)*

Notes for Guidance

FOG
In the absence of fog equipment a fine spray may be used.

DRY AGENT
Water **must not** be allowed to come into contact with the substance at risk.

V
Can be violently or even explosively reactive.

FULL
Full body protective clothing with BA.

BA
Breathing apparatus plus protective gloves.

DILUTE
May be washed to drain with large quantities of water.

CONTAIN
Prevent, by any means available, spillage from entering drains or water course.

Printed for Her Majesty's Stationery Office by Trafford Press
Dd 0239720 C250 10/86
25p per copy; £1.50 per 10 copies; £5.50 per 50 copies; £10.00 per 100 copies. Exclusive of Tax.
ISBN 0 11 340752 1

Fig. 42.2 The HAZCHEM code system aide-mémoire *card (back)*

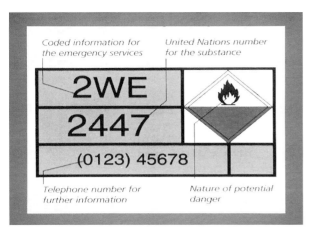

Fig. 42.3 The HAZCHEM plate

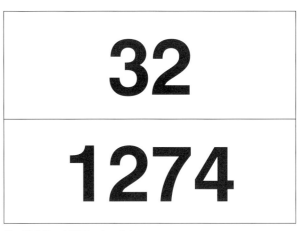

Fig. 42.4 The ADR Kemler plate

Transport emergency cards

Transport Emergency (TREM) cards exist for road and rail transportation of hazardous loads. For road transport the TREM card is a standard A4 size; it is kept in the cab of the lorry and should be changed each time the load is changed. This card gives details of the hazard, protective clothing necessary and action to be taken in the case of spillage or fire. The card will also carry first-aid information for contaminated casualties and specialist contact details. The carriage of TREM cards is not mandatory in the UK road haulage industry at the time of writing.

The information gathered at the scene from the above hazard warning systems can be supplemented and verified by the use of CHEMDATA. This is a database of many thousands of chemicals and their emergency actions provided by the national Chemical Emergency Centre at Harwell. The majority of UK fire brigades now have computer links from their control rooms to Harwell that can ensure accurate information is relayed to the fire officer in charge at the scene of the incident within minutes. With modern data modems and printers it is now possible to have hard copy information provided at the scene via a fax machine in the ambulance incident control vehicle.

Decontamination

Most fire brigades now have specialized vehicles and personnel trained in the management of chemical incidents. They will have appropriate gas-tight clothing and breathing apparatus to allow them to work in a toxic and contaminated area. The fire brigade will also provide decontamination facilities for their personnel, usually in the form of portable showers with containment of the contaminated water. The fire brigade will usually be responsible for the decontamination of casualties. In some instances this responsibility is given to the ambulance service and the hospitals. Fire brigade decontamination equipment is designed for use on firefighters in full protective clothing and breathing apparatus.

Decontamination is usually effected by stripping off contaminated clothing, which must be securely bagged in polythene bags for supervised disposal, and washing down thoroughly with water. In some situations detergent can be added. Special vacuum cleaners, or chemical absorption by fuller's earth (a dry powder) may also be used in casualty decontamination.

Emergency life-saving procedures may take precedence over decontamination and some difficult clinical decisions may have to be taken. Medical and ambulance service personnel at the scene of a chemical incident should have access to proper protective clothing suitable for the task and have undertaken joint training exercises with the fire brigade. There is a place for medical personnel capable of wearing and working in breathing apparatus.

In decontaminating casualties with running water there are real risks of inducing hypothermia. It may not be possible to decontaminate wounds effectively at the scene, and it is important that the receiving hospital staff are made aware of the potential contamination of any wounds so that they can be dealt with appropriately.

Table 42.1 The Kemler code

First digit – primary hazard	Second/third digit – secondary hazard
2 Gas	0 No meaning
3 Inflammable liquid	1 Explosion risk
4 Inflammable solid	2 Gas may be given off
5 Oxidizing substance	3 Inflammable risk
6 Toxic substancre	5 Oxidizing risk
7 Radioactive substance	6 Toxic risk
8 Corrosive	8 Corrosive risk
	9 Violent reaction risk
	X Do not use water

Accident and emergency departments should be capable of handling contaminated casualties, and both appropriate clothing for staff and a decontamination facility should be available. This area should have appropriate controlled air environment, showers and trolley baths. Thought must be given to the decontamination of the ambulances bringing casualties to the hospital, and appropriate expert advice must be sought.

Evacuation

With the release of toxic chemicals into the atmosphere, evacuation of the surrounding area may be necessary depending on the prevailing weather conditions. The decision to evacuate an area will normally be made by the police in discussion with all the other services, technical and scientific experts and the local authority. Evacuation will normally be undertaken by the police, often assisted by firefighters in appropriate protective clothing. Cordons around and security of the affected area are a police responsibility.

Local authorities will have contingency plans for such evacuations with local schools or church halls being opened as rest centres. The voluntary aid societies are often written into such emergency plans. At such incidents the medical and ambulance incident officers must become proactive once an evacuation is agreed. A medical and ambulance team should be allocated to each rest centre as many medical problems can develop over time, particularly if the evacuation was rapid and becomes prolonged. People will leave their regular medication behind in their homes, and stress levels can exacerbate previous medical conditions.

chapter forty-three:

NUCLEAR INCIDENTS

In the emergency response to an incident involving radioactivity the principles of casualty care remain the same – rapid assessment, administration of life-saving procedures, followed by stabilization and transport to a hospital able to deal with a radiation casualty. All of these procedures should be carried out without risking the safety and health of the paramedical team. Incidents involving radioactivity are fortunately rare, but whether it be an injury or illness occurring in someone working with radioactive materials or the result of an accident involving the unplanned release of radiation, the response team is unlikely to have had any training in this field, have no special protective clothing and no access to radiation meters. Nevertheless, paramedics will be expected to act rapidly and with their usual confidence. They therefore must be sure that they are not placing themselves or the casualty at unnecessary risk – or that the risk is acceptable.

The hazards to which paramedics may be exposed are the effects of penetrating radiation and contamination. Ionizing radiation cannot be detected by the human senses, but at the levels likely to be encountered in plausible accidents there is little risk and simple precautions will promote safe management of the radiological aspects of the injury. It is more likely that a threat will be posed by other hazards at the scene of the incident.

THE HAZARDS

Radioactive sources are widely used in the UK throughout industry, in hospitals and in further education establishments. Large amounts of radioactive materials are present in nuclear power stations, research establishments and military bases. Nuclear materials are transported by air, road, sea and rail, and X-ray generators are used in industry and medical care. A radiation incident could, therefore, occur virtually anywhere in the UK.

Where radioactive materials are processed on a large nuclear site, there will be contingency plans in the event of an accident,

which may require the support of ambulance, fire and local authority agencies as well as the employer's own response team. On the other hand, an incident may occur in an area where there is no local support and an ambulance is requested before radiological assessment. Radioactive materials may be discovered and cause concern at the site of an accident such as a building, fire or road traffic accident.

In this chapter 'radiation' means ionizing radiation, that is the form of electromagnetic radiation that can produce charged particles (ions) in material with which it interacts and thereby produce in human cells short-term or long-term deleterious health effects. It excludes microwaves, ultraviolet and infrared radiation, and radiowaves. The effects of high doses of ionizing radiation are well known from accidental exposures in the past. The effects at low levels are less certain and have to be deduced from epidemiological studies. However, the risk of injury at the low doses to which paramedical personnel are likely to be exposed is very small indeed.

Substances are said to be *radioactive* when they give off radiation.

Types of Radiation

The types of radiation relevant to paramedical workers are shown in Figure 43.1.

Alpha radiation

In alpha radiation a small, positively charged particle called an alpha particle is emitted; it travels a very short distance in air and is stopped by a sheet of paper, clothing, blood or dressings. It may just penetrate the superficial layers of the skin without any health effect. It is, therefore, not considered a hazard when outside the body, but ingestion or inhalation must be avoided as the particles can damage more sensitive internal organs. Examples of substances that emit alpha particles are uranium, plutonium and radon.

Beta radiation

Beta radiation is the emission of a small, negatively charged

Type of radiation	Distance travelled in air	Stopped by:
Alpha	Few millimetres	Skin
Beta	Few centimetres	Clothing
Gamma	Metres +	Lead/ concrete

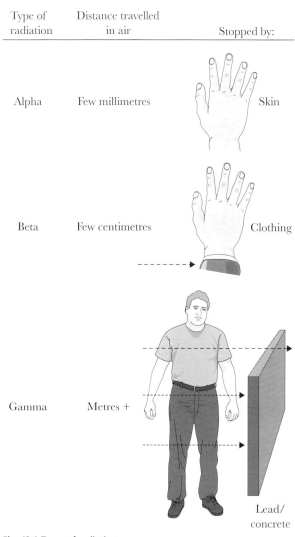

Fig. 43.1 *Types of radiation*

particle which travels a few centimetres in air, but is stopped by a thin sheet of aluminium or heavier clothing. It can penetrate the skin surface and therefore damage the epidermis and dermis to produce radiation burns. The hazard is greatest when the beta emitter is in direct contact with the skin, as may occur where clothing is saturated with a solution containing beta particles. Examples are iodine and tritium.

Gamma radiation, X-rays and neutrons

Gamma rays, X-rays and neutrons all travel great distances in air and are only stopped by thick concrete or lead. These forms of radiation can pass through the body, depositing energy and causing damage as they proceed. They are therefore still a hazard at some distance from the casualty or incident. Examples are industrial radiography sources, caesium and cobalt.

Risks of Exposure

Ionizing radiation can affect a part of the body or the whole body, causing localized effects (radiation burns) or systemic effects (radiation syndrome). It is more likely that the dose received will not cause any visible signs or reportable symptoms, but if any are present they are very significant and must be recorded accurately. Of more concern to the paramedic will be the presence of loose particles of radioactive material. This is known as contamination and is defined as the uncontrollable spread of radioactive material usually in the form of a dust, aerosol or liquid. The material will emit radioactivity, but in addition it can easily be inhaled or ingested, and precautions are needed to prevent this. There are therefore three scenarios involving exposure to radioactive materials that the paramedic will have to consider in the immediate care situation:

- The exposure to gamma rays or X-rays from a source near to the patient
- The presence or spread of contamination onto skin, hair and clothes of the patient
- The inhalation or ingestion of contamination by the paramedic or patient during rescue, resuscitation and removal

In each case simple precautions can be taken to reduce the risk to paramedical personnel and patients.

TYPES OF ACCIDENT

In an incident involving radioactivity, the treatment of life-threatening injuries or acute illness is more important than any concern about exposure to radiation. Radioactive materials may be present at road traffic accidents or construction work accidents, and the risk of further non-radiological injury should always be evaluated. There may be chemical hazards or other environmental dangers. The paramedic must consider safety a priority, and this is more important in the first few minutes than any concern about radiation exposure.

As a general rule human beings cannot detect ionizing radiation but there may be useful clues available such as a radiation identification mark on package or vehicle (Figure 43.2), bystander knowledge, or an unusual military or police presence. Such clues should alert the paramedic to the possibility of the release of radioactive materials; however, it is more likely that there will be no prior knowledge. The principles that are worth stating at this stage are:

- Any radiation dose to the attendants is likely to be small
- Simple precautions will reduce risk to personnel

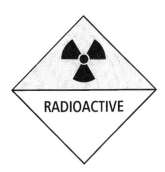

Fig. 43.2 Nuclear hazard symbol

The principles of 'ABC' (airway, breathing and circulation) still apply and must not be delayed on account of possible radiation exposure. Only when 'ABC' has been completed and life-saving procedures initiated should the possibility of radiation injury be considered.

Overexposure to Penetrating Radiation

You may be called to attend a patient who has been exposed to a large dose of penetrating radiation, such as may arise through overexposure to X-rays or gamma rays. It is important to realize that this patient is not radioactive (just as patients who have had a clinical X-ray are not radioactive) and therefore *presents no hazard to the medical personnel*. Such an incident may arise with exposure to an industrial radiography source.

External Contamination

If there has been a spread of radioactive materials, then the patient may be contaminated; this contamination may present a hazard to the patient and the paramedic, so it has to be dealt with safely. Such a release of contamination could arise in medical or research establishments from the rupture of a container or from acute illness in an employee when working with radioactive materials. Most of the contamination is likely to be on the patient's clothes.

Internal Contamination

There may have been a release of radioactivity which the patient has inadvertently swallowed, inhaled or absorbed through the skin. It may arise if the casualty has been prevented from leaving a contaminated area or has been exposed to smoke in a fire involving radioactive substances. This is unlikely to prove hazardous to attendants, but simple procedures can be used to protect both paramedic and patient.

Contaminated Wound

A patient may have an open wound which is either contaminated by radiation or has a piece of radioactive material in

it. Treatment of the injury and associated bleeding is of prime importance, but care must be taken to avoid spread of contamination around the site of the wound.

DEALING WITH A NUCLEAR INCIDENT

There are several types of accidents to which a paramedic may be called. In order to reduce potential exposure to both external penetrating radiation and reduce contamination some simple procedures need to be followed:

- Assess the risks from other hazards, e.g. buildings, traffic, smoke or chemicals, just as you would in any incident
- Position the ambulance upwind from the accident site, thereby ensuring that any contamination from a ruptured radioactive source or contaminated smoke does not pass over the ambulance
- Carry out initial survey, check 'ABC', institute immediate care and prepare the patient for movement
- Assume contamination is present and reduce risk of self-contamination by following the guidelines below
- Keep the time at the accident scene to a minimum

If there is a continued risk from radiation exposure the patient should, after resuscitation, be moved at least 10 metres from the source to reduce the dose to an acceptable level. If this is not possible, paramedics or other ambulance staff can take it in turns to monitor the patient, thereby sharing any radiation dose. If this is not possible either, an attempt should be made to reduce the level of radioactivity coming from the source. This is known as *shielding* and can be achieved by using lead or concrete, but if these materials are not available then rubble, heavy stones, sand or earth can be used.

Protection

In the emergency situations outlined above it is quite possible that personnel will have no prior knowledge of the presence of radioactive materials, but simple precautions of the type used against chemical or biological hazards will help to reduce the spread of contamination and subsequent risk to personnel.

1. Always assume that contamination is present when dealing with a casualty involved in an incident involving radioactivity.
2. Wear a simple surgical face mask and gloves. This will prevent spread of contamination to hands and face. If the clinical condition permits, a face mask can be placed on the patient.

3. Keep disturbance to the area to a minimum as this reduces the likelihood of airborne contamination. This should not, however, interfere with resuscitation and other emergency procedures.

4. If possible, cover open wounds with simple dressings. This prevents contamination entering wounds or contaminated blood spreading from the wound onto surrounding skin.

5. Remove external clothing (leaving underwear) carefully, if practicable, and place in large, sealable plastic bags. Wrap the patient in a blanket or contamination control envelope as this helps to prevent spread of radioactive materials.

6. Do not eat, drink or smoke until checked for contamination by medical physics personnel.

The above measures will help to keep spread of contamination to a minimum. It is probable that 90% of contamination will be removed with the patient's clothes, and the likelihood of spread to attendants will then be significantly reduced.

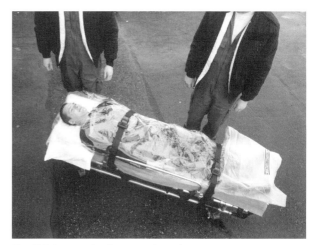

Fig. 43.3 A contamination control envelope

Management of Patients

Whether or not the patients have been exposed to radiation, it is likely that they will be concerned and anxious, and therefore reassurance is an essential part of care in this type of incident. Employees who regularly work with radioactive materials are just as likely to be affected in this way.

In all the above accidents, overexposure to penetrating radiation is unlikely to result in any specific symptoms, and other injuries will dictate the management. However, the paramedic needs to know what to look for. The onset of nausea or vomiting may indicate a significant overexposure, and the accurate recording of the time of onset is important for future hospital management. In addition, erythema may be visible on exposed skin and its distribution should be noted. The symptoms of the life-threatening complications of radiation exposure will not occur for days or perhaps weeks and therefore do not affect the initial management of the patient.

The police will be able to give information on the availability of hospital advice on irradiated or contaminated casualties under the National Arrangements for Incidents Involving Radioactivity (NAIR). The NAIR scheme is coordinated by the National Radiation Protection Board (NRPB) to provide advice in the event of a nuclear incident if advice from major plant operators (British Nuclear Fuels Ltd, Scottish Nuclear and Nuclear Electric) is unavailable.

Finally, it is most important to take the patient to the right hospital. A list of hospitals in the area prepared to accept contaminated casualties should be available to the paramedic. However, the clinical condition of the patient may make it necessary to go to the nearest accident and emergency department, and then it is essential that warning is given so that suitable preparations can be made.

Movement in the ambulance should be kept to a minimum, and staff can be expected to be directed to a specific parking area for unloading, where they should remain until screened for contamination, a task likely to be undertaken by medical physics personnel. As part of the protection available, it is recommended that ambulance crews use a contamination control envelope (Figure 43.3), thereby allowing containment of any residual contamination on the patient while permitting observation of wounds, dressings, skin colour and bruising.

FOLLOW-UP

After the patient has been transferred to hospital it may be discovered that the emergency personnel are contaminated with radiation. Decontamination is a simple process, but may need to be carried out in a special area. This could cause concern to some individuals and requires explanation.

Firstly, contaminated clothing is identified and discarded in sealable bags. All clothing is then removed and monitoring carried out by medical physics personnel using radiation monitors (Geiger counters). Areas of skin contamination are identified by skin markers and decontamination is carried out by washing with soap and water. Areas of contamination that are difficult to remove will require a mild abrasive such as dry soap powder or industrial skin cleanser of the type commonly used in engineering workshops. Continued cleansing of the skin must be done with care to avoid inflammation and must therefore be supervised by medical or nursing staff.

If contamination is present on the face or it is known that airborne spread is a possibility then it is necessary to check for inhalation, and this is normally done by checking counts on nasal swabs or nose blows. In addition personnel will be asked to produce biological samples (faeces and urine) which will be monitored for radioactive substances, or alternatively they may be monitored at a local hospital.

If it is suspected that any intake has occurred it is likely to be small and would probably not require treatment, but therapy does exist and has been used for many radioactive substances: examples are diethylenetriaminepentaacetic acid (DTPA) for plutonium exposure, Prussian blue for caesium exposure, and potassium iodate for iodine exposure.

Potassium iodate tablets are sometimes referred to as 'radiation pills' and would be recommended by public health officials in the event of a release of radioactive iodine such as might occur in an accident at a nuclear power station. The tablets provide a large amount of iodine which is taken up by the thyroid gland, blocking absorption of any radioactive iodine which is then passed out in the urine and not concentrated in the neck.

Staff who are concerned that they may have received a significant exposure to penetrating ionizing radiation may take a simple blood test. Radiation causes damage to chromosomes, which can be examined within 48 hours using cultured lymphocytes from a 10 ml sample of venous blood. In the majority of cases it is expected this test will serve to exclude rather than confirm exposure.

CONCLUSION

It is unlikely that paramedical workers will be involved in an accident involving ionizing radiation. If they are, then the principles of emergency care should be followed. The paramedic who is exposed to significant amounts of ionizing radiation will be followed up by medical physics personnel and close monitoring will establish whether any specific treatment or further examinations are necessary

FURTHER READING

Arrangements for Responding to Nuclear Emergency Health and Safety Executive (1994). London: HMSO.

ICRP (1978) *The Principles and General Procedures for Handling Emergency and Accidental Exposure of Workers.* ICRP Publication 28. Oxford: Pergamon.

Ionising radiation and its biological effects. *Occupational Health,* November 1986, 354–357.

IAEA (1978) *Manual on Early Medical Treatment of Possible Radiation Injury.* Safety Series No. 47. Vienna: International Atomic Energy Agency.

IAEA (1988) *Medical Handling of Accidentally Exposed Individuals.* Safety Series No. 88. Vienna: International Atomic Energy Agency.

IAEA (1986) *What the General Practitioner (MD) Should Know About Medical Handling of Overexposed Individuals.* IAEA-TECDOC-366. Vienna: International Atomic Energy Agency.

Planning Guidance for the NHS in Scotland, Incidents Involving Ionising Radiation.

NHS Circular GEN (1992) 32 St Andrew's House, Edinburgh EH1 3DG, November 1992.

chapter forty-four

THE SPORTS ARENA

In the affluent society in which we now live there is more opportunity to participate in an evergrowing range of sports. There has been a trend away from violent contact sports towards more individual pastimes, but it is still contact sports that attract the greatest number of players and spectators. It is a matter of some importance that the risks involved in sport are identified, so that when called upon to help, paramedical personnel can provide the best possible care. Increasingly, athletes expect their medical and paramedical attendants to be fully conversant with the treatment of sport-related injuries, and lawsuits may follow if skilled and appropriate care is not provided.

Many of the deaths that occur at sporting events are from natural causes. Examples include the spectator getting overexcited at the Cup Final, or the golfer having an infarct on the eighteenth green. Others include the tragic deaths of youngsters who have congenital heart diseases such as hypertrophic cardiomyopathy. Many, however, arise directly from participation in sports, and furthermore often occur in sports not usually recognized as dangerous (Table 44.1).

Sports injuries keep the ambulance services and the accident and emergency departments of Britain busy every weekend of the year. There are approximately a million reported sports injuries per year in Britain. Contact sports have the highest injury rate, followed by cricket and cycling (Table 44.2). This reflects the large number of participants. Other pastimes such as riding and cycling have a relatively low injury rate, but when an injury occurs it tends to be more serious.

The factors influencing sports injuries can be classified as *intrinsic* or *extrinsic*. Intrinsic factors include age, sex, physical fitness and previous injury. The age of an athlete influences the type of injury that develops; for example, younger athletes can develop stress fragmentation of bony epiphyses and can develop avulsion of bone around the hip and pelvis as a response to excessive strain, whereas older athletes tend to develop tendon tears. Additionally, younger, less experienced athletes tend to take greater risks, with subsequent increases in injury rate. No clear difference in injury rate is observed between the sexes overall, but boys over 14 years old are three times more likely to be injured than girls of the same age. Physical fitness is important to reduce the number of injuries: unfit participants are

Table 44.1 Fatal accidents in sport (UK statistics for 1 year)

Sport	Fatalities per year
Air sports	13
Horse riding	12
Mountaineering	11
Motor sports	10
Ball games	6
Water sports	6
Winter sports	5
Athletics	4
Cycling	1
Shooting	1

From OPCS, 1991

Table 44.2 Sports injuries

Sport	Percentage of all sports injuries	Estimated no. of participants (000s)
Association football	41.7	388
Rugby	9.4	87
Roller ice skating	5.5	51
Cricket	3.6	34
Riding	3.1	29
Swimming/diving	2.9	27
Netball	2.5	23
Gymnastics	2.4	22
Combat sports	2.3	21
Hockey	2.2	21
Basketball	2.1	20
Skiing	1.8	17
Athletics	1.6	14
Others	19	177

Data from DTI Leisure Accidents Surveillance System.

more likely to be injured because they do not warm up properly, and many suffer knee injuries because quadriceps muscle bulk, and hence the power to maintain stability in the knee joint, is not sufficiently developed. However, experienced athletes are more prone to recurrent sprains and strains as a result of overuse. Previous injury predisposes to further injury, and people who continue to play sport despite injuries are prone to exacerbate their problems and develop further injuries as their technique is likely to be affected.

Extrinsic factors in sports injury include the type and nature of the sport, the venue, equipment, weather and the control and conduct of the event. The nature of the sport clearly affects the injury rate. Contact and combat sports by their very nature predispose to injury. Sports that involve the elements, such as scuba diving, carry risks inherent to the hostile environment – whereas a gentle, non-contact sport such as bowls is unlikely in itself to provoke injury.

The venue for sports predisposes to certain injuries. Football players suffer more superficial injuries when playing on artificial turf than when playing on grass. A hard, frosty pitch may lead to a greater knee injury rate as players are unable to manoeuvre and change direction as freely as on a normal soft grass surface. Additionally, poor safety standards at grounds may lead to major problems for crowds of spectators, as evidenced by a number of major incidents at football grounds. Following the Taylor Report (see Chapter 56), stringent regulations have been introduced to ensure that safety is improved and that adequate medical cover is available at mass gatherings. Equipment such as rackets and hockey sticks can cause severe injury to the head and face; eyes are prone to severe injury in games using small balls, such as squash. Equipment failures, such as a collapsing bar in gymnastics or a frayed rope in climbing, also predispose to injury. The lack of proper protective clothing for goalkeepers, for instance in hockey, puts them at increased risk.

The weather can catch out mountaineers and hill walkers, the sea cruelly changes to endanger sailors, and runners can suffer heat exhaustion on hot summer days.

Finally, the control of a sport, or lack of it, can affect the safety of players. The control and conduct of a poorly refereed rugby match can result in minor disagreements spilling over into foul play and fist fights with resultant severe injury; a poorly organized cross-country ride can mean dangerous jumps and more falls from horseback, and intrusions from missile-throwing football hooligans endanger professional footballers.

NATURE OF INJURIES IN SPORT

The huge majority of sports injuries are soft tissue injuries. Injuries to the lower limbs are most common, followed by the upper limbs, head and face, and finally the chest and abdomen. The majority are minor and self-limiting; however, serious injuries such as ligament and tendon tears, fractures, spinal and head injuries and damage to viscera do occur, and paramedics must be alert to their presence. Paramedics must be able to decide whether they are dealing with a problem that must be dealt with in hospital immediately, or whether the patient can be left to arrange independently for treatment at hospital or by a general practitioner later in the day. Many injuries do not require medical intervention and can be readily treated with rest, ice, compression and elevation ('RICE').

Sports-specific Injury Profiles

Certain sports predispose to a particular profile of injury. Some of these are detailed below.

Athletics and field sports

The majority of athletes suffer soft tissue injury and sprains. Overuse predisposes them to chronic muscle and ligament problems that may be suddenly exacerbated in competition. High jumpers and pole vaulters are liable to neck injury (Chapter 26) if they land badly. Spectators are at risk from flying missiles such as hammers, shots and javelins which can cause severe injury. Heat exhaustion is a worry in warm conditions (Chapter 40). Concomitant medical problems are also common sources of illness.

Combat sports

Of greatest concern in combat sports are head and neck injuries as a result of direct blows to the head and face (Figure 44.1) or from falls following throws (Chapters 14, 21 and 26). Facial fractures and eye injuries are also common (Chapter 22). Injuries to hands and arms can occur, and in some sports involving the use of feet they too can be injured. Soft tissue injury and fractures are features of the martial arts.

Football

The majority of association football injuries are to soft tissues,

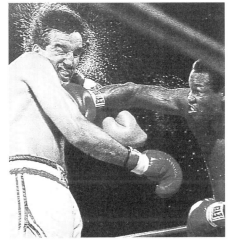

Fig. 44.1 Head injury in boxing

with strains and complete tears of leg muscles and tendons being most common. Severe knee and ankle injuries occur less frequently and fractures to the lower limb are relatively few. Head and neck injuries can occur in bad falls or clashes of heads.

Hockey

Players are prone to the same injuries as footballers; they also stand the risk of being hit by a stick or a very hard ball travelling at high speed. Facial injuries are commonly caused by follow-through of a stick. Fractures to the maxilla, mandible and nose are often seen in these circumstances. Goalkeepers are prone to soft tissue injury, and if not wearing protective face masks their facial features may be suddenly altered by a ball at over 150 km/h.

Horse riding

Falls and head injury may lead to as many as 50% of riding-related deaths (Figure 44.2). Kicking injuries and involvement in road traffic accidents (RTAs) also cause serious injury. Severe injuries to the head, neck and spine are common. Maxillofacial injuries arising from kicks can be severe and airway care may pose major problems. Crushing injury can occur if a horse rolls onto its rider, causing severe blunt chest and abdominal injury.

Motor sports

The speeds involved in motor racing and motor-cycle racing lead to horrendous injury. As in high-speed RTAs, multiple injuries will give plenty of scope for concern. Deceleration injury must always be considered, as although car safety improvements have led to the reduction of direct trauma, there is little that can be done about the deceleration forces resulting from direct contact with a brick wall. Track safety improvements have helped, but in many cases of racing on public roads, as in the Isle of Man TT races, little protection is offered to the wayward rider. Burns, fractures, and head and neck injuries are

common, and crash-helmets can lead to problems with management (Chapter 21). Spectators are at great risk from flying debris and wheels, or from direct contact with errant vehicles. Rescuers too are at risk, as unless the track is dangerously affected the race will go on.

Mountaineering and hill walking

Strains, sprains and minor fractures are the most common injuries in these sports. They take on a greater significance when they occur many miles from help in hostile terrain. The weather poses significant problems and the risk of hypothermia and frostbite (Chapters 38 and 45) is everpresent. Falls can lead to significant multiple injuries. Hill walkers often have medical conditions, and the most common cause of death on the hills is myocardial infarction rather than trauma.

> **Remember intercurrent medical illness**

Racket sports

Soft tissue sprains and strains are most common. The upper limb is more often injured in these sports. Facial injury from contact with a racket can occur. Of greatest concern in this group is eye injury. Squash balls and shuttlecocks can produce severe damage when hit into a player's orbit at close range. A familiar scenario is the unfit, middle-aged squash player collapsing on court as he attempts to recapture his youth.

Rugby football and American football

The patterns of injury in rugby and American football are very similar. Players suffer upper limb problems with fractures to the hand, arm and clavicle; lower limb problems include meniscal tear and knee ligament injury, ankle ligament damage and fractures of the tibia and fibula. Head injury with lacerations and fractures to facial bones can be associated with concussion and loss of consciousness. Neck sprains are common and severe

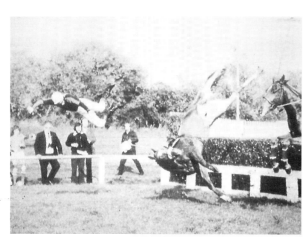

Fig. 44.2 *A typical equestrian accident*

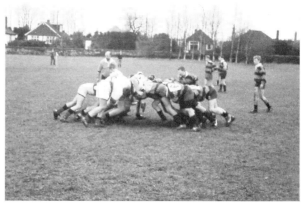

Fig. 44.3 *Collapsing rugby scrums may result in cervical spine injuries*

neck injury can occur. The majority of severe neck injuries occur in collapsed scrums or in head-on tackles where hyperflexion of the neck combined with axial loading of the spine is common (Figure 44.3). Crush injury in the regular 'pile-ups' of rucks and mauls may also occur with resultant damage to chest and abdomen (Chapters 23 and 24).

Scuba diving

The main risks to scuba divers are from faulty equipment, faulty diving practices and hypothermia (Chapter 38). Equipment can fail at depth, causing panic and a dash for the surface. Sudden pressure changes can then lead to major problems with barotrauma or the 'bends' (decompression sickness). Faulty technique on descent can lead to significant ear problems, with rupture of the tympanic membrane: cold water rushes into the middle ear and disequilibrates the balance mechanism, and as a result the diver loses all sense of direction, with drowning being a real risk. Too rapid an ascent can lead to overdistension of the lungs and air spaces resulting in barotrauma to these areas, as the enclosed air expands rapidly with the reduction in ambient pressure. Pulmonary barotrauma can lead to pneumothorax. Air embolus can also occur. Decompression sickness develops because nitrogen bubbles are released from solution in the blood when a diver ascends too quickly. The bubbles can block capillary blood vessels and cause pain, especially in the joints. Itchy skin (the 'creeps') and headache are early features. The larynx can be affected leading to the 'chokes', when the diver has the feeling of being strangled. In severe cases the circulation to the spinal cord can be disrupted, leading to a 'spinal bend' (the 'staggers') and resultant neurological damage. Nitrogen narcosis, characterized by euphoria and loss of judgement, occurs in air divers who go too deep: the mechanism is unknown. Divers can develop the bends many hours after a dive – especially if they fly in an aircraft, when the ambient pressure is further reduced resulting in an enhanced release of dissolved nitrogen; any diver who exhibits strange symptoms after a flight that closely follows a dive should be viewed with concern. Helicopter aeromedical evacuation poses theoretical risks to injured divers, although with transport at altitudes less than 1000 feet the pressure changes will be minimal.

Water sports

Hypothermia is possibly the greatest risk in water sports in the UK. Many sailors, windsurfers and canoeists are ill-prepared for sudden changes in the elements. Drowning is an ever-present risk. Head and neck injuries are common in those who dive into shallow water. Sailors can receive head injuries from flailing booms and can suffer limb injuries in falls on wet decks. The new sport of jet-skiing predisposes to head and neck injury as a result of high-speed falls and collisions. Power-boat racing poses similar risks to motor racing with multiple injuries and the extra risk of drowning for unconscious or incapacitated drivers. Water-skiers are liable to develop severe rectal and vaginal lacerations when they fall as a result of forceful injection of water into those orifices. Propeller injuries are rare but can be very severe.

THE MANAGEMENT OF SPORTS INJURIES

The most important aspect of the management and treatment of sports injuries is to recognize what has happened. An accurate history must be obtained not only from the patient, but when possible from spectators and fellow participants. The mechanism of injury will lead you to the diagnosis in most cases. A thorough examination is important to detect hidden or latent injuries. The calculation of the Glasgow Coma Scale score and if appropriate a Triage Revised Trauma Score will be helpful in further evaluations (see Chapter 56).

> It is vital that paramedics maintain a high index of suspicion

Always remember that athletes will often belittle their injuries in an attempt to continue with the game. If serious injury is suspected the player must be removed from the field of play, despite any protestations, and taken to hospital for further examination.

Many patients with soft tissue injuries may require no more than advice in accordance with the 'RICE' principle. The application of cold compresses may help considerably. If there is any doubt as to the exact nature of an injury, particularly if it involves a joint, the patient should be taken to hospital for medical examination. Dislodged teeth should be kept in milk as they can be reimplanted if stored appropriately. Always ensure, *and record*, that the patient has been advised to seek medical care if the injury deteriorates or does not resolve quickly.

All suspected head and neck injuries should be dealt with in the normal manner. In-line immobilization, a cervical collar, an extrication device and a spinal board should be used. There is *no excuse* for treating a patient with a suspected cervical injury – or indeed any other spinal injury – in any other way. Do not be fooled into allowing patients who have had a blow to the head to continue to compete; they may well be concussed or be in the latent phase after a serious head injury. Always *insist* that the patient withdraws and goes to hospital. When casualties refuse treatment either from a paramedic or at hospital, always ensure that an appropriate disclaimer is signed.

All injuries, whether they are head or neck injuries, fractures or haemorrhage, should be treated in accordance with normal practice: the *basic tenets of basic life support and advanced trauma life support must NEVER BE IGNORED* (Chapters 3–6). Airway care, the support of breathing and the maintenance of a satisfactory circulation must take priority over all other treatments. Extreme care must be maintained when head or neck injury is suspected. If these basic procedures and principles are followed then victims of injury and illness in the sports arena will be well supported.

Priorities in the management of sporting injuries

- Safety
- Airway and cervical spine
- Breathing with oxygen
- Circulation and haemorrhage control
- Disability
- Exposure

Evacuation and transportation of casualties from remote areas often cause difficulties (Chapter 45). Aeromedical evacuation may be appropriate (Chapter 46), especially when dealing with spinal injuries in remote locations. A helicopter flight may be considerably smoother and faster than a long, bumpy road journey over rough terrain.

DRUGS AND THE ATHLETE

Many competitive athletes are governed by strict rules about the use of drugs. Considerable publicity is given to those drugs that are banned, and advice is available to most athletes from their sports governing bodies. It is incumbent upon medical personnel who attend competitors to ensure that they do not inadvertently provide them with banned substances in the course of treating an injury or illness. It is possible that athletes may sue if they are banned after being wrongly advised by their attendants. Banned and restricted drugs are listed in Tables 44.3 and 44.4.

The majority of banned substances do not come into the province of the paramedic, but pain-killers and asthma treatments used by paramedics could affect athletes. A certificate is required from the administering doctor in the case of local anaesthetic agents and corticosteroids. If in doubt, do not administer any drug unless it is clear that an athlete will not continue in that competition, and even then check first if at all possible.

Table 44.3 Banned products

Type of drug	Examples
Stimulants	Ephedrine and pseudo-ephedrine in cold products
	Adrenaline
Narcotics	Co-proxamol
	Codydramol
	Nalbuphine
	Diamorphine
	Kaolin and morphine
Anabolic steroids	
Beta-blockers	
Diuretics	
Peptide hormones	Corticotrophin (ACTH)
	Human chorionic gonado-trophin
	Erythropoietin

Table 44.4 Restricted products

Alcohol
Marijuana
Local anaesthetic agents
Corticosteroids* (*inhaled, topical or intra-articular administration is allowed)

section:

8

RESCUE

chapter forty-five

RESCUE FROM REMOTE PLACES

Remote places may be defined as areas where rescue is likely to take a long time and require the help of individuals with specialist training and skills for working in such areas (Figure 45.1). This chapter covers the following topics:

- Mountain rescue
- Cave rescue
- Ski patrolling
- The lifeboat service
- Search and rescue helicopters
- Remote industrial sites

All the types of rescue work discussed in this chapter are carried out by individuals who have specialist training, physical ability and equipment for working in the remote circumstances in which they operate. Unless you possess (or are prepared to acquire and maintain) the knowledge, skills and physical attributes of these individuals, you should under no circumstances attempt to participate in their rescue activities. The only qualification for being a member of a rescue team should be the ability to perform physically at the same level as other members of the team, as you will only put yourself and other members of the team at risk if you are not able to do this.

> **Your medical skills are a bonus only if your physical skills are appropriate**

This may seem obvious with regard to mountain rescue, but it applies equally to the other services. An example is the lifeboat service, where someone who is not used to travelling in a small boat in rough seas will not be physically able to cope with such circumstances and will not be able to contribute to the patient management (and may have to be looked after by a member of the crew, thus removing this crew member from their normal essential function). People involved in pre-hospital care are encouraged not to attempt rescue from such areas without the use of such specialist teams and should not attempt to provide a service to replace these established rescue services.

It is more likely that the paramedics will be involved in meeting the specialist rescue teams to provide the treatment and transportation of the victim to an appropriate hospital.

Topics that are particularly relevant to this type of rescue are the use of helicopters, hypothermia and drowning (a Scottish study has shown helicopters to be involved in 59% of all mountain rescues). The reader is therefore directed to Chapters 38, 39 and 46. As with all pre-hospital care, the collection of as much information as possible about the mechanism of injury and the patient's medical history is vitally important. Of particular note in these circumstances will be information on the following:

- Treatment already given by the rescue personnel (rescue teams carry drugs, sometimes including injectable morphine)
- Observations (in particular, series of observations that may have been undertaken during a prolonged rescue)

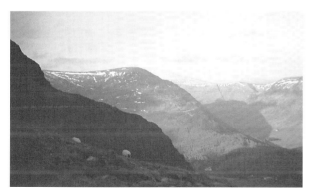

Fig. 45.1 *Remote terrain*

Most rescue teams will have members who have had training in first-aid with particular relevance to the problems they are likely to encounter: this fact should be kept in mind and their expertise used as much as possible. It is important to remember when considering situations where trauma is common that people do still suffer medical problems such as asthma and myocardial infarction, and that this may be their only problem.

MOUNTAIN RESCUE

There are a variety of publications on first-aid for mountaineers, and many mountaineering textbooks contain chapters on first-aid. It is therefore possible that the patient's companions may have applied first-aid skills at an early stage.

Mountain rescue is undertaken in this country by teams of volunteers. Such teams do not usually include a doctor, but do have members with advanced first-aid skills. Mountain rescue teams normally have a doctor as their medical adviser. These doctors do not usually take part in the rescue work, but are involved with training and may give advice to the team via a radio. It can therefore be expected that the patient will have had advanced first-aid procedures performed before arrival.

The environment of the rescue and the limitations of transport for evacuation will restrict the procedures that can be undertaken. It can be expected that initial observations will have been made, and spinal immobilization with a cervical collar and possibly a vacuum mattress may have been applied. Injured limbs may have been splinted, dressings applied to open wounds, and nitrous oxide and warmed oxygen given.

The patient will probably have been moved on a special mountain rescue stretcher; in the UK this is likely to be either a McInnes stretcher or a Bell stretcher (Figure 45.2). These are designed to provide easy transportation without the risk of the patient falling out of the stretcher, and are also suitable for lifting the patient into a helicopter. However, these design features also make it difficult to remove a patient from the stretcher while keeping the spine in a neutral position. If the team carries a vacuum mattress the patient should be enclosed in this before being put into the mountain rescue stretcher. This makes the removal of the patient from the stretcher much easier, and the patient should remain in the vacuum mattress until arrival at hospital (and probably until after X-ray examination).

The hand-over to the ambulance crew will be the first opportunity for a full patient survey. Special consideration should be given to the fact that the patient may be hypothermic, and rough handling may induce a cardiac arrhythmia. Clothing should only be removed sufficiently to allow the necessary examination, or if damp clothing is liable to cause further hypothermia. It is important to remember that a hypothermic patient cannot be certified dead until taken to hospital and rewarmed.

Hypothermia in mountain rescue deserves special consideration as it is cited as the cause of 13% of all mountain rescue incidents. It is important to remember that hypothermia can occur in both summer and winter, and that wind and damp clothing can be a cause of hypothermia as well as the air temperature. It has been suggested that where measurement of the patient's core temperature is impossible, shivering should be used as a differentiating factor. If the patient is shivering passively, then hypothermia can be considered to be mild and the patient passively rewarmed and evacuated. If the patient is considered to be hypothermic and not shivering, then the patient should be considered to be severely hypothermic, not allowed to walk and not subjected to any more movement than is absolutely necessary.

Most members of mountain rescue teams will carry aspirin, glucose and possibly tablets of a non-steroidal anti-inflammatory drug. There will also be a team first-aid pack which is likely to contain morphine for intramuscular injection, salbutamol and an antihistamine. Thanks to the efforts of a Manchester surgeon (Wilson-Hay) in the 1960s, mountain rescue teams in the UK have the facility to keep morphine, and to give it.

An analysis of mountain rescue figures shows the following distribution of injuries:

- Lower limb injuries – 46% of injured
- Bruising – 19% of injured
- Head injuries – 21% of injured

An analysis of fatalities shows the following:

- 38% were due to head injuries
- 15% were due to multiple trauma
- 18% were due to medical conditions

CAVE RESCUE

Much of what has been said about mountain rescue applies to cave rescue. The main differences are that cave systems frequently contain tunnels with diameters not much greater than that of the human body, and that caves often contain water – cavers may also therefore have been involved in diving activities. Even if skilled medical attention in the form of a doctor or paramedic can be delivered to the site of the injured caver, the only procedures that can be adequately undertaken are basic airway maintenance measures, pain relief, splinting of fractures and monitoring of the patient. It is unlikely that bulky equipment can be delivered to the patient, or that such equipment can be used on the patient in the cave.

The previous advice with regards to hypothermia applies, and patients should be wrapped in an exposure bag before being put on a suitable stretcher such as a Stokes litter or a Neil Robertson stretcher (Figure 45.3). It is important to remember

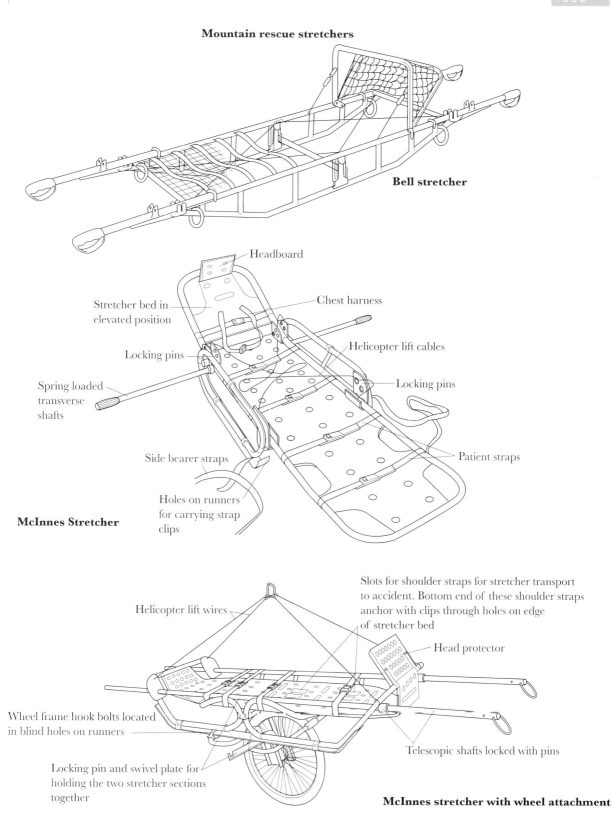

Mountain rescue stretchers

Bell stretcher

Headboard

Stretcher bed in elevated position

Chest harness

Helicopter lift cables

Locking pins

Locking pins

Spring loaded transverse shafts

McInnes Stretcher

Side bearer straps

Holes on runners for carrying strap clips

Patient straps

Slots for shoulder straps for stretcher transport to accident. Bottom end of these shoulder straps anchor with clips through holes on edge of stretcher bed

Helicopter lift wires

Head protector

Wheel frame hook bolts located in blind holes on runners

Telescopic shafts locked with pins

Locking pin and swivel plate for holding the two stretcher sections together

McInnes stretcher with wheel attachment

Fig. 45.2 Mountain stretchers. A, Bell stretcher; B, McInnis stretcher; C, McInnes stretcher with wheel attachment

A

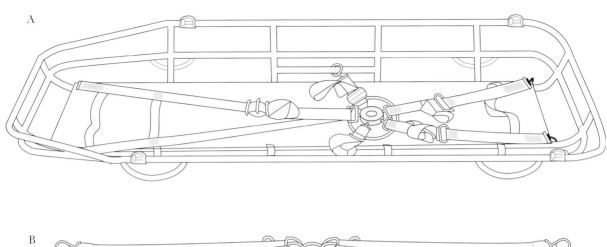

B

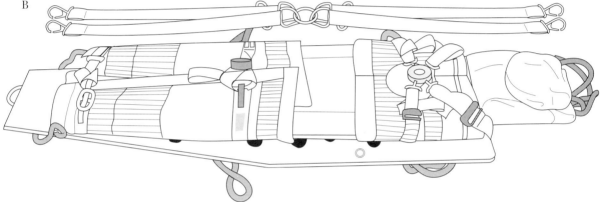

Fig. 45.3 *The Neil Robertson stretcher (A) and the Stokes litter (B)*

that an injured person who has been diving should not be given nitrous oxide inhalation (Entonox).

SKI PATROLLING

The first layer of planned medical provision on ski slopes is provided by ski patrollers. In the UK such persons may well be members of the British Association of Ski Patrollers and this organization runs courses in advanced first-aid, and further courses of Emergency Medical Technician standard. It is likely that the injured person will be brought to an ambulance rendezvous point by the ski patroller, probably on a sledge. Hypothermia and skeletal injury are likely to be major problems, and it is important to remember that areas of possible frostbite should not be actively rewarmed during the transportation phase.

THE LIFEBOAT SERVICE

Rescue at sea and around the coasts of Britain and Ireland is efficiently organized by a combined operation involving statutory organizations, voluntary organizations and the armed forces. A major contributor in this area is the Royal National Lifeboat Institution (RNLI).

Each lifeboat station has a lifeboat doctor known as the station honorary medical adviser (SHMA). This doctor has a variety of duties, including advising on the health of the crew and first-aid training, and is encouraged to attend regular lifeboat exercises and go to sea with the lifeboat in an emergency if medical services may be required. The RNLI estimates that in 10% of its calls the rescue will require medical attention, and that in 1% of its calls a doctor will go to sea with the lifeboat. The total calls for the RNLI are approximately 6000 per year.

Provision is also made for any member of a lifeboat crew who has paramedical skills to have appropriate equipment and make use of these skills when on a rescue. All crew members are encouraged to attend first-aid courses run specifically for lifeboat crews by the RNLI, which include the use of oxygen, the use of nitrous oxide inhalation (Entonox) and special techniques for airway maintenance and patient immobilization where lack of space may prohibit traditional techniques. Special reference is given to prolonged care and monitoring of the rescued as it may take considerable time for such persons to reach hospital.

If the situation warrants it the SHMA can be requested to give medical advice to the lifeboat crew via the radio. Lifeboats usually carry a basket stretcher and a Neil Robertson stretcher. As well as large lifeboats there are smaller in-shore rescue craft, and the crew on these are likely to have had first-aid training. The equipment is carried in a first-aid pouch.

SEARCH AND RESCUE HELICOPTERS

Helicopter services are mostly provided in the UK by the Royal Air Force, but in some areas are provided by civilian authorities (these are generally helicopters supplied by private companies and painted in a coastguard livery). Requests for helicopters are normally made via the police. The winch crew and winch operator will generally have advanced first-aid training. On some occasions an RAF doctor may accompany the helicopter depending on availability and whether or not the extra weight would use up critical fuel supplies. These helicopters may take on board mountain rescue team doctors if available. They can carry an extensive range of equipment, including a first-aid kit, Laerdal suction apparatus, a pneuPAC-type ventilator, nitrous oxide inhalation (Entonox), traction splints and a pneumatic anti-shock garment (PASG). It is important to remember that a PASG must not be deflated until the patient reaches hospital.

REMOTE INDUSTRIAL SITES

Certain types of work such as quarrying, oil drilling, fish farming, forestry and estate management may now take place in remote areas requiring a lengthy journey to hospital. Such activities frequently involve the use of heavy mechanical equipment, hence there is always a risk of serious injury. Regulation 3 of the Health and Safety (First Aid) Regulations 1981 requires employers to make provision for first-aid in the workplace. This involves providing equipment, facilities and suitable persons to provide adequate and appropriate first-aid to employees who are injured or become ill at work. These regulations are interpreted in different ways by employers in these industries. Some sites will be totally dependent on the emergency services. Others will have appropriate items of equipment for rendering first-aid and persons who have undertaken a standard certificate four-day first-aid course, and may have had further training directed to the particular problems of their working environment. On the better sites equipment such as survival bags, stretchers, splints, rigid cervical collars, resuscitators, nitrous oxide (Entonox), oxygen and manual suction equipment may be available. If cyanide is used a dicobalt edetate (Kelocyanor) kit should also be available.

In places that are less remote or accessible by helicopter, you may have the opportunity of treating the patient at the accident site. It is important to remember to use appropriate equipment and clothing to ensure your own safety, which may entail borrowing equipment from site personnel. Patients are at risk of spinal injury, and protection of the spine and airway while extricating and transporting the patient may be a particular problem. If, after careful assessment, the patient's need for transportation is not urgent, it is wise to take time to protect the spine and airway carefully before attempting transportation. A thorough knowledge of extrication devices and stretchers that can be used for lifting purposes is important when working in this area (see Chapter 27).

FURTHER READING

Ipswich: British Association of Immediate Care (1990) *Rescue from Remote Places – 1*.

Ipswich: British Association of Immediate Care (1990) *Rescue from Remote Places – 2*.

Gunn D (1994) *Outdoor First-aid and Safety Manual*. British Association of Ski Patrollers.

McInnes H (1984) *International Mountain Rescue Book*. London: Constable.

Steele P (1992) *Medical Handbook for Mountaineers*. London: Constable.

chapter forty-six:

AEROMEDICAL EVACUATION

Aviation and medicine may be combined in a number of different ways which encompass a complex range of treatment and transport systems. Historically, this has included the use of hot-air balloons and placing hospital beds on transport aircraft. Medical aviation is now extremely sophisticated and can be conveniently divided into *primary casualty evacuation* and *secondary patient transfer*. The expertise and equipment required for each is different.

Primary casualty evacuation (Figure 46.1) is the transport of a patient from the site of injury to a receiving hospital. This requires a medical crew which is expert in resuscitation, familiar with pre-hospital hazards and practised in cooperation with other emergency services. Equipment must be robust and specific for urgent interventions which may be required. The level of medical expertise determines the range and type of possible medical intervention. This, in turn, determines the nature of the medical equipment carried, and varies greatly between systems. The flexibility of a helicopter system makes it ideal for the primary role, allowing the medical team to take the best possible medical care to the patient's side. The helicopter can be reconfigured to take account of the specific requirements of its role.

PRIMARY CASUALTY EVACUATION: transport of a patient from the site of injury to a receiving hospital

Secondary patient transfer is the movement of a patient between hospitals (Figure 46.2). This requires a medical crew expert in the use of intensive care equipment, monitoring and drugs. Often transfers occur over long distances and it is usually quicker and more cost-effective to use fixed wing aircraft rather than helicopters for this purpose. This is a specialized subject suited to the intensive care physician, and is not normally the province of the paramedic.

SECONDARY PATIENT TRANSFER: the movement of a patient between hospitals

These two types of aeromedical system can coalesce during urgent interhospital transfer of an accident and emergency

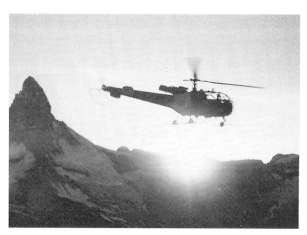

Fig. 46.1 Primary casualty evacuation

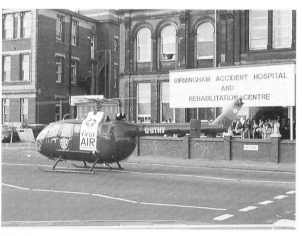

Fig. 46.2 Secondary patient transfer

department patient from a non-specialist hospital to a specialist centre. This situation can lead to role confusion, conflicting priorities and medical skill mismatch.

PRIMARY CASUALTY EVACUATION

It is a common mistake to regard all helicopter systems as a single entity. In fact, many types of aeromedical system provide this type of service, but diversity makes comparison of systems difficult, and causes much controversy. Before any judgement of value or cost-effectiveness can be made, an analysis of the aims of each system and the extent to which these aims are fulfilled is necessary in order to avoid misleading conclusions. The major objectives are discussed below.

Transport

The emphasis is on moving the patient from one location to another. Usually the casualty requires transfer from an incident scene that is remote by virtue of distance of terrain (Figure 46.3). There may be little medical expertise available (or required by the patient) and the system is cost-effective because it obviates the use of long and difficult land transport. An example of this type of service is the evacuation by an RAF Search and Rescue helicopter of a walker with a broken ankle from a mountainous area. There is no clinical imperative to use air evacuation, but it is logistically cheaper and more comfortable than the alternative: a long overland evacuation requiring time and a large number of personnel.

In areas with scanty ambulance cover owing to long distances and a diffuse population, helicopter evacuation of patients with minor illness or injury may well preserve ambulance cover and maintain response times. This type of helicopter system may be a valid use of air transport solely because of the prohibitive cost of staffing and equipping the number of vehicles that would be required to provide the same response times using a land-based alternative. The process of care may be technically improved but this is logistic rather than a clinical benefit.

Treatment

Most emergency calls to ambulance services are for relatively trivial conditions, and most of the small number of truly urgent calls can be dealt with by ambulance personnel with advanced training. However, a small number of patients, particularly following injury, require immediate medical intervention beyond the ability of the ambulance service. The patient who sustains a severe head injury (Glasgow Coma Scale score of 8 or less) urgently requires definitive airway management, yet cannot be intubated without muscle relaxants and anaesthesia. The provision of advanced medical pre-hospital life support is a scarce resource which must be matched with a rare event – the injured patient whose treatment requires more complex medical intervention than ambulance service skills allow. A helicopter can bring together the rare event and the care provider, combining high-quality pre-hospital care with advanced medical skills, delivered by experienced doctors and paramedics.

Triage

Medical services have seldom been planned logically according to the needs of the resident population. Specialist units may have arisen as a result of historical accident or the enthusiasm of individuals. The result is a hotchpotch of service provision in which highly specialized units may be on different sites from local district general hospitals. Of more significance is the rarity with which full multidisciplinary provision is available at the centre of a population mass. Bizarre geographical locations for specialist units require the pre-hospital medical team to exercise ingenuity and a high level of medical skill to determine the hospital best suited for a patient's injuries. This triage decision often taxes the trauma system, and cannot usually be achieved by the ambulance service alone.

Matching the patient to the correct hospital can result in unnecessary transport of patients to specialist hospitals. Most pre-hospital triage protocols 'play safe' by taking the patient to a multidisciplinary centre when in doubt. Transport to a specialist centre may increase the time before hospital arrival in patients with critical conditions, but decrease the time to definitive intervention. This apparent conflict is resolved if a pre-hospital medical team is able to treat critical conditions at the scene and during transport to definitive care.

If a correct triage decision is made at the first point of contact, then the patient can benefit from being taken directly to the 'right' hospital. This reduces the time to definitive management.

Concentrators

Rare conditions benefit from being seen and treated by a small

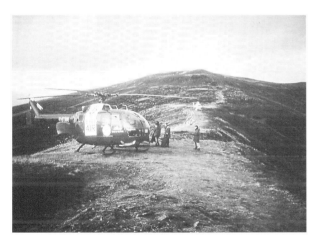

Fig. 46.3 Helicopter rescue from remote terrain

number of clinicians who become expert by virtue of this exposure. A helicopter covers large distances rapidly, and can bring patients to specialist skills from a wider area than would otherwise be possible. The patient benefits by being treated by clinicians whose skills are maintained by constant practice. The occasional practitioner of advanced techniques will be unlikely to perform as well.

Matching the Response to the Need

With the increasing sophistication of the ambulance services there are now a number of possible responses to an emergency. Standard ambulances, rapid response vehicles, motor-cycle paramedics and helicopters are all used in a stratified fashion throughout the UK. Each of these can be used extremely specifically, but must be precisely targeted at the appropriate patient. Unfortunately, response capability has developed faster than the command and control systems which target them. The emergency service response for each and every situation must be matched to the medical need of the patient. This can only be achieved with a sensitive dispatch system based on medical priority. The helicopter provides an additional resource that is available to target the appropriate treatment to each patient.

Prestige

In some parts of the world, especially in the USA, helicopters are used as statements about the hospitals from which they work. The expense of the helicopter system speaks of the prestige of the hospital and is often a 'loss leader' when considered against financial remuneration. In the UK this is less of a problem, but can still be a risk if helicopters do not adhere to their primary aims.

Clinical Indications for the Use of Air Transport

Clinical indications for the use of a helicopter as a response to an emergency must be considered separately from logistic indications, as some conditions (for example cardiac arrest or diabetic coma) are unlikely to have any better outcome when treated by a helicopter system. All paramedics ought to be well practised in treating cardiac arrest or assessing diabetic coma, so there is no additional clinical benefit to be gained from transporting a doctor or more highly skilled crew to the scene. Most hospitals are able to manage the full range of medical emergencies, so taking the patient by helicopter to a more distant hospital is unlikely to improve outcome. There may be logistic reasons for using a helicopter, for example a remote location, but medical benefits will be rare.

HELICOPTER SYSTEMS

A helicopter system comes into its own if it can provide solutions to relatively uncommon situations which require high levels of judgement and skill. The most obvious example of this sort of situation is multiple trauma.

There is still debate about the role of a helicopter in trauma management, although some early studies showed significant improvements in mortality resulting from their use. It is impossible to isolate the effect of the helicopter from the effect of the rest of the trauma system, and so it is difficult to identify which part of the system bestows the health benefit. Further, different systems use differing levels of medical, paramedical and nursing skills, making comparison of results between different systems extremely difficult. Some studies have shown an improvement in outcome, particularly with early advanced treatment followed by rapid transport to definitive care. Although lives can undoubtedly be saved, there is a cost, and the society which benefits from such a system must decide whether or not it is prepared to pay for the helicopter and all the additional facilities such as intensive care beds and rehabilitation centres that are required. In the UK, the value of a life is estimated by the Department of Transport at £860,000 (in 1995) when designing roads to reduce accidents. The London helicopter service has been shown to save 13 lives a year for about the same amount. The Department of Health would be unlikely to allow purchasers of health care such an exuberant expenditure on an individual patient basis. The value of human life is fundamental to the economic analysis of helicopter systems purchaser, but it is essentially an imponderable philosophical question, the answer to which is usually based on willingness to pay by the purchaser.

The Medical Crew

The most important factor in determining clinical outcome is the medical treatment given rather than the type of vehicle used. The composition of the helicopter medical crew therefore is of vital importance, because there is no point in using such an expensive vehicle if it does not produce the desired outcomes. The medical team must be experienced and safe in the hostile pre-hospital environment. They must be trained to cope in unusual situations including prolonged entrapments and confined spaces. There is no 'ideal' medical crew for a helicopter system, as the crew required depends on the aims and use of the system. No single individual is likely to possess all the required attributes; however, a team including an experienced doctor and paramedic will provide all the skills required. The paramedic combines a solid knowledge of safety in the pre-hospital environment with familiarity with other emergency services and their procedures, and is well versed in providing medical treatment outside hospital. The doctor contributes advanced assessment skills, and provides critical interventions that may be instantly required to treat the patient, including advanced anaesthetic and surgical skills. Any other combination of medical personnel leaves gaps in the range of skills provided. A medical team without ambulance personnel (doctor only, or doctor and nurse) may have the high level of medical skills required, but will be vulnerable to the pre-hospital environment and may have difficulty in coordinating with other emergency services. There may be a tendency to apply inappropriate in-hospital procedures to pre-hospital situations. Conversely, a 'paramedic only' team is unable to provide all the critical interventions that may be necessary. Furthermore, the paramedic may identify a problem that requires advanced medical treatment but is frustrated by restrictive protocols from performing the procedure required.

The only fully medical helicopter system in Britain with a doctor and paramedic crew, is the Helicopter Emergency Medical Service (HEMS) based at the Royal London Hospital. This combination of medical crew gives a medical specification which caters for almost all eventualities, and brings the hospital to the accident site. It provides concentrated experience of trauma management to the paramedic, encouraging ever closer links between the hospital and ambulance services.

Safety in Helicopter Operations

All personnel involved in helicopter operations must be trained to move safely around the aircraft, and obey the accepted conventions when in the vicinity of the aircraft. Any ambulance personnel who find themselves in this environment should not put themselves in a position where they might be exposed to danger. Don't pretend to know if you haven't been taught!

The primary danger when working close to a helicopter comes from the moving blades of the main rotor and the tail rotor. Never approach a helicopter from the rear. The tail rotor is not easy to see and is usually set at a height that makes resuscitation futile. The distance from the ground of both the main rotor blades and the tail rotor varies between helicopter types, and some helicopters have blades that dip at the front and do not allow access. The main rotor movement is very variable depending on wind, how fast the blades are turning, and resonance. The rule is that *a helicopter should only be approached when the rotor blades have completely stopped turning*. Always stand apart in front of the helicopter and wait for the 'thumbs up' signal from the pilot before approaching.

If a helicopter must be approached while the rotor blades are still running, wait well outside the reach of the rotor blades for a direct and unequivocal instruction from the flight crew. While approaching, duck. Do not hold any object such as a drip above shoulder height, and do not carry anything that might blow away. During starting or slowing of the rotor blades there is less centrifugal force. The blade tips tend to droop closer to the ground, and this effect may be enhanced in high winds. This is always dangerous so never approach or leave a helicopter at this time. Always await unequivocal instruction from the pilot. If a helicopter is on a slope the rotor blades are closer to the ground on the uphill side.

Rotor wash is a further hazard, throwing dust and debris into the air and blowing over light objects. If you are standing within the rotor wash, turn away and close your eyes.

The medical crew can assist the pilot in maintaining aircraft safety during flight and landing by watching out for hazards. Dark wires stretched across a dark background are particularly difficult to see. The more pairs of eyes that are on the lookout the better.

Medical crews must be well versed and practised in aircraft safety and evacuation. They must wear suitable fire-retardant clothing and approved flight helmets. Seat-belts or harnesses must be worn throughout the flight, and only released when the pilot gives the medical team clearance to leave the aircraft.

In some countries medical helicopters have a dismal safety record, with a reputation for being dangerous for patients and lethal for the medical and paramedical crew. This often stems from a desire to 'push on' in marginal circumstances. The natural enthusiasm to reach and evacuate a patient must be restrained, remembering that adding your own name to the list of casualties is foolish. A separation of medical and aviation information can be useful, allowing the pilot to make decisions in an atmosphere that is detached from any emotional pressure arising from the incident. The medical crew must never express criticism when a pilot decides that circumstances preclude a mission. The pilot must weigh up the pros and cons of mechanical failure or poor visibility within the constraints of safety. Disappointment in such cases is natural, allowed and probably mutual, but criticism or shroud-waving from the medical team can undermine the pilot's confidence and lead to an unsafe decision on the next occasion.

TRAINING OF PARAMEDICS FOR HELICOPTER OPERATIONS

The Civil Aviation Authority (CAA) controls the standards of training for all involved in medical helicopter operations. European standards are now being introduced, and will be compulsory by 1997. These regulations state that a paramedic can act either as 'medical crew' or a 'medical passenger'. If the paramedics assist the pilot with any part of the operation of the helicopter, such as navigation or using the air-band radio, they must be classified as 'medical crew'. If they play no active role during the helicopter flight they are acting as 'medical passengers'. This distinction is important, as each of these roles requires a different standard of training.

Medical crew members under the new regulations have to undergo a demanding training. They must be trained in the following subjects *to the standard required for a commercial helicopter pilot's licence*:

- Flight preparation (including fuel calculation, loading, mass and balance)
- Navigation (map reading, flight planning, navigational aid principles and use)

- VHF/RT licence
- Local air traffic control (ATC) arrangements (compilation, filing, copying down and filing ATC flight plans)
- Local meteorology
- Instrument readings, warnings and use of normal and emergency checklists
- Basic understanding of helicopter type
- Crew coordination
- Selecting required documents and extraction of information as directed
- Conducting refuelling and rotors running refuelling
- HEMS operating site selection and use
- Patient loading and unloading
- Marshalling signals
- Underslung load operations
- Winch operations
- Recurrent training on selected subjects as appropriate

These new requirements for medical crew are exacting standards that will take a number of months of full-time study to master. All single-pilot medical helicopter operations will have to train their paramedics to these standards if the paramedic is to continue to assist with the navigation.

Medical passengers do not have an active role during flight and so have a smaller training requirement. Subjects that must be covered are:

- Familiarization with the helicopter types(s) operated
- Entry and exit under normal and emergency conditions for self and patient
- Use of onboard medical equipment

In addition to the standards required by the CAA, the paramedic has to acquire the skills required for safe and effective patient care in the aeromedical environment. Training must cover safety, advanced patient assessment, advanced paramedical interventions, coordination with other emergency services, rescue in special situations (e.g. confined space, entrapment, construction site) and, if working with a doctor, the indications, rationale and technique used for medical interventions. The training period should include realistic scenarios which enable individuals to practise with a real pre-hospital team and plausible physical surroundings. This also helps a pre-hospital medical team to work together and allows the patient to benefit from a blend of jointly practised skills. This is especially important for the doctor-paramedic team because it is likely that these individuals will be used to a high level of autonomy and control.

Time spent flying as an observer with an experienced medical crew is highly desirable providing space will allow. In a busy system 2 weeks is sufficient, but in a system with few calls observer time needs to be correspondingly longer.

Aviation Medicine

The parts of aviation medicine concerned with the effects of pressure changes (e.g. exacerbation of pneumothoraces, expansion of endotracheal tube balloons) have very little relevance to the sort of systems that most paramedics will encounter. Helicopter systems involved with primary casualty evacuation in the UK are unlikely to fly at more than 450 m and at this sort of altitude pressure changes are negligible. Some transport systems do go through large altitude changes, under which circumstances the medical crew must be trained, for example, to fill balloons with water, to treat air-filled cavities prior to flying, and to know and watch for the effects of pressure changes. This is a specialist area, usually practised by an intensive care doctor. Many subtle physiological changes are produced when a patient travels by helicopter, mainly in the cardiovascular system. In practice these changes do not affect standard patient monitoring or treatment protocols. The loading of a patient may be affected by the nature of their injuries. A helicopter flies 'nose down', which has the effect of raising the patient's feet if loaded with the head forwards. This may increase intracranial pressure, so *head-injury patients are best transported with their feet forwards, to elevate the head*.

Working in the Helicopter

A number of environmental factors make a helicopter a difficult place to work in compared with a road ambulance. The noise and motion of a helicopter can be very disorienting owing to an overload of information reaching the brain from ears, eyes and the vestibular apparatus. It takes training and experience for a paramedic (or any other member of the medical crew) to develop 'air sense', in exactly the same way as it takes time to develop 'street sense'. Some people cannot or will not adjust to this environment and may remain extremely fearful of flying. It is wise for them to be channelled into other areas of work without fuss or condemnation.

The major differences from working in a conventional ambulance are discussed below.

Internal space

Many helicopters used in the medical role have limited internal space, which restricts access to the patient. This can make assessment and intervention difficult (Figure 46.4). The BK 117 has 176 cubic feet of internal space and the BO 105 has 162 cubic feet compared to 250 cubic feet in a typical ambulance. The Dauphin has 176 cubic feet of cabin space and an additional 78 cubic feet of storage space, a total of 254 cubic feet, making it similar in size to an ambulance. The internal configuration must be meticulously planned to provide the best possible utilization of the room available (Figure 46.5).

Noise

The noise level inside a helicopter is usually 90 decibels or

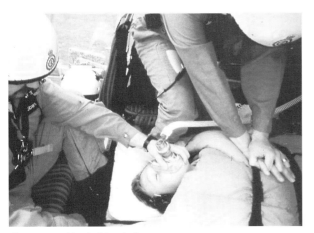

Fig. 46.4 *Working inside a helicopter*

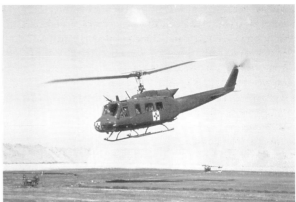

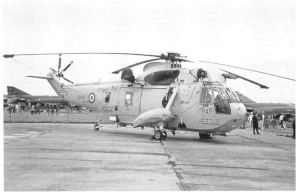

Fig. 46.5 *Different types of helicopter*

more, a level that will damage hearing over time. This is not solely a risk to the health of the crew – it also gives rise to problems of communication. All crew members must wear approved ear protection. It is essential that helmets include headsets and microphones to allow free communication between members of the team. When conscious patients are being transported, it is essential that the medical crew are able to communicate with the patient, to deliver explanation and reassurance. Some operators play music to their patients, who may wake to soothing sounds, but may draw the conclusion that they are in heaven!

Noise precludes the use of auditory alarms on monitoring equipment. Visual alarms and persistent close observation are required. Training is required so that personnel who normally rely on audible alarms have readjusted their visual and auditory senses.

Vibration, movement and air sickness

Vibration inside a helicopter is extremely variable but can be marked. This reduces the signal quality of some monitoring systems and leads to some anxiety about its effect on injured tissue.

Continual movement as the helicopter assumes different attitudes tends to cause crew fatigue as little-used muscle groups are continuously recruited in order to brace the body against a new and unnatural force.

Air sickness is closely related to movement. The vestibular apparatus of the inner ear gives dynamic and static positional information to the brain which is routinely processed to maintain balance. With movement in three planes, a mismatch of these signals with visual information will almost inevitably give rise to a feeling of nausea. Rough weather adds to the disruption and misinformation given to the brain by the position sensors making vomiting more likely. Nausea may be exacerbated by strong smells, and in particular incompletely burned fuel in exhaust fumes which are drawn into the cabin. The addition of the smell of vomit from a patient may precipitate waves of nausea. Air sickness can be minimized by adjusting air vents to give a supply of cool, fresh air. Staring at a fixed point may help but frequent changes of height may conspire to make the eyes change position, readjusting the way the object is observed. Flying with a full stomach is unwise if prone to air sickness and antiemetic medication, particularly cinnarizine (Stugeron) may be of great help to those who are prone to nausea. Frequent flying leads to some habituation and a decrease in the severity of air sickness, although some victims of air sickness cannot be desensitized.

Strength of vehicle

Helicopters are not built to the same rugged internal cabin specification as ambulances. The materials used in helicopter construction are strong where strength is of paramount importance, and the ability of the airframe and other parts to take loads is strictly defined by the CAA, but in other areas light materials are used, which tend to be fragile and do not stand up well to heavy handling by the medical crew. Helicopter doors, for example, are lightweight and can be damaged by a minor knock from a stretcher on loading the patient, or even by closure in the wrong way.

Medical management during helicopter transport

A helicopter in stable flight is possibly a less difficult place than the back of an ambulance in which to perform medical interventions. The movement does not involve sudden turns and violent road movement, and gelatin plasma substitutes such as Haemaccel do not froth as they do in the back of a fast-moving ambulance. There is advantage to moving a patient by air before critical interventions have been performed. Even if air evacuation is more rapid than ground evacuation, it may still be too long for the hypoxic, hypercapnic or hypotensive patient to be transported without critical interventions being performed at the moment of first medical contact. The quickest way to correct such physiological abnormalities is for the helicopter medical team to have the skill to perform any treatment that may be needed.

The patients who are most likely to be sensitive to pre-hospital interventions and who stand to benefit most are those with severe head injuries. To correct hypoxia and hypercapnia in these patients requires the pre-hospital medical team to give general anaesthesia with muscle relaxants. Unless the patient is already virtually dead, most will maintain laryngeal reflexes and will not accept an orotracheal tube without gagging and raising intracranial pressure. Blind nasal intubation by paramedics without anaesthetic drugs is routinely used in America, but has failed to win overwhelming support in Britain (see Chapter 5). If the helicopter medical team does not have the skills to complete the 'AB' of the primary survey in the trauma patient, and in particular the ability to give a general anaesthetic, a 'scoop and run' policy is mandatory. It seems logical that if you cannot perform the critical intervention required then you must move the patient to someone who can.

A fundamental precept of all medical treatment is to do no further harm to the patient. The patient therefore needs to be 'packaged' before transport by air. Every patient must be firmly secured and protected with spinal immobilization from further harm during transport in the aircraft. This can be achieved by using a vacuum mattress to enclose the patient in a rigid shell. It would also be possible to use firm strapping to secure the patient on a long spinal board (although this method is not currently allowed by the CAA). A particular worry with the use of a long spinal board is that the smooth surface may allow the body to slide while the head is strapped in a secure position, so causing movement of or traction on the neck.

At the time of writing military helicopters are not allowed to carry a vacuum mattress, as rupture of the mattress with release of the enclosed polystyrene beads could cause severe damage, resulting in helicopter grounding.

Selection of Receiving Hospital

A helicopter gives the pre-hospital medical team a wider choice of destinations. Hospitals have evolved with different ranges of specialities, and vary from the multidisciplinary unit with all the services on one site, to single-speciality units such as burns centres. All hospitals are not therefore equal in their ability to deal with particular conditions. As the helicopter can cover large distances in a short time the pre-hospital team are able to pick the most appropriate hospital destination for each patient. If the pre-hospital team cannot perform the necessary critical interventions then this choice may not apply, as the priority is to move the patient to someone who can perform the interventions required. This leads to a conflict between the patient's immediate need (critical interventions), and longer-term need (specialist treatment that may not be available at the local hospital).

There is good evidence that the sooner a head-injured patient receives surgery, the better the outcome (particularly in the case of traumatic extradural and subdural haematomas). The speed of a helicopter allows head-injured patients to be taken directly to neurosurgical centres, decreasing the time to definitive neurosurgical intervention.

Audit

Continuing constructive criticism of helicopter operations is essential. Medical audit is an accepted and valued way of assessing medical systems. This concept is not widely used in pre-hospital care, but is an invaluable way of examining the performance of a helicopter system. Audit should be concentrated on medical rather than logistic end-points, and so needs the supervision of a senior clinician with experience of pre-hospital care.

Psychological Effects

As a helicopter system acts as a 'concentrator', personnel working within the system will be exposed to a large number of seriously ill or traumatized patients. This method of organization makes medical sense (as outlined above), but is stressful for the staff involved. A debriefing system and regular rotation to more routine duties is essential to prevent 'burn out', post-traumatic stress, or elitism.

CONCLUSION

Aviation and medicine may be combined in a number of different ways: paramedics are most likely to be involved in helicopter primary casualty evacuation. Analysis of the effects of a helicopter system involves a complex mix of medical and logistic considerations, and there is no evidence of medical benefit from a helicopter service for non-trauma patients. Whether or not a helicopter is economically justified for trauma patients depends to some extent on the monetary value that is attached to human life.

The helicopter environment is very different from a ground ambulance. Before working with a helicopter system, comprehensive training is essential to ensure safety and to adapt existing medical skills to the new situation. To provide the best and most efficient treatment, the helicopter medical crew must be able to perform all of the medical interventions that the patient requires, and be able to decide on the most appropriate destination for each patient.

Without integration into a comprehensive medical system a helicopter cannot provide medical treatment, and becomes merely an expensive status symbol. As part of a medical system with the correct staffing, training and tasking, a helicopter can be a valuable additional resource, enabling the best pre-hospital response to be matched to each patient.

9

PREGNANCY
AND
CHILDBIRTH

chapter forty-seven

CHILDBIRTH

Childbirth is a normal, natural phenomenon, and not an illness. For the paramedic confronted with a woman in labour, the fear caused by dealing with the unfamiliar can be countered by the knowledge that human beings have reproduced and given birth without interference from doctors, midwives or paramedics for thousands of years. The old adage 'meddlesome midwifery' is as true today as it ever was, and the labouring mother should, by and large, be left to get on with labour; her attendants (be they paramedics, midwives or doctors) should stand back, not interfere, and provide moral and physical support, coupled with informed clinical observation only. The time when a paramedic may have to become involved is established second stage of labour, when the journey to hospital is too long to complete before delivery is expected.

Many of the critical decisions in childbirth relate to timing: the actual clinical execution of actions being relatively straightforward. Within the UK, there will be very few situations where the time to hospital is longer than the time to the baby's birth, and even fewer situations where the paramedic is the only medical person present at birth.

In order to make informed clinical observations and, therefore, reasoned decisions, it is necessary to be aware of the salient anatomy and physiology of normal pregnancy and reproduction, together with an understanding of the normal process of delivery. Remember, the aim is to be a safe birth attendant in an emergency situation.

In the vast majority of calls to a pregnant woman in suspected or established labour, the correct response will be to transport the patient safely and swiftly to the appropriate delivery suite. The critical question for the paramedic is, 'Can I safely get this woman to definitive care before the conclusion of second stage or delivery of the baby?' In the vast majority of cases, the answer to this question will be YES.

ANATOMY

The external female genitalia are shown in Figures 47.1 and 47.2. The layout of the female reproductive organs is shown in Figure 47.3.

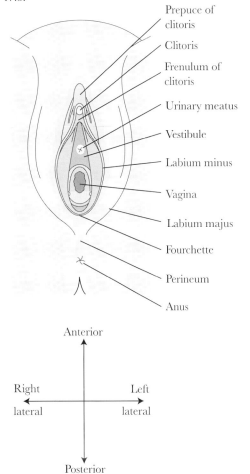

Fig. 47.1 The female external genitalia and their orientation in the dorsal position. From Miller & Callender, Obstetrics Illustrated, 4th edn, with permission from Churchill Livingstone

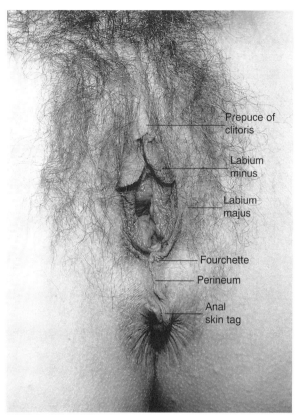

Fig. 47.2 The female external genitalia

PHYSIOLOGICAL BASIS OF PREGNANCY

To understand the process of conception and pregnancy it is necessary to have a basic knowledge of female reproductive physiology. Full details may be obtained from a textbook of obstetrics or midwifery – only the information needed for safe, effective emergency care is included here.

Women of reproductive age have monthly periods which are the manifestation of the shedding of the endometrial lining of the uterus because of falling oestrogen and progesterone levels. Hence, the first day of bleeding is the date of the last menstrual period (LMP) (Figure 47.4).

The Menstrual Cycle

Each woman has two ovaries, containing a large number of ova plus connective tissue. In the inner part of the ovary are thousands of primordial follicles consisting of an oogonium (egg) plus a single layer of stromal cells called granulosa cells. Under hormonal control, just one primordial follicle each month ripens fully to become a Graafian follicle with a proliferation of granulosa cells and an accumulation of fluid (liquor) within the follicle. Some of the stroma cells change to form hormone-secreting cells and, under hormonal influence, the follicle ripens, growing in size from approximately 0.25 mm to 8 mm in diameter. At ovulation, the follicle bursts and the ovum is expelled. Normally this enters the fallopian tube and is carried slowly down the tube, taking 3–4 days to reach the

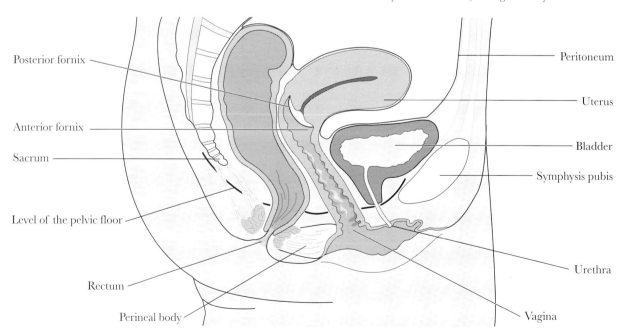

Fig. 47.3 The female reproductive organs. From Chilman and Thomas, Understanding Nursing Care, *2nd edn, with permission from Churchill Livingstone*

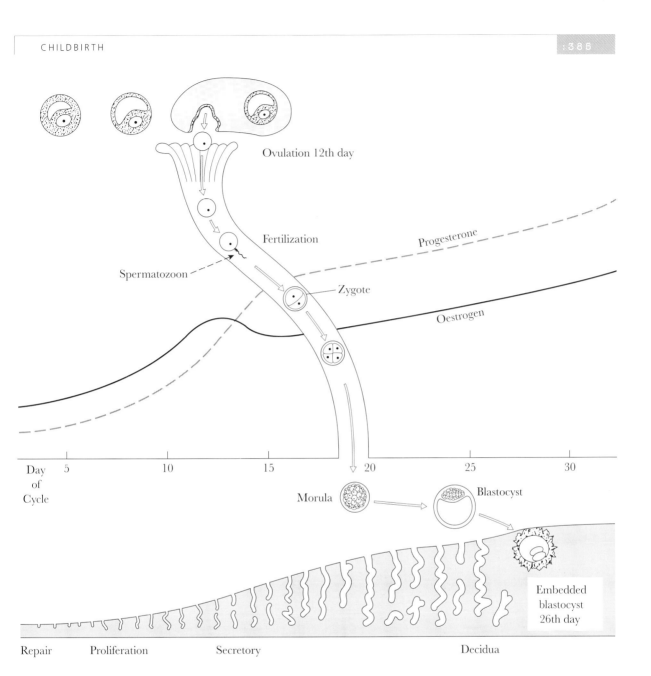

Ovulation 12th day

Fertilization

Progesterone

Spermatozoon

Zygote

Oestrogen

Day
of
Cycle

5   10   15   20   25   30

Morula   Blastocyst

Embedded
blastocyst
26th day

Repair   Proliferation   Secretory   Decidua

Fig. 47.4 *The menstrual cycle. From Miller and Callander,* Obstetrics Illustrated, *2nd edn, with permission from Churchill Livingstone*

uterus. It is while *en route* to the uterus that fertilization will occur, provided that coitus has occurred at the relevant time, and it is in the fallopian tube that the majority of ectopic pregnancies arise (Figures 47.4 and 47.5).

The remnants of the Graafian follicle develop into the hormone-secreting *corpus luteum*, providing progesterones to stimulate the proliferation of the endometrial lining of the uterus in preparation for implantation by the fertilized egg. If the ovum is not fertilized, then after about 12 days the corpus luteum ceases functioning, progesterone secretion falls, and the uterine lining – the endometrium – is shed, and the cycle starts again. The hormonal mechanisms controlling the menstrual cycle are complex.

When the ovum is fertilized, cell division follows and a *blastocyst* develops and implants in the uterine wall. Part of the blastocyst – the *trophoblast* – invades the uterine wall by forming chorionic villi (finger-like protrusions) which are the forerunner of the placenta.

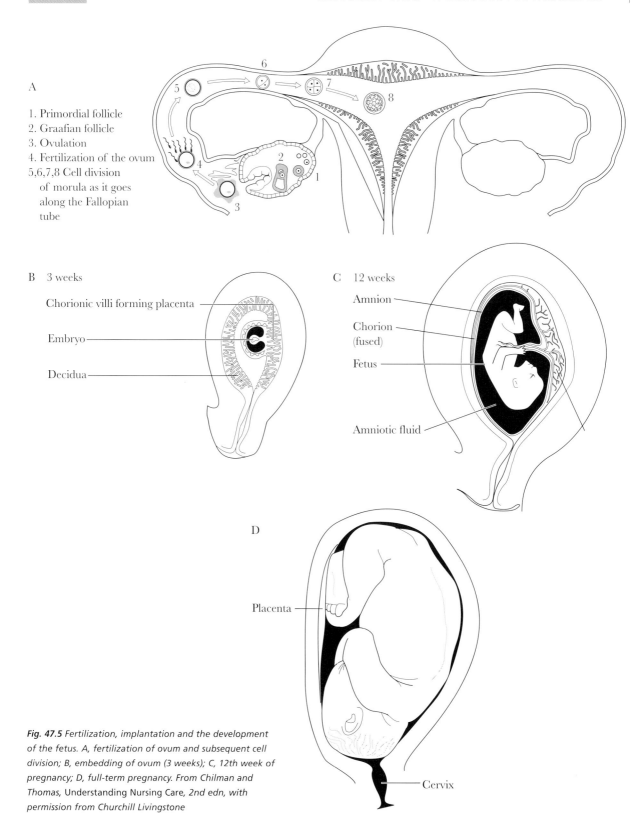

A

1. Primordial follicle
2. Graafian follicle
3. Ovulation
4. Fertilization of the ovum
5,6,7,8 Cell division
   of morula as it goes
   along the Fallopian
   tube

B   3 weeks

Chorionic villi forming placenta

Embryo

Decidua

C   12 weeks

Amnion

Chorion
(fused)

Fetus

Amniotic fluid

D

Placenta

Cervix

Fig. 47.5 *Fertilization, implantation and the development of the fetus. A, fertilization of ovum and subsequent cell division; B, embedding of ovum (3 weeks); C, 12th week of pregnancy; D, full-term pregnancy. From Chilman and Thomas,* Understanding Nursing Care, *2nd edn, with permission from Churchill Livingstone*

Gestational Dates

Most women have a menstrual cycle of approximately 28 days, although this can vary. By convention and definition, day 1 of the cycle is the first day of the menstrual bleed. The only fixed timing in the menstrual cycle is that ovulation *precedes* menstruation by 14 days. Thus, it is the proliferation phase which varies (Figure 47.6).

From fertilization to delivery is 266 days or 38 weeks, and thus the time from LMP to delivery is 280 days or 40 weeks in a woman with a 28-day cycle.

Calculation of estimated date of delivery

It is important to be able to calculate the estimated date of delivery (EDD), as many management decisions have to be made according to whether the baby is premature (born early) or post-mature (born late).

Provided that mother's cycle length is between 24–35 days, she has not been on the contraceptive pill in the past 3 months, and she is reasonably certain of the date of her LMP, the EDD is calculated by subtracting 3 months from the date, adding 1 year and then adding 7 days. For example:

LMP:	21 January 1996
Subtract 3 months:	21 October 1995
Add 1 year:	21 October 1996
Add 7 days:	28 October 1996

The EDD is therefore 28 October 1996.

Gestational calculators or even a calendar can be used to calculate the current gestation.

CHANGES TO MATERNAL ANATOMY AND PHYSIOLOGY DURING PREGNANCY

Many changes occur in maternal physiology during pregnancy to accommodate the growth of the fetus, the placenta, and in preparation for lactation. During pregnancy the mother's weight may increase by up to 12.5 kg, and there are marked changes in maternal metabolism. The most important changes as far as emergency care is concerned are those connected with the cardiovascular and respiratory systems; in short, those that affect the management of airway with cervical spine, breathing with oxygen, and circulation with posture.

As pregnancy progresses, the metabolic load increases as the fetus grows. The mother has considerably greater metabolic requirements simply to service the extra 12.5 kg of tissues a full-term pregnancy demands. From the viewpoint of emergency care, the changes in pregnancy are best viewed from the operational priorities list rather than from a formal physiological approach.

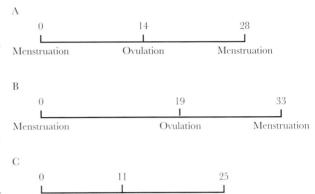

Fig. 47.6 *Menstrual cycles: A, 28 days; B, 33 days; C, 25 days*

Anatomical Factors in Pregnancy

The anatomical changes in pregnancy affecting the airway are the presence of a relatively short obese neck and engorgement of the breast tissue, especially in the third trimester, and these conspire to make airway management more difficult. In addition, the pregnant patient usually has a full dentition. As the uterus rises up out of the pelvis and into the abdominal cavity, especially towards term, it has the effect of splinting the diaphragm in the elevated position, and also causes some splaying of the ribs; these effects make ventilation and external cardiac compression difficult.

As the uterus enlarges, especially in the third trimester, the inferior vena cava is compressed when the mother lies in the supine position. Beyond 16 weeks the enlarging uterus has less bony protection and is thus at greater risk from direct trauma or deceleration forces.

In summary, the anatomical factors interfering with resuscitation techniques are:

AIRWAY

- Full dentition
- Short, obese neck
- Breast engorgement

BREATHING

- Splinted diaphragm
- Splaying of the ribs

CIRCULATION

- Vena cava compression
- Breast engorgement (affects CPR)
- Splaying of the ribs (affects CPR)

Physiological Factors in Pregnancy

Airway

The risks of reflux acid regurgitation and aspiration of stomach contents into the lungs is increased because of a relaxed gastro-oesophageal junction, delayed emptying of the stomach, and increased intragastric pressure from the compressive effects of an increasing uterine size. This is the rationale behind the recommendation for early intubation in pregnant women.

Breathing

There is an increased oxygen requirement during pregnancy because of the high oxygen consumption rates of fetal tissues and because the hypertrophied maternal breast and uterine tissue also have higher oxygen requirements. As pregnancy progresses and diaphragmatic splinting increases, although the vital capacity is not reduced, functional residual capacity is reduced, chest compliance reduces, and so to compensate there is a 40% rise in tidal volume. In short, just at the time when there is the need to satisfy a high oxygen requirement, the means to deliver this are stretched. While respiration is adequate in the fit, healthy mother, it is easily overtaxed in the ill or traumatized mother. This is the reason for early intubation, early intermittent positive pressure ventilation and high-flow oxygen at as high a concentration as possible – preferably close to 100% via a reservoir face mask in the spontaneously breathing patient.

Circulation changes

Cardiac output is the product of stroke volume and heart rate, and in pregnancy the 40% increase in cardiac output at rest is derived from cardiac muscle hypertrophy, enlargement of the cardiac chambers giving increased stroke volume, and a rise in the resting heart rate of approximately 15–20 beats per minute. Even greater cardiac output is obtained at term and in labour. Because of decreased peripheral resistance and in later weeks the arteriovenous shunt-like effect of the placental bed, blood pressure at rest drops by 5–15 mmHg. The cardiac enlargement and muscle hypertrophy may produce electrocardiographic changes with evidence of left ventricular strain and, as the heart unfolds on the aorta, inverted T waves may be seen in leads V_2 and V_3. On auscultation, as a consequence of the hyperkinetic and hypervolaemic state of pregnancy, a systolic ejection murmur may be heard, but this is not significant in pre-hospital emergency care.

Because of the hypertrophied breast and uterine tissue, the demands of the placental bed and increased renal demands, the circulating blood volume increases massively by 50%, *but there is no corresponding increase in oxygen-carrying capacity*. There is a relative *physiological anaemia* as part of the body's attempt to moderate the increased cardiac demands of pregnancy. The anaemia results in reduced blood viscosity which manifests itself as a reduced peripheral resistance and is reflected in reduced diastolic blood pressure.

In summary, the physiological changes of pregnancy are:

AIRWAY

- Relaxed gastro-oesophageal junction
- Delayed stomach emptying
- Increased intragastric pressure

BREATHING

- 40% increase in tidal volume
- Decreased functional residual capacity
- Increased oxygen requirement

CIRCULATION

- 40% increase in cardiac output
- Tachycardia
- Hypotension (systolic blood pressure reduced by 5–15 mmHg)
- ECG changes
- Circulating blood volume increased by 50%

During pregnancy the normal physiological reserves to cope with stresses are all in action to keep the demands on the heart

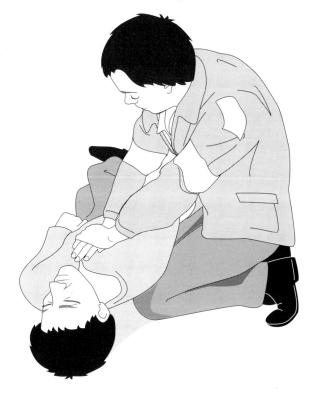

Fig. 47.7 *The human wedge*

within manageable limits. Because all the normal compensatory mechanisms are already in play, should the pregnant woman suffer blood loss of any significance, she has little physiological reserve left, and will show few premonitory signs before crashing almost immediately into often irretrievable grade III or IV hypovolaemic shock.

Within normal limits, according to Starling's law of the heart (see Chapter 10), the heart will pump out all that it is presented with. In the third trimester of pregnancy, the gravid uterus presses on the inferior vena cava reducing venous return to the heart. In the supine position the *inferior vena caval compression syndrome* reduces venous return by as much as 40%. Fully efficient basic life support only gives at best 30% of the cardiac output, and 30% minus 40% is –10%! Thus, the pregnant woman should be nursed in the left lateral position, and must be resuscitated in that position. The left lateral position may be achieved by placing a cushion or pillow under the right hip, or by a human wedge (Figure 47.7). The uterus can also be manually displaced to the left.

Other detailed changes in the physiology of the pregnant woman are not relevant to pre-hospital care, except that renal blood flow rises by 50%, occasionally glucose leaks into the urine, and protein in the urine always requires further evaluation.

THE CALL TO A PREGNANT WOMAN

A call-out to a pregnant woman is always more stressful than to a non-pregnant patient because there are two lives at stake – mother and fetus. However, in the vast majority of cases, labour is a normal, natural event which takes care of itself without sophisticated intervention from others, and there is time to transport the patient to definitive care.

The mother is the best and most natural incubator for the fetus, and therefore she is always assessed, managed and stabilized first. The main purpose of the assessment by history, examination and observation is to piece together sufficient information to answer one simple question: 'Is there time to transport the mother to hospital, or is delivery so imminent that I will have to manage it?'. The assessment may also give some warning indications of potential complications. General history-taking is outlined in Chapter 2, but more focused questions need to be asked in relation to pregnancy. Knowledge of the facts and the general mechanisms of labour will give further information on which to make a balanced, professional, but nevertheless critical decision as to whether to attempt transfer or to manage the delivery at the scene.

Definitions

Parity is the number of times that a woman has carried a pregnancy to 24 weeks. The definition has changed from 28 weeks to 24 weeks, reflecting advances in medical technology which

allows many 24-week gestation deliveries to survive in neonatal intensive care units. Similar dating changes have occurred in the definition of stillbirth and the upper limit for legal termination of pregnancy.

Gravidity is the number of times a woman has conceived and been pregnant, regardless of the outcome.

A *primigravida* is a woman who is pregnant for the first time, a *nullipara* is a woman who has never delivered, and a *multipara* (or multip) is a woman who has had two or more deliveries.

Other obstetric definitions can be found in the glossary.

THE NORMAL PROCESS OF LABOUR

At any time from 37 weeks to 42 weeks of gestation, labour is said to be at *term*. Prior to 37 weeks the labour is *premature* and after 42 weeks the pregnancy is *prolonged* (*post-mature*). Full term is 40 weeks. There are three phases of labour, but the symptoms of labour can be mimicked by 'false labour'. It is clearly important to distinguish between the two. The characteristics of each are given in Table 47.1.

Duration of Labour

Labour falls into three stages (Table 47.2). If the ambulance arrives at the end of the first stage of labour, there is almost

Table 47.1 True and false labour

	True labour	False labour
Contractions	Regular	Irregular
Intensity of contractions	Increases as time goes on	Remains at same level of intensity
Contraction-free interval	Gradually shortens	Stays long
Location of pain	Abdomen and back	Lower abdomen only

Table 47.2 The stages of labour

	Nulliparous woman	Multiparous woman
Stage 1	8–12 hours	4–8 hours
Stage 2	1–2 hours	30–60 minutes
Stage 3	A few minutes to 1 hour	A few minutes to 1 hour

always time to transfer the mother to either a consultant-led district general hospital or, failing that, to a general practitioner maternity unit. There is certainly time to summon via ambulance control a midwife and general practitioner.

Getting Help

All NHS general practitioners are required by their terms of service to respond to calls in their practice area for obstetric emergencies. General practitioners rarely practise intrapartum 'home delivery' obstetrics nowadays, but at least you will have the assistance of someone who has conducted a reasonable number of normal deliveries. These situations are never ideal, and it is important to work as a team, although the general practitioner will carry the ultimate responsibility and therefore the chain of command must be respected. It is likely that both the doctor and the ambulance paramedic will be relieved to see the midwife. Many community midwives still practise intrapartum obstetrics and are required to attend a refresher practical attachment every 12–18 months in an active labour suite, so at least one of the team will have delivered a baby in the past 18 months!

The role of the obstetric flying squad has diminished in recent years. Such squads were initially set up by teaching hospital obstetric units in the 1950s when the majority of births occurred at home. Calls were frequent, and teaching hospitals had an abundance of staff to despatch on such calls. Nowadays, most deliveries are planned for hospital or general practitioner maternity units, and there are well-established mechanisms to admit women in early labour. Additionally, most district general hospitals usually have only one obstetric team on duty, especially out of hours, and as the normal work of a delivery suite has to continue, a flying squad call simply strips the receiving unit of its staff. Therefore the despatch time for a flying squad can be up to 45 minutes while back-up staff are mobilized, either to form the flying squad or to fill the gaps on the labour ward created by the despatch of the squad. Once the travelling time is added, the flying squad can effectively be discounted in terms of practical help for normal, uncomplicated deliveries. Indeed, many obstetric units only have a flying squad in name, if at all. Find out what your local situation is.

The Normal Delivery

Unless the baby's head is about to deliver, your first action – assuming that the scene is safe – is to call for help if you feel that you cannot transport the mother in time. As in all emergency situations, the fall-back procedure if you find yourself in a clinical situation beyond your competence is to (a) recognize that fact; (b) summon help from someone competent; (c) attend to all those factors that you can deal with, i.e. airway with cervical spine control, breathing with oxygen, circulation with posture. If nothing else, prepare the area for immediate delivery, lay out your equipment so everything is to hand and, as a precaution,

set up at least one intravenous line and consider inserting a second IV cannula. The biggest threat to the mother is haemorrhage, and in this less than ideal environment, the lack of skilled pairs of hands at a crucial time will be most acute. If you cannot cope with the baby's delivery or complications arise, then as help is already *en route*, comfort the mother and attend as necessary to:

- ABC
- Posture
- Analgesia with nitrous oxide and oxygen (Entonox)

NORMAL CHILDBIRTH

Normal childbirth occurs through the process of labour which is the expulsion of the products of conception (i.e. fetus, placenta and amniotic fluid) from the uterus via the birth canal after the 24th week of gestation. It is achieved via regular and painful uterine contractions accompanied by effacement (see below) and dilation of the cervix, which can only be detected by vaginal examination. As a paramedic, you will *not* be performing vaginal examinations, as in the early stages of labour your professional role will be to transport mother (dilation of the cervix and effacement constitute part of the definition of true labour). Any one of rupture of the membranes, loss of the mucus plug from the cervix, or a 'bloody show' in addition to regular painful uterine contractions constitutes a diagnosis of true labour for the purposes of operational paramedic practice.

The Three Stages of Labour

First stage

The first stage of labour is the longest, during which the cervix (neck) of the uterus effaces and then dilates – a process taking several hours, accompanied by a pink 'bloody show' of blood-stained mucus as the plug in the cervical canal is dislodged. During pregnancy the cervix is like a long sausage with a longitudinal canal through it. *Effacement* is the process where, as the uterus changes its shape during contractions, the sausage-shaped cervix becomes compressed in its longitudinal axis, then, in the later stages of effacement, the cervix begins to dilate. Full dilation is 10 cm and marks the end of the first stage of labour. As this happens the amniotic sac containing fluid bulges through the widening cervical os; the forewaters then rupture (if they have not already done so), liberating 50 ml or more of watery fluid.

During the first stage of labour the pain of contraction becomes greater and the contractions increase in frequency, rising from one every 20 minutes to one every 4–5 minutes. During the latter half of the first stage of labour, the fetal head begins to descend into the pelvis (Figures 47.8 and 47.9).

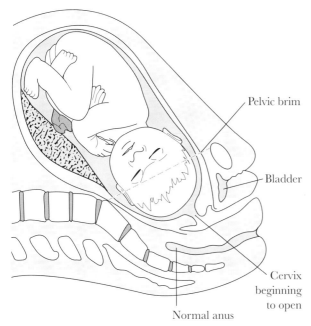

Fig. 47.8 *Birth canal, early first stage of labour. From Miller and Callander,* Obstetrics Illustrated, *4th edn, with permission from Churchill Livingstone*

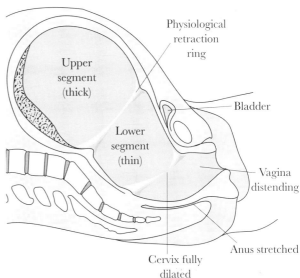

Fig. 47.9 *Birth canal at the beginning of the second stage of labour. From Miller and Callander,* Obstetrics Illustrated, *4th edn, with permission from Churchill Livingstone*

If you have difficulty in visualizing uterine activity in the first stage and early second stage, think of a chef icing a cake using an icing bag. As he ices the cake, he twists and screws up the top half of the bag in his hand, gathering up the emptying bag in his hand as the icing is expelled through the funnel and nozzle.

Second stage

The second stage of labour lasts from full dilation of the cervix (Figure 47.9) to delivery of the baby. During the second stage of labour the baby's head travels down into the pelvis where space is at a premium, and towards the end of the second stage of labour the birth canal is fully formed, but the canal outlet is at 90 degrees to the inlet. In a brief description of labour such as this there is no place for discussion of all eight of the different presentations of the vertex (head). Suffice it to say that the shape and layout of the pelvic floor musculature cause the baby's head to flex and then to internally rotate, bringing the occiput anterior (face posterior) and then allowing the head to extend at birth. All of these movements cause considerable displacement of the pelvic floor musculature, which manifests itself externally as 'crowning' (Figure 47.10A). The occiput is the first part to deliver, followed by the vertex, forehead and then face. Just after delivery of the face, the head 'restitutes', i.e. the neck untwists itself so that the head is in the neutral position relative to the shoulders (Figures 47.10B and 47.11). As the shoulders deliver so the second phase of rotation occurs. The anterior shoulder is the first to deliver followed by the posterior shoulder (Figure 47.10C). The rest of the trunk follows on by lateral flexion of the spine (Figure 47.10D).

Third stage

The third stage of delivery is from delivery of baby until delivery of the placenta is complete. Following the vacation of the uterus by the fetus, the uterus contracts in size very markedly in comparison with the placenta which stays the same size. Hence, the placenta is stripped off the uterine wall and expelled. It is at this stage that the greatest risk of haemorrhage occurs.

MANAGEMENT OF LABOUR

On first attending a woman in labour, it is important to obtain a brief general history by asking appropriate questions. An early request to see her maternity cooperation card can pay dividends, as it may possess much of the information required to decide whether there is time to reach hospital or whether delivery is so imminent that you will have to conduct it. Many women now carry their own complete maternity record with them. The layout varies from district to district, so familiarize yourself with the local one.

Ask the woman the date of her last normal menstrual period and what her EDD is (the two may not tally and you should believe her EDD). Ask whether her waters have gone or

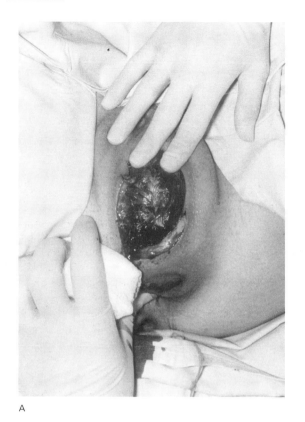

A

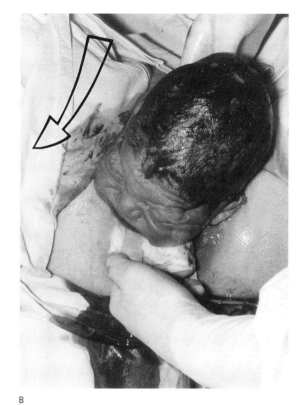

B

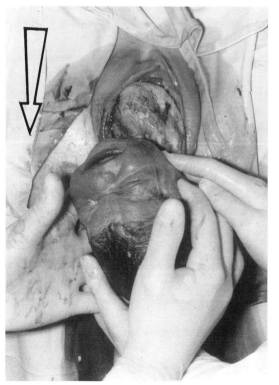

C

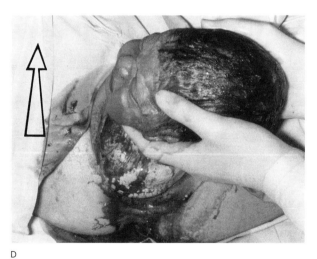

D

Fig. 47.10 The second stage of labour. (A) Normal delivery in the
lithotomy position (this patient has, in fact, had an episiotomy, but
this is not necessary for all deliveries). (B) The head is born. The
perineal pad is protecting the face from faecal contamination, and
restitution of the head has undone the twist on the neck. (C) The
anterior shoulder is being released from beneath the symphysis
pubis by directing the head and neck posteriorly. A midwife or
doctor may apply gentle traction also at this stage, but paramedics
and others without extensive formal training should not apply

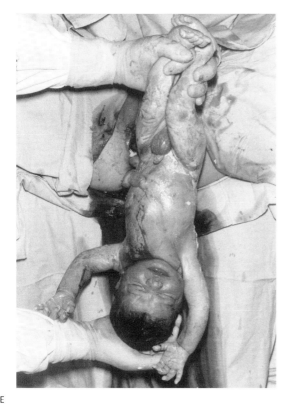

E

traction. (D) The posterior shoulder is then delivered by lateral flexion of the trunk in an upward direction. This is achieved by elevating the baby's head, neck and shoulder girdle as one fixed unit in an anterior direction. Do not apply any traction. (E) The baby is very slippery. Hold as shown in the photograph and support the head.

whether she has had a bloody show (signs of early labour). Obtain details of her pains, asking specifically:

- How long have you had the pains?
- Where are the pains?
- Are the pains getting worse or staying the same?
- Are the pains becoming more frequent. If so, how frequent are they?
- Are the pains lasting longer each time there is a pain?

According to the answers, you will be able to determine whether she is in true labour and, if so, for how long and what stage she is at. Any urge to go to the lavatory indicates rectal compression from late second-stage labour.

Enquire into the woman's past medical and obstetric history – specifically ask about:

- Previous caesarean sections – indicative of previous delivery problems
- Previous precipitate labours – indicative of very rapid labour (compare her answers with the times given in Table 47.2)
- Problems with this or other pregnancies

Clues can be obtained as to whether or not this will also be a complicated pregnancy.

Ask permission to examine the woman's abdomen and to inspect (not examine) the woman's perineum, explaining to her what you are looking for, i.e. to palpate the abdomen for contractions and observe the perineum for evidence of the waters having gone or any evidence of crowning, a prolapsed cord or abnormal presenting part, such as a foot. Auscultation of the fetal heart is almost impossible in a noisy environment, and difficult to undertake successfully without regular practice.

Unless you consider the woman to be in the later stage of labour, you should make arrangements to transport her to hospital swiftly in the left lateral position. Clinically, the order of preference for places to deliver is:

- District general hospital labour suite
- General practitioner labour suite in a community hospital
- An accident and emergency department
- A community hospital minor injuries department
- The woman's home, if enough help can be mustered in time
- A general practitioner's treatment room
- The back of an ambulance
- A public place

Most types of helicopter ambulances in the UK are not suitable places for delivering a child, as access to the mother's pelvis is difficult, if not impossible. If you are some way from a hospital and the delivery is near but not imminent, think laterally. There may be alternatives to delivering in the back of the ambulance, so call for help and arrange an alternative destination as soon as possible if there is sufficient time to move the mother but not enough to reach a district general hospital. Remember, all the hospital locations listed above have nurses, all of whom have had some obstetric training, and all can provide somewhere more spacious, warmer, and better lit than the back of an ambulance in which to conduct a delivery. Arrange medical and midwifery back-up via your control.

Preparation for Delivery

If forced to conduct a delivery, there are five phases to the preparations if you have the time. If delivery is really imminent with the head crowning, it is far more important to control the

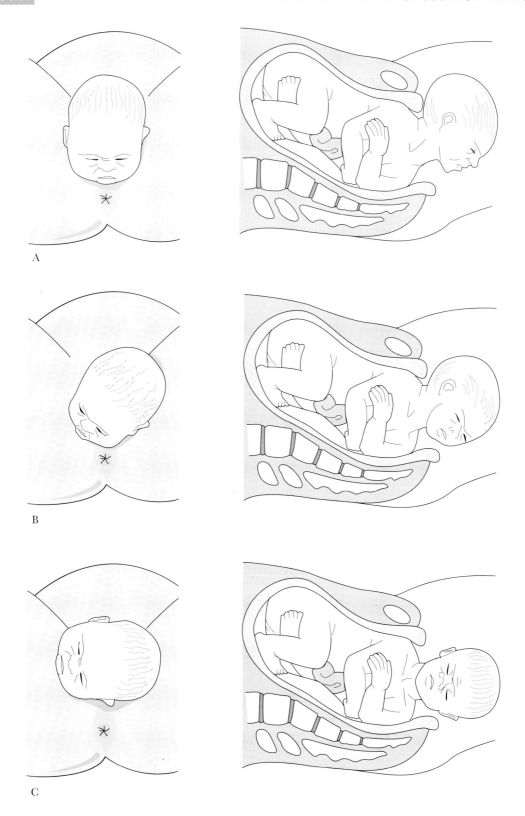

Fig. 47.11 *Delivery of the head: A, delivery; B, restitution; C, external rotation. From Miller and Callander,* Obstetrics Illustrated, *4th edn, with permission from Churchill Livingstone*

delivery than to worry about sterility, and you may only have time to put on a pair of gloves, grab a piece of gauze and place the pad over the anus with the palm of your hand, holding the gauze pad with the thumb and forefinger, pressing in the skin crease of each groin. The palm of the other hand is laid upon the crowning head, very gently providing upward pressure to encourage the head to extend and deliver. The rest of the delivery sequence is as outlined below.

If you have the time, prepare for delivery as follows.

Call for help

Call for help and back-up or, if necessary, send a reliable person with a written message to read over the telephone. Under normal circumstances your colleague should put in a call over the ambulance radio.

Preparation of the environment

Ideally, the delivery should take place somewhere warm and private, preferably with a bed or stout table on which the mother can lie. Get the maternity pack from your vehicle, together with the canvas and Incopads. Place the canvas on the bed or table, then cover the canvas with absorbent pads (e.g. Incopads) and ask mother to lie on it in the supine position and cover her with a blanket. Obtain a towel to dry the baby and preferably a second towel to wrap the baby in after drying. Additionally, if you are in a public place, move the crowds away. Wherever you are, if possible select one or two level-headed adults, preferably female; one to act as chaperone and cheerleader for the mother, and the other to act as 'gofer'. If the woman's partner is present, he can be the chaperone and comforter, but if he is too anxious to be of assistance he should be despatched to occupy himself doing something useful such as looking after the other children.

Preparation of the kit

Ensure that you have unloaded from the ambulance the maternity pack, your paramedic case, the oxygen and the nitrous oxide inhalation equipment (Entonox). Make sure everything is to hand and that the oxygen and Entonox cylinders are full and turned on. Ensure that your case is laid open in front of you so that helpers can retrieve from it any items you may require when gowned up. You may wish at this stage to cannulate the mother and have *in situ* an IV line in case of problems later.

Preparation of yourself

Remove rings, wristwatch, jacket, jerseys and other heavy clothing and remove keys and coins from your pockets. Wash your hands thoroughly, including your forearms, and get your colleague to break open your maternity pack. Depending on the contents of your pack, put on the gown. Nowadays few people bother with the mask, especially under field conditions, unless you have a cold or other infection. Put on surgical gloves.

Preparation of the mother

If there is time, have the chaperone wash the perineum with soap and water, or chlorhexidine 0.1% and water, if available. Drape the mother with sterile towels, placing one under her buttocks in a double fold. Place another towel with its edge just above the vagina with the towel lying across her abdomen. Many modern maternity packs no longer contain legging towels, but if available they may be put on. The ideal is to have sterile towels over all the field except the vagina and perineum. Your colleague can give the mother a brief tutorial on the use of the Entonox and she should be encouraged to use it at the beginning of each pain, as then the analgesic effects will be maximal at the time of maximum pain.

The Delivery

As an inexperienced *accoucheur* your aim should be simple: to achieve a safe delivery with controlled delivery of the head.

Every time the woman has a contraction she will tend to hold her breath and bear down. While preparing and in order to slow the delivery, instruct the woman to pant like a dog during pains, as this will prevent her from bearing down. In the early stages the head will come down, bulging the perineum, during contraction, but then recede during relaxation. Once the head no longer recedes during relaxations, the head has passed through the level of the pelvic floor and delivery is imminent (Figure 47.10A). If at this stage delivery of the head is not controlled, there is a risk of perineal tears. Because of the pain the woman should be encouraged to use the Entonox. It is at this stage that a doctor or midwife may consider an episiotomy, to prevent what might be an uncontrolled tear of the perineum, to protect a premature fetus or for, say, the aftercoming head in breech births. Episiotomy should not be performed by healthcare professionals without formal training in midwifery. Tears are much more likely to occur in uncontrolled, rapid births, and the risk of tears is reduced by performing episiotomy, thus increasing the size of the aperture for the head to deliver.

You should instruct the mother to pant during delivery; if she wishes to use her hands to pull her knees back onto her chest, that can be beneficial.

Take a gauze pad, preferably soaked in antiseptic, and place it in your right hand if working from the right side of mother. Hold the pad with the palm of the right hand against the anus allowing the first web space of the right hand to support the perineum with the thumb and forefinger each lying in a groin crease. Careful gentle pressure on the perineum will allow the head to deliver in a slow, controlled manner with the aim of the head delivering between labour pains. You may see a doctor or midwife at this stage applying pressure upwards using the palm of the free left hand to encourage the extension of the head on the neck to allow greater control of delivery of the head. Such additional manoeuvres are undertaken on the basis of greater experience and, often, a formal vaginal examination. To stay within National Health Service Training Directive (NHS TD) protocols, paramedics should not utilize such manoeuvres. The procedure outlined above involving only pressure on the perineum is something of a compromise in a difficult situation, but for an inexperienced *accoucheur* with only minimal obstetric and midwifery training, it is safe and allows nature to take its course. Once the head has delivered, quickly support it and then slip your fingers into the vagina and feel whether the umbilical cord is wrapped around the neck. If it is, try to slip the loop of cord off over the head. If this fails, then clamp the cord twice, cut between the clamps and unwind the cord from around the neck.

Continue by supporting the head, taking care not to put any traction on it, wipe the baby's nose and mop fluid from the mouth, clearing the face except the eyes. At the next contraction gently guide the baby's head downward towards the bed without putting any traction on the baby. This is more of a lowering manoeuvre, causing the anterior shoulder to deliver. Then, raise the baby and the posterior shoulder will deliver rapidly, followed by the rest of the trunk and legs. Allow the baby to lie on the bed and wrap it in a towel while clamping twice and cutting the umbilical cord between the clamps, close to the introitus (if this has not already been done), once the baby has cried and the cord has ceased pulsating. If the baby requires resuscitation, then double-clamp and cut the cord and proceed to resuscitation (see Chapter 50). If the baby is pinking up well and breathing, dry it off to prevent heat loss, wrap it in a dry towel and give it to mother.

At delivery of the anterior shoulder, provided it is not a multiple pregnancy, you may well see a doctor or midwife give Syntometrine intramuscularly to mother. Paramedics who have completed an emergency domestic obstetrics course may also administer this drug. Syntometrine contains oxytocin 5 units and ergometrine 0.5 mg. The oxytocin provides marked uterine contraction after approximately 3 minutes but is short-lived, and as its effects begin to wear off the ergometrine begins to act and provides longer-lasting uterine contractions, reducing the risk of post-partum haemorrhage.

Managing the Third Stage

The third stage of labour is from delivery of baby to delivery of the placenta and usually takes 5–20 minutes. Beyond 1 hour is by definition a retained placenta, which is an obstetric emergency requiring either a flying squad attendance or a transfer to an obstetric unit with anaesthetic services available. In the absence of Syntometrine following delivery, the uterus will cease contracting for a few minutes and then start contracting again regularly as the placenta separates off from the vaginal wall. Often, there is a small gush of blood and the visible length of umbilical cord will increase. The mother will then expel the placenta which should be put into a polythene bag for inspection by the doctor or midwife or at hospital. It is at this stage that haemorrhage is at the greatest risk in the absence of Syntometrine administration, and that is why a paramedic is advised if in any doubt to have an IV line *in situ*.

Doctors and midwives now manage the third stage actively, using Syntometrine, application of artery forceps on the umbilical cord, and placement of the operator's hand just above the symphysis pubis. The cord is drawn taut, but not actively pulled, using the right hand. The uterus is pushed up gently and then the left hand is pushed down onto the uterus until the placenta is seen at the introitus. The uterus is then pushed upwards and the placenta membranes will slip out of the vagina. This technique is only for experienced operators as the risks of cord avulsion or even uterine eversion are real and potentially life-threatening. As a paramedic, you must let nature take its course pending the arrival of a doctor or midwife and, in the meantime, maintain a watch for haemorrhage, acting upon the sign by instigating IV infusion rapidly, if indicated. Infuse *early* is the watchword.

After the placenta has delivered, bleeding may occur from either the uterus or the perineum or from damage to other structures in the birth canal. Place a clean pad over the vagina. If by now the doctor or midwife has failed to arrive, find out if their arrival is imminent; if not, there is a clear case for moving the woman to hospital – but there is no great urgency unless she continues to bleed.

Should the mother continue to bleed after delivery, but before the placenta delivers, then try to rub up a contraction of the uterus by vigorously massaging the uterus in a circular motion just below mother's umbilicus. Put a call out (again!) for assistance and open up the IV line which is already in place. There is a strong case for paramedics being trained and issued with Syntometrine, as post-partum haemorrhage kills. In the event of a retained placenta, or in the event of massive haemorrhage, urgent transfer to hospital will be required, although if transfer time is likely to be prolonged, medical (or midwifery) assistance (if available) might be appropriate first.

OTHER BIRTH PRESENTATIONS

By far the most common presenting part at birth is the head, but about 3% of all deliveries are breech, i.e. bottom first, and these are more common in pre-term deliveries. About 0.3% of all deliveries are shoulder presentation; another 0.3% are face presentations, and 0.1% are brow presentations. Given that the involvement of paramedics in childbirth is rare, and having to manage a delivery alone is even rarer, it is not necessary to learn the management of malpresentation in detail; such cases almost always require the skills of an obstetrician.

Breech Birth

Just occasionally, you may come across a breech birth in the second stage of labour. The management description below conforms to the NHS TD manual. As indicated earlier in the chapter, when confronted with a clinical situation to which you cannot contribute decisively, attend to those areas where you can contribute – general patient welfare, reassurance, making preparations and doing what you can to assist the maintenance of airway, breathing and circulation. Having called for help, place two IV lines and help the mother into the supported squatting, kneeling or standing position, because the aim is to have gravity aid, a much more exhausting process of delivery. If left to nature the baby will normally deliver quite easily, and should not be interfered with except to support it when free of the birth canal. A watch must be kept for a prolapsed cord where the umbilical cord drops out ahead of the baby. Alternatively, the mother may wish to labour lying down, in which case manoeuvre her so that her buttocks are at the edge of the bed. Her legs can be supported by assistants, or if there is no one, by resting them on your shoulders. Allow the baby to deliver without interference until the nape of its neck clears the pubic arch. Grasp the baby by the feet with one hand and lift the baby upright and the head will deliver. Lay the baby on the mother's abdomen. Continue as for a normal delivery, double-clamping and cutting the cord.

The method used by a midwife or doctor to conduct a breech delivery is not described, as it involves a generous episiotomy, rotation and traction of baby with Lovset's manoeuvre (see obstetric glossary) and the application of forceps to the after-coming head, and is beyond the scope of this book.

Multiple Deliveries

Multiple deliveries are not uncommon. Twins occur in about 1 in 80 pregnancies. Hopefully, with modern antenatal care, a surprise twin diagnosis at confinement is a thing of the past. Over 50% of multiple pregnancies go into premature labour, and eclampsia is three times as common, as is prolapsed umbilical cord and post-partum haemorrhage. Every effort should be made to transport to a consultant obstetric unit, or the flying squad should be called. If the first twin is delivering, then deliver as in a singleton pregnancy and set an IV line up at the earliest opportunity. If you are still on your own at this stage, wait for the second twin to deliver and then – and only then – attempt to deliver the placentae. The midwife or doctor will administer Syntometrine but *not* until the second twin delivers.

Prolapsed Umbilical Cord

Prolapsed umbilical cord is an obstetric emergency and occurs when the cord drops out of the uterus into the vagina or even outside the body ahead of the presenting part. Occasionally, the cord prolapses ahead of the presenting part with the amniotic membranes intact. Under these circumstances, there is no immediate danger. More usually, cord prolapse occurs for one of the following reasons:

- Unusual fetal presentation, e.g. footling breech or transverse lie
- Premature or abnormal fetus
- Multiple pregnancy
- Polyhydramnios (a condition where there is excessive amniotic fluid)
- Placenta praevia (see Chapter 49)

The cooling and drying effects on the umbilical cord, coupled with handling, can provoke spasm in the cord, thus cutting off the placentofetal blood supply. Occasionally, the presenting part can crush the umbilical cord against the mother's bony pelvis with a similar outcome. Out of hospital there is only one realistic course of action, and that is to obtain either gauze pads or towels soaked in warm saline, and gently replace the cord as far into the vagina as possible, with the minimum of handling. This is easier if the woman adopts the knee-elbow position. However, it is quite impossible to transport a woman in this position in a moving ambulance, especially as the doctor or midwife has to keep their gloved hand in the vagina in transit to prevent prolapse recurring. Thus, the most practical manner of transportation will be with the patient in the left lateral position. The midwife or doctor has to maintain the hand in the vagina at all times, and this means they have to jam themselves for transport in any position they can as long as their hand remains in the appropriate place. If time permits, an IV line should be inserted. Insist that the doctor and/or the midwife (if present) travel with you.

SUMMARY

The incidence of obstetric incidents in pre-hospital care is certain to rise in the UK, partly as the result of the government report on 'Changing Childbirth', which gives women much more freedom to choose where they deliver and gives the green light to midwife-only maternity units, and also because of the increasing trend towards earlier discharge from hospital. Additionally, because of the changes in the NHS concerning the free market, the purchaser-provider split and changes in hospital staffing patterns, hospital trusts are less willing and less able to provide obstetric flying squad services. General practitioners are rarely involved in intrapartum care, and apart from the time demands of such work, many are wary of undertaking work with such high medicolegal risks, especially as the falling birth rate means that even willing general practitioners will have insufficient experience of intrapartum obstetrics.

Paramedics by default are likely to transport an increasing number of obstetric cases, but the actual number requiring intervention will be small. Such is the nature of obstetric work that the only realistic approach to paramedic involvement in intrapartum care is to 'let nature take its course'. It is neither appropriate nor possible for paramedical workers to take any other approach to the problem at current resource and demand levels.

As with other areas of paramedic activity, true professionals will take the trouble to read beyond the level of their permitted practice to better understand the rationale behind that practice.

Reference to an undergraduate obstetric or midwifery textbook will pay dividends and reinforce the concept that for the inexperienced *accoucheur* the policy of letting nature take its course, coupled with skilled observation, is the only realistic approach to childbirth.

chapter forty-eight:

EMERGENCIES IN PREGNANCY

Pregnancy should be considered in any woman of reproductive age; not every woman will admit to, or even realize, that she is pregnant, for various reasons, including fear, denial or social stigma.

Pregnancy itself is not an illness, but there are medical conditions and emergencies specific to the pregnant state which must be considered in the context of pre-hospital care, as well as general emergencies that occur in any patient, for example asthma or epilepsy, which may have their assessment and management altered by pregnancy.

The most common reasons for calling the emergency services in early pregnancy are vaginal bleeding, abdominal pain, or both.

VAGINAL BLEEDING AND ABDOMINAL PAIN IN EARLY PREGNANCY

A brief history should be taken by the attending paramedic to corroborate the possibility of pregnancy in the woman complaining of abdominal pain or vaginal bleeding. A high index of suspicion can be gained simply from finding out the date of the last menstrual period (LMP). Any regularly menstruating woman whose LMP was more than 4 weeks prior to the current date is likely to be pregnant. If the LMP was normal and occurred more than 4 weeks prior to the onset of the current problems, the patient should be considered to be pregnant until proved otherwise.

Once the possibility of pregnancy is suggested by the history, or confirmed by the patient, vital signs should be measured (pulse, blood pressure, respiratory rate), to assess whether the patient is clinically hypovolaemic; if any signs suggest hypovolaemia is present, then intravenous access should be obtained, and fluid infusion started.

The most frequent cause of vaginal bleeding with or without abdominal pain early in pregnancy is miscarriage. The most dangerous cause of vaginal bleeding and abdominal pain is ectopic pregnancy, and this should be considered in any woman of reproductive age complaining of abdominal pain, especially if this is associated with collapse.

> Always consider ectopic pregnancy as a cause of collapse or abdominal pain in women of childbearing age

Miscarriage

Approximately 10–15% of confirmed pregnancies end in miscarriage. This occurs most often at either 8 weeks or 12 weeks from the first day of the LMP. There are several postulated causes of miscarriages, but most are due to a genetic defect in the fetus or uterine abnormalities. Many threatened miscarriages may settle spontaneously and lead to a normal pregnancy and subsequent delivery of a normal infant. Miscarriage may, however, cause significant uterine bleeding resulting in hypovolaemic shock.

Terminology

Threatened miscarriage In a threatened miscarriage, vaginal bleeding is associated with cramping abdominal pain; the cervix remains closed, and pregnancy may progress normally.

Incomplete miscarriage In an incomplete miscarriage vaginal bleeding may be heavy, the cervix is open and abdominal pain is caused by uterine contractions which have begun to expel the products of conception.

Complete miscarriage In a complete miscarriage, the products are completely expelled through an open cervix.

Symptoms and signs

The patient may be known to be pregnant, or admit to being late with a period. There may be a history of previous miscarriage; she will be complaining of vaginal blood loss, and may have lower abdominal cramping pain.

There may be obvious external signs of vaginal bleeding associated with varying degrees of shock; measurement of pulse, blood pressure and respiratory rate are mandatory.

Management

Many women will naturally be anxious at the prospect of a miscarriage, and gentle handling and reassurance are very important during the initial assessment and transfer into hospital for more detailed examination and management.

If signs of hypovolaemia are present or there is a history of significant blood loss, intravenous access should be established, fluid infusion started, and oxygen given.

On arrival in hospital the patient will be assessed fully by the receiving doctor, including vaginal examination and ultrasound scanning, to confirm pregnancy and determine the viability of the fetus.

Ectopic pregnancy

Ectopic pregnancy is the most life-threatening of the early complications of pregnancy; the incidence of ectopic pregnancy is approximately 1% of all pregnancies and is increasing. Ruptured ectopic pregnancies account for 13% of maternal deaths and are the leading cause of maternal death in the first trimester, although the death rate is falling due to improved awareness, early diagnostic facilities and improved management. An ectopic pregnancy normally occurs in one or other of the fallopian tubes; predisposition will occur in women with a history of pelvic inflammatory disease, previous ectopic pregnancy and in those who use the intrauterine contraceptive device (IUCD, or 'coil').

Symptoms and signs

Most tubal ectopic pregnancies occur 5–8 weeks after the LMP. Pain is a symptom in 95% of patients, and 75% complain of abnormal vaginal bleeding.

The pain is felt in the lower abdomen, and may be localized to one side early in the condition. The pain usually precedes the vaginal bleeding, unlike a miscarriage, when vaginal bleeding precedes pain (Table 48.1).

In the condition's most dramatic form the patient may present in a state of collapse secondary to hypovolaemic shock, and the diagnosis must be considered in any woman of reproductive age who presents in this way. More commonly, the patient exhibits less marked degrees of shock including tachycardia and tachypnoea, with or without hypotension. Pallor may be prominent. There will be abdominal tenderness, and a reluctance to move, since movement will exacerbate the pain.

Management

Ectopic pregnancy is a gynaecological emergency. The patient must be transferred as soon as possible to hospital for further assessment by the receiving doctor.

Table 48.1 Differential diagnosis of miscarriage and ectopic pregnancy

	Miscarriage	Ectopic pregnancy
Timing	5–12 weeks	5–8 weeks
Abdominal pain	Central, cramping Follows bleeding	May be unilateral Precedes bleeding
Vaginal bleeding	Frank blood loss May be heavy	Normally scanty Dark brown
Haemodynamic status	Shock uncommon	Shock common

Shock should be treated aggressively in a conventional manner: oxygen should be administered, two large-bore (14 G) intravenous cannulae inserted into the antecubital fossae, and fluid resuscitation commenced.

> **Do not delay transfer while struggling to obtain intravenous access**

On arrival in hospital, the patient's pregnancy will be confirmed by clinical examination and ultrasound scan and will then be managed surgically.

VAGINAL BLEEDING AND ABDOMINAL PAIN IN LATER PREGNANCY

Third trimester vaginal bleeding (antepartum haemorrhage) is bleeding that occurs from 28 weeks of pregnancy. It occurs in approximately 4% of pregnancies; the two most common causes are placental abruption and placenta praevia. All patients with antepartum haemorrhage must be assessed in hospital.

Placental Abruption

Placental abruption is the separation of a normally located placenta before delivery of the fetus. Bleeding occurs and the blood is initially confined between the placenta and the uterine wall (Figure 48.1).

Symptoms and signs

Placental abruption may present in its most severe form with painful vaginal bleeding associated with a tender, contracting uterus, shock and fetal compromise. Most women, however, do not present with so dramatic a picture; they complain of abdominal pain, usually of sudden onset, with or without vaginal bleeding.

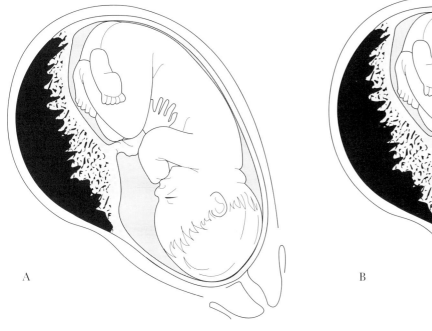
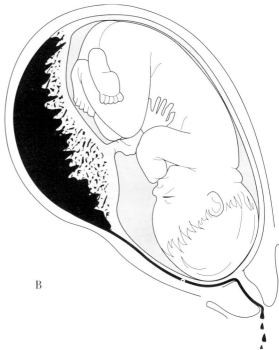

A   B

Fig. 48.1 *Placental abruption: haemorrhage may be concealed (A) or revealed (B)*

Management

Any woman in the later stages of pregnancy with abdominal pain and vaginal bleeding should be considered to have a placental abruption, since this is potentially dangerous for both mother and baby. Expeditious transfer to an obstetric unit or hospital is appropriate.

Observation of vital signs will indicate any degree of shock and the need for intravenous access and fluid resuscitation, following the administration of oxygen.

The stable patient will be fully assessed on arrival in hospital, and continued observation may be appropriate. If the patient is shocked, or has deteriorating vital signs in transit, appropriate warning to the receiving obstetric unit or hospital should be given, enabling staff to prepare for urgent delivery of the baby.

Placenta Praevia

Placenta praevia occurs when the placenta is implanted in the lower uterine segment (Figure 48.2), and subsequent separation will cause blood loss into the vagina. Patients present with vaginal bleeding, which may be heavy, but may have little or no abdominal pain. The patient should be transferred to hospital for full assessment. The need for fluid resuscitation in transit will be determined by the amount of blood loss and the vital signs.

HYPERTENSIVE EMERGENCIES IN PREGNANCY

Eclampsia

Hypertensive disorders complicate approximately 8% of pregnancies; the most severe manifestation is *eclampsia*, in which a combination of hypertension, cerebral oedema, haemorrhage and seizures may be fatal for mother and baby. It results in the death of about 1000 babies and 10 women each year in the UK.

Symptoms and signs

Clinical features of eclampsia
- Hypertension
- Cerebral oedema and haemorrhage
- Seizures
- Headaches
- Visual disturbance
- Weight gain and peripheral oedema
- Abdominal pain

Patients will normally have a known history of hypertension in

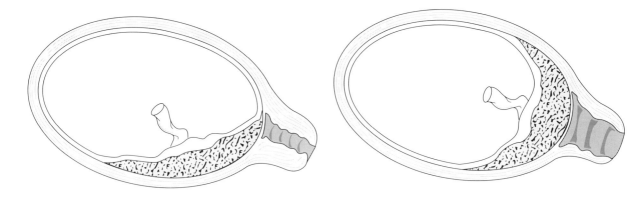

Fig. 48.2 *Placenta praevia: the placenta may partly or completely cover the uterine opening*

their pregnancy. Prior to the onset of seizures there may have been headache, visual disturbance, abdominal pain, weight gain and swelling of the peripheries. On examination, the patient may be fitting, will be hypertensive, and will have peripheral oedema.

Management

Urgent transfer to hospital is essential, since definitive treatment comprises urgent delivery of the baby. If there is fitting, the first priority is to establish an airway and ensure that the patient is adequately oxygenated for transit into hospital; in a fitting patient, often the most practical means of achieving an airway is nasopharyngeal intubation. Paramedics who have completed the emergency domestic obstetrics course are able to administer intravenous diazepam to control the fits.

Oxygen should be administered via a face mask with reservoir bag if available. Rectal diazepam (10 mg) should be given in an attempt to terminate the seizures; if fitting stops, intravenous access can be established to allow subsequent drug administration in hospital. The receiving obstetric unit or hospital should be alerted so that an appropriately experienced team can be awaiting arrival of the patient.

COMMON GENERAL MEDICAL EMERGENCIES IN PREGNANCY

A pregnant woman may have pre-existing illness which may present acutely with an exacerbation while she is pregnant; examples are asthma, epilepsy and diabetes mellitus. It is always important to bear the pregnancy in mind when managing these emergencies, but common sense and first principles apply, and these are the same whether the patient is pregnant or not.

Asthma

The effect of pregnancy on asthma is variable. The majority of patients experience less frequent attacks, but a few experience more frequent attacks. Asthma has no effect on the course of pregnancy. The management of an acute exacerbation is the same as in a non-pregnant woman, with oxygen, nebulized salbutamol and transfer to hospital for assessment.

Epilepsy

Seizures may occur in pregnancy unrelated to hypertension, simply as a manifestation of pre-existing epilepsy. Treatment regimens may have been modified prior to or early in pregnancy, and control may have been lost. Management of a seizure will be conventional and consists of prevention of harm to the patient during a seizure, attention to the airway, administration of oxygen, rectal diazepam (10 mg) if the fit is prolonged, and transfer to hospital.

Diabetes mellitus

When a diabetic woman becomes pregnant, close attention is required to maintain good control of the disease throughout the pregnancy. Hypoglycaemic and hyperglycaemic emergencies may occur and will be rapidly identified clinically using a glucose reagent strip. The most effective treatment for a hypoglycaemic emergency is intravenous glucose (in a dose of 50 ml of a 50% solution). Glucagon (1 mg) given intramuscularly is an alternative. Patients with hyperglycaemic emergencies should receive oxygen, fluid resuscitation with normal saline, and be transferred immediately to hospital.

chapter forty-nine:

TRAUMA IN PREGNANCY

A full understanding of the management of trauma in pregnancy requires complete familiarity with the anatomical and physiological changes that occur during pregnancy, and the ability to integrate the consequences of these changes into the philosophy of the consistent pattern of care expounded throughout this book – i.e. personal safety, scene safety, victim safety, primary survey and resuscitation according to the 'ABCDE' procedure, and constant re-evaluation *en route* to hospital. Because many of the physical signs of shock and haemorrhage only present late in the pregnant woman, a thorough understanding of the mechanism of trauma and a proper history are vital.

The approach to the pregnant trauma victim is exactly the same as for the non-pregnant trauma victim except that there are two victims – mother and fetus – to consider. The mother is treated directly, the fetus is treated indirectly by optimum resuscitation of the mother. The mother is the best incubator for the fetus, and in the pre-hospital situation a dead mother means a dead fetus. Trauma in pregnancy is always a highly charged emotional situation, and by adhering to the same conventional pattern of care as for the non-pregnant trauma victim, the chances of success are optimized.

According to American studies 7% of all pregnant women sustain trauma, the vast majority resulting from road accidents, followed by falls, penetrating injury and thermal injuries including smoke inhalation.

The anatomical and physiological changes in pregnancy were outlined in Chapter 47 but they are so crucial to the proper management of the pregnant trauma victim that they are restated here.

ANATOMICAL CHANGES

The anatomical factors in pregnancy include the presence of a full dentition, a relatively short obese neck and engorged breast tissue. Internally there is oedema of the upper airway, increased fat deposition especially around the face and neck, and increased

fragility of the mucous membranes making them liable to bleed. All of these features conspire to make intubation and airway maintenance more difficult and cause difficulty in the sizing and fitting of cervical collars.

As the uterus enlarges it changes from being a thick-walled organ protected deep within the pelvic cavity before 12 weeks of gestation, becoming progressively more thin-walled as pregnancy advances. Between 12 and 24 weeks the fetus is protected by the relatively large volume of amniotic fluid within the uterus, but in the third trimester as the fetus grows, the relative volume of cushioning amniotic fluid decreases and the uterine wall becomes thinner. After 34 weeks, before the fetal head engages in the maternal pelvis, the uterine fundus continues to grow, expanding further and further into the abdominal cavity until at 34 weeks the fundus is some 34 cm above the pubic bone. Under these circumstances the intestines are pushed ever further upwards, the diaphragm becomes splinted because of increasing abdominal cavity volume and the lower ribs become flared out, reducing the functional residual capacity of the lungs and the compliance of the chest wall. The splinting of the diaphragm and reduced compliance of the chest wall due to splaying of the ribs make ventilation difficult and, together with engorgement of the breasts, hinder external chest compression.

Other anatomical changes in pregnancy include enlargement of the pituitary gland which makes it more susceptible to decelerative head injuries. The urinary bladder is pulled up out of the bony pelvis during the third trimester and is therefore more liable to be damaged.

PHYSIOLOGICAL CHANGES

Relaxation of the gastro-oesophageal junction, delayed gastric emptying and increasing intragastric pressure from the compressive effects of increasing uterine size raise the potential for reflux acid regurgitation with aspiration of stomach contents into the lungs, and are part of the rationale behind the recommendation to secure the airway definitively by early endo-tracheal intubation.

Fetal tissue has a high oxygen consumption and maternal oxygen requirements are increased because of hypertrophied breast and uterine tissue coupled with the need to meet the metabolic requirements that the extra 12.5 kg of tissues of a term pregnancy demand. However, functional residual capacity and chest compliance are reduced, so demands are met by increased ventilation through a 40% rise in tidal volume, although the respiratory rate remains unchanged. Thus, just when there is a need to satisfy a high oxygen requirement, the means to deliver this requirement are stretched and while adequate in the fit, healthy mother are easily overtaxed in the traumatized mother. Thus the spontaneously breathing pregnant trauma victim must *always* receive high-flow oxygen at as high a concentration as possible, preferably close to 100% via a reservoir face mask. If there are any doubts as to the adequacy of ventilation or questions of airway compromise, then early intubation and early intermittent positive pressure ventilation are indicated. The altered chest dynamics can make observation of respiratory excursion difficult.

Always give oxygen – supplement ventilation early

In relation to trauma the most important physiological changes in pregnancy concern the cardiovascular system. The cardiac output rises by 40% through a combination of a rise in resting heart rate of 15–20 beats per minute and by an increased stroke volume achieved by hypertrophy of the cardiac muscle and enlargement of the cardiac chambers:

Physiological changes in pregnancy

- Cardiac output increases by 40%
- Resting heart rate increases by 15–20 beats/min
- Cardiac muscle hypertrophy
- Increase in cardiac chamber size
- Increase in circulating blood volume by 50%

During pregnancy the circulating blood volume increases massively by about 50% to service the increased demands of the hypotrophied breast and uterine tissue, increased renal demands and the enormous low pressure shunt of the placental bed. The placenta itself has a circulatory demand of approximately 600 ml per minute – or 10% of the maternal circulation.

Although the circulating blood volume increases by 50% there is no corresponding increase in oxygen-carrying capacity

There is thus a physiological anaemia of pregnancy. The anaemia results in reduced blood viscosity which manifests itself

as a reduced peripheral resistance (and therefore reduced cardiac work) and is reflected in the reduced diastolic blood pressure.

The normal physiological reserves to cope with stresses are already in action during pregnancy to keep the demands on the heart within manageable limits. Should the pregnant woman suffer blood loss of any significance, she has few physiological reserves to bring into play, and this is why pregnant women show few premonitory clinical signs before passing almost immediately into often irretrievable grade III or IV hypovolaemic shock.

Have a high index of suspicion for concealed haemorrhage

A high index of suspicion for both concealed and revealed haemorrhage is therefore vital, especially because initially vasodilation and increased overall blood volume cause both skin colour and capillary refill to remain within normal limits. Hypovolaemic shock in pregnancy can also cause necrosis of the anterior pituitary gland, giving rise to pituitary insufficiency with multiple endocrine problems which require lifelong replacement of thyroxine and steroid therapy.

In the third trimester of pregnancy the gravid uterus presses on the inferior vena cava reducing venous return to the heart, thus reducing cardiac output (Starling's law – see Chapter 10) by up to 40% and inducing maternal hypotension. This leads to reduced maternal cardiac and cerebral perfusion pressure and reduced uteroplacental perfusion, compromising the fetus as well. The hypotension so induced also releases catecholamines which further diminish uteroplacental circulation. When maternal resuscitation is attempted it should be remembered that fully efficient basic life support gives at best 30% of cardiac output. Thus resuscitation attempts in the pregnant woman will fail unless caval compression is relieved by nursing the woman in the left lateral or left lateral decubitus position (Figure 49.1). There are three ways that caval compression can be relieved:

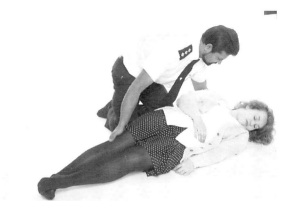

Fig. 49.1 *Maintaining the left lateral position*

- Manually, by holding the uterus over to the left
- By a sandbag or pillow under the right buttock
- By nursing the patient on a long spinal board tilted 25–30 degrees to the left

The first method will occupy an assistant who might be useful in other ways; sandbags or pillows may compromise a spinal injury; so use of a spinal board is the method of choice. A scoop stretcher is not adequate for this purpose as it is unable to take the force of external chest compressions. A tilt of 25–30 degrees is required to decompress the inferior vena cava. There is no place for the Cardiff wedge in pre-hospital care. Where access is difficult the use of the human wedge can be considered (Figure 49.2).

The patient is 'log rolled' to the left, and then one or two rescuers kneel down with their knees a few centimetres away from the patient's right side. The patient is then gently 'log rolled' back onto the laps of the rescuers. It is possible to perform external chest compressions from this position but not expired air respirations, so there would need to be at least three rescuers for this technique.

The relief of hypoxia and hypovolaemia in the pregnant trauma victim is as urgent as in the non-pregnant victim. However, by the time hypovolaemia manifests itself with clinical signs

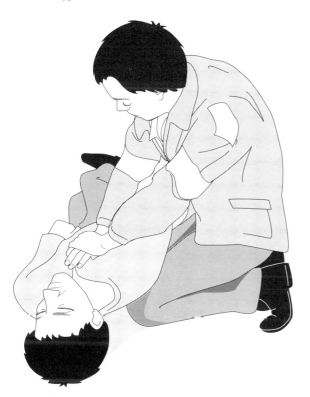

Fig. 49.2 The human wedge

(30–40% haemorrhage), the fetus will be severely compromised. Losses of only 10–20% of circulatory blood volume markedly reduce uterine perfusion, and the only sign of fetal distress may be fetal bradycardia of 110 beats per minute or less. Attempting to listen for a fetal heart at the roadside or other noisy environment is unlikely to be helpful. The chances of fetal survival fall rapidly, and unless the fetus is delivered by caesarean section within about 20 minutes of the failure of uterine circulation death of the fetus is inevitable. The practical implication of this fact is that in the severely injured, unentrapped mother whose survival may be questionable, if the hospital facility able to perform an emergency caesarean section is less than 20 minutes away, the decision must be 'load and go'. There is no justification whatsoever to 'stay and play'. Interventions including cannulation must be carried out in transit.

It is important to radio ahead so that an obstetric team can be ready on arrival. Time is of the essence; definitive treatment is not possible in the back of an ambulance, and for both mother and baby the *only* chance is immediate caesarean section. Your duty is to get the mother to a surgeon as quickly as possible in order to save the child.

THE APPROACH TO THE PREGNANT TRAUMA VICTIM

The approach to the pregnant trauma victim is exactly the same as to the non-pregnant victim. Call for help, and assess your own safety, the safety of the scene and the safety of the victim in that order. During the process of primary survey and resuscitation try to obtain an accurate history of events with special reference to the mechanisms of injury and the sequence of the accident.

- Call for help
- Safety
- Primary survey and resuscitation
- Evacuation and secondary survey

The history is important because maternal clinical signs of hypotension and haemorrhage present too late to save the fetus in 80% of cases, and unnecessary damage is caused to the mother while this haemorrhage and hypotension remain unrecognized. The only means of making such a diagnosis in the field is to think of the possible mechanisms of injury and maintain a high index of suspicion. Thus treatment precedes formal definitive diagnosis.

Treatment precedes formal diagnosis

The mother is the best and most natural transport incubator for the fetus, but physiologically the mother will always sacrifice the fetus to preserve her own life. Fetal distress will ensue after loss of only 10–20% of maternal blood volume, as at this point material compensatory mechanisms restrict blood flow to the uterus. Signs of maternal hypotension, however, will only declare themselves suddenly at 35% blood loss. The only indication of fetal distress detectable in the field is a fetal bradycardia of under 110 beats per minute, and in a noisy environment this may be difficult if not impossible to detect.

Assess and stabilize the mother first

Assessment and stabilization of mother conforms to the standard primary survey and resuscitation pattern outlined in Chapters 2 and 31, with particular attention to early oxygenation, intubation if the patient is unconscious, and relief of venal caval compression:

- High-flow oxygen
- Early intubation if unconscious
- Relief of vena caval compression

As part of the identification of life-threatening haemorrhage, look at but *do not* digitally examine the vagina and perineum. Look for bleeding or fluid from the vagina or urethra and any signs of bruising or bulging of the perineum.

Do not perform a vaginal examination

Remember that concealed blood loss is common and threatens both the fetus and the mother.

An attempt should be made to palpate the abdomen. Check for fetal parts, movements and the fetal heart rate if possible. Do not waste undue time on this part of the assessment, attend to mother's resuscitation first and seek expert help for both mother and fetus. Remember to ensure relief of vena caval compression.

Resuscitation of the mother takes precedence

It is important to remember that, except in the case of burns, pregnancy itself does not increase maternal morbidity from trauma. It is the consequence of unrecognized haemorrhage, hypovolaemia, hypotension and hypoxia which result from pregnancy masking their normal clinical signs and failure by the rescuer to understand the implications of the altered anatomy and physiology of pregnancy that increase maternal morbidity in the pregnant trauma victim.

CONSEQUENCES OF TRAUMA IN PREGNANCY

Discussion of the trauma consequences on the pregnant patient

is confined to the effects of trauma on the abdomen and pelvis; in pre-hospital care the treatment of trauma elsewhere in the body is the same as for the non-pregnant patient.

A pregnant woman sustaining *any* trauma to the abdomen and pelvis, however minor, requires specialist assessment and observation at hospital. Even small degrees of abdominal trauma can cause sufficient placental leakage for the maternal circulation to be contaminated by fetal red blood cells. As a consequence, maternal antibody formation against fetal red cells may result in fetal anaemia and problems with future pregnancies. The incidence of fetomaternal haemorrhage is raised fivefold in the face of trauma; this is the rationale behind taking samples of blood for Kleihauer testing for Rhesus status as well as for cross-matching when cannulating.

Blunt Trauma

Blunt trauma to the abdomen and pelvis is more common than penetrating trauma in UK practice, and in the pregnant woman is caused by:

> road traffic accidents
> falls
> assaults

Unsteadiness in late pregnancy increases the risk of falling. There is no doubt that any risk of injury to the pregnant passenger caused by the wearing of a seat-belt is far outweighed by the reduction in risk from ejection or impaction.

In any abdominal injury never forget the concept of concealed haemorrhage, be it from ruptured liver or spleen, retroperitoneal bleed or a concealed placental abruption. All these injuries are time critical and need a surgeon urgently.

Remember concealed haemorrhage

The three most common mechanisms of injury in blunt abdominopelvic trauma in the pregnant mother are:

- Placental abruption
- Uterine rupture
- Pelvic fracture

In each of these mechanisms of injury there is the potential for fetal injury, and in each both mother and fetus may die from unrecognized, often concealed, hypovolaemic shock resulting from haemorrhage.

Placental abruption

The uterine wall near term is relatively thin, elastic and muscular; adhering to the inside surface of the uterine wall is the placenta, which is relatively inelastic. Direct trauma to the

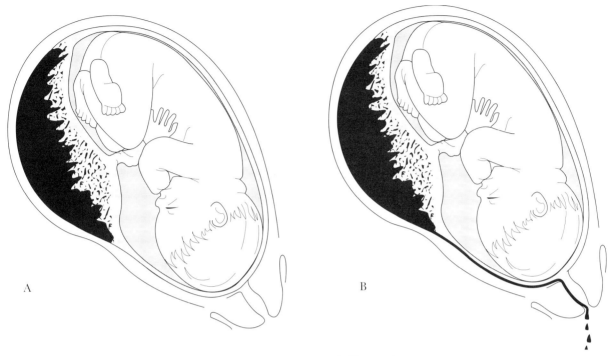

Fig. 49.3 *Placental abruption (traumatic): A, concealed haemorrhage; B, revealed haemorrhage*

abdominal wall transmitted to the uterus, or deceleration forces applied to the body as a whole, may cause the placenta to shear off the uterine wall (Figure 49.3). Haemorrhage occurs between the placenta and the uterine wall and may be concealed or revealed (*per vaginam*). This haemorrhage will strip further areas of the placenta from the uterine wall, thus increasing the bleeding.

Maternal blood flow to the placenta is approximately 600 ml per minute at term or 10% of the mother's circulating volume. At 10–20% maternal haemorrhage, blood flow to the uterus is shut down and time-critical fetal distress ensues. Beyond 20 minutes few babies will survive. At the site of placental abruption, in addition to the possibility of fetomaternal haemorrhage, substances are released into the maternal circulation which will predispose toward disseminated intravascular coagulation. Amniotic fluid embolism is also a recognized complication of placental abruption. The immediate care of both conditions is early, adequate resuscitation.

Symptoms and signs of placental abruption

- History of trauma
- Tender uterus (may feel 'woody')
- Steady (usually lower abdominal) pain
- Shock (maternal)
- Vaginal bleeding (variable)
- Fetal distress
- Premature labour
- Increasing fundal height

Placental abruption occurs in as many as 5% of episodes of minor trauma and 50% of major trauma cases, and can occur up to 48 hours after trauma. An adequate history and high index of suspicion are vital. Remember that maternal hypovolaemic shock may only reveal its presence at a late stage, and that vaginal bleeding may be absent. Premature labour may be precipitated by placental abruption.

In the late presentation of placental abruption the mother may report reduced fetal movements or no fetal movements at all. In the short period of pre-hospital care, the expanding fundal height which reflects increased bleeding into the uterus may not be seen; however, as a baseline for other carers you should mark on the abdomen the fundal height when you first assess the mother and note if the fundal height exceeds that appropriate for the gestation period.

Uterine rupture

Uterine rupture is much rarer than abruption; it requires considerable direct force, and will almost inevitably be associated with other life-threatening injuries. It is only in the absence of trauma that the milder, non-specific presentation of uterine rupture may occur.

Signs of uterine rupture include maternal shock, fetal

bradycardia (or absence of fetal heart sounds) and obvious palpable fetal parts on abdominal examination. There may or may not be vaginal bleeding or abdominal pain.

In the third trimester of pregnancy, stretching of the peritoneum by the enlarging uterus reduces its sensitivity to pain and abdominal pain, particularly in the presence of other painful injuries, may not be apparent.

Symptoms and signs of uterine rupture

- Maternal shock
- Fetal bradycardia or absence of fetal heart sounds
- Palpable fetal parts
- Vaginal bleeding (variable)
- Abdominal pain (variable)

Pelvic fracture

Even in non-pregnant patients pelvic fractures produce considerable blood loss. In the pregnant state the pelvic venous plexuses are markedly engorged and pelvic trauma may lead to massive bleeding from low-volume capacitance vessels, this bleeding being difficult to control. The usual causes of pelvic fractures are falls from a height and road traffic accidents. The signs are those of massive maternal haemorrhagic shock. This is a desperate situation. Time is of the essence and copious IV fluids are indicated, although transfer to hospital must *never* be delayed while intravenous access is attained. The standard resuscitation routine is inaugurated and consideration should be given to inflation of the leg compartments only of a pneumatic anti-shock garment. Definitive surgery (external pelvic fixation) is the patient's only hope.

Blunt trauma and pregnancy summary

All pregnant patients sustaining blunt trauma need hospital assessment. In the pre-hospital environment initial assessment should take place simultaneously with vigorous resuscitation. Under no circumstances should transfer to definitive surgical care be delayed. The priorities in the pregnant patient are identical to those in the non-pregnant patient.

Penetrating trauma

Penetrating trauma is rarer in Europe than in America. Within the UK penetrating trauma is largely from stab wounds (impalement injuries and road traffic accidents excepted). Gunshot wounds are more common in other parts of the world, and the nature of the injury will depend on the type of missile and its velocity. Nevertheless, the gravid fluid and fetus-filled uterus protects abdominal viscera and can absorb considerable quantities of kinetic energy. The usual outcome is fetal death with maternal survival. As far as pre-hospital care is concerned,

the approach is the same as for the non-pregnant woman, with a continuous watch for concealed haemorrhage and the possibility of time-critical but concealed injury to other organs. Attention to airway, breathing and circulation (ABC) and rapid transport are essential.

Burns

The management of pregnant patients with burns is exactly the same as for non-pregnant patients, except that they must be taken to a facility where caesarean section can be performed. As with all burns, check that the environment is safe for you to approach (remembering the dangers of a noxious atmosphere), ensure that the fire is out, and that any burning or chemically contaminated clothing is removed. Once the patient is removed to a safe environment the use of humidified oxygen and early intubation are essential. Remember that there may have been an explosion during the fire and the patient may also show the effects of blunt trauma. Because of the metabolic and fluid requirements of the pregnant and burnt woman, delivery by caesarean section is often the only option. The mortality rates in pregnant women depend on the body surface area burnt: in those with burns of 33–66% of body surface area, survival will depend crucially on the early management of hypoxia and hypovolaemia.

SUMMARY

The treatment of the pregnant trauma victim is the same as for the non-pregnant victim, remembering that:

- There are two patients, mother and fetus
- The only way to save both is to save the mother first
- You should always assess and stabilize the mother first
- The physiological changes of pregnancy require careful and prompt attention to oxygenation and fluid replacement
- Haemorrhage is frequently concealed in the pregnant victim and hypovolaemic shock is inevitably severe once the signs manifest
- Failure to relieve venal caval compression kills mother and fetus
- The pregnant trauma victim should always be considered to have time-critical injuries and be transported to a surgical facility quickly
- Obstetric and gynaecological diagnoses need not be made in the field

Treatment precedes diagnosis

chapter fifty

NEONATAL RESUSCITATION AND TRANSPORT

The paramedic may be faced with illness or cardiac arrest in a neonate (i.e. a baby less than 1 month old) in a range of situations: for example, a planned home delivery, an unplanned birth before arrival in hospital, or in an infant who has a normal birth and is discharged home (usually after 48 hours in a maternity unit) and thereafter becomes ill. Regardless of the situation the general principles remain the same – i.e. support of airway, breathing and circulation.

NEONATAL RESUSCITATION

The paramedic faced with a baby born outside hospital has two patients to look after – the mother and the baby. In most instances the baby will not require any advanced interventions. If the baby is active with normal respiratory rate and heart rate, then the only treatment required will be to dry and warm the baby, and to use suction as required.

However, a small number of babies will require more active resuscitative measures. In practice it is more likely that the paramedic will need to deal with an ill neonate rather than a full cardiorespiratory arrest; this chapter therefore concentrates on the approach to serious illness.

The first instance is where there has been fetal distress during labour and the amniotic fluid surrounding the baby has become contaminated with meconium from the baby. If this occurs, as soon as the baby is born, it will require active and vigorous suction to ensure that no meconium is aspirated into the trachea and lower airways, as the morbidity and mortality rates from meconium aspiration syndrome remain high.

In the second instance there is no evidence of meconium, but the baby at birth fails to respond properly and has difficulties maintaining respiration and circulation. The Apgar scoring system (Table 50.1) assesses the baby's overall condition at 1 minute and 5 minutes after birth and later if required. Resuscitative measures should be started immediately, however, and not delayed for evaluation of the Apgar score.

If the neonate has clear cardiorespiratory difficulties or a full arrest, then resuscitative measures must begin. If the child has a low respiratory or cardiac rate, then the first measure would be to stimulate the child, which occurs during drying and warming, and during suctioning. This is often enough to increase the child's respiratory rate, which as a result of better oxygenation increases the cardiac rate. However, if after a short period of stimulation the clinical situation remains grave, the next measure is to maintain the airway by placing the baby in a supine position with the neck in a neutral position, thus avoiding hyperextension. At this point supplemental oxygen via a face mask can be applied, with further suction if copious secretions are seen in the oropharynx. Again, the hoped-for result is improved respiratory effort and consequently increased cardiac output.

If the infant fails to respond to these measures it will be necessary to ventilate the baby using a self-inflating bag and mask.

Table 50.1 Apgar scoring

Sign	0	1	2
Heart rate (beats/min)	Absent	Slow (less than 100)	Greater than 100
Respirations	Absent	Slow, irregular	Good, crying
Muscle tone	Limp	Some flexion	Active motion
Reflex irritability (catheter in nares)	No response	Grimace	Cough or sneeze
Colour	Blue or pale	Pink body with blue extremities	Completely pink

Care needs to be taken not to overinflate the lungs as the infant is at risk of barotrauma, which could lead to a pneumothorax. For the neonate, the smallest self-inflating bag is used, commonly the 240 ml capacity bag. These bags have a pressure limiting valve which allows non-inflating pressures of 30–40 cmH$_2$O. The bags have a special pop-off valve which the operator can override in special circumstances, such as the infant with stiff lungs.

The paramedic should ventilate at a rate of 60 breaths per minute for approximately 15–30 seconds. The pulse is then checked to see if the rate has reached at least 100 per minute. If the neonate again fails to respond, i.e. the pulse rate remains at less than 60 per minute or ceases, then chest compressions will be the next step. These compressions are achieved as described in Chapter 35, namely two-finger compression using the ring and middle fingers on the sternum of the neonate just below the nipple line. Another technique for chest compression in the neonate is to place both thumbs on the middle third of the sternum with the fingers of both hands encircling the chest and supporting the back. In either event, the sternum should be compressed 100–120 times per minute. The normally recommended cycle for chest compressions to ventilation is 3 to 1 for a neonate as opposed to the 5 to 1 for infants and older children.

If these measures are unsuccessful and the neonate fails to respond, or indeed goes into full cardiopulmonary arrest, it will be necessary to use more advanced life support techniques. The paramedic may elect to intubate the child to improve ventilation and to secure the airway against inhalation. The usual size of an ET tube for a term baby is 3–3.5 mm. The next step for advanced life support would be to achieve vascular access either through a peripheral vein or (if the paramedic has the necessary skill) through cannulation of the umbilical vein. If vascular access cannot be achieved by either of these methods, then it is possible to insert an intraosseous needle into the tibia of the neonate and gain access by this route (Chapter 6).

Drugs that may be used in advanced life support include adrenaline: in asystole or profound bradycardia the dose is 0.01 mg/kg (0.1 ml/kg) of adrenaline 1 in 10,000 solution. This dose may be repeated every 3 minutes if required. Neonates born after showing signs of fetal distress during labour are usually acidotic and may require sodium bicarbonate at a dose of 1 mmol/kg, which is equivalent to 2 ml/kg sodium bicarbonate 4.2 solution. In addition to drugs, it is sometimes necessary to give the neonate a fluid challenge. This may be achieved by giving 10–20 ml/kg of either normal saline or a 0.45% solution if available.

Two other points worth considering in neonatal resuscitation are that the neonate has poor mechanisms of maintaining its temperature and will quickly become cold during a resuscitation attempt. This does not aid the chances of successful resuscitation and therefore care should be taken to maintain the child's temperature by using warm blankets, etc. Neonates, especially if born small for dates or preterm, have difficulty in maintaining their blood glucose levels and may become hypoglycaemic. Thus it is worth checking the glucose level in blood taken from the ear lobe; if it is low, glucose in a 10% or 25% solution can be given, usually at 2–4 ml/kg, and the blood retested for improvement.

NEONATAL TRANSPORT

The paramedic team may become involved in the transfer of a neonate from one hospital to another. This commonly occurs where babies born in peripheral units, i.e. district general hospitals, have to be transferred to specialized neonatal or paediatric units because of the need for intensive care, treatment of congenital heart disease or neonatal surgery, facilities for which are usually sited at larger units in teaching hospitals. In these instances the paramedical team will work in close association with nursing staff and doctors from the peripheral hospital who usually also travel with the neonate. The most important point is that the neonate should be stable prior to transfer, and the paramedics should work with the medical team to ensure that this is the case. It is also important that the whole transfer should be well planned by the sending and the receiving hospitals, so that it is known in advance to which part of the receiving hospital the child is to be admitted.

In most neonatal transfers an incubator rather than an open stretcher is used, chiefly to maintain the child's temperature during the transfer. Most modern incubators also allow for ventilation to the neonate. The incubator operates on a battery supply and requires the use of cylinders of oxygen and air for ventilation. When preparing for such a transfer, check the machinery prior to leaving the peripheral hospital and estimate the journey time to ensure that adequate amounts of oxygen and battery time are available. Most modern incubators can be adapted to the battery system already in the ambulance, and it is necessary to check that this is so.

Ensure that the transport team have the necessary equipment and drugs available should the child deteriorate *en route*. Remember that mishaps can happen, such as the endotracheal tube dislodging, so it is necessary for the child to be monitored during the journey, and facilities for procedures such as re-intubation should be available.

10

PSYCHIATRY

chapter fifty-one

SUBSTANCE ABUSE

Problems related to the use of alcohol, drugs and solvents are increasingly common in the UK. This reflects both an increase in incidence and greater awareness of such behaviour by medical and paramedical workers and the public. Amongst teenagers the rising incidence of substance misuse is particularly worrying. The problem is exacerbated by the availability of new 'designer' drugs, and an increase in misuse of volatile substances.

DEFINITIONS

Drug dependence is a sociopsychobiological syndrome, the key feature being the priority given to drug-seeking behaviour over other behaviours. Drug or alcohol use does not always lead to dependence and a problem substance taker is someone who experiences social, physical or legal sequelae related to intoxication, excessive consumption or dependence resulting from use of drugs, alcohol or other substances.

ALCOHOL

Epidemiology

Twenty-five per cent of men are said to be problem drinkers at some point in their lives and approximately 25% of general medical admissions involve alcohol-related problems. Two per cent of the population in the UK suffer from alcohol dependence syndrome at any time. Dependence is most common in those aged 40–54 years. There is a sharp drop in heavy drinking in men over 70 years old and in women aged 50–60 years. The male to female ratio is 4:1, but the female rate is increasing. Factors increasing risk of dependence include cheap or easily available alcohol, unsupervised work routine, unsociable working hours, and work involving separation from family or other stabilizing social constraints. Publicans, doctors, journalists and senior businessmen are most vulnerable. Alcoholism

is more likely in divorced, separated and never-married individuals.

Alcohol Dependence Syndrome

The alcohol dependence syndrome includes features such as:

- Narrowing of drinking repertoire (drinking from a smaller range of alcoholic drinks)
- Salience of drink-seeking behaviour (drinking supersedes other activities)
- Increased tolerance to alcohol (more alcohol is required to produce intoxication or stave off withdrawals)
- Repeated attempts at withdrawal from alcohol that end in failure even with professional help
- Relief or avoidance of withdrawal symptoms by further drinking (responsible for morning drinking)
- Subjective awareness of compulsion to drink (may continue long after cessation of drinking)
- Reinstatement of dependent drinking after a period of abstinence ('perhaps just one drink since we are celebrating')

Physical Consequences of Alcohol Dependence

Alcohol dependence causes problems in a number of body systems.
Gastrointestinal tract:
    liver damage
    alcoholic hepatitis
    fatty liver
    cirrhosis
    liver failure and hepatic encephalopathy
    oesophagitis and gastritis causing vomiting and retching
    Mallory–Weiss tear in lower oesophagus causing haematemesis

portal hypertension causing oesophageal varices and possible massive haematemesis

peptic ulceration

acute and chronic pancreatitis (acute has a mortality of 10–40%)

carcinoma of upper gastrointestinal tract

Cardiovascular system:

cardiac arrhythmias

cardiomyopathy

coronary artery disease, hypertension, cerebrovascular accident

Metabolic changes:

hypoglycaemia

ketoacidosis

Haematological changes:

anaemia

thrombocytopenia

Nervous system:

diffuse brain damage from cortical shrinkage and ventricular dilation

alcoholic dementia

Wernicke–Korsakoff syndrome – caused by deficiency of thiamine (vitamin B$_1$). In acute Wernicke's encephalopathy, symptoms include alteration in level of consciousness, nystagmus, external ophthalmoplegia, ataxia and peripheral neuropathy

epilepsy from withdrawal fits

Psychological Problems

Alcoholic hallucinosis

Hallucinations of voices, usually derogatory in content, occur in clear consciousness.

Affective symptoms

Affective symptoms occur in 90% of people with alcoholism.

Suicide

There is a 10–15% risk of completed suicide associated with alcoholism.

Pathological jealousy

Pathological jealousy manifests as a morbid delusional belief that a partner is being unfaithful. It is twice as common in men, and may put the partner at risk of serious violence.

Emergencies Specifically Related to Alcohol

Acute intoxication

Acute intoxication may lead to physical injury from trauma or head injury. Always look for evidence of injury or illness in intoxicated patients before putting their clinical state down to alcohol intoxication. Intoxication may cause hypoglycaemia or metabolic acidosis. Severe intoxication with alcohol can cause death, often from vomiting leading to asphyxiation, but also directly related to alcohol poisoning.

Acute alcohol withdrawal

Acute alcohol withdrawal occurs in the dependent state and is characterized by nausea, vomiting, tremors, excessive sweating and tachycardia. It may begin within 6 hours of cessation or reduction of alcohol and peaks by 48 hours, subsiding over the next 7 days. It may be associated with withdrawal grand mal epileptic seizures 12–24 hours after drinking.

Delirium tremens

Delirium tremens (DTs) occurs on days 3 to 5 following cessation or significant reduction of drinking in an alcohol-dependent person. It is characterized by confusion, disorientation, delusions, hallucinations and vivid imagery (often insects but not the pink elephants of popular belief), together with intense tremulousness. There is often a marked lability of emotions and autonomic dysfunction. There is no craving for alcohol. Admission must be to a medical ward for rehydration, sedation and nutrition. In 50% of cases DTs are precipitated by an intercurrent infection. The mortality rate is up to 10%.

OTHER SUBSTANCE ABUSE

Unlike the stereotypical image of a drug addict as a dishevelled, unwashed young man with staring eyes and an aggressive manner, people who misuse drugs or other substances come from all walks of life and there is no particular personality profile, ethnic group, class or profession that identifies characteristic substance misusers. Official figures of substance misusers in the UK relate to those seeking treatment or those notified to the Home Office and do not reflect the extent of use. In 1993 about 34,000 drug misusers were notified, a rise of one-fifth from the year before. Deaths among drug users rose by 40% in 1993 to 570.

Unusual behaviour of any sort could be due to substance misuse and it is important to note that substance misusers may often use more than one substance at a time, causing a mixture of symptoms and signs. Whenever assessing patients whose behaviour is suggestive of substance misuse, check their arms and legs for evidence of injection sites. Misusers of volatile solvents often smell of glue or aerosol propellant and may have a rash around their mouth and nose where there has been contact with an inhalation bag. Appropriate precautions against contact with bodily fluids should be taken, as the incidence of human immunodeficiency virus (HIV) and hepatitis B infection is increased in injecting drug abusers.

There are few specific antidotes for most substances of abuse and the basic 'ABC' approach is essential. Specific details of treatment are not given in this chapter unless they can be started during pre-hospital care.

In the following list of substances street names of drugs are given, but the names vary in different geographical areas and also change over time, some names becoming more popular than others. If in doubt, ask for or suggest the generic name of the substance.

Opiates

Opiates are a large group of drugs ranging from the natural substance opium to the synthetic substance fentanyl. The duration of action and toxic levels vary from drug to drug. Fatal doses (below) are given for adults: in general the fatal dose for children is unknown, but it will usually be less than the mg/kg conversion from the adult dose, since children are more sensitive to opiates. In general addicts can tolerate higher doses than non-addicts before manifesting the effects of toxicity, but beware of addicts who have had a period of abstinence (e.g. in prison) and whose tolerance therefore is markedly reduced.

Overdosage or ingestion of opiates is characterized by altered level of consciousness, respiratory depression and pinpoint pupils. Fits occur less commonly. Other signs include a euphoric or stuporous mental state, convulsions, hypotension and hypothermia.

The initial management of an opiate overdose or respiratory depression due to opiate ingestion is maintenance of the airway and oxygenation followed by the rapid administration of naloxone. Indeed, naloxone should be administered on the least suspicion of opiate ingestion. The adult dose is 1.2 mg repeated at intervals of several minutes up to a dose of 10 mg. Failure to respond to a total dose of 10 mg indicates that the respiratory depression and altered conscious level is due either to another drug, or to co-administration of another central nervous system depressant drug. It is important to remember that naloxone has a short half-life, and that recurrence of respiratory depression or altered conscious level may occur. In such cases further doses are required. The dose of naloxone for children is 0.01 mg/kg repeated as necessary.

Opium

Fatal doses

- Powder and resin 2 g
- Dry extract 1 g
- Liquid extract 27 ml
- Tincture 20 ml

Street names:
  Big 'O'
  Brown stuff
  China white
  Dust

Heroin

Heroin is produced from morphine which in turn is contained in opium, the dried sap of the opium poppy. Much street heroin is only 10% pure and costs about £60–80 per gram (1995 prices). Daily consumption is commonly in the region of 0.25–0.75 g, although the fatal dose can be as little as 0.2 g. Severe reactions, sometimes fatal, are seen when an unusually 'pure' batch of heroin becomes available for sale.

Clinical features and recognition of use Heroin acts on opiate receptors to produce analgesia, miosis, euphoria, hypotension, bradycardia and respiratory depression. Tolerance to the euphoriant action appears rapidly and dependence may occur in weeks to months.

The withdrawal syndrome appears within 4–12 hours, peaks at 48 hours and is alleviated after 1 week. Symptoms include dysphoria, aching limbs, increased perspiration with 'gooseflesh' of the skin (hence 'cold turkey'), diarrhoea, dilated pupils, shivering, yawning and fatigue. Insomnia and craving for the drug may persist for weeks. Withdrawal without supportive measures in a reasonably fit person is not dangerous or fatal.

Street names:
Black tar	Persian
Boy	Rock
Chinese (rock)	Smack
Dana	Stuff
'H'	TNT
Harry	White elephant
Horse	White stuff
Noise	

Morphine

The fatal dose of morphine is as little as 100 mg.

Street names:
  Cube juice
  Dreamer
  Hard stuff
  Hocusmorf
  Morpho

Methadone

Methadone is a synthetic opiate that can be taken orally or intravenously and has a half-life of 15 hours. This longer half-life increases the time of onset of withdrawal symptoms and when used therapeutically to wean addicts off heroin it is administered as a once daily dose.

Street names:
  Doll
  Dollies
  Dolophine

Dipipanone (Diconal)

The fatal dose is unknown. Diconal is a combination of dipipanone and cyclizine. It produces intense euphoria when used intravenously but presents a danger of arterial closure and gangrene.

Street name:
  Dike

Pethidine

The fatal dose of pethidine is about 1 g.

Street name:
  Meperidine

Fentanyl

The fatal dose of fentanyl is unknown. It is a potent drug with a short half-life, and therefore doses near the therapeutic range may be fatal.

Street name:
  China white

Dextromoramide (Palfium)

The fatal dose is about 500 mg.

Street name:
  Peach palf

Codeine

The fatal dose of codeine is more than 1 g.

Street name:
  Schoolboy

Dextropopoxyphene napsylate (co-proxamol)

The fatal dose is 1–1.5 g.

Hallucinogens

Lysergic acid diethylamide (LSD)

Lysergic acid diethylamide is a synthetic psychedelic drug of low toxicity. Symptoms include confusion, agitation, hallucinations, dilated pupils, coma and respiratory arrest. Supportive measures only are required.

Street names:

Acid	Green caps
Beast	Paper acid
Blotter acid	Pink drops
Blue caps	Purple haze
Blue drops	Sunshine
Boy	White lightning
Dome (dots)	Yellow caps

Dots	Yellow drops
Ghost	

Psilocybin (magic mushrooms)

Ingestion of magic mushrooms is a seasonal problem, usually well known in particular localities where the mushrooms can be picked. Cases may occur in small epidemics. The fatal dose is unknown.

Euphoria, anxiety, depression, illusions and psychosis are all common manifestations. Hyperthermia, tachycardia, tremors and dilated pupils are characteristic. There is no specific treatment in the pre-hospital setting but efforts should be made to calm the victim by giving reassurance that the effects are self-limiting.

Street name:
  Shrooms

Phencyclidine

Phencyclidine is a psychedelic drug, fatal dose unknown. Symptoms include anxiety and psychosis, ataxia, paraesthesia, catatonic movements, fits, coma, hypotension, respiratory impairment, Cheyne–Stokes breathing and respiratory arrest. Treatment is supportive.

Street names:

Angel dust	Mist
Aurora borealis	PCP
Busy bee	Peace weed
CJ's	Seccies
Cycline	Sherman
Dust	Snorts
Embalming fluid	Superkool
Fuel	Supergrass
Happy sticks	Superjoint
Hog	Superweed
Horse tracks	Surfer
Joy sticks	TAC
Killer weed	TIC
KJ	White powder
LBJ	Zoom

Cannabis

Cannabis is a common drug of abuse considered by many to be a 'recreational' drug (i.e. without serious consequences from its use). Of relatively low toxicity (unless ingested by children when coma may ensue), it may be smoked or eaten. The symptoms of toxicity include excitement, euphoria, drowsiness, panic attacks, toxic psychosis and, rarely, coma and dilated pupils. There are no specific treatments required in the pre-hospital setting apart from supportive measures.

Street names:

Acapulco gold	Joy sticks

Bhang
Charas
Dope
DP
Ganja
Grass
'H'
Hagga
Happy sticks
Hash (oil)
Homegrown
Joint
Mary Jane
MJ
Paki
Pot
Red oil
Reefers
Resin
Roaches
Shit
Smoke
Tea
Thai sticks

Amyl nitrate

Amyl nitrate is toxic by ingestion and inhalation. Its principal mode of toxicity is by the formation of methaemoglobin. The fatal dose is unknown, but even small amounts can cause symptoms. Symptoms occur within a few seconds of inhalation, but may be delayed by ingestion. Headache, nausea and vomiting occur along with sweating and flushing. Tightness of the chest is common as is confusion and occasionally fits. Cyanosis due to methaemoglobinaemia may occur. There is no specific pre-hospital treatment apart from maintenance of the airway and administration of oxygen to treat cyanosis.

Street names:
   Poor man's cocaine
   Poppers
   Snappers
   Sweat

Stimulants

Amphetamines

Illicit amphetamine sulphate may only be 20–30% pure and costs around £10–15 per gram (1995 prices). A heavy user may use several grams a day. Dexamphetamine (Dexedrine, 'dexies') and amphetamine-like drugs such as methylphenidate (Ritalin) and diethylpropion (Tenuate), are also taken.

Acute effects include euphoria, anxiety, increased energy, miosis and tachycardia. Amphetamine psychosis mimics acute symptoms of schizophrenia and manifests with paranoid delusions, auditory, visual and tactile hallucinations and increased arousal and irritability. Consciousness is impaired.

Withdrawal effects include dysphoria, fatigue, lassitude and depression.

Street names:
   'A'
   Amphet
   Speed
   Splash
   STP
   Sulp
   Sulphate
   Uppers
   Ups
   Wake-ups
   Whizz

Cocaine

Cocaine is a local anaesthetic agent, which is still used in some clinical areas (such as ear, nose and throat surgery). The fatal dose is approximately 1 g when taken orally and 10 mg when injected. Symptoms include tachycardia, sweating, hallucinations, increased respiratory rate, increased temperature, fits, arrhythmias and rarely cardiac arrest. There is no specific treatment; fits should be controlled with diazepam and general supportive measures instituted.

Street names:
   Base
   Bazooka
   Big 'C'
   Blow
   'C'
   Candy
   Cake
   Charlie
   Coke
   Crack
   Dose
   Dust
   Dynamite
   Flake
   Freebase
   Gold dust
   Happy dust
   Heaven dust
   Hit
   Ice
   Koks
   Paradise
   Pimp's (drug)
   Smack
   Snort

Ecstasy (MDMA)

A semisynthetic amphetamine (3,4-methylenedioxymethamphetamine), Ecstasy has become notorious in recent years as the cause of deaths which have occurred in otherwise healthy teenagers. Two causes of death are commonly recognized: early deaths are due to arrhythmias and late deaths are due to an effect on muscles associated with a fatal rise in body temperature (a similar condition, neuroleptic malignant syndrome, occurs rarely as a side-effect of antipsychotic drugs). Deaths can occur after exposure to doses previously tolerated and are thought to be due to an idiosyncratic reaction. Symptoms range from mild to life-threatening and include muscle spasms, dilated pupils, anxiety, tachycardia, increased temperature, abdominal pain, hypotension, fits, coma and stroke. The fatal dose is unknown, but is near to the 'therapeutic' dose. There are no specific treatments other than supportive measures in the pre-hospital setting.

Street names:
   Acid
   Adam
   AKA
   Bart Simpson
   Dennis the Menace
   Disco biscuits
   'E'
   Ecsta
   Red and black
   White burger
   White dove
   XTC
   Yellow burger

Ephedrine

Ephedrine is a sympathomimetic drug with a fatal dose of

200 mg in children and over 2 g in adults. It causes restlessness, tachycardia, dilated pupils, arrhythmias and hallucinations. Apart from treating fits with diazepam there is no specific pre-hospital treatment required and supportive measures should be instituted.

Street names:
   Uppers
   Ups

Caffeine

Caffeine has similar side effects to ephedrine; the fatal dose is 10 g. Treatment is as for ephedrine.

Street names:
   Uppers
   Ups

Sedatives

Barbiturates

The barbiturates are a group of drugs that include:

- Amylobarbitone (Amytal)
- Barbitone
- Butobarbitone (Soneryl)
- Pentobarbitone (Nembutal)
- Phenobarbitone
- Quinalbarbitone (Seconal)
- Sodium amylobarbitone (Sodium Amytal)

Symptoms include ataxia, dysarthria, decreased conscious level, coma, respiratory depression, hypothermia and hypotension. There are no specific treatments apart from general supportive measures. Withdrawal seizures may occur and should be controlled with diazepam.

Street names:

Barbs	Love drug
Bennies	Love pill
Black Beauties	Meth
Bluebirds	Mollies

Blues	Peace
Crank	Pep pills
DOM	Rippers
Downers	Rocks
Ice	Serenity
LA turnarounds	Sodies

Volatile Solvents

Glue

Toluene is the most common solvent in glues available over the counter. Effects include excitement, chest tightness, fits, coma, arrhythmias and death. Supportive measures should be instituted with particular emphasis on oxygenation to reduce the likelihood of arrhythmias.

Butane

A colourless, odourless gas, commonly used as the propellant in 'ozone friendly' sprays but also available in cigarette lighters, butane is generally inhaled from a bag. Symptoms include respiratory depression, coma, hypotension and arrhythmias. Treatment is supportive only.

Butyl nitrate

An industrial solvent, butyl nitrate is also used as a room deodorizer. Fatal when ingested in even small quantities, the fatal dose is unknown. Symptoms include flushing, tachycardia, hypotension, confusion, shortness of breath and cyanosis (from the formation of methaemoglobin), coma and fits. Treatment is supportive.

Street names:
   Liquid incense
   Locker popper
   Locker room
   Room deodorizer
   Rush

FURTHER READING

Robson P (1994) *Forbidden Drugs*. Oxford University Press.

chapter fifty-two:

THE UNCOOPERATIVE OR VIOLENT PATIENT

When an ambulance is called to the scene of an accident or emergency, the crew will find that the majority of members of the public are friendly and helpful. There will be occasions, however, when you arrive at the scene of a call to find an uncooperative or violent patient. This chapter focuses on assessing the scene and the patient, managing the person (or persons) and the legal rights of the patient and ambulance personnel. Each individual will have his or her own background, culture, standards and beliefs. These characteristics will affect the manner in which you deal with a situation.

PRIOR TO ARRIVAL

Information before arrival at the scene may suggest the environment you are about to enter. It is essential to take care of yourself in the first instance, to prevent injury to yourself, a colleague or the patient. The attendant should think of a plan of action before you arrive. The driver must concentrate on the driving!

Think about equipment on your person that may be used against you or your colleague, for example:

- Hand-held radio sets or pagers
- Torch
- Equipment bags
- Scissors, pens, pencils
- Stethoscope

Check all communication equipment, including hand-held devices. The last thing you need is a communications breakdown when you need help.

ON ARRIVAL

On arrival you should:

- Position the vehicle safely and with an exit
- Survey the scene
- Ask if there are other services present. Who is in charge?
- Determine whether you need support
- Clear bystanders

The person you are called to may feel that it has taken a long time for you to arrive. Feelings you may be faced with include:

anger
fear
frustration
joy
relief

To deal with these feelings in the best way possible it is important to remain alert and flexible in your approach to care.

BASIC PRINCIPLES OF ASSESSMENT

Survey the scene:

- Is it safe to enter?
- Where is the person: are they standing, sitting or lying?
- Is the person calm, upset or angry?
- Are there objects nearby they could use to hurt themselves, or you?
- If there are, discreetly remove the objects to a safe distance.

Do not rush in and try to make everything all right. Be prepared to spend time with the person. Ensure you have an exit in case the situation deteriorates. Treat the person in the same manner in which you would like to be treated, with respect and maintenance of dignity. Address the person as 'Sir' or 'Madam' until told otherwise.

Verbal and Non-Verbal Communication

Verbal

When speaking to an aggressive (or potentially aggressive) or uncooperative patient, speak more slowly than normal, but at a normal volume – *do not shout*. Ideally the pitch of the voice should be slightly higher than normal to increase clarity.

Non-verbal

Non-verbal communication is often referred to as 'body language'. It is the signs and signals that we give out to others. At times we are aware of what we are communicating non-verbally, but at other times we need to take care. This is especially important when dealing with people in personal crisis. Some of the forms of non-verbal communication that we use are:

- Facial expressions
- Movement of arms, hands, legs
- Body stance
- Distance from the other person
- Touch

Appropriate use of non-verbal behaviour is given in Table 52.1.

Establishing a Rapport

Basic skills of communication are vital in establishing a rapport with the person. Encourage reality and orientation, e.g. awareness of place, date and time. First, gain eye contact. Do not stare, break eye contact regularly but always keep the person in your sight. Introduce yourself:

'Hello sir, I'm John, a paramedic with the ambulance service.'

If necessary repeat your introduction – you may not have been heard. Ask the person if it is all right to approach. If the answer is yes, then approach slowly, stopping at arm's length. Any closer to the person would be encroaching on their 'personal space', and may provoke an aggressive verbal or physical response. If the answer is no, then stay where you are, and be prepared to discuss the person's fears or worries. Try to get the person to sit down:

'Would you like to sit?'

Give choices to the person rather than orders. If the person chooses to sit then you too should find a suitable chair to sit in. Position your chair at an angle of 45 degrees, allowing yourself and the person enough room to stretch their legs.

Establish ground rules

'I am here to help, not to hurt you.'

Explain to the person it is all right to show emotion, e.g. cry or scream, but it is not all right to harm themselves, or harm you or others. Put to the person that you will be honest with them: do not lie! Trust can be lost easily. Seek confirmation that the person has heard what you say.

'Do you understand what I have said?'

If necessary, be prepared to reiterate what you have said.

Identify the Problem

Open the questions by allowing the person to speak, give a story and ventilate his or her feelings. For example:

'You appear to have been crying, can you tell me what has been upsetting you?'

Do not use closed questions, i.e. those requiring a response of only 'Yes', 'No' or 'I don't know'. Firstly they give you no information, and secondly they cause frustration for the person being interviewed, as well as the interviewer. For example, do not simply ask:

'Are you upset?'

Do not ask leading questions, as these can give a false reflection of what is happening. An example of a leading question is:

'Is it your neighbour who is causing the problem?'

Do not interrupt. If there are silences, appear supportive by remaining alert and attentive:

verbally – '. . . *and then what happened?*'
non-verbally – maintain eye contact; nod the head.

If the person shows emotion, say that it is all right to do so:

'It is all right to cry.'

If necessary offer support, for example tissues or a drink of water. Allow the person enough time to regain control and composure.

Table 52.1 Appropriate use of non-verbal communication

Appropriate behaviour	Inappropriate behaviour
Expression showing acknowledgement of crisis	Laughing inappropriately
Appear relaxed, arms by your side	Arms and legs crossed
Stance side-on to person	Stance exposing your front
Arm's length from person	Within arm's length

'Telling the story' may be traumatic. It is important to clarify the 'story' by repeating key phrases and asking if what you have repeated is correct. This demonstrates that you value the person, firstly by spending time with them and secondly by listening to what they have said.

The following steps summarize the systematic approach to the uncooperative or violent patient:

- Maintain safety
- Introduce yourself
- Establish a rapport
- Set the ground rules
- Seek a history
- Seek clarification

Assessment and identification
of the problem is vital:
It gives you a clear history
It prevents frustration
It prevents violence and non-cooperation
towards yourself and others

RIGHTS OF THE PATIENT

Unless requested to attend a call to a person placed under the care of the Mental Health Act 1983, you must treat all patients as voluntary.

Voluntary Patients

Voluntary patients have the choice of receiving or not receiving care. They should always be given the choice. If the person declines, the options are:

- Give the person all reasonable help and advice
- Inform ambulance control that the person has refused treatment
- Ask the person to sign the journey sheet next to the appropriate entry, stating they are refusing treatment
- If you are unhappy to leave the person, e.g. they appear to be at risk, then request the police to attend (who can section the patient for involuntary treatment)

Compulsory Admission

The majority of admissions to psychiatric hospitals are voluntary. Approximately 10% are by formal admission, i.e. under the Mental Health Act 1983 (see Chapter 53). This Act in the first instance sets out to provide appropriate care for the mentally disordered, and secondly provides a safeguard for those people who are not mentally disordered, against wrongful detention.

As discussed earlier, you should find out who is in charge. This may be an approved social worker (ASW) or the responsible medical officer. Talk with the person in charge to help assess the situation. You should see all the relevant documentation for the appropriate section. All parts of the forms must be completed satisfactorily. If in doubt seek advice from the person in charge or with ambulance control.

The person's rights according to the section that they have been placed under would have been explained to them by the ASW. It must be remembered that during this time the person is in personal crisis. There may be family or friends involved, who are also distressed at the situation. Time, patience and diplomacy are vital in caring for these people. In the case of a female patient, a woman ambulance crew member, ASW, doctor or police constable must be in attendance at all times. This also means during transport to the hospital.

If the person wishes to speak then follow the guidelines for assessment. Do not enter into the person's delusions or hallucinations; try to maintain reality. If the person does not accept reality, then you will have to accept the situation. If the person chooses not to speak then respect that decision. Do not force conversation.

Persons expressing suicidal thoughts should be treated with care. It is not your role to decide whether or not they are serious. Be aware they may try to deceive you to carry out their intentions. These persons should not be left alone but supervised at all times.

If patients refuse to go to hospital then a minimal amount of force may be used under the Mental Health Act 1983, to transport them safely. If after assessing the situation it is felt that the support of the police is required, then explain to the family or friends the reasons for this decision.

RIGHTS OF AMBULANCE PERSONNEL

You must be responsible for your actions at all times. If an incident takes place, inform your senior officer immediately. Document the event fully. If the incident is reported to the police, then a criminal investigation will take place to see if there is sufficient evidence to prosecute. Prosecution could result in a fine or imprisonment. This in turn may lead to dismissal. In a civil proceeding, action would be undertaken by the person or their relatives against you, when they would present their evidence. The High Court would decide whether or not to allow the prosecution to continue. Prosecution could result in payment of damages to the person or the person's family.

If you are attacked by someone then you should seek legal advice. You may be able to claim compensation for injuries from the Criminal Injuries Board (Criminal Justice Act 1988). Dealing with mentally ill persons forms part of your job description. You must therefore expect to be given appropriate training in this area. When dealing with persons placed under Sections 2, 3 or 4 of the Mental Health Act 1983, Section 139 protects you from criminal or civil proceedings when carrying out your duties in accordance with the Act unless it is done without reasonable care.

The Role of the Police

Your own personal safety and that of your colleagues must come first. There is no point in becoming a casualty yourself. If the situation appears to be threatening and the police have not been contacted, then a decision must be taken as to whether their assistance is required. The role of the police is to uphold and enforce the law. Good communication skills are vital. Cooperation and respect for each other's role must be maintained.

The police may request a transfer of a person from the police station to the accident and emergency department for treatment. All such persons must be escorted by a police officer.

MANAGEMENT OF VIOLENCE

Before reading this section, re-read the sections 'Prior to arrival' and 'On arrival' above.

People may become violent for a number of reasons:

- Crowd incidents (e.g. shooting, stabbing)
- Drug and alcohol abuse (use of, or withdrawal)
- Illness (e.g. hypoglycaemia, sepsis, electrolyte imbalance, raised intracranial pressure)
- Mental disorder (mania, psychosis)

You must be continuously alert for any sign that the situation is deteriorating.

Verbal signs of a deteriorating situation

- The person's attitude towards you changes
- The person becomes more demanding
- Volume of voice rises
- Sarcasm features strongly in conversation
- The person demands help from others

Non-verbal signs

- The person becomes restless, e.g. pacing the floor, tapping feet, wringing hands
- Difficulty in concentration

The following approach will help when dealing with a violent patient:

remain calm

ensure you have an exit

maintain a 2-metre distance from the person

side-on stance

maintain non-threatening eye contact

seek extra help (have support in the background, e.g. in another room)

remain in control of your talking

try to negotiate and so defuse the situation

do not lie, or promise outcomes you cannot keep

recognize the need for rapid intervention if the situation deteriorates further

Once a situation has deteriorated into violence, your first priority must remain your own safety and it is essential to call for appropriate assistance. Personal heroics are not appropriate. The following approach should ensure an optimal safe outcome:

immediately call for police assistance

use only the minimum of physical restraint to control the situation

never restrain a person in a way that could impair breathing, e.g. pushing the person's face down or sitting on their chest

never restrain the person around the neck

when restraining use only the large limbs, i.e. legs and arms

check pulses in these limbs to ensure circulation

reassure the person at all times

keep calm, avoid threats

negotiate with the person

when the person is calm, slowly release the physical restraint

liaise with the police to decide appropriate management – hospital care or police custody

Transportation of the Uncooperative or Violent Person

When arranging transport, consider whether you need a police officer to accompany you to hospital and ensure that ambulance control is fully aware of the situation. Before you enter the ambulance, make sure that any potentially dangerous objects are stowed securely away. Once such patients are in the ambulance, if carried on a stretcher, use the adjustable straps to ensure that they do not harm themselves during transit. If the patient is sitting, consider the seating arrangements, bearing in mind the patient's potential for violence or escape and your own safety.

If the person is to be admitted under the Mental Health Act 1983 then you should satisfy yourself that all documents are completed. An Application for Admission, including the appropriate medical recommendations, is required for the person to be transported to hospital. The applicant is normally the ASW. Normally the ASW follows in his or her own transport to the hospital; however, you can insist that the ASW or an approved escort accompanies you in the ambulance. If male ambulance personnel are transporting a disturbed woman, then a female chaperone is necessary. This will protect the crew from allegations of misconduct.

What to do after an Incident

After an incident involving violence has occurred:

1. Inform ambulance control of the incident.
2. Document the facts of what happened at the incident: the predisposing factors and the action taken then and afterwards (good record-keeping helps with debriefing and identifying training needs).
3. Violent incidents can leave people feeling angry, guilty, tired or upset; the policies relating to violent incidents (verbal and/or physical) should be adhered to. Included in such a policy should be a provision for debriefing staff following an incident.
4. Speak to other professionals involved. Sharing thoughts and feelings can reduce stress (see Chapter 54).
5. Nobody in the caring profession enjoys being involved in violence. Help and support each other.

FURTHER READING

Jones RM *The Mental Health Act 1983*. London: Sweet & Maxwell.

Wright R (1993) *Caring in Crises – A Handbook of Intervention Skills*, 2nd edn. Edinburgh: Churchill Livingstone.

chapter fifty-three:

PSYCHIATRIC EMERGENCIES

Psychiatric emergencies differ from medical emergencies in that admission to hospital is not always indicated. Most psychiatric emergencies are not immediately life-threatening and there is usually time in which to plan a coordinated and careful response. Unfortunately, perhaps owing to ignorance, there is a tendency to overreact and to look on hospital admission as the only option; this may result in the unnecessary use of expensive resources, but more importantly may have a profound and long-lasting detrimental effect on the patient. Prejudice against mental illness remains rife, as does stigma associated with psychiatric hospitals. Immense efforts are being made in many areas to promote the use of alternative, community facilities for the management of people with mental disorders and it is likely that many people who in the past would otherwise have been admitted to hospital can now be managed at home or in an alternative community facility. Unfortunately community facilities may carry with them the same prejudice that is linked to more traditional psychiatric settings. This applies equally to patients presenting as an apparent emergency, who are often subject to the fear and apparent helplessness of carers or authorities, who in turn may have become blinded by their desire to react quickly and remove the person from the crisis situation without first considering other options that may be available. On the other hand, severe mental illness must be taken seriously, and hospitals are the first choice for those patients who require intensive support, treatment and supervision. Admission to hospital should never be avoided because of ideological considerations.

Most psychiatric emergencies involve patients who are distressed and helpless and who may appear dangerous or at risk of harm. Most psychiatric patients are not dangerous, and it is important to bury the myth that they are. It is particularly important to be aware that as a result of their behaviour (if they are deemed to be a risk to themselves or others) mentally ill patients may be admitted to hospital involuntarily under the Mental Health Act. This results in their loss of liberty and may have a profound effect on how they are treated both immediately and in the long term.

Dealing with psychiatric patients requires important skills of counselling, empathy, negotiation and ability to liaise with different professional groups (the police, social workers, nurses and doctors). The general public too have a role, as their concerns may have precipitated the response from health or social services and it is especially important to support and inform relatives who are often bemused and upset at the situation. They may harbour strong feelings of anger, guilt and sadness, and require reassurance and understanding.

WHAT IS A PSYCHIATRIC EMERGENCY?

A psychiatric emergency can be defined as a situation involving someone exhibiting psychological distress that exceeds the coping strategies of that individual, the carers or society, and that may involve a possible risk to themselves or others.

The causes of psychiatric emergencies are manifold. Some are described below. However, it is important to note that many apparent emergencies can be resolved without resorting to the powers of the Mental Health Act or the facilities of the local hospital. Problems often arise out of particular social difficulties (e.g. financial problems, lack of electricity, homelessness, lack of food), breakdown in relationships or altercations with the police. Some may occur as a result of a physical disorder or be related to medication or the use of illicit drugs. All require an assessment that may be prolonged and may involve psychiatrists, social workers and relatives; at the end of this assessment the result may be the loss of liberty of a person who is admitted to hospital against his or her will.

ESSENTIALS OF ASSESSMENT

The essentials of assessment of a psychiatric emergency are to engage the patient and to gather detailed information in a sensitive manner; to undertake mental state and physical examinations; to support any relatives or carers; and above all to remain patient and unflustered. Ensuring the safety of everyone involved is paramount, and if there is any doubt as to the level of risk towards those undertaking the assessment no attempt should be made to continue without further reinforcements.

Gather Information from Patient and Informant

All psychiatric assessments should begin with gathering as much information as possible about the patient. The nature of presenting symptoms (whether gradual or sudden onset), past medical and psychiatric history including substance misuse, present medication (both prescribed and non-prescribed) and level of support at home are essential elements of an accurate assessment and should be obtained both from the patient and from an informant. This initial assessment may not be straightforward. For example a patient may not allow access to the house. In this case it may be possible to conduct a reasonable appraisal of the situation through the letterbox, thereby persuading the patient to open the door or gathering enough information to make a decision that there are likely to be grounds for admission under the Mental Health Act. Neighbours can be extremely useful informants who, as well as providing background information about the patient, will often have noticed recent changes in behaviour. Close relatives are often available to give detailed information.

Mental State Examination

Mental state examination is the term given to observation of the patient's behaviour, mood and speech in order to gather evidence of mental disorder. It is important that a mental state examination is objective and not subjective or based on supposition. A comprehensive mental state examination should be carried out in all cases. The usual procedure is to subdivide the examination into the following categories:

- Appearance and behaviour
- Speech form (i.e. coherence) and content
- Beliefs and thoughts expressed
- Overall mood state and whether it is congruent with the thought content
- Observable abnormal perceptions or experiences (e.g. hallucinations)
- Assessment of level of consciousness, orientation in time, place and person, concentration and short-term memory
- Presence of insight (the acknowledgement by the patient that there are psychological problems that require to be resolved)
- Suicidal ideation

Physical Examination

Physical examination should be carried out in every case as far as possible, even if there appears to be no apparent physical disorder. Common organic causes of psychiatric emergencies (such as hypoglycaemia, infection, cardiac failure, delirium tremens and subdural haematoma) should be rigorously and systematically searched for. Breath odour may reveal solvent or alcohol misuse, and recent skin puncture marks suggests drug misuse.

PSYCHOSIS: RECOGNITION AND TREATMENT

Psychosis refers to disturbances in thinking and behaviour usually involving delusions, hallucinations and thought disorder. Where these symptoms are sufficiently recognizable and characteristic, they may be attributable to a diagnosis such as schizophrenia, mania or psychotic depression. However, psychiatric diagnosis is complicated and bedeviled by problems of definition and applicability and it is usually simpler just to describe symptoms expressed and signs observed.

Assessment of Psychosis

Delusions
A delusion is a firmly held but false belief that is out of context with the person's social and cultural background, unamenable to any logical argument that is presented to refute it, and based on spurious and inappropriate evidence. There is often an element of persecution that accompanies the belief, but patients may express delusions that they have special powers or are invested with great authority or fame. Examples include delusions that they are being persecuted or hounded by others (often the police or other authority figures); that others are watching or listening to them through bugging devices; that presenters on the television are referring directly to them, or items in newspapers or the media have special significance to them; beliefs about bodily malfunctions (e.g. bowels seizing up or interference with particular organs), or excessive guilt or self-blame for particular life circumstances. Often it is impossible even to attempt to confront the reality of the belief, and there is a danger of losing rapport with the patient resulting in argument.

Hallucinations
Hallucinations refer to the experience of perceptions (e.g. hearing voices or noises, seeing vivid images, or tasting particular flavours) in the absence of stimulus causing the perception. They can occur in any sensory modality. They are not imagined experiences and to the patient appear real. Often a delusional explanation of the hallucination may be put forward. For example, voices may be explained in terms of transmitters

through the electric cable or bugging devices in the pipes. Hallucinations are often frightening and distressing, and the patient may be observed to be responding to apparent hallucinations – especially if the patient appears to be distracted, preoccupied or talking or muttering inappropriately. Rarely patients may act on their hallucinations in an impulsive manner.

Psychotic behaviour

Psychotic behaviour is often the reason why emergency services have become involved. Patients suffering acute psychological distress may act in unusual, bizarre or even frightening ways. They shout and swear, gesticulate in a threatening way and indulge in antisocial behaviour. Their speech may be incoherent and their thoughts disjointed. They may be preoccupied with delusions and responding to hallucinations. They may attempt to harm themselves or appear to be endangering others. On the other hand, they may become withdrawn and uncommunicative.

Dangerous behaviour

It is important early in the assessment of a psychotic patient to be aware of any propensity to dangerous behaviour. It is a common fallacy that all psychotic patients are dangerous. While this is not true for the overwhelming majority, a few have a tendency to be violent usually as a direct consequence of their illness. Part of the initial assessment should include an appraisal of the presence of any such aggressive or violent behaviour. Pointers towards whether a patient is likely to be violent are a past history of violence, whether violence has already occurred, the patient's appearance and behaviour, whether the patient is intoxicated by alcohol or drugs, and the content of any delusions. Clearly it is inadvisable to enter a situation that puts the paramedic in physical danger and if there is a likelihood that this will occur the police should be involved.

As a general rule it is inadvisable to assess an acutely psychotic patient alone because of the risk of unpredictable behaviour that may lead to injury. The assessment should be carried out in an area that is easy to escape from and the paramedic should remain between the patient and the exit. Although it is sufficient in many cases to defuse the situation by sitting down, if necessary the interview should be conducted standing up. It should be noted that much aggression in these situations is born out of fear, and it is helpful to be as reassuring, empathetic and non-confrontational as possible to try to establish a rapport.

Management of Psychosis

The key to managing an acutely psychotic patient is to be able to control behaviour. This can often be achieved by use of good interpersonal skills of empathy, reassurance, a non-threatening posture, an air of calmness, and confidence. For any patient – and particularly for patients who are paranoid (believing fervently that individuals or groups are against them), distressed and reacting to threatening hallucinations – the use of inappropriate force, verbal aggression and impatience is distressing and may be seen as confrontational. This may invite retaliation, further compromising any established therapeutic relationship and resulting in a greater use of force. Worse still, the display of aggression by the patient is very likely to be attributable to 'illness' and this will colour others' assessment and will label the patient as aggressive and perhaps a troublemaker.

If sedative medication is required this will usually take the form of antipsychotic drugs (also called neuroleptics or major tranquillizers) of which there are several different groups.

Antipsychotic drugs

Antipsychotic drugs have an initial sedative action that precedes any antipsychotic effect. They are not available for use by a paramedic, and are included here for information. The safest group to inject are the butyrophenones (haloperidol 2–10 mg or droperidol 5–10 mg). It may be necessary to repeat the dose if the initial dose has been ineffective. Haloperidol can be given in doses up to 30 mg for emergency control. Chlorpromazine has been associated with fatal cardiovascular collapse when given by intramuscular injection and should not be given by this route. However, it is the most sedative neuroleptic and effective when given orally in doses of 25–100 mg. Thioridazine in doses of 25–100 mg is effective for severe psychomotor agitation. It is important to be aware that neuroleptics can precipitate severe 'extrapyramidal' side-effects in the form of acute dystonia (a bizarre combination of abnormal rigid posturing, eye rolling and pelvic thrusting), tremor, muscular rigidity or motor restlessness. This can be treated symptomatically or prophylactically with procyclidine 5–10 mg intramuscularly. One rare but potentially fatal consequence of using antipsychotic medication is *neuroleptic malignant syndrome*. This is characterized by a rapid onset over 1–3 days of acute autonomic instability (with marked swings in blood pressure, tachycardia, excessive sweating, salivation and urinary incontinence), hyperpyrexia and muscular rigidity. The mortality is 1–15%. Treatment is symptomatic. The patient should be cooled and fluid balance maintained. Often there is an intercurrent infection that should be treated.

PARASUICIDE: RECOGNITION AND TREATMENT

Evaluating suicide risk is one of the hardest yet most pertinent parts of any psychiatric assessment. In an emergency (e.g. following a suicide attempt), the first consideration must be safeguarding the physical welfare of the patient and this will usually entail transportation to the nearest accident and emergency department. Be alert to the suspicion of a suicide attempt, especially if the patient has a past history of psychiatric contact, is drowsy or unconscious, or is drunk. Do not be deceived by any apparent evidence that only a small quantity of tablets have been ingested or the patient's protestations that the overdose was not life-threatening. A significant proportion of those who attempt suicide will make a further fatal attempt, and often patients are unaware of the lack of toxicity of the medication that they have taken and believe that the quantity ingested was sufficient to cause death. In particular, do not be side-tracked by the responses of others who may minimize the importance of a person's actual or threatened attempt at self-harm and give explanations or interpretations of behaviour (most commonly in terms of manipulativeness, acting out or attention-seeking). More violent methods of attempted self-harm (e.g. hanging, shooting or deep lacerations) should always be assessed by a psychiatrist. Think of attempted suicide when you attend a single-occupant road traffic accident and the conditions of the accident are unclear.

It is important to be aware that self-harm is not in itself a mental illness and the majority of people who harm themselves have no psychiatric illness. Moreover, there is no good evidence that psychiatric treatment will prevent the repetition of self-harm behaviour in the absence of psychiatric illness. Nevertheless, the most important intervention in the management of the suicidal patient is the treatment of any psychiatric illness.

If a person has not made an attempt at self-harm but is expressing suicidal ideation then a thorough assessment should be made as outlined above. Risk factors of eventual suicide such as present or past psychiatric illness (especially depression, schizophrenia and eating disorders), personality disorder, family history of suicide, single status, unemployment, social isolation, problem drinking, previous attempts at self-harm, recent 'loss' events and older age should be noted. If the person agrees to admission to hospital and this is appropriate then it should be expedited. If the person does not agree, but is detainable under the Mental Health Act, then the appropriate procedures should be followed with the patient being closely supervised until admission takes place. The paramedic has no powers under the Mental Health Act. The police may take an individual to a 'place of safety' (psychiatric unit) under section 136. Alternatively, the patient's general practitioner can arrange an emergency admission for assessment and treatment under this Act. Before leaving the emergency the paramedic should supervise the patient until an appropriate professional can take over. If the person is deemed not to be detainable under the Mental Health Act but still expresses suicidal ideation, then there is an ethical dilemma. Strictly speaking the patient cannot be prevented from leaving. However, persons who appear to be actively attempting to end their own life, or seem to be about to do so, can be restrained from doing so (under common law), pending a further psychiatric assessment.

Risk factors in suicide

- Past or present psychiatric history of depression, schizophrenia or eating disorder
- Personality disorder
- Family history of suicide
- Single status
- Unemployment
- Social isolation
- Problem drinking
- Previous attempts at self-harm
- Recent 'loss event'
- Older age

DEPRESSION AND MANIA

Suicide is most commonly associated with depression, although people with serious and long-standing mental disorders such as schizophrenia, manic depression, alcohol dependence and chronic anxiety, are at risk of suicide. Clinical depression refers to a persistent and debilitating disorder of mood characterized by sadness, an inability to derive pleasure from any activity, low self-worth, lethargy and lack of motivation. Other common symptoms include disturbed sleep and appetite, lack of libido, anxiety symptoms and thoughts of guilt and self-blame. Patients may neglect themselves and become physically at risk through not eating or drinking. Often depressed mood is associated with poor social circumstances and deprivation.

Occasionally patients with a history of depression may become elated and overactive with increased speed of thought and excessive, expansive speech. They may appear to be excessively cheerful or irritable, or their mood may swing between the two emotional states. They may express grandiose delusions of excessive self-importance or unwarranted ability, and there is often a history of increased spending (sometimes extravagantly) and sexual excesses or disinhibition. They may see themselves as being famous or having particular powers, and may experience hallucinations which reinforce their behaviour. This is a presentation of mania and is often difficult to manage outside hospital. Such individuals may become so preoccupied with their beliefs and behaviour that they neglect their appearance – or dress in florid but totally unsuitable clothing – stop eating and drinking, and pay little attention to their living conditions. If their mood state progresses unchecked they may develop a manic stupor in which they appear mute and motionless, although fully conscious. Stuporous states can also occur in depression.

ANXIETY DISORDERS

Anxiety disorders include anxiety states, phobias and obsessive compulsive disorder. These disorders rarely present as a psychiatric emergency, but anxiety commonly accompanies other psychiatric disorders and may exacerbate a patient's distress. Anxiety can be defined as the combination of psychological symptoms of fearfulness, irritability, difficulty in concentration, sensitivity to noise and feelings of restlessness, with physical symptoms or sympathetic nervous system overactivity such as sweating, increased heart rate, churning stomach and dry mouth.

Acute anxiety is extremely distressing and may occur in normal people, especially victims of (or witnesses to) traumatic events. It is manifested in a psychological and physiological response of which the most important feature is hyperventilation. Hyperventilation is the result of excessive breathing from the upper chest (rib cage) and results in hypocapnia, which causes tinnitus, tetany, tingling, weakness and chest pains. The experience of these physical symptoms may exacerbate the feeling of anxiety, causing more hyperventilation. An explanation of the symptoms and reassurance that the patient will not come to any harm as a result of them is the first step, and may need frequent and authoritative repetition. Hyperventilation is effectively managed by getting the person to breathe into a large paper bag for several minutes, or until the breathing begins to regulate. Ensure that the patient is sitting or lying in a supported posture, and stress the need to regulate the breathing by breathing more slowly and taking shallower breaths (not deeper ones) ideally until the patient can breathe through the nose. Demonstrate how the patient can breathe using the diaphragm by placing one hand on the chest and one on the abdomen. The hand on the abdomen should move more than the one on the chest. Continue to offer explanations for the symptoms and give reassurance.

These measures may obviate the need for pharmacological treatment. If treatment is required, benzodiazepines are the drugs of choice for acute short-term anxiety. The intravenous or rectal route is the most effective for administration. Diazepam should not be given by intramuscular injection because of its variable absorption rate, but can be given intravenously in the form of diazepam emulsion (Diazemuls). Doses vary considerably between patients with a range of 2–20 mg. Lorazepam (25–30 µg/kg) is a short-acting benzodiazepine and is effective for panic attacks (episodes of acute anxiety associated with overpowering thoughts of dying or imminent physical ill-health and desire to escape). Only in the rarest circumstances should anxiety disorders be treated with benzodiazepines out of hospital.

PHYSICAL CAUSES OF PSYCHIATRIC EMERGENCIES

There are numerous physical causes of psychiatric emergencies which manifest as an acute toxic confusional state. The cardinal features of this state, also called delirium, are clouding and fluctuation of consciousness (patients have periods of drowsiness, poor concentration and lack of lucidity), increased arousal (often manifested in acute anxiety and fearfulness), disturbances in perception (in the form of illusions or hallucinations) and disorientation in time, place and person. As a result of these experiences a person may become extremely distressed and be liable to misinterpret the actions of others. Often elderly people present as an emergency in this way and it is important to be aware that many drugs to which the elderly are sensitive can precipitate delirium. An elderly person suffering from dementia may develop a toxic confusional state as a complication. Differentiation of dementia and delirium is not difficult – the latter has an acute onset with an abrupt change in behaviour, whereas dementia is altogether a more gradual deterioration in functioning and behaviour and does not fulfil the criteria for delirium.

Features of acute toxic confusional state (delirium)

- Clouding and fluctuation of consciousness – drowsiness, poor concentration and lack of lucidity
- Acute anxiety and fearfulness
- Illusions or hallucinations
- Disorientation in time, place and person

Alcohol and Illicit Drugs

The assessment and appropriate management of intoxicated individuals poses particular problems for all health service staff. It may not be easy to decide whether an intoxicated individual requires hospital assessment or (if causing a disturbance) whether police custody is more appropriate. On the one hand, intoxication is not uncommon, is sanctioned by society and in most cases leads to no harm; on the other, intoxicated individuals may be a considerable risk to themselves, especially if they have a history of alcohol dependence, and may therefore require assessment in a hospital setting. If it is felt that intoxicated patients are likely to suffer from physical effects of the intoxicating substance (e.g. delirium tremens, withdrawal fits or septicaemia) to the extent that they need to be monitored in hospital, then they should be taken to an accident and emergency department, if necessary against their will. However, as soon as they are no longer at physical risk, they must be allowed to leave unless they are liable for detention under the Mental Health Act. Admission to a psychiatric hospital may be indicated for assessment of a suspected underlying mental disorder. In this case it may be possible to detain the patient under the Mental Health Act. Certain hallucinogens (e.g. LSD or magic mushrooms) can trigger off a psychotic reaction in a previously undiagnosed or vulnerable person, or may worsen pre-existing states of psychosis.

Delirium tremens, which occurs hours or days after the cessation or reduction of drinking, is characterized by tremulousness, disorientation, vivid hallucinations or illusions, and autonomic overactivity, is associated with a mortality of 10% and should always be managed in a general hospital. Acute withdrawal can be managed with long-acting benzodiazepines such as chlordiazepoxide. However, it should be noted that many problem drinkers will supplement benzodiazepines with alcohol and only a small quantity should be prescribed at any one time. Chlormethiazole (Heminevrin) should not be used for outpatient detoxification or treatment of withdrawal.

PERSONALITY DISORDER

One of the most difficult categories of patient to assess are those with a diagnosis of personality disorder. The validity and meaning of this term are a matter of some debate and it is often used as a perjorative and demeaning label (along with other discredited terms such as 'manipulative', 'hysterical', 'attention-seeking' and 'inadequate'). These patients often harm themselves or express suicidal ideation, and have often been frequently admitted to hospital. They may be hostile and impatient, and lack the ability to form a rapport. They appear to induce feelings of irritability and antagonism in staff and it is easy to lose an objective approach to their problems. This may result in an inadequate assessment and a failure to recognize serious psychiatric illness. There may be a tendency to minimize these patients' risk of eventually committing suicide because of the number of previous attempts which are often not life-threatening. However, a proportion of these patients do succeed in ending their lives, and it is important therefore to be aware that personality disordered patients do develop other psychiatric disorders (e.g. depression) which may predispose them to making a more serious attempt to end their life. Thus it is vital that patients with personality disorders are assessed thoroughly if they are expressing suicidal ideation. Other professionals who may be involved include social workers, community psychiatric nurses and the patient's general practitioner, as well as family and friends or voluntary agencies. It often benefits the patient if these other professionals are involved sooner rather than later, as they are likely to be extremely familiar with the patient's history and may obviate the need for hospital assessment.

THE MENTAL HEALTH ACT 1983

If after assessment it is felt that a patient needs to be in a psychiatric hospital, a patient who refuses admission can be admitted compulsorily under the provisions of the Mental Health Act 1983. The sections that are most likely to be used in an emergency are Sections 2, 3 and 4, and Sections 135 and 136. The section papers must be filled in before the patient is taken to hospital but it should be noted that the section only comes into force when all the forms have been accepted by or on behalf of the hospital managers after the patient arrives in hospital.

It is important to note that the Mental Health Act does not apply to persons who are intoxicated by alcohol or drugs. However, if it is felt that there is an actual or possible underlying mental disorder in someone who is intoxicated, and that person is a risk to self or others, then admission under the Act may be appropriate.

Section 2: Admission for Assessment

Section 2 is for assessment in hospital, or for assessment followed by treatment, and it is usually applied when a patient has no past history of mental disorder, or is not known to the local psychiatric service. The grounds for detention are that the patient must suffer from a mental disorder that warrants the patient's detention in hospital, and that admission is necessary in the interests of the patient's own health or safety or for the protection of others. A specific diagnosis is not a prerequisite for detention – indeed the rationale for detention is to make a diagnosis. The section is valid for 28 days. The procedure requires an application by an approved social worker or nearest relative, and medical recommendations by two doctors, one of whom must be approved under the Act (usually a consultant psychiatrist). The approved social worker must have seen the patient within the last 14 days and should, so far as is practicable, consult the nearest relative. The approved social worker can be contacted at the local social services department.

Section 3: Admission for Treatment

Section 3 allows the compulsory admission of a patient and treatment for up to 6 months. It is usually applied when there is a known diagnosis. In order for this longer-term order to apply, the patient must suffer from a mental disorder – specified as mental illness, severe mental impairment – psychopathic disorder or mental impairment – that is of a nature or degree which makes it appropriate for the patient to receive medical treatment in a hospital. In the case of psychopathic disorder or mental impairment, treatment should alleviate or prevent a deterioration of the patient's condition. In addition, in all cases, it must be necessary for the health or safety of the patient or for the protection of others that such treatment should be given, and that it cannot be provided unless the patient is detained under this section. The application is made by the patient's nearest relative or an approved social worker. The latter must, if practicable, consult the nearest relative before making an application and cannot proceed if the nearest relative objects. The medical recommendations are as for Section 2. In addition, the recommendations must state the particular grounds for the doctor's opinion, specifying whether any other methods of dealing with the patient are available and, if so, why they are not appropriate. The doctor must specify one of the four types of mental disorder (see above).

Section 4: Admission in an Emergency

If there is difficulty in obtaining a second medical application from an approved doctor to detain the patient under Section 2 and the situation is an emergency, then an emergency order for assessment (Section 4) can be completed by the approved social worker and a doctor who need not be approved under the Act. Application is made by the approved social worker who must have seen the patient within the previous 24 hours, or the nearest relative. The patient must be admitted within 24 hours of the medical examination or application. The duration of the order is 72 hours and is expected that it will be converted to a Section 2 order as soon as possible after the patient has arrived in hospital.

Section 135

A social worker who believes that someone is suffering from a mental disorder and is unable to care for himself or herself, or is being ill-treated or neglected, may apply to a magistrate for a warrant for that person's removal to a place of safety.

Section 136

It is possible that some emergency situations (e.g. road traffic accidents) will necessitate the removal of apparently mentally ill people to a place of safety without being able to obtain applications from social workers or psychiatrists. With Section 136, police constables have the power to remove to a place of safety a person whom they find in a public place who appears to be suffering from a mental disorder and to be in need of care and control for his or her own interests or for the protection of others. The person should be taken to the nearest convenient place of safety (usually a hospital or police station) to be detained for a period not exceeding 72 hours for the purpose of examination by a doctor and interview by an approved social worker. An accident and emergency department is not a place of safety – a psychiatric ward is.

COMMON LAW AND INFORMED CONSENT

Any interaction between a health service worker and a patient is assumed to occur with the patient's informed consent. If a patient does not give consent for a particular examination or intervention, however minor, and is capable of consent, then the worker can be charged with assault. If a patient is unable to give consent because of mental illness then a health worker can act against the patient's wishes, but only in certain circumstances: the treatment or investigation must be seen to be life-saving or necessary to prevent immediate serious harm to the patient or others, and should be given in good faith. If at all possible, treatment should be given under the provisions of the Mental Health Act 1983. However, in certain circumstances this will not be possible, and emergency treatment (usually an injection) can be administered against the patient's will. It is good practice always to make a note at the time as to the reasons for any treatment given without the patient's consent, as well as recording the names of witnesses.

CONCLUSIONS

Assessment and appropriate management of a psychiatric emergency requires time, patience and common sense. It is a dynamic process in which negotiation and arbitration may have to take place not only between the patient, relative or carer and professionals, but also between the professionals involved. Time should be taken to gather information and decisions should be reached as a result of objective appraisal of that information, as opposed to arbitrary, hasty and ill-informed opinion. A knowledge of psychiatric disorders and the psychopathology that accompanies them, and an understanding of the risk of psychiatric patients losing their right of autonomy and advocacy as a result of misplaced stigma and prejudice, will increase the likelihood of a thorough assessment.

At the end of the assessment, it should be possible to decide whether the patient has an organic, functional or predominantly social problem. The decision then needs to be made as to whether the patient requires further assessment in hospital or a local community facility or whether it would be more appropriate for other agencies (e.g. social services) to review the situation. It may be more appropriate for the patient to make contact with voluntary agencies or self-help groups. These have been established for many of the problems that can present as psychiatric emergencies and include substance misuse groups such as Alcoholics or Narcotics Anonymous, Aquarius; helplines for drug addicts, rape victims or battered wives; church organizations; and marriage guidance (Relate).

Patients who appear to require further assessment and agree to go to hospital should be taken there. Patients who refuse, and appear to be a risk to themselves or others, either can be taken by the police to a place of safety (if they are in a public place) or a Mental Health Act assessment can be arranged by the local social services team. Where patients do not appear to be at immediate risk but remain distressed, it would be appropriate to contact their general practitioner.

chapter fifty-four:

COPING WITH STRESS

Men are not disquieted by things themselves but by their idea of things

Epictetus

This chapter offers practical ways of coping with stress. The origins and evolution of the stress response are outlined, as are the physiological and psychological responses of individuals. An overview of the principles of dealing with excessive stress and a detailed, practical account of stress-reducing techniques are provided. Throughout the chapter it is emphasized that it is not events that are stressful but our reaction to them. Coping with stress involves changing our reactions, thereby altering how stressful we feel. Stress is not all bad – it can have positive effects too.

WHAT IS STRESS?

Stress is a nebulous term. It is subject to individual interpretation and experience, and cannot be rigorously defined. However, unless there is common understanding of what stress means there is little worth in discussing ways of coping with it, because successful stress management starts with its recognition. When considering 'psychological' stress two themes emerge. Firstly, stress is an experience that occurs when people are faced with situations that they perceive as threatening to their physical or psychological well-being. Secondly, dealing with those situations engenders a degree of uncertainty. The psychological component to stress has its origins in the way the body reacts in response to immediate danger. However, whether this psychological response is activated depends on a cognitive evaluation by the individual of what demands are being made and what resources are available to deal with them.

Stress and Health-Care Professionals

Health-care professionals are particularly likely to be affected by adverse stress. The fact that they deal with people in crisis about whom decisions have to be made often in emergency situations heightens the degree of pressure upon them. Frequently they have to practise within time and resource constraints, both of which limit their ability to deal effectively with the situations with which they are faced. Most experience an intense sense of responsibility and personal involvement in their work, and all of these factors increase stress. However, health-care professionals also show a remarkable reluctance to seek help when faced with the results of adverse stress. Whether this is due to a sense that they will let themselves or the service down, professional machismo or just plain ignorance has not been established. However, it is clear that among health-service workers there are high rates of substance misuse, psychological distress and suicide. It seems peculiar that in a profession that experiences such a high degree of stress at all levels there is such apathy when it comes to recognizing and dealing with it.

ORIGINS AND EVOLUTION OF STRESS RESPONSE

Biological Adaptivity to Threat

The origins of stress lie in the process by which the body mobilizes its capacity for dealing with danger through the 'fight or flight' response. When an individual is faced with what is perceived as a threatening situation, that individual can either stay and confront it or make good an escape. Both of these options depend on the body's ability to prepare itself for immediate physical exertion. The 'fight or flight' response is a description of these physical changes: they include an increase in heart rate, diversion of blood to major muscle groups, dilation of airways with increased rate of respiration, slowing of the digestive system, increased acuity of senses (e.g. pupil dilation), and release of endorphins, cortisone, adrenaline, thyroid hormones and glucose into the blood stream. Normally a period of intense activity would ensue which would end when the threat was no longer present. The subsequent release of tension at the end of physical exertion comprises the relaxation response. The source of many stress-related health problems is that the 'fight or flight' response is triggered many times a day but there is no resulting physical exertion. This results in the production of tension which is not released, the relaxation response is not activated and the body chemistry does not return to normal.

Good Stress and Bad Stress

Stress results from the interplay between demands and resources. Tension results from the non-resolution of stress. If the resources are equal to the demands stress may still be experienced, but in a positive way leading to greater productivity and a sense of satisfaction. Even when the demands increase, provided they are within capabilities, the stress induced may be pleasurable. Stress that results in better achievement is associated with well-being and satisfactory relaxation. However, if the pressure becomes a little greater, individuals may be pushed beyond their ability to cope and start to become fatigued. Similarly, stress resulting from a situation that is unresolved creates tension that leads to ill-health. If a situation has been resolved satisfactorily – or if not resolved is accepted as being a satisfactory conclusion – this is a healthy response, but if the outcome of the situation is not accepted this leads to tension that is destructive.

Stress and Personality

Research has shown that certain personality types are more likely to be affected adversely by stress. Individuals known as type A personalities demonstrate behaviour such as having high levels of energy, doing several things at once and being unable to delegate. They have high ideals and expectations and are very conscientious. These individuals are unable to deal with the stress that they encounter and are prone to physical consequences of excessive stress – in particular there is a strong association between heart disease and type A personality.
Burn-out is a phenomenon that describes the fatigue and frustration brought about by devotion to a cause, way of life or relationship that fails to produce the expected reward (Freudenberger and Richelson, 1980). Burn-out too is associated with type A personalities.

Stress and Physical Illness

A number of physical symptoms or disorders have been linked with stress. These range from minor rashes and food sensitivities to more disabling and serious conditions such as hypertension, peptic ulcers and irritable bowel syndrome. Musculoskeletal, cardiovascular and gastrointestinal systems can all be affected, and there is some evidence that stress and fatigue can weaken the action of the immune system and predispose to the development of cancer, multiple sclerosis and rheumatoid arthritis.

Stress-related illnesses comprise almost 75% of conditions for which people seek medical attention.

Stress and Psychiatric Illness

Substance abuse
Individuals who have difficulty coping with stress may resort to artificial relaxants in the form of alcohol or prescribed anxiolytics such as diazepam (Valium). These are central depressants that induce relaxation at the cost of dependence. The cost is high, causing physical, emotional and social damage. Not only do these substances fail to deal with the source of the stress (i.e. the stress-producing circumstances), they also provide extra unforeseen stresses such as physical ill-health, employment compromises (e.g. through drinking and driving, accidents, poor work record), relationship difficulties and increased anxiety.

Depression and anxiety
Chronic unresolved stress can predispose to the development of clinical depression. If a situation is habitually interpreted as threatening or the resources for dealing with it as being inadequate, then not only will that situation induce stress but also the ability to deal with the stress is likely to be compromised. This may result in persistent low self-esteem and predispose to the development of a depressive illness. Similarly, neutral events that are interpreted in a negative way are thought to contribute to the onset of depression. Continued, unresolved stress can predispose to the development of an anxiety disorder.

Post-Traumatic Stress Disorder

Post-traumatic stress disorder is an established psychiatric condition. First recognized in the Vietnam war this psychological reaction to a horrific, exceptionally threatening and catastrophic situation is not uncommon in both victims and witnesses. The situation can cause pervasive distress in almost anyone, and the disorder manifests itself after a short time in 'flashbacks' consisting of intrusive memories or nightmares of the trauma, a sense of numbness and detachment, lack of enjoyment, heightened anxiety levels and avoidance of cues that remind the sufferer of the original trauma. The onset follows the trauma usually with a delay of several weeks. The course is fluctuating but recovery occurs in the majority of cases. Most are treated with psychotherapy but it is important to exclude the possibility of a depressive illness.

COPING WITH EXCESSIVE STRESS

Principles of Stress Management

The principles of coping with stress (here meaning excessive stress, i.e. stress that is stressful) are recognition of tension, deciding that 'something needs to be done', knowing what is causing the stress, and dealing with it by either taking action against the stressor, or if this is not possible making a positive decision to ignore it or adapt to it.

Coping with stress

- Recognize tension
- Decide that 'something must be done'
- Identify the stressor
- Deal with it

Recognizing the effects

Signs of bodily tension include ankle bending or tapping of feet; coiled legs; hair-twirling; arms folded tightly across the chest with abdomen drawn in; nail-biting; tight, hunched shoulders; clenched fists with tight knuckles and a gripped thumb; clenched teeth with jutting jaw; worry muscles of the forehead contracted. Tension may become apparent through the development of symptoms such as headache, neckache or stomach problems (Table 54.1). More serious manifestations such as anxiety, depression or physical symptoms have been described above.

Recognizing the causes

The most effective way to deal with actual or potential stress is to anticipate it. By looking at the common causes of stress and the effects of particular demands on individuals it should be possible to recognize the origin of stress. It may be related to the nature of a job, or may be closer to home and more personal.

General causes Many of the general causes of stress relate to how work is structured. Poor organization, lack of appropriate supervision and long or unsociable hours can all contribute to devaluing a person's role at work and chip away at their self-esteem. Frequent changes in policy, lack of communication and a perceived lack of direction from superiors contribute to poor morale, lack of status and job dissatisfaction. The necessity to

conform with bureaucratic procedures ('paper pushing') that are inappropriate to the level of training affects performance ('the harder I work the more I have to do and the less efficient I become'). Poor pay and promotion prospects lead to financial pressures and frustration of ambition.

Life events Research has shown that stressful events can have both positive and negative effects. Holmes and Rahe (1967) in their study in the USA found that 80% of those who experience many dramatic changes in their lives can expect a major illness within the next 2 years. They identified and rated 43 changes in lifestyle ranging from death of a partner (100 points) to minor violation of the law (11 points). Marriage was set at 50 points, with 73 points for divorce. If the total score was over 300 in 1 year there was likely to be major illness. A score over 100 indicated the need to take some remedial measures. Effects were cumulative such that events from 2 years previously could still produce effects (Table 54.2).

Specific causes Specific causes of stress at work comprise those that relate to how individuals tackle their roles. Uncertainty about one's role causes uncertainty in decision-making. There may be problems deciding on how far one's responsibility extends. There may be a conflict of interest regarding patient care and loyalty to colleagues or family. Those with perfectionistic and obsessional qualities (clearly necessary to some degree in health-care workers) may have difficulty knowing when to stop and how to delegate. An inability to influence those making decisions (powerlessness) may produce high levels of frustration. Difficult relationships with colleagues, especially superiors, will be detrimental to performance.

Task-related causes Being at the forefront of health care, especially being first on the scene at emergencies, produces its own problems. Difficulties may arise with patients or their relatives who may be obstructive, violent, verbally abusive or just in need of copious reassurance. An inability to help or act immediately coupled with demonstrable suffering may lead to doubts about professional effectiveness. The responsibility entailed by

Table 54.1 Signs and symptoms of stress

Signs	Symptoms
Ankle bending or tapping of feet	Headache
Coiled legs	Neckache
Hair twirling	Nausea and
Arms folded across chest	vomiting
Clenched fists with tight knuckles	
Gripped thumbs	
Clenched teeth	
Furrowed forehead	

Table 54.2 Life events

Event	Score
Death of a partner	100 points
Divorce	73 points
Marriage	50 points
Minor law violation	11 points

working in an increasingly litigious health service for an increasingly sceptical, informed and querulous public conscious of their rights may lead to overcautiousness and 'defensive' practice. Emotional involvement with patients may colour judgement and compromise objectivity. The requirement to be impartial and avoid being caught up in a patient's distress may be difficult for some individuals.

Stress in the home Domestic stress is a powerful means of destabilizing efficiency at work, whether caused by a partner, children, domestic arrangements or environmental pressures upon the home (e.g. noisy neighbours, financial worries or insecurity of accommodation).

Personal causes Stress involves the personal response to a demand or situation. How we react when faced with a particular circumstance governs how stressed we feel. The more we know about our likely or actual responses, the more we can minimize feelings of tension. Thus becoming aware of ourselves, our personalities and our patterns of reacting to situations and circumstances allows a more appropriate response to demands upon us. Being aware of our temperamental characteristics, our degree of obsessionality and the extent to which we indulge in risk-taking is important in recognizing when we are stressed. Similarly, ways in which we may blame ourselves unnecessarily for a set of circumstances or overidentify with a particular outcome may be relevant in the development of stress.

Managing the Stressor

Once excess stress has been recognized and there is motivation to deal with it, the next step is to make a list of likely causes. Doing this not only entails a process of self-evaluation but also starts a process of solution. Identifying possible stressors allows the possibility of resolution of the stress, and list-making in itself seems to reduce tension. Once the list has been formed, choose the stressor that is easiest to resolve and break it down into objective parts. For example, if 'unclear role' has been identified as a source of stress, look at your present activity and compare it with what you think you ought to be doing. Identify which part of your role is unclear, and give examples. If you recognize 'poor communication' as being stressful, analyse why this is the case, with whom and in what circumstances. Having made a list and objectified the problem it is important to decide whether this requires immediate action or should be left for the future, and also whether the circumstance is likely to be resolved or will be impossible to resolve and should be ignored or adapted to (e.g. pay, promotion aspects). It must be realized that choosing to ignore or adapt to stress is a positive outcome. If there is difficulty arriving at a solution try thinking creatively, perhaps putting yourself in the place of some hapless manager, and do not forget to use humour. A lighthearted approach to difficulties can immediately reduce their intensity and threat.

The steps in coping with stress are:

- Make a list
- Think creatively
- Objectify the problem
- Use humour
- Decide on immediate or future action
- Ignore or adapt to the stress

PERSONAL MANAGEMENT

Self-Awareness

Unless we are able to get in touch with our physical, emotional and spiritual states, any attempt to modify them will be bound to fail. Self-awareness is the process by which an individual undergoes such analysis. Understanding how we ourselves react gives an insight into how others see us, and that in itself may go some way to solving hitherto intractable problems.

Time Management

Much of the cause of non-specific stress lies in personal inefficiency and poor time management. Clearly, there will be unavoidable demands on one's time, and the wider organization may be inefficient and time-consuming. However, throughout the day there are pockets of time that can be used effectively. Thinking about how you spend your time and why you are spending time in this way, setting yourself goals and plans, listing priorities and being assertive are all techniques that will make you an effective time user rather than a time-waster. Beware of meetings, overavailability on the telephone, poor communication, indecision and lack of self-discipline. These are all potential causes of time-wasting.

Meditation

Meditation and relaxation are valuable skills to help cope with stress. A full discussion of meditation is beyond the scope of this chapter. However, a simple method is to sit in an upright position, undisturbed, for 5–10 minutes each day. When comfortable, close your eyes and allow your attention to focus gently upon your breathing. At the same time any thoughts that arise are denied attention. Attention instead is focused on a particular object or experience, such as the air rushing in through the nostrils or a repeated word or phrase (a mantra). In this way it is possible to train attention and increase control over thought processes. Subsequently there is an improved ability to handle emotions and physical relaxation is more effective.

Relaxation

The relaxation response was first described by Walter Hess in 1957. The psychological changes that accompany it are:

- Decrease in muscle tone, heart and respiratory rate, blood pressure, and blood lactate and cortisone levels
- A noticeable decrease in oxygen consumption and carbon dioxide elimination
- Increased blood flow to major internal organs
- Improvement in peripheral circulation
- A rise in skin temperature
- An increase in basal skin resistance

One way of measuring the extent of relaxation is by use of biofeedback machines. These monitor the physiological processes within the body that usually are unnoticed (e.g. muscle tension, skin temperature, blood pressure and heart rate) and can give a visual or audible reading of them. The different subjective feelings of relaxation can then be related to the accompanying physiological changes. Moreover, this monitoring of psychological processes helps bring them under voluntary control so that individuals can learn what brings about body relaxation, what disrupts it and how to apply relaxation at times of stress.

There are several different types of relaxation technique. The thread that runs through them all, however, is that they have to be learned to be effective. This requires an effective understanding of the technique to be used, the achievement of satisfactory relaxation on each occasion, and frequent (at least daily) practice. It is no good attempting to learn relaxation in an environment that is not peaceful or is liable to interruption or other disturbance. Clearly, once effective relaxation has been learned it is valuable to apply it in any situation. Types of relaxation include the use of breathing techniques, graded muscle relaxation and graded imagery.

Breathing techniques

Overbreathing is common in anxiety and usually takes place in the upper chest. Breathing exercises are effective in reducing anxiety, depression, irritability and fatigue, and most systems of relaxation include emphasis on breathing. Breathing exercises can be done either sitting upright on a supportive chair with legs uncrossed, or lying on the floor with knees bent and spine straight. Start by scanning the body for tension, especially in the throat, chest and abdomen, and allow the release of tension. Next, place one hand on your chest and one on your abdomen. Inhale slowly and deeply, feeling your abdomen rise with each inhalation. There should be very little movement in the upper chest but plenty in the lower. Exhalations should be slow, allowing the air to leave the body with a slight sigh through the mouth. Inhalation should be through the nose. Focus should be kept on the sound of your breath, the slow rhythm of breath-

ing and the gentle abdominal rise and fall. Be conscious of your deepening sense of relaxation and continue for 5–10 minutes at a time. At the end of each breathing session scan your body for tension again and note whether it is different from before.

Graded muscle relaxation

Graded muscle relaxation involves tensing groups of muscles and relaxing them, making note of the difference in tension.
Lie on the floor, flat on your back with your feet about 30 cm apart and your hands resting by your side. Begin by gently breathing in through your nose and out through your mouth. Now put all your attention into the muscles of your face: screw up all the muscles as tight as you can. Hold that tension for just a few moments . . . then relax. Now focus on the muscles in your shoulders. Hunch your shoulders up as high as you can . . . hold the tension in them for a few moments . . . and relax, allowing your shoulders to drop and allowing your shoulders to broaden and make greater contact with the floor. Now clench both fists tightly . . . then stretch both your arms downwards, towards your feet . . . hold the tension for just a few moments . . . and allow your hands and arms to relax completely. Then focus your attention on the muscles in your stomach. Take a deep breath and as you breathe out, allow the muscles of your stomach to be pulled in. Hold the tension for just a few minutes . . . then relax them completely and breathe normally . . . allow yourself to feel more and more relaxed. Finally, focus your attention on your legs and feet. Point both feet downwards as far as you can . . . allow your legs to push forward as far as you can . . . hold the tension for a few moments . . . then relax both feet and legs. Allow yourself to relax completely. Feel how much heavier your body now is and allow your body to sink further into the floor. Appreciate what it feels like to have all your muscles relaxed. Breathe gently and easily and remain in the relaxed position for a few minutes.

Graded imagery

Using graded imagery entails closing your eyes, scanning the body for tension and releasing it, and then visualizing a scene either that you know well or that you can imagine clearly. It should be a pleasant scene in which there is plenty of detail. Examples include a garden, a beach or a picture. Once the vision has been established start to envisage details; be as accurate as possible without straining too much. Pick out colours, scents, noises and touch sensations as you pass through or scan the vision. Feel the physical sensations associated with it – the warmth of the sun, the gentleness of the breeze, the sparkling of water and the softness of touch and noise. As you become part of the scene, become also part of the tranquillity within it. No deadlines, no demands, no pressures . . . just the feeling of being at one with the peace around and within you. Stay in this state for as long as you wish and then gradually let yourself sink back into the surface on which you are lying or sitting. Let the scene gently dissolve, and then open your eyes and reorient yourself.

Diet, Fluids and Physical Exercise

Some of the physiological effects of stress result in dehydration. Moreover, people who are stressed tend not to eat or drink regularly, thereby compounding the problem. It is recommended that four pints (approximately 2 litres) of fluid per day are taken in addition to that in food and added to cereal. Tea and coffee are diuretics and contain caffeine so should be avoided. Excessive intake of caffeine during the week can lead to weekend withdrawal symptoms of headache, nausea and tremor. In order to combat stress the body requires more energy, and a healthy diet is important. Cut down fat intake, especially saturated fat, e.g. red meat, hard cheese, cream, butter and eggs. Increase the quantity of fruit, vegetables and absorbable fibre; reduce sugar and salt intake, and watch your weight. Exercise regularly, and remember that each time the body becomes stressed it is gearing itself up for exercise. If this is met by actual physical exercise on a regular basis, the subsequent release of endorphins aids relaxation.

Role of the Team

The team has an important role in helping to cope with stress. By recognizing the signs of stress in team members and being aware of demands on individuals, support can be given to encourage resolution of problems. Group activities such as debriefing and staff councils allow presentation of problems at an early stage. Lines of communication can be drawn up, allowing effective dissemination of news and management changes.

REFERENCES

Freudenberger HS & Richelson G (1980) *Burnout: The High Cost of Achievement*. Garden City, NY: Anchor Press.
Holmes TH & Rahe RH (1967) The social readjustment rating scale. *Journal of Psychomatic Research* 2: 213–218.

11

MAJOR INCIDENTS

chapter fifty-five

THE MAJOR INCIDENT:
AN OVERVIEW

Events in Britain and elsewhere have highlighted the need for contingency planning and preparation to cope with possible disasters. In the 1980s the UK suffered a flurry of major incidents, including the King's Cross Underground fire, the Clapham rail crash (Figure 55.1), the sinking of the *Marchioness* and the Kegworth air crash. The combined effect of these was to generate a surge of activity in the field of emergency planning. Greater importance was given to the roles of health authority and ambulance service emergency planning officers. Local authority emergency planning departments are now allowed a role in civil emergencies, rather than remaining restricted to their former wartime contingency planning. Practical experience has raised awareness of the need for an integrated interservice cooperation in response to disasters.

The key players from each service must be aware of each other's capabilities and responsibilities, and effective lines of communication must be established long before they are put to the test at a major incident.

While these encouraging developments within the emergency services and local authorities have been taking place, the health service has been subjected to considerable organizational restructuring. The development of trusts, both for the health and ambulance services, has fundamentally changed the provision of health care. The purchaser-provider split has further confused the ground rules for the response to major incidents. As the statistical chances of a disaster occurring in any given area is remote, it is often difficult to raise the motivation to provide for an adequate response to such incidents.

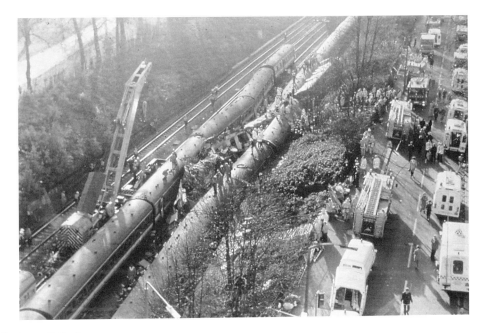

Fig. 55.1 The Clapham rail disaster

Maintaining stockpiles of equipment that are unlikely to be used does not seem cost-effective to a management that responds on a 'just in time' principle.

Lessons of past disasters are rarely learned and incidents tend to repeat themselves. For the paramedic the major incident is a challenge. Few are likely to attend more than one in their entire professional career, and most will never be involved at all. The developing role of paramedics in the modern efficient ambulance service requires them to be prepared to cope with the disaster around the corner. The old saying is as true today as ever: *'Failure to plan is planning to fail'*.

DEFINITIONS

The health service defines a major incident as:

> 'Any occurrence which presents a serious threat to the health of the community, disruption to the services, or causes or is likely to cause such numbers of casualties as to require special arrangements by the Health Service.' (HC90 25)

Major incidents can and do occur without producing live casualties. The Lockerbie plane crash, when a passenger aircraft was blown up by a terrorist device as it flew over a small Scottish border town, caused minimal disruption to the health service. For the police, fire service, military and local authorities the impact was enormous, and involvement spanned weeks and months. On the other hand, a food poisoning epidemic would have major repercussions for the health service, but little or no effect on the fire service. While all the services are not fully engaged in all disasters, integrated 'all hazards' planning with the other emergency services may produce a simpler and better definition of what constitutes a major incident:

> 'Any situation which develops or threatens to develop which is beyond the local resources and requires the special mobilization of the emergency services to deal with it.'

Major incidents can be classified into simple or compound, and compensated or uncompensated. A *simple* incident is one in which the structure of the community in which it occurs remains intact, for example a train or air crash. A *compound* incident destroys the whole structure of the surrounding community, for example the Los Angeles or Japanese earthquakes. In a *compensated* incident there are sufficient local resources to deal with the incident, whereas in an *uncompensated* incident the medical and other responding emergency services are destroyed or totally inadequate. Almost all British major incidents have been simple and compensated. However, the risks of a major incident on a far greater scale have to be considered from storms, floods, terrorism or disease. Earthquakes, common in some parts of the world, are a remote consideration for Britain. Teams of British paramedics and other rescuers have attended uncompensated major incidents in other parts of the world, and it is useful for training to include these worst-case scenarios. An uncompensated major incident is synonymous with a 'disaster'.

COMMAND, CONTROL AND COMMUNICATION

The 'three Cs' – command, control and communication – are the management tools of a successful major incident response. It is vital that time is spent initially in establishing good command, control and communication, because without these essentials the incident cannot be handled effectively. The first principle is to provide the greatest good for the greatest number of casualties. To be side-tracked into heroic resuscitation for the first casualty found, who has no hope of survival, may have fatal consequences for others whose survival is dependent upon rapid airway intervention alone.

The first crew on scene have enormous responsibilities for the future smooth management of the incident. The driver of the vehicle should remain by the radio to provide constant updates to ambulance control. The attendant must make a quick reconnaissance of the scene, identifying hazards and approximate casualty numbers, and report these details back to the driver for transmission to control. Additionally, the attendant must establish contact with the senior officers of the other emergency services present, and become the initial ambulance incident officer (AIO). Until other resources arrive the attendant cannot be side-tracked into the care of casualties. It may be necessary to utilize 'buddy aid' (basic medical care provided to each other by victims of a disaster), bystanders, police and firefighters to provide initial care.

Command – Control – Communicate

To assist the first crews on scene, many services provide action cards based on the 'CHALET' mnemonic

C	>	Casualties – approximate number and types
H	>	Hazards – present and potential
A	>	Access routes for other emergency service vehicles
L	>	Location of incident – exact point on map
E	>	Emergency services additionally required
T	>	Type of incident (train crash, explosion, etc.)

The principal role of the ambulance service is, in conjunction with the other emergency services, to save life, promote recovery and, as the Americans sometimes say, return casualties to full taxpayer status! This is achieved by promptly providing sufficient ambulances, staff and equipment to deal with readily accessible casualties. Vehicles must arrive in a steady flow and be able to leave the scene without delay. Ambulances are the only emergency vehicles which need to come and go from the incident. It is most important that access and egress routes are established early and maintained by police officers. An *emergency services rendezvous point* or *ambulance parking point* may also need to be established. The ambulance service will determine, in conjunction with medical personnel, the priority for treatment and evacuation of casualties. A dynamic system of triage is essential. *A casualty clearing centre* will act as the focus to which patients should be brought. This should be managed by an experienced, senior paramedic or doctor, depending on availability. Hospital-based mobile medical teams should normally also work from this point. Adjacent to the casualty clearing centre, an *equipment dump* should be prepared under the management of a suitable officer. An *ambulance loading point* should also be established nearby (Figure 55.2).

Traditionally, ambulance service efficiency at a major incident has been judged by the speed at which the first casualties are removed from the scene. This marker is no longer appropriate. The first five ambulances arriving at a major incident should probably be used to provide equipment and personnel to the scene rather than for the transport of patients. In a multiple casualty incident 'stay and stabilize' is now considered normal best practice. Patients can be stabilized at the incident before

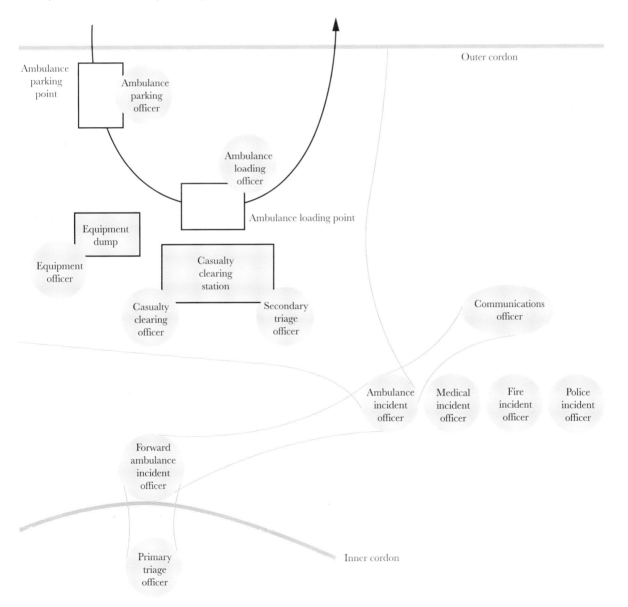

Fig. 55.2 *Organization of the ambulance service at a major incident*

transport, thus reducing the emergency need for rapid transport. The first few crews arriving provide a triage and treatment team. Some paramedics may work at the 'sharp end' with trapped casualties if the incident requires it. Trained and experienced doctors from local immediate care schemes or local hospital mobile medical teams will be of considerable support to paramedics and should always be mobilized to assist at the scene according to local protocols. On the other hand, doctors who turn up or who are plucked out of a local hospital or surgery just because they happen to be on duty may well be a liability to the ambulance service. This is certainly true if they are not properly trained, equipped and in appropriate protective clothing. Bogus doctors have often been attracted to the scene of major incidents. If the identity and experience of a doctor cannot be verified the ambulance service must decline their assistance and have them escorted from the scene.

CONTROL ACTIVITY

As soon as reports of a possible major incident are received, the ambulance control should automatically bring into action a prepared response to cope with the incident. Once the incident is confirmed as genuine the plan should continue to resource the scene. Initial reports may be very vague and sketchy, and later become confused and contradictory. Eventually control will be bombarded with information which needs careful documenting and coordinating. It is important to remember that control staff are completely blind to the incident. They rely totally on graphic and descriptive reports from personnel on scene. The media response to a disaster is often rapid. Many controls now rely on television, especially cable or satellite continuous news reports, to obtain a better understanding of the situation at the scene. Accident and emergency departments are also blind to the scene. They too are initially relying on rumours, media reports, and impressions from patients and staff arriving at their department.

Most areas have adopted the 'gold', 'silver' and 'bronze' system of management. The *Gold Command* is the chief officer or deputy at headquarters, who dictates overall policy and delegates the incident strategy to the *Silver Command*, the senior ambulance incident officer at the scene. The Silver Command determines tactics and delegates specific tasks to *Bronze Level* officers, who undertake the various operational functions at the scene (Figure 55.3).

The mobilization of paramedic managers by ambulance control to the scene should be automatic. They should perform the various management functions initially undertaken by the first few responding paramedics, freeing them to undertake their normal treatment functions. It is vital to remember the importance of integrated response from all the emergency services. The ambulance service must not act in isolation from the others. A briefing meeting of incident officers responsible for the management of the incident should be established as soon

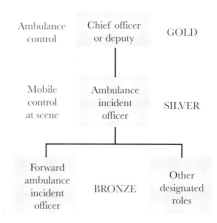

Fig. 55.3 The Gold, Silver and Bronze Command. 'Other designated roles', include parking, loading, safety, casualty selection, triage, equipment, hospital liaison etc.

as practicable. It should be possible to ensure that the first meeting takes place within 60 minutes. This meeting of Silver Commanders will need to be documented (logged). It will normally take place near to the incident. The first priority is to share intelligence and establish what has happened. What are the main priorities for the next hour? What difficulties need to be resolved? Are other resources required? Which are the casualty receiving hospitals? Where is the survivor reception centre and who is resourcing it? Do any of the services present have particular problems or difficulties that another may be able to help with? All major incidents are a potential scene of crime. They need to be treated as such, with maximal preservation of evidence. What about any dead? Are body collecting points or even a temporary mortuary going to be required.

A *joint emergency services liaison and control point* should be established by locating the command vehicles from each service at a suitable point adjacent to the incident. Where a Gold, Silver and Bronze Command system is used this point is where the Silver level is situated. Command vehicles must not be so close together that radio communications are interfered with, but should be close enough for officers to meet easily (Figure 55.4).

CORDONS

As soon as sufficient police and fire service resources are available, it is essential to establish cordons. Traditionally the inner cordon surrounds the incident site itself, and an outer cordon surrounds the assembled emergency vehicles. Members of the public and the media are held outside the outer cordon. Personnel permitted to work within the inner cordon must be strictly controlled. Nationally a variety of local systems are used, varying from cordon control cards that are deposited in a box in a method similar to the fire service tally system, to an armband system. Whatever system is used it must be possible at all times to know

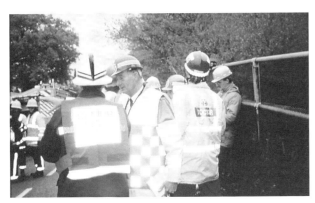

Fig. 55.4 Interservice liaison at a major incident

who is inside the inner cordon in case of a secondary incident or a requirement for evacuation. Early in the incident there may well be members of the public doing a useful first-aid function, who should tactfully and slowly be withdrawn and replaced with professionals once the cordon can be effectively controlled. The fire service traditionally takes responsibility for safety issues within the inner cordon, but each service should appoint its own safety officer. For the ambulance service an officer must assume responsibility for the health and safety issues for all health service personnel on site. Hard hats with visors, high-visibility protective clothing and appropriate protective footwear and gloves are the minimum requirements. Goggles and respiratory filter masks may be necessary.

In large incidents the traffic police may establish an outer ring of traffic diversions away from the scene and away from priority routes for ambulances going to and from the receiving hospitals.

ON-SITE MANAGEMENT STRUCTURE

Depending on the size and complexity of the incident a series of management functions have to be achieved. The attendant of the first vehicle will be relieved by an officer who assumes the tabard of Silver Commander or ambulance incident officer. This officer will then order other staff to fulfil the other key roles. A medical incident officer (MIO) should be dispatched to the scene by the ambulance control as soon as it becomes apparent that a major incident has occurred. Forward ambulance officers and forward medical incident officers are established as deputies. They will function at Bronze level and will operate within the inner cordon, acting as the eyes and ears of the Silver Commanders. The command vehicles will normally be parked between the two cordons.

The *casualty clearing centre* may be just a series of fire brigade salvage sheets on the ground, a series of inflatable tents or a local building commandeered for the purpose. A senior ambulance officer or immediate care doctor should supervise this location. All live injured casualties should pass through this point. A triage officer should assess quickly each casualty on arrival, allocating an appropriate triage category label for each person. A treatment and stabilization team of paramedics, doctors and possibly nurses from a hospital mobile team should be working here to stabilize and 'package' patients for transport to hospital.

An Ambulance loading officer should be nearby, selecting the appropriate casualty mix to load on each ambulance. It will normally be necessary to convey priority 1 casualties on their own, especially if attention is required *en route*. A suitable mix of priority 2 and priority 3 casualties may be possible in the same ambulance to ensure all available space is utilized. The process of triage has never been really effectively used at a major incident in the UK; this is because the triage labels do not arrive on scene early enough. For triage to be performed effectively there must be about a dozen sets of labels on every front-line vehicle. It is not satisfactory for them to be kept on major incident control or equipment vehicles. Whichever system is used it must be dynamic. At the scene of the incident two triage stages are necessary: the first stage is for immediate treatment aimed to stabilize and 'package' the patient. The second triage stage is for transport. Transport triage dictates whether the patient travels on a stretcher, ambulance seat or non-ambulance transport, and to which of the receiving hospitals they are to be transported.

The destination of each vehicle and the numbers and sex of the casualties leaving the scene are recorded by the ambulance loading officer. In some districts ambulance control will determine the destination; in others that choice is made at the scene and the control informed of where the vehicle is going.

In large-scale disasters there may be difficulty in obtaining enough personnel at the scene. It should be considered that paramedics may not be best using their skills by driving ambulances. Other drivers from the community transport services, the police or voluntary aid societies can in extreme situations be utilized, freeing paramedics to use their resuscitative skills. It is normally considered appropriate to dispatch priority 1 casualties first from the scene. This may not always be sensible. If there are a large number of 'walking wounded' cluttering the site it may be sensible to move them away from the scene first. Buses, coaches, police vans or Patient Transport Vehicles (PTS) could all be utilized. Each vehicle used, however, should have at least one ambulance attendant and a police officer on board. Patients with multiple or serious injuries, especially those who are trapped, will take longer to release, and priority 1 casualties may be dispatched over a period of some hours.

COMMUNICATION WITH HOSPITALS

Communications with hospitals have been a problem area for many years. Traditionally the hospitals have considered their representative on scene to be the medical incident officer (MIO). The hospital staff will have a natural curiosity about the scene and want to have as much detail as possible. It is difficult for those not on site to understand the inevitable confusion. Casualty numbers are usually only wild guesses to start with. Important information really needs to flow in the opposite direction. The management team of the MIO and the ambulance incident officer (AIO) need to know the casualty capacity of the receiving hospitals. How many theatres can be staffed? How many intensive care unit beds are available? How many general beds are there? Are there adequate blood supplies? How many more minor injuries can they cope with in the next hour? The site management team will use as many receiving hospitals as appropriate. It is unnecessary for one hospital to try to cope with all casualties. The ambulance service should aim to achieve an even distribution of the injured to several hospitals. To aid communication between hospitals and the scene, the ambulance control should despatch a liaison team to each receiving hospital. One officer should ensure smooth turnaround and re-equipping of ambulances, and document the number of casualties. The other should join the hospital coordination team to advise and update the hospital staff on progress at the scene. It is vital that these ambulance officers have radio communications to the scene and to ambulance control. Traditionally, hospital beds are freed by the early discharge of convalescent patients. In the 1980s this was easy and produced a substantial number of free beds; however in today's surgical wards patients are discharged very quickly, almost as soon as they can stand up. The potential pool of available beds has disappeared. While there are often wards closed, they are not staffed and would take a long time to make useable. Moving patients from one hospital to another has transport implications for the ambulance control who may well have to seek aid from neighbouring services and voluntary aid societies. In extreme circumstances military resources might be requested.

Facsimile (fax) machines are a useful means of communication between hospitals and ambulance controls, particularly for lists of casualties. They substantially save air time on radio channels, which are always overloaded and prone to being overheard by scanners used by the media. Mobile phones, on the other hand, are rarely much use as the media reporters overload the cells when they keep lines open continuously. Unless special arrangements are invoked by the police, mobile phones cannot be relied on. These arrangements are known as ACCOLC, or access overload control, whereby only mobile phones operating on a protected number of cells will continue to function. This requires a modification to the 'phone, which must have been authorized previously by the Cabinet Office.

If the incident scene is complex or extensive, agreement should be reached by all the emergency services on 'sectorization'. In a rail accident, each carriage might be considered as a sector. If different buildings are involved, again each may be considered as a separate sector. In multiple motorway crashes each vehicle should be allocated a number. The location of each casualty released can then be recorded in terms of vehicle number. As staff become available each sector can be supervised and the activity to release and free trapped casualties can be monitored and reported back to the Silver Control.

Requests for drugs and equipment must be kept under careful control and a clear chain of communication established. Past experiences have shown that messages can easily become duplicated and confused. Often the equipment is already on scene but not identified. Equipment officers can be invaluable in keeping control over the utilization of equipment, the provision of oxygen, nitrous oxide (Entonox), masks and drugs. If controlled drugs are required, careful control and documentation is necessary. If emergency blood is required on scene, requests should always go via the ambulance Silver Control to the hospitals, with the MIO being involved. Independent requests direct to hospitals by mobile phone or via police officers are a recipe for disaster, confusion and duplication.

On occasions amputations and other surgical procedures may be considered. To keep control over this it is suggested that two doctors must agree with the attending paramedic(s) that this is the best course to take. The MIO and senior police officer present should also agree, and whenever possible photographs should be officially taken for evidential purposes.

THE DEAD

In England and Wales the dead are the responsibility of the coroner, and in Scotland of the procurator fiscal. In practice the police act as the coroner's agents and will control all further management of the deceased. As bodies will provide forensic evidence, liaison with the coroner's officer will be essential at an early stage. Initially those casualties believed to be dead by paramedics should be labelled as such and covered with a blanket where they are found. Subsequently, when the pressure of the incident is reduced, a doctor accompanied by a nominated police officer should formally confirm death. An attached label should indicate the date and time, location found and the name of the doctor and police officer. Photographs of the body *in situ* should be taken, before it is removed to a body collecting point or temporary mortuary.

TERRORIST INCIDENTS

The major incident plan needs to be capable of modification to cope with the specific problems that terrorist incidents can cause. Bomb explosions result in devastation over a wide area (Figure 55.5). Secondary devices are a common hazard, and all attending emergency service personnel need to remember the basic rule – *protect yourself*. The location of the rendezvous point for attending vehicles should be chosen with great care. A search of this area to confirm safety is of paramount importance. A minimal number of personnel should be deployed in

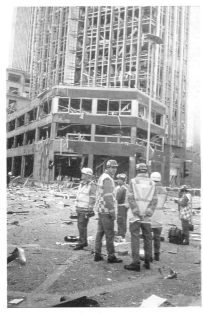

Fig. 55.5 *The City of London bomb*

the explosion site, at least until safety has been established. The preservation of life and rescue of live casualties has to be balanced carefully with the risks to the rescuers. There is considerable importance attached to the preservation of forensic evidence after a bomb explosion. The dressings, clothing and other belongings of the casualties may well be required to be preserved for forensic examination. Pieces of shrapnel must also be preserved. It goes without saying that the scene should be disturbed as little as possible. Dead victims should not be moved until after full forensic investigation and photography *in situ*. The only exception to this rule is if the body must be moved to gain access to a live patient, or there is imminent danger of loss of the body from fire or further explosion (*this rule holds true for all major incident settings*).

CIVIL DISORDER

Civil disorder can present special challenges for the paramedic. The key to a successful operation in a civil disorder situation is neutrality. The paramedic must not take sides with the police or with demonstrators, with left-wing or right-wing political protestors, or with racial groups. Three distinct patterns of civil disorder can occur. Firstly, a prearranged demonstration may have potentially violent overtones. The demonstrators muster at a predetermined point, and move along a prescribed route to a known destination. Police intelligence should allow for pre-planning and preparation for the paramedic ambulance service. Secondly, there can be static confrontation: demonstrators against the police, or rival factions with police intervention, usually with an area of conflict fairly clearly defined. Advanced

warning of such an incident is usual and sensible plans can be prepared to contend with difficulties. The third scenario, with rampaging hordes and no set pattern or direction, is much more difficult to manage. Innocent persons or property may be attacked, with vehicles overturned and set alight. There may be a changing focus of casualties.

With other major incidents the casualties occur all at once and usually in a defined place. With civil disorder casualties may continue to occur for hours or even days. The point at which it becomes a major incident is debatable. No-one can predict the casualty numbers in the next few hours. Rioting casualties can cause mayhem in accident and emergency departments. Rival groups must be taken to separate hospitals. If the police form a third group then they too must have a dedicated accident and emergency department. In rural areas or small towns this can cause problems, but whenever possible this principle must be adhered to.

Treatment facilities at a static point may avoid the need for a large number of people with minor injuries being moved to hospital. Minor dressings and treatment for strains and bruises should, where possible, be available on site. Additionally supplies of drinking water and minor analgesics such as paracetamol should be available. Paramedics should consider these minor treatments an important part of their role. Seriously injured casualties should be recovered and evacuated to a place of safety. Battlefield medicine principles may apply. Police should recover their own personnel, evacuating them to *paramedic forward aid points*. Full riot protective clothing and in some situations flak jackets may be required by crews. Foot patrol teams are most useful. Ambulances should have a crew of three whenever possible. The flashpoints and the continuing production of casualties make pre-planning difficult. At times it may not be possible to reach an incident safely. An ambulance liaison officer in the police control room is vital in informing paramedic teams of police tactics to ensure their safety when working among demonstrators or rioters. Similarly, ambulance liaison officers have a major role at the receiving hospitals. Hospital staff are often frightened by what is happening in the community and will be seeking advice about safe routes in and out of the hospital. Intelligence reports should be shared with hospital staff. To preserve neutrality it is essential that ambulances are not seen to be used to transport police officers, even if they are only given a well-intentioned lift from a hospital back to the incident.

UNDERGROUND INCIDENTS

Major incidents underground may present special problems. Communications can be particularly difficult. For caves and coal mines specialist rescue teams are usually available, but in the underground railway system ambulance paramedics will be required to work in conditions of very high temperatures. In the London underground railway system, temperatures regularly rise to 40 °C. Evacuation of trains with over a thousand passengers is often necessary. On occasions the scene may have to be approached from two different stations either side of the incident.

CHEMICAL INCIDENTS

Chemical incidents (see Chapter 42) may also require modifications to major incident plans. The fire service will of necessity take a lead role in ascertaining safety. Only fire officers normally have the appropriate protective clothing and breathing apparatus. Decisions about evacuation of areas affected by a chemical plume can be very difficult. It may often be preferable to keep members of the public inside buildings with windows and doors closed, rather than expose them in the street to a higher level of contamination while effecting their evacuation.

RADIATION INCIDENTS

Nuclear installations all have detailed on-site and off-site plans to cope with major incidents (see Chapter 43). Considerable fear and anxiety are created by radiation, based largely on ignorance of its nature. It cannot be seen, felt or smelt and is only detectable with sophisticated monitoring instruments. Acute and long-term effects can be considerable. The paramedic needs to understand the nature of radiation, know the details of locally produced plans and be informed about the workings of the National Arrangements for Incidents Involving Radiation (NAIR) scheme as applied locally.

DEBRIEFING

When paramedical staff have finished their duties at the scene of a major incident it is most important that a senior officer takes the trouble to thank them personally and check that they are safe to travel home. Fatigue and soiled or damaged clothing may mean they need assistance to get home. Words of encouragement and thanks go a long way to prevent post-traumatic stress. This 'hot debrief' can either occur at the scene or back at a suitable station. It should not last for very long and be directed towards welfare issues.

Within a few days it is necessary to arrange a more formal debrief for those involved. This should be directed to fact-finding. Who did what, and when? What went well, and what went wrong? What lessons can be learnt, and how can the plans be modified for next time? Requests for written reports from all those with a specific role should be requested. A final, full written report can then be prepared for all interested parties. This meeting provides another opportunity to spot those with post-traumatic stress and inappropriate reactions who may need the

offer of professional support and help. It must always be remembered that these meetings are never for personal recriminations and 'mud-slinging'. Nobody does less than their best at an incident. Any criticism must be utilized in a positive way to modify and change responses next time.

A further interservice debrief to assess the level of successful integration and cooperation in working together is essential. Similar debriefs with casualty receiving hospitals provide a useful forum for further discussion.

Nobody does less than their best at a major incident

Major incidents will always subject the emergency services to intense public scrutiny. The inevitable public enquiry will follow. Documentation and recording of all times and decisions are essential. Every choice or action made will be dissected with the benefit of hindsight and alternative activities considered. A detailed log must be kept at the ambulance control, at the incident Silver Command vehicle and at forward Bronze controls if necessary. All radio messages must be tape-recorded and transcribed as soon as possible after the incident. Pocket tape recorders are useful jotter systems for some officers but it is important to dictate the time of the note for future transcription.

CONCLUSION

Major incident planning for the ambulance service must be based on the question 'What if . . . ?' Any paramedic could play a part in a major incident response and so requires a detailed knowledge of the local centres likely to be involved. Railway stations, airports, sports stadia, industrial and chemical works, shopping centres and motorway complexes are all potential hazard spots. Each front-line ambulance should carry maps and plans of such locations in their normal operational area. These maps should show normal access and egress routes for ambulances, predetermined rendezvous points and joint emergency service controls.

The clinical care of casualties from a major incident is relatively straightforward, with the paramedics utilizing all their skills to provide the greatest good to the greatest number of patients. The real challenge is in the organizational aspects of command, control and communications. Regular exercises to test major incident responses should be targeted towards interservice liaison and multiagency working, rather than the clinical aspects that are used every day.

FURTHER READING

All ambulance services, local authorites and hospitals have major incident plans which can usually be obtained on request.

National and Local Emergency Plans for the UK

Ambulance Service Major Incident Plans.
County or Borough Emergency Plans.
Local Hospital Major Incident Plans.
Health Service Arrangements for Dealing with Major Incidents, HC90(25).
Home Office (1995) *Dealing with Disaster*, 2nd edn.
Home Office (1994) *Dealing with Fatalities During Disasters*, Working Party Report, October 1994.
CIMAH Site Plans for local installations.
Health Service Arrangements for Dealing with Accidents Involving Radioactivity. The NAIR Scheme. HC(89)8.
Health Service Responsibilities in Civil Defence. HC(88)31.
HMSO (1994) Arrangements for Responding to Nuclear Emergencies. HSE.
Ministry of Defence (1989) Military Aid to the Civil Community, 3rd edn.
The Responses of the Faith Communities to Major Emergencies: Some Guidelines. (Available from the Board for Social Responsibility of the General Synod of the Church of England.)
HMSO (1991) Disasters: Planning for a Caring Response. The Disasters Working Party.
BMJ Publications (1995) Major Incident Medical Management and Support: The Practical Approach. Advanced Life Support Group.

General Reading

Baskett P & Weller R (1988) *Medicine for Disasters*. Bristol: John Wright.
Hines K & Robertson B (1985) *Guide to Major Incident Management*. BASICS.
Murray V, ed. (1990) *Major Chemical Disasters: Medical Aspects of Management*. London: RSM.
Neal W (1992) *With Disastrous Consequences: London Disasters 1870–1917*.

chapter fifty-six

TRIAGE

Triage is a casualty assessment process and as such is a key part of the clinical care of patients. It is at least as important as treatment – triage errors can be very detrimental to patient outcome. Triage often involves choices about order of intervention, and unlike treatment, a single error may affect a number of patients.

Triage should be undertaken whenever the number of casualties exceeds the number of skilled helpers available. Thus a two-vehicle collision involving four people attended by one ambulance with two crew members is just as appropriate a place for the application of triage as a major incident with hundreds of casualties and many paramedical and medical staff.

Triage principles can be applied to individual patients to assess the urgency of their problem. Specific criteria can be applied to determine where patients should be taken – in particular the decision about where to take victims of trauma needs to be soundly based if there is tiered care available.

HISTORY OF TRIAGE

The sorting of casualties into priorities considerably predates the use of the word 'triage', and there is evidence of the triage process in ancient Egyptian drawings. The term itself is derived from the French word 'trier' meaning to sieve or sort. It was used by Surgeon-Marshal Larrey (Napoleon's Chief Medical Officer) to describe a system of sorting wounded French soldiers into priority for treatment – in this case the minor wounds receiving quick dressings while the more serious wounds waited. The first written English language usage was again military and described the area of an American World War I dressing station that dealt with the sorting of casualties. By common usage it has come to mean the sorting process itself. Triage has been adopted in the day-to-day management of most civilian accident and emergency departments, and remains a key element of military medicine.

TRIAGE PRINCIPLES

Triage is intended to establish the relative urgency of each casualty. In its purest form the result of the triage process would be an exact ordering of patients by urgency – thus 30 patients would be ordered from number 1 to number 30. This approach, although superficially attractive, is impractical for a number of reasons. Firstly, it is difficult to establish sufficient information about each casualty to make such a fine judgement about relative order; this is especially so in the chaos of a major incident. Secondly, it is impossible for anyone (however skilled) to collect and collate the available details with any degree of consistency of accuracy. Finally, the clinical state of patients is constantly changing – either because of interventions that have been made or because they have deteriorated further. To overcome these problems the end-point of the triage process is not an ordering of patients, but the allocation of a triage priority. These priorities must be standard and must be assigned according to set criteria. The actual method used to decide the priority will vary according to when and where the decision is being made, and will depend on the skills of the person making the decision.

Triage must reflect the changing state of the casualty and is therefore a dynamic rather than a static process. Casualties may be re-triaged repeatedly at a given stage of care, and must be re-triaged whenever they enter a different stage of their care. Thus triage may occur a number of times at the site of an incident and will be repeated on reception at hospital.

It is essential that the current priority of a given casualty is known to the staff making decisions about interventions. To achieve this there must be an agreed method of indicating the priority. Triage labelling is one method of achieving this.

PRIORITIES

The end-point of the triage process is the allocation of a priority.

This priority is then used in conjunction with other factors to determine optimum care.

The systems of priorities in common use are referred to as the treatment (T) system and the priority (P) system (Table 56.1). The words describing the priorities and their associated colours are as important as the numbers from the two systems. In the past different words have been used to describe priorities, different triage criteria have been applied, and different colours have been associated with the categories.

As can be seen from Table 56.1, the only difference between the T and P systems is the additional category (expectant) included in the former.

Definitions

It is essential that at each stage all staff involved in triage use the same criteria for categorizing patients into defined priority groups. Failure to do this can lead to significant errors. An understanding of the definition of each priority category is essential if triage is to be performed correctly. The definitions are deliberately broad, because they must be applicable in a range of situations, from an initial sorting of casualties at the scene of an incident to the allocation of priorities for surgery. The triage category definitions are given in Table 56.2.

Use of the fourth category

Whether or not the *expectant* category is used is a decision for the senior personnel involved (the ambulance and medical incident officers at the scene, and the chief triage officer at the hospital). The decision must be based on an overall assessment of the situation, and must take into account both the patient load and the resources available. It must be emphasized that failure to institute the use of this category as soon as it becomes necessary will result in higher overall morbidity and mortality rates. The undoubted difficulty of making the decision to leave seriously ill or injured casualties without treatment cannot be used as an excuse for not making it at all.

Many triaging labelling systems do not include an expectant label and a local solution to this problem needs to be found. Standard approaches would be to use the green (delayed) category and ensure that the patients are placed in a separate area, or to use the red (immediate) category and mark the card 'hold'.

TRIAGE METHODS

A sorting of casualties according to an exact description of their injuries with an informed estimation of the overall severity of injury is impractical (and unnecessary) for most triage decisions. The method used for triage must be varied according to the time available for decision-making, the location of the patient, the nature of the treatment being considered and the experience of the person performing triage. It should not be changed to reflect the number of patients, nor the resources

Table 56.1 Triage groupings

Description	Colour	T system	P system
Immediate	Red	1	1
Urgent	Yellow	2	2
Delayed	Green	3	3
Expectant	Blue	4	
Dead	White		

Table 56.2 Triage category definitions

Category	Definition
1. Immediate	Casualties who require immediate life-saving treatment
2. Urgent	Casualties who require treatment within 6 hours
3. Delayed	Less serious cases who require treatment but not within a set time
4. Expectant	Casualties whose injuries are so severe that either: they cannot survive despite treatment; or the degree of intervention required is such that, in the circumstances, their treatment would seriously compromise the provision of treatment for others

available – except that the fourth (expectant) category may come into play as discussed earlier.

The information gathered to make triage decisions will reflect the particular decision being taken – thus primary triage at a major incident will be based on different information from that used to decide whether a patient should be taken to a trauma centre. Decisions about single patient urgency should be based on yet another group of observations. Some situations and the appropriate methods of triage are discussed below.

Primary Triage at Major Incidents

There may be a large number of casualties at a major incident, and thus an enormous number of decisions need to be made as quickly and efficiently as possible. The method used must therefore be fast, easy, safe and must give the same result whoever carries it out. Since the accuracy of any method depends on the amount of information used to reach a decision, and gathering information takes time, there is a trade-off between speed and accuracy. All patients will be re-triaged after the first look and any necessary refinements can then be made.

Triage sieve

The aim of the triage sieve is to convert the absolute chaos at the site of the incident into some sort of medical order. Since the greatest number of patients are likely to have minor injuries, the most effective first step in establishing order is the separation of the priority 3 (delayed) patients from the rest. At this stage it is reasonable to assume that patients who can walk do not require urgent or immediate treatment, and all such patients are therefore categorized as priority 3 (delayed). Once this has been done, the state of the airway, breathing and circulation is considered in the remainder.

Patients who remain after the mobility sieve has been applied must be priority 1 (immediate), priority 2 (urgent) or dead. They are sorted into the appropriate category by looking at simply assessed aspects of airway, breathing and circulation.

Airway patency (not security) is assumed in conscious patients, and is assessed in the unconscious by performing a simple opening manoeuvre (chin lift and jaw thrust) and seeing if breathing occurs. Patients who cannot breathe despite an open airway are dead. Some patients may need a simple airway adjunct to maintain airway patency, which can be inserted at this stage.

Those who can breathe have their respiratory rate counted. If the respiratory rate is low (10 breaths/min or less) or high (29 breaths/min or more), then the casualty is priority 1 (immediate). If the rate is normal (11–29 breaths/min) then an assessment of circulation is carried out.

An assessment of circulation is difficult even in hospital, and no single measure will reliably give an accurate overall picture. Despite this reservation, the capillary refill time fulfils other criteria in that it can be measured simply and quickly in the nail bed. Pressure is applied over the quick of the nail for half a second and then released – the time taken for the colour to return is the refill time. If this time is greater than 2 seconds then the patient is assigned to priority 1 (immediate); if it is less than 2 seconds then the casualty is assigned to priority 2 (urgent).

In the cold the capillary refill time is reduced even in patients with a normal circulation. This can be overcome to some degree by 'resetting' the circulatory sieve cut-off point to the rescuers' own refill time; thus if the triage officers find that their own capillary refill times are 3 seconds, then patients with times of over 3 seconds should be categorized as priority 1 and those with times of under 3 seconds as priority 2. In extreme conditions peripheral perfusion of the digits may be so slight as to render capillary refill useless; in such circumstances the pulse rate should be measured and a cut-off of 120 beats per minute used to differentiate between the priorities.

Every effort should be made to stop frank external exsanguinating haemorrhage at this stage. Time is of the essence and this task must be left to follow-up treatment staff if it is not accomplished rapidly.

The triage sieve should take no more than 20 seconds for each non-ambulant patient, and first-look triage can therefore be done very rapidly. This 'broad brush' approach gives some urgently needed direction to the health service response which can then be focused on the priority 1 patients (Figure 56.1).

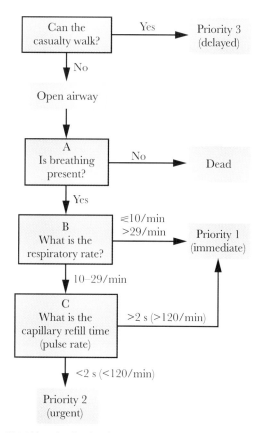

Fig. 56.1 Aide mémoire *for the triage sieve*

Triage Sort

Following the triage sieve, on arrival in the casualty clearing centre patients are triaged using a more detailed method: this is the *triage sort*. The triage sort is based on three parameters:

- Respiratory rate
- Systolic blood pressure
- Glasgow coma scale

A score for each of these is assigned to the patient (Table 56.3). The score derived from the table is the *triage revised trauma score* (TRTS). This method can be used to assign triage priorities (Table 56.4).

Remember that patients can deteriorate – or get better! If this occurs, reassessment of the triage category will be required.

Although more time-consuming than the triage sieve, the triage sort is more accurate and can be used to prioritize further treatment and evacuation.

Triage is dynamic

Table 56.3 Physiological parameters of the triage sort

Physiological parameter	Measured value	Score
Respiratory rate (breaths/min)	10–29	4
	> 29	3
	6–9	2
	1–5	1
	0	0
Systolic blood pressure (mmHg)	90	4
	76–89	3
	50–75	2
	1–49	1
	0	0
Glasgow coma scale score	13–15	4
	9–12	3
	6–8	2
	4–5	1
	3	0

Table 56.4 Priorities assigned using the triage revised trauma score (TRTS)

Category	Priority	TRTS
Immediate	T1	1–9
Urgent	T2	10–11
Delayed	T3	12
Dead	T4	0

Crams

An alternative triage system used by some UK ambulance services is the CRAMS system.

C	>	Circulation
R	>	Respiration
A	>	Abdomen and thorax
M	>	Motor response
S	>	Speech

The CRAMS score is calculated by adding the five values together (Table 56.5).

The triage category is then assigned as shown in Table 56.6

TRIAGE LABELLING

It is essential that everyone involved in the response is kept aware of the current triage status of the casualties. This simple

Table 56.5 Calculating the CRAMS score : the values for each of the five assessments are added together

Circulation

2 Normal capillary refill or systolic BP more than 100 mmHg
1 Delayed capillary refill or systolic BP 85–99 mmHg
0 No capillary refill or systolic BP less than 85 mmHg

Respiration

2 Normal respiration
1 Laboured, shallow or rate above 20/min
0 Respiration absent

Abdomen thorax

2 Abdomen not tender
1 Abdomen tender
0 Abdomen rigid, flail chest or penetrating injury

Motor response

2 Normal (obeys commands)
1 Responds only to pain
0 Postures or no response

Speech

2 Normal speech (oriented)
1 Confused or inappropriate
0 Nil or unintelligible sounds

Table 56.6 Triage category using the CRAMS system

Priority	CRAMS score	Mortality (%)
Immediate (red)	< 6	15–100
Urgent (yellow)	7	3
Delayed (green)	8–10	0–0.5

measure will reduce needless duplication of effort, and will ensure that the overall management plan (which will be heavily dependent on the triage status of the patients) does not go awry. The best cards currently available are cruciform (i.e. in the shape of a cross – Figure 56.2). Folding the corners of the cross into the middle causes the card to become rectangular; the colour and markings that remain visible depend on the way in which the folds are made, thus the card can show any priority. If the priority changes it is simple to adjust the card so that it shows the appropriate colour and markings. This system

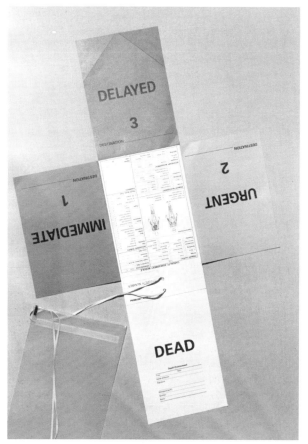

Fig. 56.2 The cruciform triage card

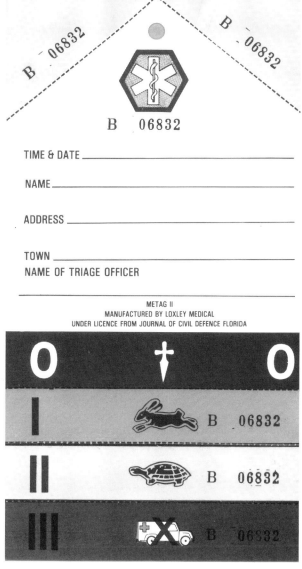

Fig. 56.3 The Mettag triage card

elegantly overcomes the problems inherent to dynamic triage in that category changes are simple, and clinical notes are secure since only one card is ever used for each patient. Additionally, there is no reason why the card initially placed on the patient during or immediately after the triage sieve cannot be used at all subsequent stages of triage.

The disadvantage of the cruciform card is that becuase the categories are so easily changed, the method is open to abuse by the patients and their relatives.

The Mettag triage card is in widespread use in Europe (Figure 56.3). A disadvantage of this system is that patients can only deteriorate on the same card, as the category is indicated using a tear-off strip: any improvement in the patient's condition requires a new card.

chapter fifty-seven

THE AMBULANCE SERVICE AT MASS GATHERINGS

Mass gathering medicine is a new development in pre-hospital care and is only a modification of our routine work, frequently providing light relief, a training opportunity (particularly for contingency planning) and a wide range of new experiences. A mass gathering is defined as a collection of 1000 people or more, and the emergencies that may occur depend on the people, the venue and the climate. Some mass gatherings, such as political marches, rallies and local derby sports matches, may give rise to outbreaks of violence, often exacerbated by alcohol. Peaceful gatherings, even if attracting crowds in their millions such as papal masses, may be totally uneventful. However, in any mass gathering the individual members of the crowd are at risk from both day-to-day minor and major medical crises, as well as accidents associated both with the venue and the sheer volume of the crowd.

Casualty figures reported at mass gatherings range from 0.11 per thousand to 9.0 per thousand. Surprisingly, the lower figure relates to a Rolling Stones concert in 1982 with an audience of 92,000. A low figure (1.6 per thousand) was also reported for the estimated 3,500,000 people who attended the Los Angeles Olympic Games (despite the length of the latter event). The higher figures relate to the US Air Show and the US Open Golf Tournament – at first this was thought to be because it attracted an older population, but this would not account for a New Zealand music festival reporting a casualty rate of 9 per thousand in 1973. Part of the difference may be due to the absence of a standard method of recording casualty statistics; but weather conditions and other factors cause wide daily variations at similar events.

Contingency planning for such events should always include major incident planning, working closely with venue owners, the organizers of the gathering, the police and local authorities. As a member of the ambulance service you may well be aware of existing plans, but familiarizing yourself with the local geography, evacuation routes and specific amendments to baseline plans for a specific event is mandatory. An empty stadium is easy to memorize, but once filled to capacity it offers a great challenge if trying to evacuate part of the crowd (or even a single casualty).

In the UK interest in mass gatherings has been spurred on by several football tragedies, notably the Bradford fire in 1985 and the report of the subsequent inquiry undertaken by Mr Justice Popplewell, and the Hillsborough stadium disaster in 1989. The latter was seen by millions of people worldwide through the media and caused public outcry. Lord Justice Taylor chaired the public inquiry and made many wide-reaching recommendations in his comprehensive report. Many measures to ensure safety were not medical, and the Football Licensing Authority (which had first been set up under Section 8 of the Football Spectators Act 1989 as a direct result of the Heisel stadium tragedy, in order to oversee the introduction of the Football Membership Scheme) was asked to take the lead in ensuring the implementation of certain key Taylor report recommendations concerning safety at football grounds. These included the operating of a licensing scheme for grounds at which designated football matches were played, advising the government on the introduction of all-seater stadia and keeping under review the discharge by local authorities of their function under the Safety of Sports Grounds Act 1975. The football membership scheme itself was shelved after the final Hillsborough report. Until the Popplewell and Taylor reports were published, the bible for mass gatherings was the HMSO publication known everywhere as the 'Green Guide': *A Guide to Safety at Sports Grounds*, first produced in 1975 and regularly updated since, the latest edition being in 1994.

In the Taylor report, overall responsibility for medical matters at football stadia was given to the ambulance service. After the report was published, Mr Myles Gibson, honorary medical adviser to the Football Association, was asked to make recommendations on the implementation of the spirit and the letter of Lord Justice Taylor's recommendations concerning first-aid, medical facilities and ambulances. He consulted with medical, ambulance and voluntary aid society colleagues and the recommendations were interpreted as follows.

Recommendation 64:

'There should be at each sports ground at each match at least one first-aider per 1000 spectators.'

The club should have responsibility for securing such attendance. As first-aiders are trained to work in pairs and have rest needs too, a minimum of three first-aiders at any match is required. A first-aider should be defined as a person who holds the standard certificate of the voluntary aid societies. Local knowledge may decree that on occasions such as local derbies, more first-aiders may be needed.

Recommendation 65:

'There should be at each designated sports ground one or more first-aid rooms. The number of such rooms and the equipment to be maintained within them should be specified by the local authority and subject to minimum standards.'

To provide a guide to the equipment needed, the Gibson report looked at the list of items agreed by the Scottish Football Association (predominantly the dressings needed to equip a first-aid room) and added to this further equipment needed for resuscitation as well as a list of emergency drugs, including those to be carried by the crowd doctor.

Mass gatherings worldwide seem to produce medical statistics that are surprisingly similar: about 20–25% of the work is caused by pre-existing disease (such as diabetes mellitus, bronchitis, epilepsy and ischaemic heart disease), and 20–30% is due to trauma such as sprains, strains and abrasions, burns and scalds, foreign bodies in the eye and the inevitable blisters at events that involve walking around all day. Environment-related illnesses are common – heat stroke and exhaustion in the warmer zones, hypothermia (especially associated with alcohol excess) in colder climes. The occasional collapse due to cardiac arrest, stroke or a drug-related incident is seen at many events, and equipment for treating a full cardiac arrest is mandatory. Minor complaints such as headache, allergic conjunctivitis, sore throats and non-specific maladies make up the rest. The voluntary aid societies keep statistics on the ailments they see, which is a useful guide when planning dressing and drug requirements. Just as conditions seem to vary little from event to event, the same applies from year to year. However, if you are to be responsible for an event lasting several days, plans must be in place to refurbish supplies. Doctors often establish arrangements with the local pharmacy rather than carry a large supply.

Recommendation 66a:

'At every match where the number of spectators is expected to exceed 2000, the club should employ a medical practitioner to be present and available to deal with any medical exigencies at the ground. He should be trained and competent in advanced first aid. He should be present at the ground at least an hour before kick off and should remain until half an hour after the end of the match. His whereabouts should be known to those in the police control room and he should be immediately contactable.'

Recommendation 66b:

'At any match where the number of spectators is not expected to exceed

2000, the club should make arrangements to enable a medical practitioner to be summoned immediately to deal with any medical emergency at the ground. The arrangements made should be known to those in the police control room.'

Although the requirement is for the club and police to be aware of the doctor's whereabouts, it is more important that the ambulance service knows too, and works closely with the doctor, maintaining contact (preferably through the ambulance radio network) and cooperating on the ambulance plans for the match, including any exercises.

Since these recommendations came out, more than 250 doctors have gone through a one-day introductory course for football crowd doctors, some more than once, and other doctors from other mass gathering events have joined them. A more detailed refresher course is also held and doctors are expected to attend every 3 years. This may not produce a cadre of doctors highly skilled in resuscitation techniques, but they are competent and aware of the role of the ambulance service and their place in the medical response. More and more doctors are taking the Diploma in Immediate Medical Care under the aegis of the Royal College of Surgeons of Edinburgh. Such doctors have to demonstrate their skills in many medical and surgical emergencies and major incident management. Many are already known to their local ambulance service as members of the British Association for Immediate Care (BASICS), having worked together at the roadside.

Recommendation 67:

'At least one fully equipped ambulance from or approved by the appropriate ambulance authority should be in attendance at all matches with an expected crowd of 5000 or more.'

Recommendation 67 allows a busy ambulance service to delegate attendance to an appropriate private or voluntary ambulance service, but the responsibility remains with the statutory ambulance service. It is usually when this service deems that more than one ambulance is required that other non-service vehicles are used. The vehicle should be equipped to paramedic standard and have at least one paramedic in the crew. In the event of a major incident this vehicle may initially be used as the control vehicle rather than for patient transport. However, many Premier and First Division football grounds have excellent multidisciplinary control rooms, equipped with adequate communications, including ambulance control, where the 'Silver' control can be established.

Recommendation 68:

'The number of ambulances to be in attendance for matches where larger crowds are expected should be specified by the local authority after consultation with the ambulance service and should be made a requirement of the safety certificate.'

It is important that services are aware of this and do not have arbitrary numbers dictated to them by the local authority through the safety certificate.

Recommendation 69:

'The need for liaison between the various people in ensuring safety is encouraged by recommending a liaison meeting each season and before each match.'

This meeting should include representatives from the club, preferably the club secretary and safety officer, a representative from the local authority, all the statutory services, the accident and emergency consultants from the hospitals designated to take casualties in the event of a major incident, and the club and crowd doctors. This is a vitally important meeting and must take place at a time when all senior people can attend, rather than sending deputies. This meeting sets the standards, deals with problems from the previous season and reviews any changes – structural, managerial or legislative. The future events in the season should accommodate both pre-match and post-match meetings where day-to-day strategy can be reviewed.

Recommendation 69:

'A Major Incident Equipment Vehicle designed and equipped to deal with up to 50 casualties should be deployed in addition to other ambulance attendance at a match where a crowd in excess of 25,000 is expected.'

Again, this is left to the discretion of the local ambulance service, and many feel the major incident vehicle should be present at smaller gatherings where trouble may be expected.

Although this chapter has concentrated on sports grounds, particularly football, the lessons learned are providing guidance for other events. Courses relating to mass gatherings have been held at the Civil Emergencies Planning College at Easingwold and a useful series of publications and resources are held at the college library. The college's publication on crowd-related disasters draws on experience gained from a wide range of disasters.

With these recommendations in place and the analysis of the morbidity and mortality rates of the many mass gathering events worldwide, mass gathering medicine is becoming a recognized and rewarding aspect of paramedical work.

FURTHER READING

A Guide to Safety at Sports Grounds, 4th edn (1994). London: HMSO (The 'Green Guide').

Emergency Planning College (1992) *Lessons Learned from Crowd-Related Disasters*. Home Office Emergency Planning College, Easingwold, Paper 4.

Football Club Contingency Planning FLA 1994 *A Guide to Safety Management and Practices and Appointment, Training and Duties of Stewards at Football Grounds*. Football Licensing Authority, FA Premier League, Football Association, Football Safety Officers Association and the Football League.

Report of the Committee of Enquiry into Crowd Safety and Control at Sports Grounds (Popplewell Report, 1985). London: HMSO.

Safety of Sports Grounds Act 1975. London: HMSO.

Stadium Control Rooms. London: Sports Council/Football Stadia Development Committee.

The Hillsborough Stadium Disaster 15th April 1989 (Taylor Report, 1990). London: HMSO.

12

ADMINISTRATION, ETHICS AND THE LAW

chapter fifty-eight

RECORD-KEEPING IN PRE-HOSPITAL CARE

Record-keeping is viewed as a major chore by both paramedics and doctors involved in pre-hospital care. The acknowledged stresses faced in the field by these individuals pale into insignificance compared with the sight of the non-user-friendly A3 sheet, at the end of a difficult patient care episode.

'No-one ever looks at them', 'They throw them straight into the bin', 'I've already given them a complete verbal report', are all familiar complaints that are expressed while completing the pre-hospital record. The importance attached by paramedics to keeping a good and accurate record is not high, and as a result the information generated is frequently incomplete and of questionable accuracy. However, the real value of accurate pre-hospital record-keeping must not be underestimated.

The report form is a statement of one's professional attitude to practice. A well-documented and accurate patient record creates the immediate image of a competent and professional practitioner in the eyes of the reader. An incomplete and poorly completed record creates the opposite impression. The absence of any report form for the incident at all leaves one even more vulnerable, as it questions the very professional basis of one's clinical practice.

Remember that the hospital copy is retained within the patient's hospital file, and may well be referred to for information hours to weeks after admission by hospital medical and nursing staff. On occasions, that report form will contain the sole information of injury circumstances, mechanism of injury and scene findings and interventions for these clinicians.

The report form can be your closest ally when, for example, a solicitor's letter arrives 2 years after the incident threatening legal action because of an apparent omission of care. The incident itself will now be a faded memory, but unearthing the completed report form can aid greatly in refuting allegations, and refreshing one's memory of the event.

> **Good notes – Good defence**
> **Poor notes – Poor defence**
> **No notes – No defence**

Conversely, if procedures have not been recorded, it will leave one vulnerable to the allegation of 'if it is not written down it was not done'. The form must therefore be viewed as a legal document, and stored safely for future recall.

> **If it is not written down, it was not done!**

Because the report may act as a record for future recall of an incident, it is worth noting any peculiar aspects, especially in incidents likely to result in police or other legal action, such as fatal road accidents and assaults.

The report form is an integral part of the clinical record, and merits time and commitment to record accurately all relevant pre-hospital data.

Many pre-hospital care practices have never been subjected to scientific scrutiny. Similarly, the benefits of many procedures used in accident and emergency departments have yet to be scientifically proved. It is important in the advancement of pre-hospital care to evaluate the aspects of care that produce the best survival outcomes for the patient.

Audit is the process used to assess the effectiveness of a particular clinical intervention, and to compare the results with an established standard. Once that comparison has been made, suggestions for improvement can be implemented and the process reassessed in the wake of these changes to see if improvement has occurred.

This process, along with scientific research into areas of pre-hospital practice, is central to any scientific evaluation of pre-hospital care. It can be used to prove or disprove whether our impressions of the effectiveness of practices in our system are correct. It further allows reassessment after changes in practice, to ensure changes bring about the improvements hoped for.

Audit and research are impossible without accurate, consistent and reliable pre-hospital data. Virtually all these data will originate from the patient report form, and omissions and inaccuracies will minimize the validity of any research. This is not just a minor problem for those who try to analyse the inadequate

BASIC OBSERVATIONS							INTERVENTIONS
TIME ≻≻≻≻≻≻							OP Airway ☐ NP Airway ☐
1	AIRWAY	Clear					Suction ☐ ET ☐ NT ☐
		Obstructed					Attemps ....Success ☐
2	**BREATHING RATE** ≻≻						Man C-sp immob ☐
3	Breathing Qual.	Normal					C-sp collar ☐
		Shallow					Red ☐
		Deep					Spinal board ☐
		Laboured					Traction splint ☐
4	Breath Sounds	Present					Mask ☐ B&M ☐ Assisted ☐
	Left	Absent					Mechanical ☐
		Clear					Oxygen ☐ .... %
		Noisy					
5	Breath Sounds	Present					*Needle cricothyrotomy* ☐
	Right	Absent					Cannula size.......... Time..........
		Clear					
		Noisy					*Chest decompression* ☐
6	**BREATHING RATE** ≻≻						Cannula size.......... Time..........
7	Pulse	Strong					Left ☐ Right ☐
		Weak					Site ....
		Regular					*CANNULATION*
		Irregular					Size / No att / Site / ✓ / ✗
8	Pulse Site	Radial					☐ ☐
		Brachial					☐ ☐
		Femoral					☐ ☐
		Carotid					*INFUSION*
9	Skin Condition	Normal					Fluid / Time / Finish / Total
		Pale					
		Perspiring					
		Flushed					
10	Capillary Refill	Normal					
		Delayed					
11	Blood Pressure ≻≻≻						*DRUGS*
12	LOC	Alert					Name / Time / Dose / Batch #
		Voice					
		Pain					
		Unresponsive					
13	Pupils N=normal D=dilated R=reactive	L:	L:	L:	L:		
	c=constricted U/R=unreactive	R:	R:	R:	R:		
14	Oxygen Saturation ≻≻≻						
15	Peak Flow Reading ≻≻≻						
16	Blood Gluc (mmol) ≻≻≻						

Fig. 58.1 Patient report form

data. Accurate and scientifically valid proof of the effectiveness of pre-hospital care is critical if service provision and funding for pre-hospital ambulance and medical care is to be successfully sought from increasingly cash-limited health authority purchasers. In effect, the security of paramedical jobs in the future may depend on careful recording of patient data and information now.

As an example, the Major Trauma Outcome Study (MTOS) has a data set for pre-hospital patient recordings. The use of data and evaluation of the pre-hospital component of the care of most of these patients has been frustrated since the outset by the frequent omission of key data such as respiratory rate from report forms.

Trauma scoring as a method of field triage has a number of practical problems, mainly related to time, particularly in major trauma cases. The use of the primary survey as a basic field triage tool in trauma cases appears to work in practice, as any major 'ABCD' problem merits a 'critical' category and consideration for trauma unit admission.

However, retrospective gathering of trauma scoring data is the key to the effective assessment of the potential merits of pre-hospital care procedures.

Recognition of training deficits within an ambulance service can also be highlighted by accurate and coordinated report form audit. Without this, training efforts may be wasted or misdirected.

Finally, patient safety depends on well-completed report forms. Verbal information about fluid volumes and drug administration given to the accident and emergency department doctor during the hand-over may not be passed on to doctors who care for the patient subsequently. Overdosage of opiate drugs and overinfusion of intravenous fluids have occurred because of the lack of a written report at the hand-over of a patient, and omissions in the verbal reports.

The completion of paperwork is undoubtedly a burden for pre-hospital carers, but it is one of the most important tasks of the professional paramedic or doctor. The patient's well-being and the professional integrity of the paramedic or doctor may depend on the time and effort spent on completing an accurate patient report form, and therefore few tasks in pre-hospital medicine can rate more highly than precise record-keeping.

An example of a section of a patient data collection form, designed to collect data in the order that the paramedic clinically assesses the patient, is shown in Figure 58.1.

chapter fifty-nine:

COMMUNICATIONS AND DISPATCH

Communications are the cornerstone of a successful emergency medical services operation. Accessibility of the service to the public is the first essential requirement, and in this respect the national 999 emergency telephone system is well known to the population as a whole.

THE 999 CALL

It is vital to have well-trained call-takers, and an effective handling system for emergency and urgent calls within the ambulance control centre. Emergency calls must be readily identified on receipt in the control room, and details passed directly into the ambulance computer-aided dispatch (CAD) system. This permits rapid dispatch of an emergency ambulance as soon as the dispatcher knows the location of the incident. The call-taker will still be taking further details while the ambulance mobilizes, and an update message to confirm location and clinical details is passed by the ambulance controller to the vehicle as it is *en route* to the emergency.

Additional resources such as paramedical or medical support may be dispatched to the scene depending on initial information received. The initial information-gathering by the call-taker has to be of the highest quality if appropriate care is to be provided for every emergency.

The new generation of computerized telephone exchanges can provide an enhanced service to emergency service controls, identifying on receipt of the call the call-back number and subscriber details. This information can be put directly into the CAD system via an interface, which speeds up mobilization since the call-taker has only to confirm these details with the caller.

Pre-arrival instructions to the caller about life-saving first-aid procedures should be a feature of every ambulance control centre's service to the public. There is evidence of the effectiveness of 'telephone CPR', and the case for prolonging the period of ventricular fibrillation with early basic life support is now convincing.

The ambulance service must concentrate on reducing the time taken for well-trained and well-equipped crews to reach patients with life-threatening problems. If all life-threatening emergencies were attended within 8 minutes by a defibrillator-equipped ambulance crew, and telephone-advised CPR were widely used, cardiac arrest survival in the UK could well improve significantly.

Medical Priority Dispatch

Two systems are in use which provide enhanced ability to judge the medical priority of incoming emergency calls to the ambulance control centre. These systems allow structured and thorough questioning of the caller, so that more medical detail can be obtained from the initial emergency call. This has a number of advantages. Firstly, it allows better information to be passed to crews *en route* to emergency calls; this reduces stress, and allows the crew to make decisions about the correct approach and selection of appropriate equipment prior to reaching the patient.

Secondly, a better judgement may be made as to the dispatch priority for the ambulance. Where it becomes apparent that this is not a life-threatening emergency, the ambulance crew can be advised by radio to attend without using blue lights and siren, reducing the risk to both the public and the crew. In rural and quieter urban areas, blue light and siren progress makes little time difference in reaching the casualty, but in traffic-choked inner cities the difference is significant. The dispatch system must be both safe and accurate, and the tendency of both systems is to err on the side of an emergency response. There will, however, be a significant reduction in unnecessary emergency responses with these systems.

In the UK, the ambulance service will be effectively an all Advanced Life Support (ALS) service by the end of 1996, with a paramedic on each emergency ambulance. Another current function of a medical priority dispatch system is to differentiate between calls requiring an ALS or Basic Life Support ambulance, which will become inapplicable in the UK.

Finally, a major feature of the systems is the provision of pre-arrival instructions to emergency callers. This scripted advice extends from looking out for the ambulance and restraining the family dog, to basic life support (BLS) instruction. Undoubtedly, lives have been saved by advice on BLS and the relief of choking given over the telephone. Ambulance services in the USA have suffered lawsuits as a result of failing to provide pre-arrival instructions to callers.

There are two prioritized dispatch systems which vary in principle. The Advanced Medical Priority Dispatch System (AMPDS) is protocol driven, and is designed for use by emergency medical dispatchers without paramedical training. The second, the Criteria Based Dispatch System (CBDS), is designed as an advisory system for paramedic use in the control centre.

There are extensive quality assurance procedures involved in the AMPDS, which have been refined over some 15 years of operation, and the majority of top-line, high-performance ambulance systems in the USA use the AMPDS (Figure 59.1). Both systems are based on a set of cards, one for each important condition, with its own specific questions. A base information set including age, sex, breathing status and conscious level precedes each condition-specific card. The ability to proceed to a computer-based system integrated into the CAD is a feature of both systems. Quality assurance is much easier on the computer-based system, as is the recording of morbidity data.

These systems are an essential part of any modern control centre, and the advantages of medical information-gathering, better prepared crews, fewer unnecessary emergency responses and life-saving telephone instruction cannot be overstated.

RADIO AND PAGING SYSTEMS

The alert message must reach the ambulance without delay. Telephone contact with an ambulance station and turnout from the station probably takes at least 1–2 minutes. Direct radio alert to a vehicle at a standby location achieves mobilization in around 30 seconds.

Taking longer than 8 minutes to reach a cardiac arrest costs approximately 7–10% of lives per minute of lateness. Saving 90 seconds by more rapid mobilization will literally save lives. Ambulance stations are usually in or near town centres. The majority of the population live in the outlying suburbs, where most emergencies occur. Positioning ambulances around these population centres will frequently reduce attendance times.

Ambulances use very high frequency (VHF) radio systems, both fixed in the vehicle and as lower-powered portable handsets. These handsets may be VHF, or ultra-high frequency (UHF) from a UHF repeater radio linked to the vehicle VHF set (Figure 59.2). Communication is greatly enhanced with the handsets, as crew to crew and crew to vehicle communication is possible in addition to contact with the control centre.

Many services use an automatic updating system, with status

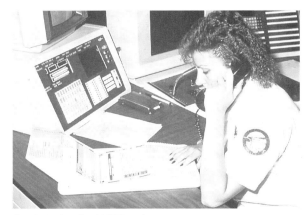

Fig. 59.1 *Using the AMPDS card set*

codes sent by radio to update the control centre on vehicle status, without the need for repeated speech updates. This makes for a largely speech-free radio system, and saves much time in recording times in the control centre. Ambulance mobile radios can travel with muted radios until the control centre opens up the vehicle radio for a call. The disadvantage of this system is the absence of awareness of the operational situation in the service by crews; they are unable to offer help if nearer to an emergency than a tasked unit, or to offer assistance in finding a location to a crew operating in an unfamiliar area.

Most ambulance services are in radio communication with local accident and emergency departments. This is a vastly better system than telephone relay of information by the control centre. Ambulance crews should have direct 'talk-through' of their own priority messages with the receiving senior nurse or doctor in the accident and emergency department. Reluctance of hospital staff to use a radio, and the siting of the sets in the reception area and their operation by reception staff, are the only major problems in the use of this facility. Crews must present a brief but comprehensive alert message, and ideally a pro forma for these reports should be provided in conjunction with the accident and emergency departments.

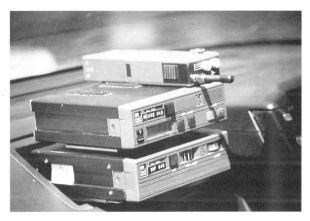

Fig. 59.2 *Vehicle fixed and portable radio sets*

One system in use is ASHICE

A	>	Age
S	>	Sex
H	>	History
I	>	Injuries/illness
C	>	Consciousness
E	>	Estimated time of arrival

The scarcity of radio frequencies available to ambulance services is a major constraint in providing even more elaborate ambulance–hospital communications. Medical guidance for on-line advice would be far more practical if more radio frequencies were available.

The development of digital trunked radio systems for emergency service use will provide both higher speech quality and more efficient use of radio channels. Interlinking with more elaborate facilities via the CAD system will also be easier with a digital radio system. Laptop computer-based patient report forms are now in use and can be linked to the CAD via the vehicle radio. Direct entry of the call details into the laptop and download of patient data to the receiving accident and emergency department during transport of the patient are both feasible.

Paging

Paging is often used as a duplicate or reserve alerting system for emergency ambulance crews. Alphanumeric paging offers rapid alerting with location and call details as a parallel alert to the radio; it allows a location confirmation if this is in doubt, and allows updates to be passed by control without the need to use radio (Figure 59.3). By issuing personal pagers to all crew members, operational messages can be passed at any time, for instance if extra personnel are needed for a major incident to cover shifts. Paging also provides a medium for sending discreet messages to crews, where open channel radio would allow the patient or relatives to be aware of the nature of the message.

These pagers can be linked through the CAD to an internal paging system, or linked to a commercial paging agency. This facility, along with other communication services, also provides a basis for the ambulance service to fulfil the communication needs of other NHS agencies.

Cellular telephones offer a useful facility for major incident management, now that the access override system will provide preferential access in these situations for the emergency services. Certain specialist functions can be performed using cellular telephones, including fax and electrocardiograph transmissions, but variable performance and recurring costs may inhibit more widespread use.

Automatic Vehicle Locating Systems

A variety of automatic vehicle locating systems (AVLS) are commercially available and in use by UK ambulance services. They are based either on triangulation of transmitted radio signals or on positioning derived from the global positioning satellite system (Figure 59.4).

These systems use vehicle locator transmitters and a mapping system to demonstrate the vehicle location on a visual display unit (VDU) screen. Additional data transmission is possible, including status reporting using keypads in the vehicle. These status and location reports can be integrated with the CAD system. Vehicle location, status and even speed can be demonstrated on screen, and the system can further locate incidents on the mapping screen using six-figure map references incorporated in the system gazetteer. This can use the CAD facilities to locate the incident and nearest vehicle on the mapping screen, enabling rapid deployment of the most appropriate ambulance.

Effective communication with the public, ambulance vehicles and staff, and other emergency services is the key to a respon-

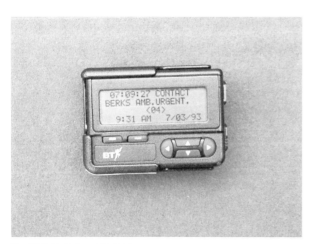

Fig. 59.3 Alphanumeric pager

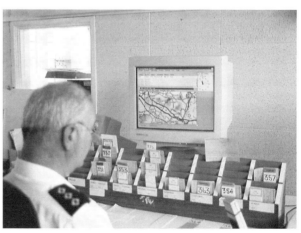

Fig. 59.4 Automatic vehicle location system

sive ambulance service. If the service is to meet the medical priorities of the community it serves it must become increasingly responsive to their medical needs by medical direction. Many services are satisfied with fulfilling outdated and inadequate performance targets, which in no way reflect current medical practice, or knowledge of the needs in particular of life-threatening emergency cases.

Operational performance must be geared to providing a rapid response (under 8 minutes in urban areas) to life-threatening emergencies. This is only possible with a rapidly accessible 999 system, medical priority dispatch, and high-quality radio and pager communications. It also requires innovation in redesigning ambulance systems to enable ambulance numbers to be tailored to fluctuations in demand and vehicles to be located in areas of maximum call density. These changes will enable the service to fulfill its commitment to the public.

chapter sixty:

ETHICAL AND LEGAL ISSUES

In the UK paramedical staff are fortunate that litigation has been relatively rare. However, litigation is now on the increase, and far more responsibility is placed on ambulance trusts for the financial liability resulting from successful actions than was the case in the past.

While it is generally true that an employer is legally liable for the actions of its employees, it would be unwise for an individual paramedic to feel immune from legal action. Civil law allows anyone to sue anyone else, whether their claim is justified or not. Regardless of whether you win or lose, or whether you or your employer are liable, the experience of having your actions questioned and dissected under the microscope of a court is never pleasant. This chapter aims to identify those areas where you can plan your conduct to aid in avoiding such an experience.

ETHICS AND MORALS

Definitions

A dictionary definition of *ethics* is 'A system of moral behaviour', with *ethical* being defined as 'That which is morally good'.

Moral is defined as 'Of or based on the difference between good and evil or right and wrong. Pure and honest in character and behaviour'.

Discussion

It is necessary to be 'moral' to be 'ethical'. The problem of the definitions provided is that they do not actually state what conduct constitutes these behaviours. Who defines what is good or evil, right or wrong? Essentially society does, and the actions and responses of everyone around us defines what is acceptable and what is not. A consensus is developed through an unwritten process of precedent set over many generations, passed on

through the teaching and example of parents, schools and, where appropriate, religious institutions.

An important consideration is the concept that society is a product of culture; because cultures vary in different parts of the world, it is not surprising that each culture's perception of what is moral and ethical will be different. As a paramedic you are privileged to be involved in working intimately with people from many different ethnic communities, and it is important that you are aware that there may be differences in their moral and ethical beliefs. You must respect these, and not judge these individuals by the standards that you have adopted for yourself. Remember that each society generates its own perceptions and rules of good and evil, right and wrong, and that none of these necessarily represents the correct or only one. In some cultures the relationship between men and women and the individual roles of each sex are seen as being very different from that generally accepted by Western society. When you encounter the different behavioural patterns that arise from your own society's norm, you may feel that you are encountering prejudice or sexism. In reality some cultures do not share what is after all a Western concept, and should not therefore be judged adversely if they do not subscribe to your own culturally based beliefs.

On the other hand, it is our own ethical and moral values which we should use to measure our personal behaviour. They are what form our conscience and provide us with guidance as to what is right and wrong in our own actions. Generally, if you listen to your conscience, you will feel comfortable about what you do, but if you ignore it and act against that nagging voice of doubt or self-criticism you may find yourself plagued by second thoughts. If it feels wrong, then it probably is!

Ethical Dilemmas

The most basic ethical dilemmas arise from a conflict between conscience and ego. This occurs when you 'know' something is wrong, but the desire for personal gain suggests that you should break your own internal rule system. What happens most commonly under circumstances such as this is that we rationalize 'good' reasons for deviating from our normal code of moral conduct. For example, it is not unusual to be offered 'tips' by grateful patients. Unfortunately this generosity is most often displayed by those least able to afford it, such as the elderly whose only income is a small pension.

The argument most often voiced for accepting tips is that patients only offer what they can afford, and would be offended if refused. In reality this is unlikely to be true. The offering of tips is probably an unconscious response to the pressure of another norm: that of providing gratuities to those in 'service' occupations, who were traditionally poorly paid. There are many logical reasons as to why acceptance of money could be judged by society at large as unethical:

- Ambulance paramedics earn far more than most pensioners
- Patients have already paid for their use of the ambulance service (and hence the wages of its employees) via their National Insurance contributions, and by tipping they are in effect paying again
- Ambulance paramedics have the controlling stake in their relationship with subsequently vulnerable patients and should not abuse this
- Employing ambulance trusts typically have rules relating to employee conduct that state staff should not accept gratuities
- Patients who give gifts may feel that they subsequently have the right to preferential treatment, and if this is not forthcoming can become upset or angry. This type of manipulative behaviour can be very difficult for ambulance staff to cope with, and may unfairly prejudice the interests of other patients who are unable or unwilling to give tips

Nurses and firefighters are rarely offered gifts of money in gratitude for their services, nor do they expect them. The reasons for this difference are likely to be complex but may possibly centre around the view of the ambulance professional as a 'driver' (particularly common among the elderly), which is the very image the modern ambulance service has tried to avoid. Other ethical dilemmas are more complex and occur when a society's unwritten guidelines for personal conduct are unclear or at conflict with each other.

Case history 1

You attend a road accident involving a car which has hit a bridge. The passengers consist of a family of three: father (who was driving), mother and 6-year-old daughter. On arrival everyone is out of the car and lying around the wreckage, and you take care of the father. During your examination you discover a needle and syringe in his clothing. You challenge him and he admits that he is a heroin addict and had 'shot up' prior to getting in the car.

Should you inform the police? The driver has clearly broken the law, and by his actions endangered the life of his family and other road users. The information you have received has come to you as part of your therapeutic relationship: are you bound by the rules of confidentiality?

There is probably no right or wrong answer to this or other similar dilemmas. Opinion will be divided based on an individual's life experiences and cultural background, and society's current standards of behaviour. Perhaps the best approach is to focus, as a care-giver, entirely on the patient, addressing his immediate needs and maintaining confidentiality. It is not appropriate for paramedics to stand in judgement on others, and we must therefore avoid imposing our standards of behaviour and world view of what is right or wrong on others. However, if the information you receive indicates to you that future harm may be caused by the behaviour of your patient, and furthermore that such harm may be prevented by timely action on your part, it may well be appropriate to inform the doctor in charge of the patient's case, who can then consider what action is appropriate.

Field Trials

Paramedics are occasionally asked to participate in the field trials of new drugs (or new applications of drugs in the field) and medical devices. These trials must be approved by both the local paramedic steering group and an ethics committee. Many ambulance services do not have access to an ethics committee of their own, and subsequently approval may be sought from a group attached to a local hospital. The role of an ethics committee is primarily to act as the patients' advocate. Its members must ensure that, where possible, the consent of each patient to participate in the study is gained, or if this is not possible, that consent is given by the patients' immediate relatives. 'Consent' requires that patients fully understand:

- That they are being invited to participate in a study
- That they have the right to refuse to take part
- The purpose of the study
- The potential beneficial effects (if known) of the drug or device
- Any potential risks
- Any side-effects that have occurred in previous usage of the drug or device

The ethics committee must also ensure that patients are given no inducement to participate in the study. Inducements may include financial reward, gifts or a promise of speedier treatment. The committee must ensure that the study is reasonable in its design and that in their best judgement is likely to produce a valid result. It is a primary responsibility to ensure that the risk involved for consenting patients is minimal.

The membership of ethics committees will typically consist of physicians, nurses, scientists of appropriate background, and representatives of the community at large. It is generally accepted that the community representatives should outnumber the medically trained and that the chairperson of the group should be drawn from their ranks. Where possible patients should be included in the committee. For a study in which ambulance personnel are participating the membership of a paramedic instructor would be invaluable, although this individual should probably be drawn from the ranks of a service not directly involved in the trial. Ethics committees also have the potential to contribute positively to the development of ambulance service policy in other matters discussed later in this chapter.

The process for approval of studies is necessarily bureaucratic in order to protect the interest of patients. It would be highly unethical for ambulance paramedics to introduce new equipment or drug regimens on a trial basis without this type of approval, and would almost certainly result in a breach of both protocol and their contract of employment.

Making Assumptions

Circumstances often tempt paramedics to judge the integrity of certain types of patients or the validity of their complaint. We hate to see our service 'abused', and often justify our attitude with a stated desire to reserve resources to those patients 'who truly need them'. Unfortunately, attempting to filter out the so-called 'abusers' without careful checks and balances (such as physically examining the patient) will also result in inadvertently and inevitably filtering out those who demonstrably need emergency medical aid. It is a common feature of all emergency services all over the world that they spend much of their time responding in emergency mode to what turn out to be non-emergency calls. Nevertheless, it is undoubtedly better to overrespond than to underrespond.

It would be unreasonable to expect ambulance personnel to be entirely free from personal prejudices and preconceptions; however, it is essential to prevent these attitudes affecting clinical practice. All personnel should identify their own prejudices clearly, and make a consistent and disciplined effort to avoid being influenced by them. For example, the common distaste for individuals who abuse alcohol and who make a public nuisance of themselves has led to many problems. Patients have died in police cells from airway obstruction or alcoholic poisoning because ambulance staff did not wish to burden themselves or hospital staff with their treatment. Even in hospital, this prejudice can lead to inappropriate care (or lack of care) for patients who appear to be drunk, but are actually suffering from medical or traumatic conditions.

In order to protect yourself and your patients from the results of your human preconceptions and prejudices you should discipline yourself never to judge the integrity of the patient, relatives, bystanders or other professional care-givers.

Case history 2

You are summoned by a 999 call to a man who is unable to talk. On arrival you are met by a colleague of the patient. The colleague appears friendly and sympathetic, and tells you that the patient is a malingerer with a poor attendance record and a multitude of complaints. 'Now he's pretending he can't talk!'

The patient indicates by vigorous and theatrical hand signals that he is unable to utter a sound. He appears unconvincing, and when you give him a piece of paper and a pen attempts to explain that he is unable to write either. You are convinced he is a fraud, but take him to hospital anyway.

Two months later you receive a letter of grateful thanks from the same patient who tells you that he has just been discharged from hospital following a stroke which affected the speech centre of the brain resulting in expressive dysphasia – inability to talk. Interestingly, this area of the brain also controls other forms of expression such as writing skills.

THE LAW

Living Wills

The legal status of 'living wills' in the UK is vague and needs clarification. Living wills (also known as 'advance directives') are documents in which people state their wishes for restricted medical care should they become seriously ill in the future. It is a method of withholding consent to treatment in the event that any future illness incapacitates them to the extent that they cannot express their wishes.

The legal issues associated with 'living wills' have been the subject of much discussion. A precedent was set regarding the validity of advance directives by a ruling by the House of Lords in the Tony Bland case. This stated that it would be unlawful to give treatment against the previously expressed wishes of the patient. Consequently, although no statutory legislation exists, this precedent implies that advance directives will have force in common law. As a result, if a care-giver fails to follow the clear instructions of a patient regarding limitation of treatment, even if the instructions are given in advance, that patient will have a right of action for trespass against the person. Additionally, the Law Commission published a consultation paper in March 1995 which included draft legislation regarding 'living wills'. Some or all of its recommendations will eventually find their way into law, conferring statutory rights on patients enacting advance directives and providing further guidance for healthcare workers.

The circumstances in which an advance directive will have the greatest impact for paramedics are where an individual with a 'living will' suffers a cardiac arrest out of hospital. Ethically, it would probably be generally agreed that the wishes of the victim should be honoured; it is not a pleasant thought that we as citizens potentially have no control over our destiny, even in death. On the other hand, as the legal status of these directives is so vague, there may not be incontrovertible evidence available in an emergency that such a document is genuine or does indeed represent the patient's current wishes. There is a potential for unscrupulous or even well-meaning relatives to produce 'fake' documentation. Withholding resuscitation attempts under these circumstances may not represent the patients' wishes and is unlikely to be in their best interest.

There is no universal answer to the problem of how paramedics should respond when presented with a 'living will'. The most important step is for each service to establish a clear written policy on how they would wish their staff to act. This should be formulated by either the local paramedic steering group or the ethics committee, and in any event must have medical as well as managerial approval. The British Medical Association has produced guidelines for doctors which will form a useful reference point. Any ambulance service policy would also need to encompass the delivery of telephone cardiopulmonary resuscitation (CPR) instructions, as provision of this type of aid is becoming increasingly common in ambulance controls.

The State of Florida in the USA has issued legislation to mandate how 'living wills' should be enacted, verified and responded to. It recognizes the right of individuals to determine their fate and the medical care they receive, and provides a standard form for documenting their wishes in this regard. This has to be signed by the person and a physician, who must confirm that the patient is of sound mind at the time the document is enacted. Medical staff are required to honour 'living wills', with the strict provision that they must see the signed original form and evidence that this relates to the patient concerned. Despite this, telephone CPR instructions are normally given prior to the arrival of medical care at the incident, as dispatchers are of course unable to see these documents; however, relatives are not obliged to follow these instructions. Once reasonable proof of the veracity of a document has been provided to personnel at the scene, failure to comply with the patient's wishes as set down in the document is viewed as assault. There is a need for similar legislation in this country, not only to protect patients' interests and wishes, but also to define the role and actions of responders. Until this has been enacted the most important action for individual ambulance services is to establish a written policy.

'Do Not Resuscitate' Orders

'Do not resuscitate' orders take the form of written and signed instructions from the physician responsible for the care of the patient concerned. They are developed after discussion with, and the consent of, the patient (where possible), relatives and other health-care professionals associated with the individual affected. Paramedics are not practitioners in their own right (that is, they are practising under the licence of a doctor) and they are therefore required to follow the medical instructions of a patient's physician. As such, if they are shown written, signed instructions from a medical practitioner stating that a patient should not receive resuscitation or other treatment, then

paramedics must comply. If possible these orders should be confirmed with the doctor face-to-face, and clarification sought as necessary. 'Do not resuscitate' orders must always be in writing in order to protect the interests of care-givers other than the physician making the order.

Pronouncing Death

In law the ability to certify death is confined to registered medical practitioners. This should not be confused with the pronouncement that death has occurred. Paramedics and technicians are not legally entitled to 'pronounce' patients dead, nor are other medically unqualified persons. However, this does not impose a requirement on them to start treatment when, according to the definition of a medically approved and established policy, the patient has a non-salvageable condition. Unfortunately very few services have established written policies addressing this issue, and therefore paramedics, to be entirely free of the risk of criticism, should theoretically attempt to resuscitate all patients in cardiac arrest regardless of their condition or circumstances. This could potentially lead to ludicrous situations and paramedics will often exercise their own judgement, but a written policy is far more appropriate to protect the interests of staff and patients. Such a policy should be developed cautiously by the paramedic steering committee or an ethics committee, and medical approval is essential. It can sometimes be difficult to reach agreement as to what exactly constitutes 'obvious' death beyond hope of successful resuscitation, and it is important to avoid potential ambiguities. Certain ambulance services in the UK have now introduced protocols which allow paramedics to pronounce death. Examples of findings used by some ambulance services in the USA to define 'obvious death' (with appropriate caveats) are given in Table 60.1.

Whatever local policy is established, any pronouncement of death by a paramedic must be unquestionable. If errors occur they must be in the direction of patient safety, to maximize the potential for survival. If in doubt, the best advice is to resuscitate and let a doctor at the receiving hospital make the decision to stop.

Stopping Resuscitation

Few if any services in the UK allow paramedics to terminate resuscitation attempts on their own initiative. This is unfortunate, as a study in the USA demonstrated that few patients receiving full advanced cardiac life support in the field who did not develop a perfusing rhythm prior to transportation responded to hospital treatment, and none survived to discharge. Similar findings have come from research in the UK. This suggests that provided adequate and comparable treatment regimens are provided by paramedics for the victims of medical cardiac arrest (as opposed to trauma-related death), failure to respond in the field implies irreversible death.

Table 60.1 Findings defining 'obvious' death

Finding	Caution
Decomposition	Requires clear definition
Rigor mortis	Beware of muscle rigidity as a result of parkinsonism or hypothermia
Dependent lividity (post-mortem staining)	Can be an uncertain finding
Expected death from a terminal disease	Presence of a written 'do not resuscitate' order preferred
Decapitation	
Total incineration	Death is not always immediate in these circumstances
Complete separation of the entire heart, lungs or brain from the body	Requires clear definition and some experience to determine
Submersion confirmed as being greater than 24 hours	A very rare event (if a submersed body is visible for 24 hours, why has no-one taken action during that time?)
The duration of the absence of both carotid pulses is confirmed as being greater than 30 minutes, in the absence of any CPR	Again, a very unlikely circumstance (if a professional whose judgement we are willing to accept has been with the victim for this period of time, why have they not started CPR?)

Subsequent removal of non-responsive patients to hospital is potentially hazardous as it requires rapid transportation with the use of lights and sirens and with unrestrained staff providing treatment in the patient compartment. It prolongs the period for which an ambulance is unavailable and inappropriately ties up medical and other resources at the receiving hospital. The whole process of transportation of the patient may be distressing for relatives as it may raise their expectations unfairly and could be perceived as depriving the victim of their dignity.

There appears to be no legal bar to paramedics stopping resuscitation in the field, although if the patient is 'in the public eye' such an action could cause unnecessary concern and distress for onlookers. However, if the patient is at home it would appear reasonable that, in the presence of an appropriate ambulance service policy which has medical approval, paramedics could be authorized to abandon resuscitation attempts after a particular point in their protocol has been reached. This would have to be defined by the local paramedic steering group, but is most likely to refer to cases of persistent asystole where the protocol loop has been applied at least three times without response.

If resuscitation is stopped in the field it will be necessary to call the patient's general practitioner (or rarely the police surgeon if the former cannot be identified) to certify life extinct, and the police to act for the coroner's officer.

In modern times the technology available to paramedics to confirm death is often greater than that which the attending physician can bring. Electrocardiographs with time stamps on their printouts and end-tidal carbon dioxide monitors can provide reliable evidence, although this is not always acceptable to the physician.

Confidentiality

Although there is no legal requirement to maintain patient confidentiality and paramedics are not required to swear a duty to this ethic, there are sound reasons for doing so. Firstly, confidentiality is a general rule of all professions where a practitioner has a privileged relationship with a client. Secondly, it is a generally accepted standard and expectation amongst the population at large that health-care personnel do not discuss confidential matters outside their own profession, and only within it for educational purposes and (wherever possible) with the patient's consent; hence it is reasonable to assume that a breach of confidentiality will be considered 'unethical' by the public. Thirdly, such a breach would prejudice the relationship with the person concerned, who would be unlikely to trust or consent to treatment by that practitioner in the future. Finally, most ambulance services have rules that define conduct and prohibit discussion of confidential patient-related matters. If any such rule is broken it could be judged as a major breach of contract and dismissal may follow. Indeed, a wise employer must consider this level of action: if they fail to do so and the breach of confidentiality is repeated, the employer could be liable for a negligence suit.

It is not always as easy to maintain confidentiality as one would imagine. Inadvertent slips are very possible, such as when relaying patient information to a nurse or physician within earshot of other patients or their relatives. A further risk occurs with radio and telephone transmissions. It is easy and cheap for members of the public to buy a scanner that will allow monitoring of ambulance frequency radio transmissions and analogue mobile phones. Inevitably, much patient information passes via these media with a subsequent risk of loss of privacy. Many services, in addition to providing the address of incidents, will pass details of the patient's medical condition over the radio, and sometimes even the patient's name. It would be worthwhile to consider if a name is of any real value to responders prior to their arrival at the scene, and if any such value outweighs the patient's right to privacy.

A number of strategies could be employed to reduce the risk of loss of confidentiality. Firstly, where possible call details should be passed via telephone land line, which while not entirely secure is far less prone to amateur interception. The use of analogue mobile phones should be avoided as far as possible, as these are as susceptible to being scanned as radio transmissions. One method of increasing the privacy of data transferred from the ambulance control to responders is to send it as text to a mobile data terminal. Although these devices are not widely used by UK ambulance services, they have been in regular use in the USA for a number of years with considerable success. Another advantage of this technology is that it reduces transcription errors when crews take down details of incident locations.

The next technological leap in communications will be the introduction of digital technology. Digital mobile phones and their associated networks have been available in the UK since the end of 1994, and a working group led by the Home Office is investigating the potential application of digital (800 MHz) trunked radio systems for the ambulance service. Digital communications technologies have a far higher level of security than conventional analogue systems, as they encode voice data and select from a large number of available frequencies on a random basis before effecting each transmission. While it is theoretically possible to monitor calls sent in this way the equipment required would be prohibitively expensive and extremely complex. Another advantage with these systems is that portable and mobile devices can be remotely turned off from the control centre, thus providing security in the event of their theft.

One area of constant concern to paramedics is the threat of infection with human immunodeficiency virus (HIV). This very real fear has, on occasion, led to what was assumed to be a 'justified' breach of confidentiality. The rationale where confirmation that a patient has aquired immune deficiency syndrome (AIDS) has been transmitted over the radio is to allow ambulance staff to 'protect' themselves or to 'take precautions'. In reality this is no justification at all. All services should by now have policies in place that require paramedics to take universal precautions against direct contact with any body fluids from any patient. This implies that whenever a member of staff is in a position of risk of infection with HIV they will already be protected. It also implies that, logically, there will be no additional necessary precautions that they can take. Consequently the knowledge that any specific patient has HIV should have no effect on the handling of that particular person, and the information is therefore unnecessary to protect crews' safety.

Infection with HIV undoubtedly wrecks lives; however, it is AIDS that kills people. The majority of the HIV-infected population do not have AIDS; but their lives can be effectively destroyed long before their physical condition deteriorates, as a direct result of breaches of confidentiality by health-care staff. Infection with HIV carries an appalling stigma, and the knowledge that an individual has the virus dramatically affects how others respond to them. Sufferers often become isolated, and may be subjected to behaviour from people with ill-informed prejudices, which can be so unpleasant that they are obliged to move house in order to avoid threats of harm. They may have difficulty getting work or keeping a job, even when their illness is no threat to colleagues. Obtaining insurance can become impossible. Health-care professionals should not, by infringing confidentiality, allow this type of prejudice to occur.

Consent

Patient consent is required before providing any form of treatment to the victim of a medical illness or trauma incident. What is more, this must be *informed consent*, which implies that patients will understand their right to refuse treatment, and have been informed of the foreseeable benefits and possible side-effects of the treatment concerned and, most importantly, of the foreseeable effects of refusing the treatment offered. Failure to obtain consent or, more explicitly, providing treatment against a patient's will is, in legal terms, an assault, and such an action brings with it the risk of prosecution. As a minimum the patient whom you force to have treatment has the right of action against you for 'trespass against the person'. Even threatening to provide treatment against a patient's will constitutes the criminal offence of battery.

In the event that a patient is unconscious, or is under 16 years old (i.e. a minor) and no legal guardian is present, health-care practitioners may assume implied consent. The measure of whether or not this is a reasonable implication is to ask if an ordinary person would, given the opportunity, consent to the treatment being provided under the same or similar circumstances.

It is vital to ensure that patients are fully aware of the possible consequences of their rejection of treatment. Ideally, written evidence should be recorded that this is the case. It is helpful to include a section on the patient report form to allow documentation of this. Patients should be asked to sign a statement to the effect that they have refused treatment and that the ambulance personnel have informed them of the possible consequences of this action. Their signature should be witnessed by someone other than the ambulance personnel who can confirm the veracity of this statement. In the event that the patient refuses to sign, two witnesses should be asked to provide their signature. Ambulance control should be informed of the incident, and any further information carefully documented on the patient report form. This procedure is not designed to threaten patients or to attempt to force them to change their minds. Technically, health-care staff must demonstrate that the patient has given informed consent to refuse treatment, and this process may help provide that evidence when necessary.

It is not always possible or practical to obtain consent in emergencies where time is crucial, even if the patient is conscious or relatives are present. In a situation where seconds count, and provided your actions are reasonable and justifiable, it is likely that any treatment carried out to save life would be considered to be associated with implied consent. However, explanations can help prevent distress for relatives and avoid serious misunderstanding.

Restraint or Assault

Ambulance personnel have no legal right to restrain a patient over and above that of the ordinary citizen, even if the patient is being admitted under a relevant section of the Mental Health Act on the orders of a doctor. As a result, any attempt to restrain a patient under any circumstances is a criminal assault. The only exception to this rule is the right to make a citizen's arrest, and this is only lawful if you know beyond doubt that a criminal act has taken place. Being mentally ill is not a criminal act, nor is refusing treatment for any other reason. Therefore should restraint or forced transportation be necessary for any reason, the assistance of the police should be requested. In addition to assisting with the enforcement of a section of the Mental Health Act, police officers may also order on their own initiative that a person should be removed to a place of safety if they are a risk to themselves or others. They are naturally somewhat reluctant to apply this power to confused aged persons who are refusing to go to hospital for treatment for their fractured neck of femur, but who have not injured themselves as the result of a criminal act. However, with a little tact and diplomacy, the police can usually be persuaded to do so.

Should you be assaulted you do have a legal right to defend yourself, but again your power to do so does not extend beyond that granted to the general public. In effect this means that you can only use 'reasonable force' to prevent harm being inflicted on you.

Ultimately the best approach to an attack on you is to avoid it happening in the first place. This may appear easier said than done, but it is generally true that most attacks are preceded by a threat. Your attitude to both the assailant and the circumstances can have a great deal of impact on whether the violence remains a threat or is actually realized. If you are threatened, avoid responding in an aggressive manner at all costs. Aggression provokes further aggression, and this cycle of emotion always escalates. As a professional your aim should be to break this cycle. Avoid cornering your attacker, either physically or verbally. Always leave them room to manoeuvre and allow them to feel they are in control. When it is possible and safe to do so, let them have their own way (hence the philosophy of giving the mugger your money). If they feel they have the upper hand they will also feel safe and are far less likely to attack you physically. The sense of control reduces the feeling of fear or threat and hence the desire of the assailant to attack you to defend themselves or to establish territorial rights or dominance. Your attitude and interpersonal skills are far more likely to prevent you being assaulted than any physical techniques.

Medical Errors and Negligence Claims

Negligence can be defined as: 'The failure to exercise that degree of care which a person of ordinary prudence with the same or similar training would exercise in the same or similar circumstances'.

What this means for paramedics is that in the event of a negligence claim, their performance or actions would be judged against that of their peers, who are other similarly qualified paramedics. Comparison is not made against the care a physician might be expected to provide. Care would, however, be expected to exceed that provided by a first-aider or member of the public (provided appropriate equipment was available).

Negligence claims can arise as a result of a perceived act of commission or one of omission. Negligence can be very difficult to prove; 'proof' requires evidence that the following four components are all present:

1. Duty to act – this is evidence that an individual was reasonably required to act in the situation found. For instance, if you report to work as a paramedic for your ambulance service and respond to emergency calls you have a duty to provide care to patients.
2. Breach of duty – failure to act appropriately where you have a duty to do so. If you respond to a patient with severe external haemorrhage but make no attempt to control the bleeding, you are in breach of your duty as a paramedic. Similarly, if you apply a tourniquet to a patient with a minor haemorrhage and they lose their arm as a result of the lack of a blood supply, you will also be in breach of your duty.
3. *Damage – it is necessary to demonstrate that damage or harm occurred to the* individual.
4. Causation – the requirement to demonstrate that the damage or harm resulted from the breach of duty.

Remember that to prove negligence it is necessary to provide evidence that all four of the above elements were in place.

Drug Security

To the author's knowledge there is only one ambulance service in the UK that authorizes its paramedics to administer a drug that is classified as a controlled substance (diamorphine). Drugs so classified must, by law, be kept in a locked cabinet within a locked cabinet fixed to an immovable surface. While it could be argued that an ambulance is anything but an immovable surface, it does apparently suffice for legal purposes.

Common sense and safety precautions suggest that all drugs carried by ambulance personnel should be afforded some form of security. Although there is no legal requirement to keep non-controlled prescription-only drugs locked up, there have been many instances of the theft of these substances from ambulances. The drugs can be dangerous if administered inappropriately and it could be argued that there is a moral requirement to minimize the chances of such thefts occurring. In the USA ambulance crews working in inner city areas will typically lock all the doors of their vehicle when leaving it to treat a patient. This is a perfectly practical procedure if both members of the team have keys and the vehicle is fitted with well-designed locks. Some modern ambulances are even being fitted with remote control central locking devices to facilitate both security and easy access. Failure to secure drugs could potentially result in a charge of negligence if a child gained access to them and was harmed as a result, and the prevention of theft will at least help to ensure your ability to treat patients when drug therapy is indicated.

Drug Administration and Invasive Techniques

The November 1992 amendment to the 1983 Medicines Order finally provided legislation regarding the administration of a limited list of prescription only medications (POMs) by paramedics. This was valuable in that it provided legal protection for ambulance staff who were authorized to give drugs and perform invasive techniques, which are also addressed in the same act.

Equally importantly was the provision of statutory guidance on what actually constituted a 'paramedic', at least in terms of the Act itself, restricting its meaning to those holding a certificate of proficiency in ambulance paramedic skills issued by the Secretary of State. This effectively excludes persons not having this qualification from administering POMs or performing invasive techniques such as intubation or venepuncture, unless they are medically qualified. It does not, unfortunately, restrict the use of the word 'paramedic' to those with the National Health Service Training Directive (NHS TD) qualification. The most important implication of this Act for legitimate ambulance service paramedics is that they must keep their qualification current in order to be able to practise their skills. 'Bogus' paramedics are an increasingly common problem. If you are unable to recognize someone at the scene of an accident, ask them to identify themselves to you: doctors who are members of BASICS (British Association for Immediate Care) or a valid immediate care scheme will carry identification. If necessary individuals who are unable to prove a genuine reason for attendance should be escorted from the scene by the police.

The Health and Safety at Work Act

The Health and Safety at Work Act establishes a duty on your employer to take all reasonable precautions to ensure your safety and minimize risks to you resulting from your employment. Resulting activity should include a formal assessment of potential risks, the development of policy and procedure to guide you in reducing risk and coping with hazards, and the provision of safety equipment and relevant health care to protect you from identifiable or predictable risks.

The Act also places a statutory duty on you to minimize risk to yourself. Failure to follow policy, to use safety equipment provided or to identify hazards to your employer will place you in breach of this duty. For example, if you fail to follow a written policy that requires you to wear gloves provided by your employer whenever you encounter body fluids you are technically breaking the law, and would certainly have no redress if you contracted an infectious disease as a result of your omission.

Breaking and Entering

Unlike the police and fire service you have no legal rights to force entry into private property, even if you suspect that an individual's life is at risk. However, in practice, it seems unlikely that anyone would press charges if your suspicion proved correct. A prudent paramedic would ensure that there was sound evidence that a patient was indeed at risk before using force to make an entry.

In all other instances you should request the assistance of the police and await their arrival before forcing an entry.

Accidents While Driving

Ambulance personnel have the same duties under the Road Traffic Act if involved in an accident as the general public, regardless of whether they are responding to an emergency call or not. This Act requires that the driver stops, and provides to persons having reasonable grounds for requesting the information:

- Name and address
- Name and address of the owner of the vehicle
- Registration number of the vehicle
- Insurance certificate or relevant exemption document (i.e. the certificate of crown ownership affixed to the windscreen)

If you are unable to give this information because the relevant person is not present or would be unable to understand this information, you must report the accident to a police officer as soon as possible and within 24 hours. Note that 'I was responding to an emergency call' is never an acceptable reason for not stopping and providing the required information.

In the event that an injury occurs to a person other than you (as the driver of the vehicle) you should report this to the police within 24 hours of the accident occurring, although prudence suggests that you should request police attendance at the scene immediately.

All ambulance services have policies setting out their expectations of their employees should they be involved in a road traffic accident. These steps should be followed precisely in order to protect yourself, and will almost certainly include the requirement that you complete an NHS Traffic Accident Report form. Note that it is most unwise to say anything that might indicate that you accept liability for an accident, and that to do so would almost certainly be in breach of your service's policy.

Responding to Emergency Calls

Drivers of ambulances are able to claim exemption from certain specific sections of the Road Traffic Act when responding to an emergency call or, if appropriate, when transporting a seriously ill patient to a hospital. More accurately, these exemptions are considered to be applicable when observance of the referenced sections of the Act 'would be likely to hinder the use of the vehicle for the purpose for which it is being used on that occasion'. Theoretically this leaves space for interpretation as to what constitutes hindrance of the vehicle and for precisely what uses of the vehicle the exemptions would apply. For example, it may well be considered in a court of law that exceeding the statutory speed limit while transporting someone with a twisted ankle to a hospital does not warrant the application of the relevant exemption.

The following are the specific exemptions that drivers of ambulance vehicles engaged in true emergency duties may reasonably expect to be able to claim:

- You may exceed the statutory speed limit
- You may treat red traffic lights as a 'give way' sign rather than an instruction to stop and wait
- You may pass on the offside of a refuge (including those with 'keep left' or 'keep right' signs)
- You may turn right at junctions where this is normally banned or restricted to buses
- You may use bus lanes during their times of restricted operation
- You may stop and park on clearways
- You may stop and park in a pedestrian crossing controlled area or on the crossing itself
- You may park at or near to double white lines

- You may use white lights (e.g. floodlights) other than reversing lamps and may show these to the rear while stationary
- You may use audible warning devices at night when necessary
- You may leave the engine running when your vehicle is stationary

Note that all of these exemptions are worded in such a way that if you are involved in an accident while claiming them they cease to apply and you cannot claim their protection. In other words the accident may subsequently be considered to be your fault. For example, if you were involved in a collision while exceeding the speed limit it is perfectly possible that you could be charged with dangerous driving.

If you were involved in a collision while proceeding through a red traffic light a subsequent charge might relate to your failing to observe a 'give way' sign or driving without due care and attention. Similarly, if an accident resulted from your passage through a red traffic light without any direct involvement of your vehicle you could still be liable. So if a car runs into the back of another vehicle which has stopped to allow you to progress through a red traffic light, even though your ambulance is not struck your action in proceeding through the light could legitimately be considered to be the cause of the accident as you did not give way to all vehicles. The policy of the police is to refer all such cases to the Director of Public Prosecutions who could decide to bring an action against you.

Interestingly the exemptions listed here are defined as applying to vehicles 'used for ambulance service purposes', and are therefore not restricted to ambulances.

The following are a few of the many non-exemptions that you should be aware of, and apply under all circumstances, including when engaged on emergency duties:

- You may not park dangerously
- You may not drive without reasonable consideration for other road users
- You may not ignore one-way signs
- You may not ignore stop signs
- You may not drive against the flow of traffic at a roundabout
- You may not cross double white lines (other than as described in the Highway Code)

Always use good defensive driving practices; claim exemptions only when responding to emergency calls or when transporting to hospital the very, very small percentage of patients whose condition suggests that a few seconds or minutes saved will positively affect outcome; and proceed with the utmost caution when claiming these exemptions.

CONCLUSION

There are some surprising inadequacies and oversights in the legislation of certain areas of paramedical practice. However, where such guidance is either vague or not available it is important to apply sound ethical practices by following the example set by colleagues in the medical profession. Always refer to your employer's policies, and if you find these to be inadequate or missing, you should lobby for written directions to guide you as you carry out your challenging duties as a paramedic.

appendices:

GLOSSARY

a- Prefix meaning without or absent.

ab- Prefix meaning away from (e.g. abduct).

abdomen The portion of the body between the thorax and the pelvis containing the majority of the organs of digestion as well as the liver and spleen.

abduct To move away from the midline.

aberrant Deviating from the normal path or site.

ABO blood groups One of a number of classifications of blood types based on the presence of the protein groups A or B on the red corpuscles. Groups are divided into A (the presence of group A proteins), B (the presence of group B proteins), AB (both A and B present) or O (no antigens present). Normally blood requires cross-matching into at least a similar blood group between patient and donor before transfusion, though in a desperate emergency blood from group O may be given to any patient.

abortion The termination of a pregnancy before the fetus is viable. This may be a pathological process related to disease of the fetus or disease of the mother, or a deliberate attempt to terminate a pregnancy.

abruptio placentae Separation of the placenta from the uterine wall prior to the commencement of labour, normally associated with massive haemorrhage. It more frequently occurs during the third trimester.

absolute refractory period Period of time when cardiac muscle cells or neurons are completely refractory to depolarization however large the depolarizing stimulus is.

acetabulum The socket of the hip joint in the pelvic bone.

Achilles tendon The major tendon of the gastrocnemius muscle running down from the midcalf to insert in the heel on the calcaneal bone; it can be easily felt posteriorly at the ankle.

acidosis The condition of an excess concentration of hydrogen ions in the body. This may be as a result of either a metabolic problem or a respiratory problem. Treatment relies on treating the cause to correct the imbalance. This is the opposite of alkalosis.

acoustic Related to hearing and the ear.

acromion The tip of the scapula articulating with the clavicle.

activated charcoal A compound used in the treatment of acute poisoning where it is given orally to prevent further absorption of ingested poisons from the gut.

acute abdomen The condition of acute onset of severe pain within the abdominal cavity. It may indicate a condition that requires urgent surgery and therefore normally requires rapid assessment by a doctor.

acute confusional state Confusion caused by interference with the normal brain activity by drugs or metabolic insults.

acute epiglottitis Rapid progressive bacterial infection of the upper airway in young children. One of the key features is a markedly swollen and infected epiglottis which may actually cause sudden airway obstruction and respiratory arrest.

acute hypoxia Sudden fall in oxygen concentration within the blood stream. It may be caused by airway obstruction, lung failure or cardiac failure. Signs may be subtle such as confusion, or more obvious such as acute loss of consciousness.

ad- Prefix meaning towards (e.g. adduct)

addiction Condition characterized by physical and psychological dependence on a substance.

adduct To move towards the midline.

adeno- Relating to a gland.

ADH (antidiuretic hormone) Hormone secreted by the posterior pituitary which has a water-retaining effect on the kidney. It affects the permeability of parts of the kidney leading to water being removed from the urine, concentrating the urine and reducing its volume.

adhesion A fold of scar tissue which causes abnormal tethering of tissue. Most problematic within the abdominal cavity, where it may cause obstruction of the bowel.

adipose Pertaining to fatty tissue.

adrenal glands Two glands each lying superior to the two kidneys in contact with the upper surface. Anatomically they are divided into two distinct regions: the medulla and the cortex. They are responsible for secreting a variety of compounds such as adrenaline and noradrenaline (from the adrenal medulla) and cortisol and androgens (from the adrenal cortex).

advanced life support (ALS) The combination of basic life support (BLS) with advanced and invasive techniques including drug therapy and defibrillation.

afebrile Without fever (i.e. normal physiological temperature)

afterbirth Placenta

after-load The resistance against which the ventricle has to pump.

agitation Restlessness and anxiety; may be pathological, as part of a psychiatric illness.

agonal rhythm The terminal dysrhythmia recorded before death, normally consisting of broad-based bradycardic tracing with no cardiac output.

AIDS Acquired immune deficiency syndrome. A disease characterized by a deficiency in the cell-mediated part of the immune system. It is caused by the human immune deficiency virus (HIV) which is transmitted either through exposure to contaminated blood or blood products or via sexual contact. There is an increased risk of infection in these patients, particularly recurrent infection. Certain cancers such as Kaposi's sarcoma and non-Hodgkin's lymphoma are more common in these patients.

air embolism The presence of pockets of air within the cardiovascular system. If the volume is large enough this results in the obstruction of normal flow of blood.

air hunger Dyspnoea: shortness of breath and rapid, laboured breathing.

airway The passage allowing free movement of air into and out of the lungs. The term is also used to describe clinical devices for maintenance of a patent airway; these may range from simple devices such as Guedel airways to endotracheal tubes.

alcoholic 1) One who has a physical and psychological dependence on alcohol. 2) Mixed or diluted with alcohol.

aldosterone A mineralocorticoid secreted by the adrenal glands that are responsible for the reabsorption of sodium ions from the urine sweat and gastric juice. In the kidneys this is accomplished by the exchange of sodium ions for potassium; the latter is then excreted instead.

aliquot A small measure of a substance.

alkalosis The condition of a decrease in the body's concentration of hydrogen ions or an increase in bicarbonate ions. Like acidosis, this may be caused by respiratory (hyperventilation) or metabolic causes (the ingestion of excess bicarbonate or loss of excess gastric acid following vomiting.)

allergy Abnormal sensitivity to normally harmless antigens. In the severest form this may result in an anaphylactic reaction.

alveolus (Latin, a small hollow) the small sac-like terminations of lung tissue at which level gas exchange takes place.

ambulatory Able to walk. Often refers to patients who are not hospitalized e.g. day-case surgery is often referred to as 'ambulatory' surgery.

amnesia Loss of memory induced by severe physical or emotional trauma.

amniotic fluid The fluid surrounding and cushioning the fetus within the mother's womb.

amputation The loss of a digit, limb or appendage, either deliberately (surgically) or as a result of trauma, vascular disease or infection.

anaemia An abnormally low haemoglobin concentration in the blood.

anaesthesia (Greek, absence of feeling) A loss of normal sensation, particularly pain. This may be as a result of disease or induced deliberately. Anaesthesia may be local (by injecting local anaesthetic drugs around an area), regional (by blocking a nerve or nerves supplying a region) or general, which normally involves reducing a patient to a state of unconsciousness.

analgesic A pain-relieving drug.

anaphylactic reaction An extreme reaction to an allergen characterized by release of histamine from cells of the immune system and resulting in generalized itching, angi-oedema, collapse, tachycardia, bronchospasm and (in the worst cases) death.

anastomosis The surgical joining of two tubular structures.

aneurysm A saccular swelling of a blood vessel.

angio- Relating to blood vessels.

angina (Latin, choking distress) a term primarily used to describe chest pain of myocardial origin relating to insufficient coronary blood flow. This may be stable, occurring only in episodes of excitement or exercise, or may be unstable, preceding a myocardial infarction.

angle of Louis The prominence of the sternum opposite the second intercostal rib space.

antecubital The anatomical area at the front of the elbow (e.g. antecubital fossa).

antepartum Referring to the period before delivery.

anterior In front of or at the forward limits of the body (see Figure 1).

antiarrhythmic A drug that may be used either to control a cardiac dysrhythmia or to prevent it occurring.

antibiotic A drug with antibacterial actions

anticoagulant A drug that delays or prevents the normal clotting of blood.

anticonvulsant Drug with antiepileptic activity used to stop fits or to prevent their occurrence.

antihypertensive agent A drug designed to lower a raised blood pressure.

aorta The main arterial supply to the body. It commences at the outflow of the left ventricle as the ascending aorta and arches within the chest cavity (aortic arch) to give off the main vascular supply to the head. It then descends through the thorax (thoracic aorta) and into the abdomen (abdominal

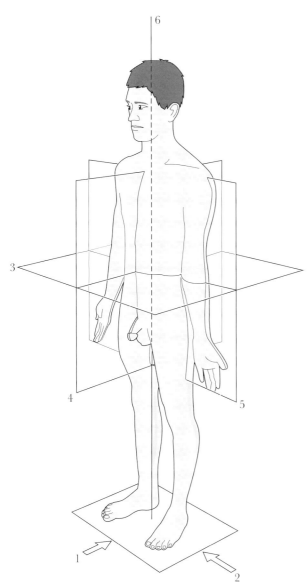

Fig. 1 *Anatomical position: 1, anterior aspect; 2, lateral aspect; 3, transverse plane; 4, sagittal plane; 5, coronal plane; 6, median line*

aorta) to supply the intestines before splitting into two terminal branches (the common iliac arteries).

apgar score An assessment of the newborn infant based on five factors (irritability, heart rate, respiratory effort, colour and muscle tone), each of which is scored between 0 and 2 at 1 minute and at 5 minutes after delivery.

aphasia A feature of a disease resulting in problems with speaking and understanding speech.

apnoea Absence of breathing.

appendicitis Inflammation of the appendix; normally requires surgical removal of the appendix.

appendix A small blind-ending sac at the junction of the

ileum with the caecum. It may become inflamed giving rise to the condition of appendicitis, and may go on to perforate leading to peritonitis.

ARDS Acute (or adult) respiratory distress syndrome. A sudden onset of respiratory failure often associated with the critically ill patient and may frequently require ventilatory support.

arrhythmia *see* Dysrhythmia.

arterio- Relating to an artery or arteries.

artery Blood vessel supplying tissues with oxygenated blood.

arthritis Inflammation of one or more joints.

arthro- Pertaining to the joints.

articulation The junction between ends of bones or cartilage which form joints.

artificial respiration The artificial maintenance of respiration when normal breathing has ceased. This may be from basic respiration as mouth-to-mouth respiration up to respiration via an endotracheal tube and ventilator.

ascites The abnormal collection of fluid within the peritoneal cavity which may lead to problems with fluid balance. It is a complication associated with malignancy, cirrhosis and cardiac failure.

assisted ventilation The boosting of tidal volume in a spontaneously breathing patient.

asthma A disease characterized by episodes of narrowing of the small airways (bronchospasm) resulting in difficulty with breathing, wheeze and mucus plugging of the small airways. In its severest form it may be fatal without rapid medical aid.

asystole Complete absence of a heart-beat and a straight-line ECG.

ataxia The inability to coordinate muscles.

atheroma The deposition of fatty material within the walls of the arteries, leading to narrowing and the conditions of stroke, coronary artery disease or peripheral vascular disease, depending on the area affected.

atlas The first cervical vertebra supporting the head (after Atlas, the Greek god who held up the world).

atrial depolarization The process of electrical depolarization and contraction of the atria.

atrial fibrillation The rapid and disorganized contraction of the atrium. In response the ventricles capture only some of the beats but this still results in an increase in the cardiac rate of up to 150 beats/min. These contractions are irregularly irregular in their timing and also in their pumping ability.

atrial flutter A state of rapid but organized and regular contraction of the atria, resulting in a subsequent increase in the cardiac rate, often associated with varying degrees of block between the atrial rate and the ventricular rate.

atrioventricular block Hindering or prevention of the passage of impulses from the atrium to the ventricle.

atrioventricular dissociation Complete lack of coordination of the electrical activity between the atria and the ventricles.

auditory Pertaining to hearing.

auscultation Listening and interpreting sounds as heard through the stethoscope.

avulsion Injury that tears tissue away from its anatomical connections, e.g. a finger may be avulsed from the hand.

axilla The armpit.

bacteraemia The presence of bacteria within the blood stream (*see also* Septic shock).

baroreceptor Specialist receptor within the aortic arch and carotid sinus detecting the changes in pressure within the vascular system.

barotrauma Injury as a result of pressure change across a body or organ, such as may occur with rapid ascents following diving, etc.

basic life support The maintenance of airway, breathing and circulation without any equipment.

Battle's sign Bruising behind the ear over the mastoid region due to a basilar skull fracture.

Beck's triad The three principal physical signs of cardiac tamponade: muffled heart sounds, hypotension and neck vein distension.

bends The formation of bubbles of nitrogen within the blood stream as a result of rapid decompression.

benign neoplasm A tumour with limited potential to grow. It does not invade local tissues or metastasize, and is frequently surrounded by a capsule. Its dangers lie in its site of expansion and the damage it may do by this.

benign prostatic hypertrophy An expansion of the prostate seen characteristically in elderly men and a common cause of acute retention of urine. It may be preceded by a history of frequency of passage of urine, nocturia and poor stream.

bi- Prefix meaning two.

biceps (Latin, two heads) one of the main muscles in the upper arm responsible for flexion of the elbow.

bifurcate To split in two.

bigeminy An abnormal cardiac rhythm with two rapid beats followed by a longer pause. Caused by every other beat being premature.

bile duct The terminal part of the biliary tree, which leads from the junction of the cystic duct (which drains the gallbladder) and the common hepatic duct (draining bile from the liver) through to open in common with the pancreatic duct into the duodenum.

bilirubin A yellow pigment excreted by the liver and giving rise to the yellow colour of the skin in jaundice, when it is inadequately excreted by the liver.

biopsy The surgical removal of a small piece of tissue for histological (microscopic) analysis.

blood pressure The pressure exerted by the circulating blood on the arteries as it is pumped around the circulation.

blood glucose The concentration of glucose within the blood. In diabetic patients who lack adequate insulin secretion the blood glucose level would be expected to be raised

(hyperglycaemia) owing to lack of control. It may become dangerously low (hypoglycaemia) as a result of excessive amounts of insulin relative to the oral intake of food.

bone marrow The contents filling the cancellous bone, responsible for the maturation and production of red blood cells.

bounding pulse A peripheral pulse which when palpated seems to be of excessive volume.

brachio- Relating to the arm.

bradycardia An unusually slow pulse rate, generally understood to be less than 60 beats/min, though this may be normal in a fit young individual.

breech birth Delivery where the presenting part is a foot or the buttocks.

bronchiectasis A pathological dilatation of the small airways, forming chambers within which infection may pool and multiply.

bronchitis Infection or inflammation of the bronchi.

bronchopneumonia Acute infection of the lungs, particularly the bronchioles. Patients are severely ill with fever and rigors; the condition may result in pleural effusions and empyema as complications.

bronchospasm Severe constriction of the bronchial tree.

bronchus (plural bronchi) The division of the trachea leading down to the alveoli; the two first divisions after the trachea are known as the right and left main bronchi.

bulla A large fluid filled blister or thin walled air containing space within the lung.

bundle branch block Disturbance in electrical conduction through either the right or left bundle branch of the heart's conducting system.

burn An injury caused by extremes of temperature – hot or cold. Classified as full-thickness or partial-thickness, depending how deep is the extent of tissue damage. Other causes of burns include chemicals and electricity.

bursa A synovial-lined cavity whose function is to enable the passage of tendons, muscle and soft tissues over bony points to be smoothed and effectively lubricated. The most common and well-known are the infrapatellar and prepatellar bursae which may become inflamed in the conditions of clergyman's knee and housemaid's knee respectively.

caecum The first segment of the colon at the site of the junction of the ileum and the appendix.

caesarean section The delivery of a baby through an abdominal incision into the uterus.

calcaneus The heel bone.

caput medusae The pattern of veins on the abdomen seen in such conditions as advanced cirrhosis.

carbon dioxide retention An increase in the concentration of carbon dioxide within the blood stream, often secondary to respiratory failure. Care must be taken in treating these patients with oxygen as this can precipitate a sudden respiratory arrest in these patients if this condition is chronic.

carbon monoxide A colourless, odourless gas. It has the

ability to combine with haemoglobin in an almost irreversible manner, displacing oxygen and causing anoxia of the tissues.

carboxyhaemoglobin The product of combination between carbon monoxide and haemoglobin.

carcinoma A malignant neoplasm which has the ability to grow and metastasize, and eventually kill.

cardiac arrest Sudden stop to effective circulation. It may be caused by a variety of arrhythmias, including electromechanical dissociation, asystole and ventricular fibrillation.

cardiac output The volume of blood pumped out by the heart in 1 minute. It is derived from the stroke volume (the amount of blood pumped per heart beat) multiplied by heart rate.

cardiac tamponade A collection of fluid within the pericardial sac that leads to a reduction in the output of the heart.

cardio- Relating to the heart.

cardiogenic shock Normally due to the effects of a myocardial infarction where sufficient ventricular damage has taken place such that the heart cannot maintain an adequate perfusion of tissues.

cardiogram *see* ECG.

cardiomyopathy A pathological condition of the muscles of the heart. It may take the form of the heart cells becoming weak and unable to pump properly, or they may multiply in number, obstructing the outflow of the heart.

cardioversion The use of an electrical shock synchronized to the heart's rhythm to change an abnormal heart rhythm.

carotid arteries (from Greek *Karos*, heavy sleep) The two major arteries that can be felt in the neck giving arterial supply to the face and brain.

carotid sinus massage The use of pressure over the carotid sinus to stimulate a vagal mediated reflex that slows the heart. It also can be used to try to convert certain supraventricular tachyarrhythmias into normal sinus rhythm.

carpo- Relating to the wrist.

cartilage (Latin, gristle) A supporting tissue found in a number of anatomical sites, e.g. joints, trachea and ear. It varies in its make-up depending on its anatomical site, e.g. fibrocartilage or articular cartilage. In the joints articular cartilage provides the smooth gliding surface to allow smooth movement between joints.

cataract An opacity of the lens of the eye. A common condition in the elderly.

catheter Any flexible tube that may be placed within a body cavity to drain or instil fluids, e.g. urinary catheter for draining the bladder.

cephalo- Relating to the head.

cerebellum The part of the brain responsible for coordination of voluntary motor activity; it resides within the posterior/inferior portion of the cranial cavity.

cerebral haemorrhage Bleeding into the cerebrum – a form of stroke or cerebrovascular accident (CVA).

cerebral oedema An increase in the fluid around the cells in brain tissue with resultant swelling. A number of causes include head injury (the commonest). It may present with signs of raised intracranial pressure owing to the closed nature of the skull.

cerebral perfusion pressure A measure of the circulatory pressure to the brain. It can be calculated as the mean arterial pressure minus the intracranial pressure.

cerebro- Relating to the brain.

chest lead One of six conducting leads placed on a patient's chest in predetermined positions during twelve-lead electrocardiography.

chest pain A physical complaint, symptomatic of many differing disorders, some extremely serious such as myocardial infarction, others less dangerous such as hiatus hernia or indigestion. It should be taken seriously until investigated thoroughly.

Cheyne–Stokes respiration An abnormal pattern of breathing characterized by slow, shallow breaths, building to deep, rapid breathing, and finally dying away to a period of apnoea lasting up to 20 seconds before the next cycle begins.

cholecystectomy The surgical removal of the gallbladder, often performed by 'key hole' or laparoscopic surgery.

cholecystitis Inflammation of the gallbladder (may present as an acute abdomen).

chondro- Relating to cartilage.

chronic bronchitis A common respiratory disease, with increased sputum production for at least 3 months of the year for 2 years.

chronic obstructive pulmonary disease (COPD) A blanket term for the three chronic diseases (chronic bronchitis, emphysema and asthma) that may cause obstructive problems with the airways.

circum- Prefix meaning surrounding, around.

claudication Pain felt in a limb or muscle group (particularly the calves) on exercising the muscle group. Caused by poor arterial circulation to the muscle, leading to ischaemic pain when the muscle action outstrips the blood supply to it.

clavicle The supporting bone articulating between the scapula and the sternum.

coagulation factors Thirteen named factors circulating in the blood stream, which are responsible for the successful and efficient clotting of blood.

coagulopathy An abnormal condition characterized by a decreased ability of the blood to clot. In trauma this may be caused by continual bleeding and an inadequate replacement of coagulation factors after large blood loss.

coccyx The small bone at the base of the spine joined to the sacrum.

colic A pain, originating from a tubular structure, that characteristically comes in waves; it may be caused by obstruction, or spasm of the muscular coat of the structure. Typical organs that may produce colic include the gut and the ureter.

colitis *see* Ulcerative colitis.

collateral Running alongside (e.g. collateral ligament).

colloid A solution used to increase circulating volume by intravenous transfusion, which contains proteins and large molecules, e.g. hetastarches, dextrans or albumin.

colon The large bowel reaching from the caecum to the rectum. Divided into four parts: the ascending, transverse, descending and sigmoid colon.

colostomy The surgical creation of an opening of the large bowel on the abdominal wall after resection or decompression of the bowel.

coma Deep unconsciousness with no response to vocal or painful stimuli or spontaneous eye movement. Causes are many and include trauma, infection and metabolic states.

compensatory pause A longer than normal interval between heart beats. Often associated with premature ventricular contractions.

complete heart block A block anywhere between the atria and the ventricles to electrical conduction. Thus the ventricles are driven by an ectopic pacemaker at some level below the block, at a slower than normal rate.

concussion The injury (used with regard to head injury) following a violent jar or shock.

condyle A rounded projection at the end of a bone (e.g. femoral condyle at the distal femur).

congenital Any condition acquired before or present at birth.

congestive heart failure (CHF) Also known as congestive cardiac failure. Pathological condition most frequently related to a myocardial infarction or to ischaemic cardiac disease where the heart does not pump efficiently enough to clear fluid around the circulation. It is characterized by peripheral oedema and shortness of breath; the symptoms that predominate depend on whether the right or left side of the heart is most affected.

conjunctiva The membrane that lines the eyelids and the sclera of the eye.

contaminated Infected with bacteria (or viral or fungal organisms); this may apply to a wound, or to any substance or area.

contra- Prefix meaning against.

contracoup The head injury sustained on the opposite side of the head to the site of the blow. It results from the movement of the soft brain against the cranium on the opposite side.

contralateral On the opposite side.

contusion The result of a blow to the body which fails to break the skin but produces swelling, bruising and pain.

coracoid A bony projection from the scapula that can be felt below the clavicle.

cornea The transparent covering over the anterior part of the eye.

coronary 1) Referring to the heart or to its encircling vessels, e.g. coronary vessels.

2) Alternative term for myocardial infarction, as in coronary thrombosis.

coronary artery bypass The surgical reconstruction of the coronary arteries with vein or graft in order to bypass areas of narrowing.

coronary artery disease A common affliction, particularly of the Western world. The coronary arteries become narrowed owing to the deposition of atheroma within their walls. This results in symptoms of angina or may lead to thrombosis and further narrowing of the artery which may clot off completely, producing a myocardial infarction.

coronary care unit Hospital unit equipped and staffed to deal with the acute problems associated with coronary disease, particularly relating to myocardial infarctions.

cor pulmonale Heart disease arising secondarily to lung disease.

corpuscle (Latin, a small body) One of the cells suspended within the blood stream, e.g. white or red corpuscles.

costo- Relating to the ribs.

coup injury Head injury occurring on the side of the blow.

CPR Cardiopulmonary resuscitation: the provision of cardiac massage and artificial ventilation during attempts to resuscitate patients in a state of cardiac arrest.

cranio- Relating to the skull.

cranium The bony framework of the skull.

cricoid (Greek, ring-like) The last complete ring of cartilage in the upper airway before the horseshoe-like cartilages of the trachea.

cricothyrotomy Puncturing of the cricothyroid membrane in order to create an emergency airway. This may be done using a thick needle, or a formal surgical incision may be made.

cruciate Crossed (e.g. the posterior and anterior cruciate ligaments which stabilize the knee and cross each other).

crush syndrome The life-threatening condition seen after massive crush injury to the body which results in haemodynamic instability and potential renal impairment.

crystalloid Solution used for intravenous fluid replacement, containing only electrolytes and water.

CSF Cerebrospinal fluid: the fluid surrounding the brain and spinal cord.

cubital Relating to the elbow (e.g. antecubital fossa).

cutaneous Pertaining to the skin.

cyanosis The blue colour seen at the periphery or centrally caused by the inadequate oxygenation of blood, which thus contains too much deoxyhaemoglobin which has a bluish colour.

cyst- Relating to the bladder.

dead space The area of the lung that is in contact with oxygen but is not being perfused with blood; also applied to the volume of air that is contained within the trachea and the bronchi which never reaches the gas exchange surface.

death   The absence of palpable heart-beat and spontaneous respiration.

decerebrate   A condition of profound brain dysfunction associated with a classical posture of extension of both arms and legs and internal rotation of the arms.

decorticate   Similar to decerebrate; a severe brain dysfunction but owing to the difference in area affected the posture is different with flexion of the upper limbs and extension of the legs.

deep vein thrombosis   The development of a blood clot within the deep venous system (normally within the lower limb). It may be detected clinically by swelling of the calf and accompanying tenderness. It may be complicated by fragments of the clot breaking off and clotting to the lungs as a pulmonary embolus.

defibrillate   To use an electric shock to convert an abnormal rhythm of the heart (fibrillation) to a normal rhythm.

definitive care   In-hospital management of the trauma victim, usually surgical.

dehiscence   A separation. Used to describe a healing surgical wound breaking apart (wound dehiscence).

delirium tremens (DTs)   The stage of agitation and hallucination sometimes experienced in uncontrolled withdrawal from alcohol.

deltoid   A muscle clothing the shoulder and linking scapula and clavicle to the humerus.

dementia   A deterioration in mental function, frequently associated with old age although it may occur in younger age groups as a result of pathological processes.

dermato   Relating to the skin.

dermatome   An area of skin supplied by sensation by one particular spinal root.

dermis   The skin.

dextrose   A sugar used in intravenous nutrition and in some crystalloid solutions.

dia-   Prefix meaning through.

diabetes mellitus   The disorder of metabolism clinically due to inadequate secretion of insulin by the pancreas. A variety of classifications exist. Treatment may range from a diabetic diet through tablet therapy to insulin therapy.

diabetic coma   The lapsing into unconsciousness by a diabetic patient. Though occasionally this is due to an excess of sugar in the blood stream (hyperglycaemia), it is much more frequently a result of low blood glucose levels (hypoglycaemia).

diabetic ketoacidosis   The condition where by dehydration high blood glucose levels and an increased quantity of fat breakdown leads to the state of extreme illness which may slide into coma and eventual death if untreated.

dialysis   *see* Haemodialysis.

diaphragm   The musculotendinous sheet that separates the thoracic cavity from the abdominal cavity.

diastole   The period of time during the cardiac cycle when the heart is relaxed and blood enters the atria or ventricles.

diastolic blood pressure   The systemic blood pressure during diastole. It rises slightly in the early phases of hypovolaemic shock.

digit   A finger or toe.

digitalis toxicity   The condition associated with overdosage of digoxin.

dilatation and curettage (D&C)   The scraping of the endometrium of the uterus after dilating the cervix. This may be performed to correct heavy periods or to remove the products of conception.

diplopia   Double vision.

dislocation   The displacement of any joint from its normal anatomical site and relationship with the surrounding tissues and bones.

distal   Further away along the body or a limb from a reference point.

diuretic   A drug used to aid the excretion of urine; particularly useful in conditions of fluid overload such as heart failure.

diuresis   The excretion of a quantity of urine; normally used to describe the response to a drug or fluid load.

diverticulitis   Inflammation of a diverticulum. This may lead to abdominal pain and may even perforate, leading to peritonitis.

diverticulum   A small out-pouching through the muscular wall of a tubular organ, most commonly referring to those found in the colon (e.g. diverticular disease).

dorso-   Relating to the back or posterior aspect of the body or limb.

dorsum   A structure on the back of a body or limb (e.g. the dorsum of the hand).

duodenal ulcer   The common type of peptic ulcer.

duodenum   The first segment of small bowel linking the stomach to the jejunum. Contains the entry of the common bile duct and the pancreatic duct.

dura mater   One of the three layers of membrane that surround the brain and spinal cord. In the head this layer is fused to the cranial vault and is indistinguishable from the periosteum. Bleeding between the dura and the bone following head injury may lead to an extradural haematoma which may have potentially fatal results.

dys-   Prefix meaning painful.

dysmenorrhoea   Pain that accompanies menstruation.

dyspepsia   Epigastric discomfort associated with eating, heartburn and bloating.

dysphagia   Difficulty in swallowing or painful swallowing.

dyspnoea   Shortness of breath whether as a result of disease or as a result of excessive exercise.

dysrhythmia   An abnormal cardiac rhythm: may be a tachydysrhythmia or a bradydysrhythmia.

dysuria   Pain on passing urine.

ECG   *see* Electrocardiogram.

eclampsia The onset of fits associated with pregnancy; these may occur before or after delivery.

-ectasis Dilatation of a tubular structure or sac.

ecto- Prefix meaning on the outside.

ectopic The development of tissue away from its normal site – particularly ectopic pregnancy, when fetal growth begins in an abnormal site such as the fallopian tube. Other tissues such as bone may form in ectopic sites.

electrocardiogram (ECG) A trace of the electrical activity of the heart normally taken as 12 differing views of the heart. Used to diagnose abnormalities of the heart such as arrhythmias and previous myocardial infarction.

electromechanical dissociation (EMD) The state of cardiac arrest where electrical activity is maintained but no cardiac output results. Common causes include pulmonary embolus, cardiac tamponade, tension pneumothorax and hypovolaemia.

embolism The passage through the blood vessels of a substance (e.g. clot, amniotic fluid, plastic particles) not normally found within the blood stream. Finally the embolus impacts within the vascular tree.

embryo The human fetus from conception to the first 8 weeks.

emphysema A chronic disease where there is destruction of the parenchyma of the lung and distension of other parts of the lung. Alternatively described as chronic obstructive pulmonary disease.

encephalitis An inflammation of the brain.

endo- Prefix meaning innermost.

endocrine Relating to glands or cells that release their secretions into the blood stream or lymph rather than into the digestive tract or onto the skin.

endometrium The lining of the uterus into which the fetus implants.

endothelium The lining epithelial cells of the serous cavities, lymphatic vessels and blood vessels.

endotracheal tube A large-bore tube used to secure an airway or to administer positive pressure ventilation. Apart from those used in small children, all tubes have an inflatable cuff at one end to secure the tube within the trachea.

epidemic The occurrence of a disease in a large number of people over a large area.

epidermis The superficial layers of the skin: the outer cornified layer and a deeper living layer.

epiglottis Protective structure that overhangs the larynx and hinges backwards during swallowing to prevent food entering the larynx.

epiglottitis A childhood disease characterized by swelling and inflammation of the epiglottis. A sudden obstruction of the upper airway may occur without warning resulting in respiratory arrest.

epiphysis The proximal or distal part of a long bone that is separated from the shaft by the epiphyseal plate that allows growth of that bone.

epistaxis A nose bleed.

erythrocyte A red blood cell.

exercise ECG An ECG which is performed while the patient exercises in an attempt to disclose latent ischaemia.

exo- Prefix meaning outermost.

exsanguinate To bleed to death.

extension Movement between two bones, generally in a direction to increase the angle between them.

external chest compressions The application of rhythmical mechanical compression of the chest wall, compressing the ventricles and maintaining a cardiac output during a state of cardiac arrest.

extradural Literally, outside the dura; particularly refers to the cerebral bleed associated with a temporal fracture where the middle meningeal artery bleeds into the extradural space compressing the cerebral substance.

extrasystole A cardiac contraction that is outside the timing of the normal cycle.

fascia (Latin, a band or sash) Fibrous connective tissue found in a variety of sites in the body, often wrapped around structures such as muscle or as a lining below fat and skin.

femur The thigh bone.

fever An increase in body temperature above the normal value of 37 °C.

fibula The small outer (lateral) bone of the lower leg.

Fio$_2$ The concentration of oxygen that a patient is receiving normally expressed as a fraction or percentage, e.g. Fio$_2$ 0.56 or 56%.

fistula An abnormal connection between two organs: this may take the form of a bowel-to-bowel fistula, a join between two blood vessels (arteriovenous fistula) or a connection between an organ and its surroundings (bronchopleural fistula).

flail chest A chest cavity that as a result of trauma has two rows of multiple rib fractures leading to paradoxical movement of the chest wall.

flexion Movement between two bones, generally in a direction to decrease the angle between them.

flutter waves Regular sawtooth waves on the ECG diagnostic of atrial flutter.

Foley catheter A rubber or Silastic catheter that is inserted into the bladder via the urethra and is left *in situ* to drain urine. It has a small balloon on the end which is inflated once the catheter is in the correct site in order to prevent the catheter falling out.

fontanelle A space between certain of the cranial bones in the newborn, covered by tough membranes.

foramen A small space or opening.

fracture An injury to the bone at which the continuity of the bone is broken. There are a variety of classifications, but one important feature of note is whether the skin has been broken over the fracture site (compound or open fracture) or not (closed).

frostbite The damage to tissues caused by subjection to freezing temperatures.

gag reflex The reflex occurring in response to irritation of the pharynx.

galea The fibrous fascial layer that connects the frontalis muscles on the forehead to the occipital muscles of the posterior aspect of the head (the scalp).

gallbladder A small sac linked to the bile duct and to the hepatic ducts of the liver whose role is to concentrate bile from the liver, store it and when required release it into the common bile duct, whence it flows into the duodenum to aid in digestion.

gallop rhythm A description of an abnormal heart rhythm where there is an extra heart sound (either a third or fourth sound).

ganglion 1) in anatomical terms, a group of nerve cells outside the central nervous system; 2) in pathological terms, a small cystic swelling associated with a tendon.

gangrene Death of tissue, often due to inadequate blood supply as the main cause, though a variety of other conditions such as cold injury may also cause gangrenous changes. Often divided into wet or dry gangrene: typically, wet gangrene follows major tissue damage such as crush injury.

gas gangrene Infection of tissues with a particular genus of bacterium (*Clostridium*), characterized by aggressive infection accompanied by bubbles of gas formation within the tissues. If untreated, may rapidly become fatal.

gastric Pertaining to the stomach.

gastric ulcer Ulceration of the lining of the stomach which may present with pain and indigestion responsive to milk or antacids. It may also present as a perforation of the stomach wall or with an acute bleed and vomiting blood.

gastrocnemius The most superficial muscle of the posterior aspect of the calf.

gastrointestinal bleed Any bleeding that originates from the gastrointestinal (GI) tract. It may frequently be due to upper GI causes such as peptic ulcers or oesophageal varices, or lower GI causes such as bleeding from diverticuli or bleeding due to cancer.

gastrointestinal obstruction Any obstruction of the GI tract. Causes may be manifold. Symptoms are predominantly colic pain, decrease in bowel opening and vomiting.

geriatrics The section of medicine that specializes in the care and medicine of the elderly.

gestation Pregnancy.

glands Collections of tissues or an organ which produces substances to excrete or secrete that are not primarily related to their normal metabolism.

Glasgow Coma Scale A swift method for assessing and monitoring the conscious level of a patient. It is based on the verbal response, the motor response and eye opening.

glenoid The socket part of the scapula against which the humeral head articulates.

glomerulus (Latin, a small ball) The first part of the nephron where small blood vessels allow filtering of plasma to start the production of urine.

glosso- Relating to the tongue.

glucose A simple sugar, important as an energy source, whose metabolism is disturbed in diabetes.

goitre An abnormal swelling of the thyroid gland. This may represent an overactive or an underactive gland, or a growth (malignant or benign) within the gland.

graft A portion of tissue or complete organ taken from one site in a body and placed in another site or into a different patient to correct a deficiency or absence of tissue.

grand mal seizure Generalized motor seizure, a form of epilepsy.

gravidity The number of pregnancies that a woman has had.

greenstick fracture An incomplete fracture, usually in children, where the bone cortex is bent and deformed rather than disrupted.

guarding The contraction of the abdominal muscles to protect a painful area from the pressure of an examining hand.

gynae- Referring to woman or female reproductive organs.

haematemesis The vomiting of bright red blood, normally signifying rapid upper gastrointestinal blood loss such as an ulcer or oesophageal varices.

haemato- Relating to blood.

haematoma A collection of blood within the tissues; this may be as a direct result of trauma or of surgery.

haematuria Passage of blood in the urine.

haemodialysis The procedure necessary in patients with renal failure to remove the toxic products of metabolism from the blood stream. Blood is taken through a large-bore cannula from an arteriovenous fistula or from a central line and passed through a dialysis filter to remove the toxins before being returned to the body.

haemoglobin The red pigment found in red blood cells that is responsible for the carriage of oxygen around the body.

haemoptysis The coughing up of blood in the sputum.

haemorrhage The loss of blood – a term normally referring to rapid loss of a large quantity of blood either internally or externally.

haemorrhoids (piles) An abnormal dilatation (or varicosity) of the lower rectal veins: may present with rectal bleeding or protrude through the anal rim and become thrombosed.

haemothorax The filling of a pleural cavity with blood, usually after trauma to the chest or following thoracic surgery.

hallux The great toe.

head tilt The act of hyperextending the head to open the airway.

heart block Illness where the passage of electrical impulses from the atria to the ventricles is delayed or prevented. Varying forms exist: first degree block is characterized by a prolonged PR interval; second degree block is where a variable percentage of the P waves are not followed by a QRS complex; third degree block is a complete failure of impulses to reach the ventricle from the atria and an ectopic focus takes over (see complete heart block).

heart failure *see* Congestive heart failure.

heat cramps Muscular cramps resulting from dehydration and salt loss following exercise.

heat exhaustion A state of nausea, muscle cramps and eventual loss of consciousness due to excessive exertion in hot conditions resulting in loss of fluid and electrolytes.

heat stroke A disturbance of the ability to thermoregulate resulting in extreme fever and dry skin, eventually progressing to coma.

hemi- Prefix meaning half.

hemiplegia (half paralysis) Paralysis of one half of the body; this may be as a result of congenital illness such as cerebral palsy, or due to such causes as stroke.

hepatic, hepato- Pertaining to the liver.

hepatitis An inflammation of the liver which normally results in jaundice, abdominal discomfort and loss of appetite. There are many potential causes including infections (such as hepatitis B, hepatitis A) parasitic infections, drugs and alcohol.

hernia The abnormal protrusion of an organ through the muscular wall surrounding it; may be congenital or acquired later in life. If in the abdomen, may present with obstruction due to incarceration or strangulation of the bowel by the margins of the hernial sac.

hormone A chemical produced within the body that regulates cell activities, often at a distant site.

humerus The long bone of the upper arm and shoulder.

hyaline Glassy and smooth (e.g. hyaline cartilage).

hyper- Prefix meaning increased.

hypercapnia (hypercarbia) A high level of carbon dioxide in the blood.

hyperglycaemia A higher than normal concentration of glucose in the blood stream.

hyperkalaemia A high level of potassium in the blood, normally as a result of administration of drugs affecting the excretion of potassium or the failure of the kidney to adequately excrete potassium. In excess this may result in cardiac dysrhythmias.

hyperlipidaemia An excess of lipids within the blood.

hyperpyrexia An extremely elevated body temperature. Malignant hyperpyrexia, a condition of rapidly rising temperature, is a complication of general anaesthesia.

hypertension Disorder of blood pressure control that results in an elevated blood pressure.

hyperventilation A rate and volume of breathing above that normally required for adequate gas exchange. The removal of carbon dioxide from the blood stream as a result of this may cause dizzy spells, numbness of the periphery and chest pains.

hypervolaemia A larger than required circulating volume, generally the result of overtransfusion, though overdrinking (particularly in the presence of reduced renal function) may also give rise to it.

hypo- Prefix meaning low or inadequate.

hypoglycaemia An abnormally low blood glucose level. In extremes it may cause faintness, then unconsciousness and coma.

hypokalaemia Low or adequate levels of potassium in the blood. In extreme cases this may lead to flaccid muscles and an abnormal ECG.

hyponatraemia A low or inadequate concentration of sodium in the blood.

hypotension A low blood pressure which is inadequate for perfusion of the vital organs. This may be as a result of abnormalities of the heart, side-effects of drugs in excess or loss of circulating fluid.

hypothermia A pathologically low body temperature (normally defined as below 35 °C), most frequently due to exposure to cold conditions.

hypovolaemia A state of low blood volume. *See also* Hypovolaemic shock.

hypovolaemic shock The state of inadequate perfusion (and therefore oxygenation of the tissues) due to a fall in the circulating volume (usually due to blood loss) and a subsequent fall in blood pressure. Excessive loss of body fluids due to other causes (e.g. diarrhoea) can also occasionally cause this.

hypoxaemia Low level of oxygen in the blood.

hypoxia A fall in the concentration of oxygen in cells. This may result from inadequate oxygenation due to a decrease in the atmospheric oxygen, inadequate respiration (due to a reduction in the respiratory drive, an obstruction of the respiratory tract or lung injury) or inadequate circulation (e.g. shock).

hystero- Relating to the uterus.

idiopathic Of unknown cause.

ileostomy The surgical creation of a connection between the ileum and the abdominal wall.

ileum The terminal part of the small bowel linking the jejunum to the caecum.

iliac Referring to structures around the inguinal and pelvic region or the ilium, e.g. the iliac vessels.

ilium Upper portion of the hip bone.

incisor A cutting tooth.

incomplete abortion A spontaneous abortion that does not result in the complete expulsion of the products of conception and may result in haemorrhage from the vagina needing surgical intervention.

incontinence The inability to control the excretion of urine or faeces. This may be due to congenital problems or to problems ranging from damage to the nerve supply of the bladder or bowels to direct damage to the organs themselves.

inevitable abortion A spontaneous abortion which is imminent and cannot be avoided. Bleeding, abdominal pain and cervical dilatation are major features.

infant   Child of less than 1 year old.

infarct   An area of cell death that results from the interruption of the blood supply. Examples include myocardial infarction and some types of stroke.

infra-   Prefix meaning below or beneath.

infusion   The introduction of a drug or fluid into the venous system directly.

inguinal   Pertaining to the groin (e.g. inguinal hernia, a hernia that passes through the inguinal region of the body).

inotropic   Affecting the force of cardiac contraction.

insulin   A hormone secreted by the B cells of the pancreas which is responsible for the lowering of blood glucose levels.

inter-   Prefix meaning between.

intermittent positive pressure ventilation   Ventilation of a patient who is not breathing, using a positive pressure system.

intestinal obstruction   *see* Gastrointestinal obstruction.

intra-   Prefix meaning within.

intravenous   Into a vein (administration of fluid or drugs).

intraventricular block   The slowing or stopping of the cardiac excitatory impulse within the ventricles; it can be seen on an ECG and identified as a left or right bundle branch block.

intubation   The passage of an endotracheal tube through the mouth or nose to secure an airway to the trachea or allow the passage of an anaesthetic agent.

ion   An atom or molecule in its charged state; e.g. chlorine naturally exists as a negatively charged chloride ion (Cl⁻), ammonia exists as the ammonia ion (NH_4^+).

ipsi-   Prefix meaning the same (e.g. ipsilateral, on the same side).

ischaemia   Pain within an organ or tissue caused by a lack of blood supply, e.g. angina, which is due to a decrease in the supply of blood to regions of the heart.

isotonic   In medical terms, having the same osmotic pressure as extracellular fluid.

jaundice   A yellow colour first noted in the mucous membranes and sclera, caused by excess circulating bilirubin.

jaw thrust   A manoeuvre to open the airway by pushing the mandible forward, normally with the fingers behind the angle of the mandible.

jejunum   The intermediate portion of the small bowel linking the duodenum to the ileum.

joint   A junction between two bones. This may be classified in a number of ways, for example by its structure (e.g. a ball and socket joint such as the hip) or by its type (e.g. fibrous, cartilaginous or synovial).

jugular   Pertaining to the neck (e.g. jugular vein, the major vein running on the right and left of the neck alongside the carotid artery draining blood from the face and head).

jugular veins   The veins lying either side of the neck that return blood to the heart. They may become full and visible when central venous pressure increases as in cardiac failure.

junctional rhythm   A cardiac rhythm initiated by the atrioventicular node.

junctional tachycardia   An automatic rhythm of greater than 100 beats/min that is controlled from the atrioventricular node.

ketoacidosis   A complication of diabetes mellitus where excessive blood ketone levels (products of uncontrolled metabolism) create a metabolic acidosis which can result in nausea, vomiting, dehydration and eventually coma and death.

lactic acid   One of the waste products of protein and carbohydrate metabolism. It may accumulate in certain conditions to cause a metabolic acidosis which may lead to a loss of consciousness: this may be one of the causes of coma in diabetic patients.

landmark position   The correct position of the hands during CPR.

laparotomy   The surgical exploration of the abdominal cavity.

laryngo-   Relating to the larynx.

laryngoscope   A tool for examining the larynx or for aid in viewing the larynx to assist the passage of an endotracheal tube.

larynx   The upper part of the windpipe.

lateral   A position on the body further from the midline relative to another point.

latissimus dorsi   A large muscle running from the iliac crest posteriorly over the back to insert in the upper arm.

lavage   To wash out (e.g. gastric lavage to remove contents of the stomach).

left heart failure   Limited function of the left ventricle leading to back pressure in the pulmonary artery and veins, pulmonary oedema and breathlessness. Often accompanied by some degree of right heart failure. *see also* Congestive heart failure.

leuco-   Prefix meaning white.

leucocyte   A white blood cell. May be further differentiated into types such as neutrophil, eosinophil, etc., according to histological appearance and function.

leukaemia   A malignancy of the bone marrow cells characterized by the replacement of the marrow with immature white cells which are released into the circulation.

ligament   A band of connective tissue connecting bones and cartilages together and stabilizing these structures.

ligate   To tie off.

lipid   The fat of the body. This term includes the structural fats in the membrane of cells through to the layers of adipose tissue.

lipo   Relating to fat.

lobar pneumonia   Bacterial infection of one of the five lung lobes. It passes through a series of stages eventually ending with consolidation of that lobe.

log roll   Manoeuvre to move a patient to expose the back but maintaining in-line stability of the whole spine.

longitudinal   Along the long axis of the body.

lumbar   (Latin *lumbus*, the loin) General term referring to the lower back between the thorax and the pelvis, e.g. lumbar spine.

lunate bone   One of the small bones in the wrist.

lymph   (Latin *lympha*, clear water) Fluid produced by the seepage of plasma through the intercellular spaces and drained into the lymphatic vessels.

lymphatics   The series of hollow tubes responsible for draining lymph from the periphery back into the circulation.

lymph nodes   Small round or oval structures responsible for production of cells of the immune system and for filtering lymphatic fluid.

macro-   Prefix meaning large.

malignant neoplasm   A tumour with the characteristics of growth, metastasis and invasion.

malleolus   (Latin, a little hammer) Rounded, bony protuberances found on the inner (medial) and outer (lateral) aspect of the ankles.

Mallory-Weiss tear   A partial-thickness tear of the oesophageal lining following an attempt at stopping vomiting by keeping the glottis closed, leading to a raised intraoesophageal pressure that tears the oesophagus.

mammo-   Relating to the breast.

mandible   The lower bone of the jaw.

medial   Towards the midline.

mean arterial pressure (MAP)   The mean of the systolic and diastolic blood pressure.

median   In the midline of the body.

mediastinum   (Latin, a middle partition) The middle cavity of the thorax within which the heart, the trachea (and its bifurcation), the great vessels and the oesophagus are contained.

medulla   The marrow cavity of long bones, a useful site for gaining emergency vascular access in children using an interosseous needle.

meninges   The membranes surrounding the brain substance, which become inflamed in meningitis. They comprise the pia mater, dura mater and arachnoid.

meningitis   Any infection or inflammation of the lining membranes of the brain. The condition presents with headache, photophobia, neck stiffness and vomiting.

meniscus   (Greek, a crescent) The half-moon-shaped cartilages found within the knee joint; may be damaged by sporting accidents.

mesentery   The fold of peritoneum that surrounds parts of the large and small bowel, tethering them to the posterior abdominal wall but allowing considerable mobility. May be torn by sudden deceleration injuries and result in intra-abdominal bleeding.

metabolite   The product of any form of chemical reaction or process within the body. This may refer to the production of carbon dioxide (a metabolite of respiration) or to the breakdown of drugs.

metaphysis   The junction between diaphysis and epiphysis.

metastasis   The product of a malignant tumour seeded to a site distant from the original tumour, where it multiplies.

micro-   Prefix meaning small.

micturate   Urinate.

midclavicular line   The imaginary line that runs vertically downwards from the midpoint of the clavicle.

migraine   A severe headache caused by vascular spasm. It may be heralded by visual disturbance and a prodromal feeling, and may be accompanied by vomiting and nausea.

military anti-shock trousers (MAST)   A garment for application to the legs and abdomen that may be inflated to provide autotransfusion from the lower extremities and some degree of tamponade in cases of hypovolaemic shock.

minute volume   Volume of air expired (or inspired) in 1 minute.

missed abortion   A condition where the fetus dies but is not actually expelled for 2 or more months.

mitral valve   One of the four heart valves. As such it can be afflicted by the same disease processes as the other valves and become excessively tight (stenosis) or not close properly (incompetence), each condition being accompanied by its own characteristic sounds at varying times of the heart cycle.

mono-   Prefix meaning single.

morbidity   Illness or features of a disease.

mortality   Death.

mouth-to-mouth resuscitation   A procedure to supplement inadequate ventilation or absent breathing in a patient by exhaling air into the patient's lungs via a mouth-to-mouth seal.

multigravida   Woman who has had at least two pregnancies.

multipara   Woman who has had at least two deliveries.

murmur   Sound heard with a stethoscope over the heart, indicating that one of the valves is leaking or narrowed.

myelo-   Relating to the spinal cord.

myo-   Relating to muscle.

myocardial infarction   The blockage of a coronary artery by a thrombosis leading to death of some of the tissue beyond. Also known as a heart attack or coronary artery thrombosis.

myocardium   The muscle that is unique to the heart; it contracts to pump the circulating blood.

myoglobin   Protein contained within the muscle structure. Its release into the circulation following a crush injury may result in renal failure.

myotome   A group of muscles supplied by one spinal segment.

narcotic   A drug that has pain-relieving properties and causes sleep.

nasal airway (nasopharyngeal airway)   A flexible piece of tubing designed to pass through the nose into the pharynx to maintain an airway.

nausea   The sensation often preceding vomiting.

navicular   A small bone in the forefoot, the equivalent of the scaphoid in the hand.

nebulize   To break up a drug or liquid into fine droplets in order for it to be inhaled and absorbed. Particularly useful for treating conditions of the lung such as asthma.

necrosis   The death of tissue, often due to ischaemia.

neonate   A young child between birth and 28 days old.

neoplasm   The benign or malignant new growth of tissue.

nephron   (Greek, the kidney) The basic unit of the kidney comprising the glomerulus and the renal tubule.

neurogenic shock   The condition of low blood pressure due to an injury to the spinal cord resulting in widespread dilatation of blood vessels.

neuron   The basic nerve cell of the central and peripheral nervous system. Comprises the cell nucleus and one or more processes which extend and link with other neurons via synapses.

neutropenia   The state of an abnormally low number of circulating neutrophils in the blood stream; if low enough may result in immunosuppression.

nocturia   The need to get up at night to pass urine.

normal sinus rhythm   The state of normal conduction of the electrical impulses in the heart with progression of depolarization from atria down to ventricle.

nucleus   The central part of the cell responsible for storage of DNA and regulation of the cell's activity. Also applied as a collective term to groups of nerve cells in the central nervous system with a common and integrated role.

nystagmus   Involuntary oscillations of the eye. This may be as a result of neurologic ear or eye disease. The oscillations may be in a vertical, horizontal or circular plane, or may be a combination. They may be accompanied by other features of the disease such as nausea or vomiting.

oculomotor nerve   The third cranial nerve.

oculogyric crisis   A state where the eyes are held in one position of gaze, often upwards, due most frequently to drug side-effects.

oedema   The abnormal collection of fluid around tissue and cells or within tissue spaces.

oesophagus   The muscular structure that carries food from the oropharynx to the stomach, linking the two structures.

olecranon   The bony protuberance on the posterior aspect of the elbow formed by the proximal end of the ulna.

oliguria   A reduced output of urine resulting in a failure to detoxify the blood.

omentum   A large fatty sheet derived from a fold of peritoneum within the abdomen. It may have a role in limiting the spread of inflammation within the peritoneal cavity in such illnesses as appendicitis.

oncology   The branch of medicine specializing in the study of tumours and their treatment.

oophoro-   Relating to the ovary.

open fracture   *see* Fracture.

open pneumothorax   The collapse of a lung with entry of air into the pleural space and direct communication of the pleural space with the external environment. Also known as 'sucking' chest wound.

ophthalmo-   Relating to the eye.

ophthalmoplegia   Paralysis of the oculomotor nerves. This may affect just one particular muscle (and thus lead to an inability to look in one direction) such as following a nerve injury, or be more widespread affecting all eye muscles leading to an inability to move the globe at all (for example in some neuromuscular conditions such as myasthenia gravis).

-opia   Suffix meaning vision or visual.

opiates   Morphine and related drugs which may be used for pain relief. They have a tendency to cause respiratory depression and nausea. They may be administered subcutaneously, intramuscularly or intravenously.

oral airway   A plastic or rubber device such as the Guedel airway designed to maintain an open airway in the unconscious or anaesthetized patient. Also known as an oropharyngeal airway.

orthopnoea   Severe dyspnoea that occurs when lying flat but which may be relieved by sitting upright. Often a sign of left heart failure.

orthostatic hypotension   A fall in the blood pressure that occurs when changing from a supine to a standing position.

osteo-   Relating to bone or bony.

osteoarthritis   Arthritis of any joint in which degeneration of the joint takes place. There is loss of the cartilage and the articulation of the bone on bone causes thickening and hardening of the bone (sclerosis).

osteomyelitis   Any bacterial infection of the bone, usually as a result of trauma, surgery or extension of local infection, or carried to that site by the blood stream.

osteoporosis   The thinning of bone mass seen in the elderly or immobile, also caused by certain drugs such as steroids. Common complications of this are fractures as a result of very little stress or force.

oximeter   A device that measures the saturation of the blood stream with oxygen by attaching a light transmitting and receiving probe to the skin.

oxygen   A colourless and odourless gas which is vital for cellular metabolism. In conditions of shock and respiratory deficiency its supplementation forms an important part of the therapy.

oxygen mask   A device which is strapped to the face and used for administering supplementary oxygen.

pacemaker   The sinoatrial node or other collection of specialized cells within the heart which is responsible for the initiation and maintenance of the heart rhythm. Also an artificial device which is implanted under the skin and linked to the heart in order to maintain a heart rhythm in cardiac disease. It may be set to fire only when the heart fails to initiate a beat, or set to drive the heart rhythm permanently.

packed cells   The red cells from a bag of donor blood separated from the plasma (which is used for other purposes) so that the transfusion with packed cells is of a smaller volume.

paediatrics   The branch of medicine specializing in the study and care of sick children.

pain   A sensation mediated by sensory nerve endings that is representative of tissue damage and inflammation.

palate   The dividing tissue forming the roof of the mouth separating the oral and nasal cavities. It is split into the hard (bony) palate anteriorly and soft palate posteriorly.

palpation   To examine a patient by feeling for differences in tissues.

palpitation   A sensation of racing of the heart, often associated with emotional excitement, or a premature ventricular contraction.

pancreas   A large, glandular structure lying across the posterior midline of the abdomen which provides enzymes (exocrine secretions) for digestion of food; these enzymes are secreted into the pancreatic duct which drains into the duodenum. The pancreas also produces insulin and glucagon which are secreted into the blood stream (endocrine secretions) for regulation of the blood glucose level. It may become inflamed either acutely or chronically (pancreatitis).

pancreatitis   Inflammation of the pancreas; may be acute or chronic, and may be caused by damage to the biliary tree, drugs, alcohol and certain infections. There may be severe pain and jaundice, and if chronic the decrease in enzymes produced by the pancreas may lead to malabsorption.

paracentesis   The insertion of a needle or drainage tube to drain fluid or blood from the abdominal cavity.

paradoxical breathing   Generally associated with traumatic damage to the chest, resulting in instability of the chest wall such that on inspiration the chest wall collapses in and the lung fails to expand.

paraesthesia   The sensation of 'pins and needles' or tingling in the extremities.

paralysis   An abnormal loss of muscle function due to a variety of conditions.

paralytic ileus   A lack of peristalsis in the gastrointestinal tract occurring because of a whole variety of conditions including local trauma, operations on the gut or painful conditions in the thorax or retroperitoneal space. There is retention of secretions in the bowel and therefore abdominal distension but there are no bowel sounds.

parasuicide   A deliberate act of self-harm but without the intention of committing suicide, the act of parasuicide is associated with a high probability of suicide owing to the acts often performed during the parasuicide attempt.

parity   The obstetric way of classifying a woman by the number of live births or stillbirths after 28 weeks.

Parkinson's disease   A chronic neurological disease characterized by tremor, mask-like face and rigidity of movement.

paronychia   An infection of the skin of the nail fold.

parotid   The largest of the salivary glands, lying between the posterior aspect of the mandible and the external ear canal.

patella   The bone forming the kneecap; it is a sesamoid bone (i.e. it forms within a tendon).

patent   The condition of a tubular structure being open and not blocked.

pathological fracture   The fracture of a bone secondary to the bone being weakened by disease.

$P\text{CO}_2$ The concentration of carbon dioxide within the blood stream.

pectoral   (Latin *pectus*, the breast) Relating to the breast – usually the muscles (e.g. pectoralis major).

pelvic inflammatory disease (PID)   An inflammatory condition of female pelvic organs, often a bacterial infection. There may be an offensive vaginal discharge, abdominal pain over the uterus or fallopian tube, and signs of bacterial infection such as fever.

pelvis   The lowest region of the trunk of the body, generally understood to be surrounded by the pelvic bones as its boundary (anterior, posterior and lateral). It contains female reproductive organs, bladder, coils of small bowel and the lower reaches of the colon and the rectum.

peptic ulcer   Any ulceration, normally of the stomach or small intestine, which has as a major part of its causation acid damage to the bowel mucosa. Ulcers may be aided in their formation by mucosal damage due to a variety of factors including certain drugs and bacterial infections.

perfusion   The passage of blood through a tissue at a rate adequate to supply it with the necessary nutrients and remove toxic metabolites.

peri-   Prefix meaning around.

pericardial tamponade   A collection of blood within the pericardial sac which prevents effective contraction of the heart. A cause of EMD cardiac arrest.

pericardiocentesis   The aspiration of fluid or blood from a pericardial effusion.

pericardium   The fibrous sac that surrounds the heart. Fluid collecting within this sac but outside the heart as a result of either inflammation of the sac or trauma may lead to pressure on the heart and reduction in cardiac output, and in severest cases an EMD arrest.

perineum   The area between the anal opening and the urethra perforated by the vaginal opening in the female.

peripheral vascular disease   The development of vascular damage due to calcification and fat deposition within the arterial walls in any part of the arterial supply excluding the heart's arteries. It may result in local effects to the tissues supplied by the vessels that may be noted on the use of the limb (e.g. claudication) or may present with acute loss of blood supply and gangrene.

peritoneal dialysis   The removal of toxic metabolites from the body by fluid washed in and out of the peritoneal cavity.

peritoneum   The lining membrane of the abdominal cavity, enfolding all the abdominal cavity. Organs in the abdomen may be within the peritoneal cavity or retroperitoneal (behind the peritoneal cavity): examples of the latter are the kidneys and pancreas.

peritonitis   Inflammation of the abdominal cavity due to bacterial, chemical or other causes. Commonest causes include appendicitis, perforation of an ulcer or perforation of a large bowel diverticulum.

petit mal Momentary loss of concentration and awareness but with no motor symptoms. This form of epilepsy is seen in children.

pH The measure of acid and base balance within the body. It is a measure of the concentration of the hydrogen ions present in the blood (the log of the reciprocal of the hydrogen ion concentration). Normal body pH is 7.4. In cases of acidosis (metabolic or respiratory) the pH falls. In alkalotic conditions (metabolic or respiratory alkalosis) the pH rises.

pharynx The throat. It is divided into the nasal cavity (nasopharynx), the oral cavity (oropharynx) and the larynx (laryngopharynx).

phlebitis Inflammation of the veins, often accompanied by a clot within that segment of vein (thrombophlebitis). This may affect the superficial veins or the deep veins (deep venous thrombosis, DVT).

phlebo- Relating to veins.

phrenic nerve The nerve supplying the diaphragm (motor and sensory).

pituitary gland A small gland attached to the hypothalamus in the brain. It secretes a number of hormones vital to normal functioning including adrenocorticotrophic hormone, thyroid stimulating hormone and follicle stimulating hormone.

placenta The fetal organ through which the fetus absorbs nutrients and oxygen from the mother and excretes its waste products.

placenta praevia An abnormal position of the placenta such that it occludes the exit of the uterus. If labour commences it may cause a dramatic and exsanguinating haemorrhage.

plantar Relating to the sole of the foot.

plasma The watery solution of salts and proteins that suspends the cellular components of the blood.

plasma expander A substance given intravenously that is used to expand the plasma volume or increase the oncotic pressure.

pleura The lining tissue that coats the inside of the thoracic cavity, the mediastinal contents and the lungs, allowing movement of the lungs relative to the thoracic cavity.

pleuritic pain Chest pain worse on coughing or deep breathing, representative of pleural inflammation.

pneumatic anti-shock garment *see* Military anti-shock trousers (MAST).

pneumonia Acute infection of the lungs: often refers to bacterial infection although pneumonia may well be due to viral or other organisms.

pneumonitis Acute inflammation of the lungs: may be due to viral infection, hypersensitivity to dust or allergens, or chemical contamination of the lung.

pneumothorax A collection of air within the pleural space leading to collapse of the lung. This may be caused by a spontaneous leak from the lung or from perforation of the thoracic wall, e.g. in stabbing. When a leak exists with a 'one-way valve' effect the pressure of the pneumothorax may increase, leading to distortion of the mediastinum, decreased venous return and collapse: this is known as a tension pneumothorax.

Po$_2$ The concentration of oxygen within the blood stream.

podo- Relating to the foot.

poisoning The absorption in some manner of a substance that has toxic effects on the body.

polydipsia Excessive drinking; this may indicate a variety of pathologies including diabetes mellitus.

polymorphonuclear leucocyte A white blood cell with a lobulated nucleus.

popliteal fossa The fossa found at the back of the knee through which in its depths the major vascular and nervous tissues run to the calf and foot.

portal hypertension An increase in the venous pressure within the portal vein, resulting in spleen enlargement and oesophageal varices among other effects.

postero- Prefix meaning back.

post-ictal Relating to the state seen after a grand mal seizure.

pre- Prefix meaning in front of.

precordium The area over the front of the heart. In some resuscitation protocols the area that should be hit in a precordial thump.

pre-eclampsia An abnormal condition associated with pregnancy of hypertension and limb swelling, preceding eclampsia.

pre-load The pressure that causes ventricular filling.

premature Description of an infant born before 37 weeks of gestation.

presenting part The first part of the baby to be delivered.

priapism Persistent penile erection usually secondary to spinal cord injury.

pro- Prefix meaning before.

proctitis An inflammation of the rectum and anus; may be due to local trauma, drug administration or a variety of disease processes, and may be acute or chronic.

procto- Pertaining to the rectum or rectal.

proprioception The perception of the position in space of the body and limbs.

prostate A small gland in the male urogenital tract responsible for the addition of certain key secretions to semen. In elderly men it may enlarge as a result of either benign or malignant change causing a decrease in urinary stream and eventual urinary retention.

prostatectomy The surgical removal or partial removal of the prostate gland. This may be by either an open approach through the abdominal wall or an endoscopic approach via the urethra.

proteinuria   The presence of unusually high quantities of protein in the urine; this may signify renal tract disease or renal involvement secondary to some other disease, for example diabetes mellitus.

proximal   Usually referring to a point on a limb which is closer to the trunk than another point, e.g. the elbow is more proximal than the fingers.

psychiatrist   A doctor who specializes in psychiatry.

psychiatry   The study and treatment of mental illness.

psychosis   An extreme form of behavioural disturbance, whether organic or mental in origin, normally requiring hospitalization for its treatment and characterized by severe changes in the behaviour of an individual.

PTCA   percutaneous transluminal coronary angioplasty: an effective form of treating coronary artery disease where a small catheter is inserted through a small opening in a major artery and threaded into the coronary arteries. At the site of narrowings in the artery a small balloon can be inflated to stretch the constriction, allowing greater blood flow to the tissues of the heart.

pubis   One of the three paired bones (including the ischium and ilium) that constitute the pelvis.

puerperium   The period during which the reproductive organs return to their pre-pregnant condition – usually regarded as an interval of 6 weeks after delivery.

pulmo-   Relating to the lung.

pulmonary   Pertaining to the lungs and respiratory system.

pulmonary embolism (PE)   The obstruction of a pulmonary artery, most commonly by a blood clot, though fat, air or amniotic fluid may also cause obstruction. It may present with chest pain, shortness of breath, cyanosis, tachycardia and shock.

pulmonary oedema   The accumulation of excess fluid, firstly within the interstitial tissues of the lung and in severe cases within the actual alveoli of the lungs. Most commonly caused by congestive cardiac failure, though also associated with other acute conditions such as following acute head injury, near drowning, and following inhalation injuries.

pulmonary vein   One of two blood vessels that transmit oxygenated blood from the lungs back to the left side of the heart.

pulse   the expansion and contraction of an artery as a result of the intermittent flow of arterial blood; can be detected by palpation or other means.

pulse pressure   The difference between the systolic and diastolic blood pressure. A reduction in the pulse pressure as a result of an increase in the diastolic pressure may be one of the first and subtle signs of shock.

pus   A thick, creamy liquid of varying colour, a result of tissue or bacterial necrosis. Its main constituent is the polymorphonuclear white cell.

P wave   The upward deflection on an ECG preceding the QRS complex and representing atrial depolarization.

pyloric stenosis   Obstruction of the outflow tract of the stomach, resulting in a reduction of flow of food to the small bowel. This presents with vomiting which may be enough to cause systemic alkalosis.

pyrexia   *see* Fever.

QRS   The complex of electrical activity seen on an ECG that represents ventricular depolarization.

quadri-   Prefix meaning four.

quadriceps   The group of four muscles that comprise the front (anterior) part of the thigh.

quadriplegia   The condition of paralysis of all four limbs, normally below the level of a spinal cord injury.

radial pulse   The pulse of the radial artery which can be felt in the wrist; because of the ease with which it can be felt, it is the most frequently palpated.

radiograph   An X-ray image.

radiotherapy   The branch of medicine concerned with the treatment of disease using ionizing radiation.

rebound tenderness   The pain felt on sudden release of a hand palpating the abdomen. It is seen in conditions of inflammation of the peritoneum.

rectum   The terminal portion of the large bowel where faeces are stored prior to evacuation.

reduce   Surgical term used to describe the manipulation of tissues back into their original position after they have been moved abnormally. Particularly refers to fractured bones being brought back into alignment.

referred pain   Pain felt at one site but caused by disease or illness at another anatomical site, e.g. hip disease may present with knee pain.

regional anaesthesia   Loss of feeling in an area of the body by injection of local anaesthetic solution around the sensory nerves supplying that area.

renal failure   Failure of the kidneys to perform their normal function of waste product filtration, concentration and excretion. This may be a manifestation of disease affecting only the kidney, or may reflect the kidneys' involvement by other disease.

reno-   Relating to the kidney.

reservoir bag   A component in anaesthetic or resuscitative apparatus that is used as a store for ventilatory gases between ventilatory cycles.

respiration   1) The process of inhaling oxygen-rich atmospheric air and exhaling carbon dioxide-enriched air. This may be affected pathologically by central factors such as in Cheyne–Stokes respiration or by the degree of acidosis or alkalosis within the blood stream. 2) At a cellular level, the process of cellular exchange of oxygen as a fuel, metabolizing it into carbon dioxide and excreting it.

respiratory acidosis   The condition of increased carbon dioxide and carbonic acid (thus an increased hydrogen ion concentration) due to failure of excretion of carbon dioxide by the lungs. This may be due to suppression of the respiratory centre in the brain (head injury, drugs, etc.) or lung disease.

respiratory alkalosis A condition characterized by a decrease in the concentration of carbon dioxide in the blood stream. Like respiratory acidosis it may be caused by lung disease, through hyperventilation and excess excretion of carbon dioxide (e.g. asthma or pneumonia). Other causes may include drugs and a variety of medical conditions.

respiratory arrest A sudden cessation of respiration which if not corrected by artificial respiration may progress to cardiorespiratory arrest.

respiratory centre A group of neurons in the brain that control the rate of respiration in response to the circulating levels of oxygen, carbon dioxide and hydrogen ions.

respiratory rate The number of breaths taken per minute. Normally this is between 12 and 15. Slower rates may be due to drugs or head injury. Higher rates may be due to a range of acute medical conditions, pain or anxiety.

respiratory tract infection Any infection (bacterial, viral or with any other organism) that is harboured within the upper or lower respiratory tract.

retained placenta The retention of all or part of the placenta following delivery.

retina The light-absorbing surface within the eyeball.

retinopathy The degeneration of the retina, seen particularly in diabetic patients, which may be complicated by the occurrence of haemorrhage and visual loss.

retro- Prefix meaning behind.

retrograde A movement in the opposite direction to that considered normal.

retroperitoneum The potential space lying behind the peritoneum in which the retroperitoneal organs may be found (e.g. the pancreas and kidneys).

Reyes' syndrome An acute condition characterized by disturbed liver and brain function. Viral illness and aspirin have been implicated as causative agents.

rheumatoid arthritis A chronic and destructive inflammatory disease particularly characterized by swelling of the synovium of the joints and joint swelling. It may have an autoimmune element to it.

rhino- Relating to the nose.

rhinorrhoea The passage of cerebrospinal fluid from the nose following a head injury.

right heart failure A condition characterized by impairment of the right ventricle and a subsequent increase in the systemic veins and capillaries.

rule of nines An approximate formula that may be used to calculate the surface area of a body affected by thermal injury; 9% is allocated to each arm and the head; 18% (2 × 9) to each leg and the front and back of the trunk; and 1% to the perineum.

sacrum The penultimate segment of the lower spine. It lies between the two hip bones, articulating with them via the sacroiliac joints.

sagittal Anatomical term describing the plane that runs from the front to the back of a body.

salpinx (Greek, a tube) Any tube, though normally used to describe the tubes leading between the ovary and the womb in a female.

scaphoid bone One of the small bones of the wrist. May be broken and then fail to unite properly, leading to chronic disability; this is related to the blood supply of the bone which enters from the far end and may be disrupted by the fracture.

scapula The bone forming the shoulder blade.

sciatica The presence of leg pain often with back pain due to a prolapse of an intervertebral disc which through either direct pressure or other mechanisms leads to irritation of the nerve roots to the lower limbs.

segmental fracture A fracture where the bone breaks into more than one large fragment.

semi- Prefix meaning half.

septic arthritis The bacterial infection of a joint, normally by haematogenous spread or direct contamination of the joint, presenting with acute pain, swollen joint and fever as the main constituents.

septic shock A form of shock secondary to the release of toxins from certain bacteria when they infect a patient. These cause decrease in the vascular resistance and a drop in blood pressure. Fever, an increased respiratory rate and confusion may also be features.

serum The thin clear fluid that is left behind after blood has clotted or after plasma has been allowed to form a clot.

shock Reduced perfusion of tissues inadequate to maintain their metabolic rate and oxygenation. It may have many causes, which fall into five main groups: septic, cardiogenic, spinal, hypovolaemic and anaphylactic.

sickle cell anaemia A severe, chronic inherited condition, characterized by low haemoglobin levels as a result of an abnormal haemoglobin (Hb-S) within the red cell. The abnormality predisposes to fragile red blood cells which break down or distort blocking capillary flow and lead to painful infarcted areas. This occurs sporadically, and such blockages are known as crises.

sick sinus syndrome The presentation of a variety of cardiac diseases with a combination of varying cardiac arrhythmias, all of which contain some kind of bradycardia (this may be alternated with tachycardia or atrioventricular block).

sigmoid S-shaped; applies to any S-shaped bodily curve, in particular the terminal part of the colon before it joins the rectum.

sigmoidoscopy The inspection of the rectum and sigmoid colon with a sigmoidoscope.

sinus arrhythmia The slight variation in pulse rate caused by breathing changing the resting parasympathetic tone.

sinus bradycardia Sinus rhythm less than 60 beats per minute.

sinus tachycardia Sinus rhythm greater than 100 beats per minute.

skin traction   A method for attaching bandage or material (either adhesive or non-adhesive) to the skin of a limb in order to apply a corrective force reducing a fracture or orthopaedic deformity.

sphincter   (Greek, a tight binder) A controlling band of muscle surrounding a hollow, tubular structure such as the gut or urinary tract.

sphygmomanometer   A device for measuring the arterial blood pressure.

spinal cord injury   Traumatic damage of the spinal cord. The results depend on the level of the cord that the injury occurs at and the severity of the cord damage. Cord damage below C5 and above T1 is associated with quadriplegia, while damage below T1 produces paraplegia. The effects depend on the severity of the damage and may range from temporary to permanent. Transection of the cord is associated with spinal shock characterized by warm peripheries, low blood pressure and absence of sensation and movement below the level of the injury.

spine   The collective term for the group of bones which articulate together to form the backbone.

splanchnic   (Greek *splanchnos,* an entrail) Relating to the viscera.

spleen   A vascular organ in the upper left quadrant of the abdomen. Its role is primarily producing cells for the lymphoreticular system. Traumatic damage may result in severe haemorrhage owing to its vascular nature.

spleno-   Relating to the spleen.

splint   Any device that may be used to immobilize an injured part of the body.

spondylo-   Relating to the vertebrae.

spontaneous abortion   The expulsion of the fetus and placenta before the 24th week of gestation.

sputum   The products coughed up from the lung. These may be expectorated into a specimen container to gather a sputum sample.

Staphylococcus aureus   A natural bacterial inhabitant of the skin which may infect open wounds or may cause infection of internal organs if it enters the blood stream.

status asthmaticus   A particularly severe and prolonged asthma attack.

status epilepticus   A prolonged and continuous epileptic fit with no regaining of consciousness between the seizures.

stenosis   An abnormal narrowing of a tubular structure. This term may be used in relation to the gut, blood vessels or bony canals such as the spinal column.

sternum   The breastbone.

stillbirth   The delivery after the 24th week of gestation of a baby showing no spontaneous signs of life at delivery.

stoma   Literally, a pore or orifice on the surface. Generally refers to the artificial surgical creation of a communication between an internal organ and the skin.

strangulation   The constriction of a tubular structure within the body preventing effective function.

stroke   A sudden onset of neurological deficit corresponding to an area supplied by a cerebral vessel, normally caused by obstruction of the vessel and loss of blood supply.

sub-   Prefix meaning under.

subacute bacterial endocarditis   A chronic bacterial infection of the heart valves presenting with fever and heart murmur.

subarachnoid haemorrhage   The presence of blood within the subarachnoid space. This may be due to the rupture of a small aneurysm of the arteries of the brain with resultant leakage of blood into the space.

subcutaneous emphysema   The presence of free gas within the subcutaneous tissues. The gas originates from airway or alveolar damage and tracks through the soft tissues to the subcutaneous plane.

supination   The movement of a limb or body towards the supine position, i.e. flat on the back with hands in a palms upward position.

supra-   Prefix meaning above.

suprarenal   Above the kidney.

supraventricular tachycardia   An abnormal tachycardia that can be identified as originating from a focus above the ventricles, but more precise identification of the focus of origin may not be possible.

sural   Relating to the calf or leg. The sural nerve supplies part of the lower limb with sensation.

surgical emphysema   The presence of gas in the subcutaneous or deep tissues of the body that has been forced there due to a leak of air from the lungs (rarely the gut). It may indicate the presence of a penetrating neck wound or a pneumothorax, for example.

suture   A material used to join surgical wounds or damaged tissues.

syndrome   A collection of symptoms or clinical signs that are recognized to exist together in certain disease states.

synovial   Relating to synovia, the fluid secreted by the synovial membranes which lubricates joints and tendon sheaths.

systole   The part of the cardiac cycle in which the heart contracts and blood is expelled into the aorta.

tachycardia   An abnormally fast pulse rate, generally defined as a pulse rate above 100 beats per minute.

talus   (Latin, ankle) The small bone that fits into the mortice formed by the tibia and fibula at the ankle joint.

tendon   The connective tissue that joins muscle to bone.

tension pneumothorax   *see* Pneumothorax.

term   Pregnancy from 37 weeks up to 42 weeks.

tetanus   A potentially fatal infection affecting the central nervous system, caused by the release of a toxin from the bacterium *Clostridium tetani.* The bacterium is a common inhabitant of the soil and a normal commensal of the gastrointestinal tract of cows and horses, and infects wounds that contain dead tissue. The disease consists of fever, headache and muscular spasm, eventually affecting all the muscles of the body.

tetanus immunoglobulin an effective injectable antibody originating from humans immune to the tetanus toxin and used in the treatment of tetanus and protection following possible exposure.

tetanus toxoid The material used for conferring active immunity to tetanus by production of an antigenic response within the body.

tetany A state of cramps, muscular twitching and (at its worst) convulsions. It is due to an abnormality of calcium metabolism.

thenar Relating to the palm of the hand. The hypothenar eminence is the small group of muscles over the little finger side of the palm and the thenar eminence is the group of muscles at the base of the thumb.

thermoregulation The natural physiological ability to maintain heat production and loss.

thoraco- Relating to the chest.

thoracostomy The formation of a hole in the thoracic wall to enable the passage of a chest drain. In the emergency setting this may be performed by the insertion of a needle (needle thoracocentesis).

thoracotomy The surgical incision and opening of the thoracic cavity.

thorax, thoracic cage The upper body cavity containing the principal organs of respiration and circulation. Bounded by the sternum at the front, the thoracic vertebrae at the back and the ribs around the sides.

thready pulse A pulse that is weak or difficult to feel; may be related to a small pulse volume secondary to shock.

threatened abortion Uterine bleeding and abdominal cramps suggestive of a miscarriage occurring before 24 weeks of gestation.

thrill A palpable disturbance indicating underlying disease of either blood vessel or heart.

thrombocytopenia An abnormally low level of platelets circulating in the blood. This may present as a tendency to bleed, particularly from small cuts or into the subcutaneous tissues.

thromboembolism The blockage of a blood vessel by an embolus which has been carried within the vessel from upstream. This may result in an ischaemic periphery in the region normally supplied by the vessel, or in the event of a pulmonary embolus, chest pain, cough and tachycardia.

thrombolytic The dissolving of a thrombus; the term is normally used to refer to drugs that cause breakdown of an established clot.

thrombophlebitis The inflammation of a vein, often accompanied by formation of clot within the vein wall. In deep venous thrombi this may be indicated by calf pain and swelling.

thrombus The collective constituents of a blood clot (fibrin, red blood cells, white blood cells, clotting factors, etc.) adherent to a blood vessel wall; thus it is possible to have an arterial or a venous thrombosis.

thrush Candidal infection of tissues, usually the mouth, vulva or gastrointestinal tract.

thyroid (Greek *thyroeides*, like a shield) The small gland found in the neck, consisting of two lobes joined in the middle (the isthmus), responsible for secreting a mixture of hormones which control and influence the metabolic rate and growth. It may be overactive or underactive in disease states.

thyroid function test Biochemical tests used to assess the activity of the thyroid gland.

tibia The main weightbearing bone of the lower limb below the knee joint.

tidal volume The volume of air breathed in and out during normal respiration.

tinnitus Ringing heard in one or both ears; it may be associated with acoustic trauma or as a feature of disease such as Ménière's disease.

tonsil A small quantity of lymphoid tissue found in the oropharynx, commonly inflamed in the condition of tonsillitis.

torsades des pointes A form of ventricular tachycardia.

torsion fracture A spinal fracture, usually the result of a twisting injury.

total joint replacement Surgical treatment of severe arthritis of joints such as the hip, knee, elbow and shoulder.

total peripheral resistance The overall peripheral resistance to blood flow caused by the constricting effects of the peripheral vessels.

toxicity The results of exposure to a toxin which in smaller quantities gives rise to no such effects.

toxin A substance which may act as a poison.

trachea The main air passage connecting the lungs to the oropharynx and nasopharynx.

tracheostomy The surgical creation of an artificial airway by incising the trachea. This may be performed to aid long-term ventilation on an intensive care unit or as an emergency to circumvent an airway problem.

traction The placement of a limb or body part under tension; often used in orthopaedics to correct deformity, realign broken bones and as a temporary method of pain relief at a fracture site.

trans- Prefix meaning across or over.

transfusion The replacement of lost blood with stored blood. This is most commonly from an unrelated donor and as such the blood requires cross-matching prior to transfusion. Occasionally in routine surgery the blood may be given by the patient in advance of the operation and stored until the procedure.

transfusion reaction The response of the body to a transfusion of unmatched and incompatible blood. Fever, bronchoconstriction and renal failure may result. At its worst profound shock may develop.

transient ischaemic attack The occlusion or partial occlusion of a cerebral vessel, with symptoms related to the area supplied by that vessel (often called a 'mini-stroke');

symptoms resolve within 24 hours or else they are classed as a stroke. Often the eyes are affected, with disturbance of vision.

transplant The movement of tissue from one anatomical site to another, or from one (donor) individual to another individual (recipient). In the case of the movement from one individual to another they require to be as closely matched as possible with regard to blood groups and immunological typing.

transverse At right angles to the long axis of the body (this plane is also at right angles to the coronal and sagittal planes).

transverse lie An abnormal presentation of the fetus within the uterus.

tri- Prefix meaning three.

triage The classification and sorting of casualties into groups based on the severity of injury and chance of survival. Successful triage aims to do the most for the most, even if resources are limited.

triceps The large muscle on the posterior aspect of the upper arm whose main action is to straighten the arm at the elbow.

trimester One of the three periods that pregnancy is divided into.

truss A belt or device used to prevent the passage of abdominal contents into a hernia.

tubal pregnancy An ectopic pregnancy where the embryo implants into the uterine tube; this may be predisposed to by previous uterine infection or injury.

tuberculosis (TB) A chronic disease caused by infection with the bacterium *Mycobacterium tuberculosis*. Histologically this is characterized by granulomatous areas in the tissues. Primarily the lung is affected, though infection may spread from the lung to other tissues.

tumour A swelling or enlargement of tissues, which may be a result of local inflammation or a new growth. The latter may be a benign or malignant neoplasm.

ulcerative colitis Chronic inflammatory disease of the large bowel: a relapsing and remitting disorder. During attacks there is diarrhoea with blood, pus and mucus. There is a higher than average risk of developing carcinoma of the large bowel in the long term.

ulna The long bone of the forearm that runs on the inner aspect of the forearm from the elbow to the wrist. At the elbow it forms the olecranon.

ultrasound High-frequency sound waves (> 20,000 Hz). There are numerous applications in medicine, from imaging to physiotherapy treatment.

umbilical cord The flexible link between the fetus and the maternal circulation (via the placenta).

umbilicus (Latin, the navel) The site of the junction of the umbilical cord in the newborn with the abdominal wall.

unconsciousness The inability to sense and respond to external stimuli, due to a variety of causes.

undisplaced fracture A fracture which although completely across the cortices has failed to displace away from the anatomical position of the bone.

uni- Prefix meaning one.

universal donor The blood group O Rh negative which can be given to almost any individual with minimal risk of a transfusion reaction in the event of an emergency.

ureter The muscular tubes responsible for passage of urine from each kidney into the bladder. They originate from the continuation of the renal pelvis and terminate by passing obliquely through the bladder wall, forming a one-way valve into the bladder.

urethra The terminal passage from the bladder for voiding of urine. In females it is a short tube that lies anterior to the vagina; in males it is about 20 cm long and passes through the middle of the prostate before running the length of the penis to the external meatus.

urinary retention The inability to pass urine; in the male, it may well be preceded by the symptoms of frequency, poor stream, nocturia and dribbling.

urology The branch of medicine concerned with the study, treatment and surgery of disorders of the urinary tract.

vaccination The injection of organisms attenuated so that they cannot cause disease but are capable of stimulating a body reaction and active immunity.

vagus A nerve lying next to the carotid artery on either side of the neck. Its sensory fibres are wide-ranging and supply sensation to the thoracic viscera and motor supply to the gut from the soft palate to the splenic flexure of the colon.

valgus The abnormal deformity of a joint away from the midline.

Valsalva manoeuvre Breathing out against a closed glottis to increase intrathoracic pressure. This may be used as a method for testing the physiological mechanisms that control the blood pressure.

valvular heart disease Congenital or acquired disease of heart valves; may take the form of stenosis of the valve or incompetence. Features may include cardiac failure, arrhythmia and more chronic features such as weight loss and anorexia.

varicose veins Abnormally tortuous and dilated veins. Although occurring in other anatomical locations they are most common in the legs.

varus The abnormal deformity of a joint towards the midline.

vascular insufficiency The inadequate flow of blood through a periphery owing to stenosis of the vessels by arteriosclerosis. Symptoms may consist of pain on use of the limb (e.g. intermittent claudication), and in severe disease the skin may have reduced capillary return and be pale.

vaso- Relating to a vessel.

vasoconstriction The narrowing of the blood vessels, particularly the arterioles and veins. This may be accomplished by a variety of stimuli and is useful in the response to shock or to control blood pressure.

vasodilatation The widening of the various small vessels (see vasoconstriction) brought about by relaxation of the smooth muscle in the walls of the vessels.

vasovagal attack Loss of consciousness due to a sudden decrease in blood pressure following bradycardia, decrease in cardiac output and vasodilatation, causing cerebral ischaemia. This may be triggered by a variety of stimuli, including pain or fright.

ventilation The process of exchanging gases from within the lung to the atmosphere.

ventilator A device that may be used either to provide ventilatory support or to perform complete ventilation.

ventricular fibrillation A cardiac dysrhythmia with rapid and disorganized depolarization of the whole ventricle resulting in no effective organized electrical signal and no cardiac output. Unless CPR and subsequent defibrillation take place, death occurs.

ventricular tachycardia A cardiac dysrhythmia originating normally from the Purkinje fibres of the ventricle.

Venturi mask A mask that is designed to mix atmospheric air with oxygen to create fixed oxygen concentrations.

vertebra One of the constituent bones of the spinal column. It may be a cervical, thoracic, lumbar, sacral or coccygeal vertebra.

virus A micro-organism smaller than a bacterium that may only replicate by infecting another organism. The key constituent is a core of DNA or RNA which provides the information necessary for replication.

visceral Relating to any internal organ in a body cavity. Though often referring to organs of the abdominal cavity it can also refer to those of the thoracic cavity.

vital capacity The maximum amount of air that can be expelled slowly after full inspiration.

vital signs The pulse rate, blood pressure, respiratory rate and temperature.

volume expander Any form of intravenous fluid that stays within the intravascular space, expanding it (normally refers to colloid, though blood is also classified as a volume expander).

volvulus A twist of the bowel upon itself causing intestinal obstruction.

Weil's disease (leptospirosis) An infectious disease caused by the organism *Leptospira icterohaemorrhagiae*. Most commonly caught from contaminated water, clinical features include jaundice, haemorrhages, kidney and liver failure.

wheeze A whistling sound produced by bronchoconstriction.

whiplash injury Forced flexion extension injury of the neck often seen following a road traffic accident.

xiphoid The lower part of the sternal bone, generally cartilaginous in nature. It may be used as an anatomical reference point to decide where to place the hands for CPR.

X-ray A form of electromagnetic radiation that penetrates soft tissues more than bone and therefore can be used in conjunction with an appropriate film to show structures of the body.

zygoma An extension of the temporal bone of the head which forms the prominence of the cheek.

GLOSSARY OF OBSTETRIC TERMS

abortion The process by which the products of conception are expelled from the uterus via the birth canal before the 24th week of gestation.

accoucheur Deliverer of babies, midwife (originally male).

abruptio placentae (accidental haemorrhage): Bleeding from a normally situated placenta causing its complete or partial detachment after the 24th week of gestation. The diagnosis is confirmed by the demonstration of an old retroplacental clot after delivery.

antepartum haemorrhage Bleeding from the birth canal in excess of 15 ml in the period from the 24th week of gestation to the birth of the baby.

Apgar score A numerical scoring system usually applied at 1 minute and 5 minutes after birth to evaluate the condition of the baby, based on the heart rate, respiration, muscle tone, reflexes and colour.

bradycardia Fetal heart rate below 120 beats per minute.

Brandt–Andrews method Method of delivery of the placenta from the uterus: controlled cord traction is applied with one hand while the contracted uterus is pushed upwards away from the placenta with the other hand on the mother's abdomen.

Braxton Hicks contractions Spontaneous, painless uterine contractions described originally as a sign of pregnancy. Occur from the first trimester onward, and probably promote uterine blood flow and transfer of oxygen to the fetus.

breech presentation
  Complete: the fetus is flexed and buttocks, genitalia and the feet present;
  Incomplete: (frank breech) the legs are extended and buttocks and genitalia present;
  Footling: one or both feet present; there is a 10% risk of cord prolapse.

caesarean section Surgical removal of the uterine contents by the abdominal route after fetal viability (24 weeks).

cord presentation The cord is below the presenting part with the membranes intact.

cord prolapse As for cord presentation, except that the membranes have ruptured, and pressure on the umbilical cord vessels is more likely to occur.

corpus luteum The yellowish body formed from the graafian follicle after ovulation which produces oestrogen and progesterone.

crowning of the head Visualization of the fetal head as birth becomes imminent. The widest diameter has passed the bony pelvic outlet and emerged from under the pubic arch.

delay in the second stage of labour More than 1 hour in a nullipara, or 30 minutes in a multipara.

delivery The process of expulsion of the fetus at the time of birth.

dystocia Difficult or abnormal labour due to cephalopelvic disproportion, or a primary disorder of uterine action.

eclampsia (Greek *eklampein*, to flash forth) A clinical state characterized by convulsions, not attributable to cerebral conditions such as epilepsy or cerebral haemorrhage, and usually superimposed on preceding severe pre-eclampsia.

ectopic pregnancy Implantation of the fertilized ovum outside the uterine cavity. The most common site is the fallopian tube.

effacement of cervix Thinning of the muscle of the cervix with shortening of the cervical canal prior to delivery.

embryo The name given to the conceptus up to the 10th week of gestation (8th week post-conception); after which the word fetus is used.

endometrium The mucous membrane lining the uterus which responds to ovarian hormones during the menstrual cycle.

engagement The fetal head is engaged when its maximum diameters have passed the pelvic inlet.

engorgement of breasts Full, red, hard, sore breasts due to increased blood flow before milk secretion commences.

episiotomy An incision of perineum and vagina that enlarges the introitus and lessens the curve of the birth canal.

ergometrine The active oxytocic principle derived from ergot.

face The area of fetal head below the root of the nose and the orbital ridges.

fertilization The union of one sperm and the mature ovum; usually occurs in the outer half of the fallopian tube.

fourchette The fold of skin formed by merging of the labia minora and labia majora posteriorly.

generalized oedema Excessive accumulation of fluid in the tissues demonstrated by the swelling of the legs, hands and face; one of the definitive signs of pre-eclampsia.

grand multipara Para 4 or more; a patient likely to have powerful uterine contractions – hence the risk of uterine rupture if there is cephalopelvic disproportion.

gravid Pregnant; a primigravida is a woman pregnant for the first time.

hyperemesis gravidarum Vomiting during pregnancy sufficient to warrant admission of the patient to hospital.

hypertension A blood pressure of 140/90 mmHg or above, or a rise of 15–20 mmHg systolic and 10–15 mmHg diastolic. Essential hypertension is diagnosed when hypertension is known to be present before or during early pregnancy.

implantation Penetration of the endometrium by the early fertilized ovum (blastocyst) which becomes completely surrounded by decidua. Occurs 6–8 days after ovulation.

introitus Entrance to the vagina.

inversion of the uterus Uterus turned inside out, usually due to pulling on the cord with the uterus relaxed.

labour The process by which the products of conception are expelled from the uterus via the birth canal after the 24th week of gestation.

Left lateral position The preferred position for rest in bed in late pregnancy; when a patient turns from the supine position to her right side, cardiac output increases 10%; from supine to her left side, the increase is 20%.

lie of the fetus Relationship of the long axis of the fetus to the long axis of the uterus. Usually longitudinal, but can be transverse or oblique.

lightening Usually occurs after 36 weeks and is commoner in nulliparas; the presenting part enters the pelvis, and thus reduces the pressure on the diaphragm; the mother notices that it is easier to breathe. Lightening is not synonymous with engagement; often 3–4 cm of the head remains palpable abdominally.

lochia The discharge from the uterus during the puerperium; it is initially red (lochia rubra), then yellow (serosa), and finally white (alba).

Lovset manoeuvre Rotation and traction of the fetal trunk during breech birth to facilitate delivery of the arms and shoulders.

lower uterine segment The thin, expanded lower portion of the uterus which forms from the isthmus in the last trimester of pregnancy; it provides the usual method of approach to the baby in the operation of caesarean section.

manual removal of the placenta Removal of the placenta by means of a hand inside the uterus; it is performed when other methods fail.

maternal death Death occurring during pregnancy, childbirth or in the first year following birth or abortion, from any cause related to or aggravated by the pregnancy or its management. The maternal mortality rate ranges from 10 to 40 per 100,000 births in developed countries.

meconium Greenish-black, fetal faeces composed of cellular debris, bile, lanugo and vernix caseosa.

moulding Alteration in shape and diameters of the fetal head during labour. The fontanelles and sutures permit the force of contractions to compress the head against the bony pelvis and adapt its shape to that of the birth canal.

multigravida A woman who is pregnant for the second or subsequent time.

neonatal death A liveborn infant who dies within 28 days of birth.

normal labour A labour in which the fetus presents by the vertex, the occiput rotates anteriorly, and the result is the birth of a living, mature fetus with no complications, the duration of labour ranging from 4–24 hours.

occiput The back of the fetal head behind the posterior fontanelle.

operculum The plug of mucus that occludes the cervical canal during pregnancy.

ovulation Extrusion of the ripened ovum from the graafian follicle in the ovary to the peritoneal cavity (and then into the tube).

oxytocic An agent that hastens the birth of the fetus and/or placenta by stimulating contractions of the uterine muscle; by definition may accelerate first, second or third stages of labour.

parous Having delivered a viable (28 weeks or more) child. A nullipara is a woman who has never reached 28 weeks in a previous pregnancy, although she may have been pregnant more than once (multigravida).

perineal body A triangular wedge of tissue based on the perineum, separating the lower third of the posterior vaginal wall from the anal canal.

period of gestation The number of completed weeks from the first day of the last menstrual period to the date in question.

placenta The organ of communication (nutrition and products of metabolism) between the fetus and the mother. Forms from the chorion frondosum with a maternal decidual contribution.

positive signs of pregnancy Signs that are infallible: fetal heart sounds, palpable fetal parts or movements, X-ray and tests for the presence of chorionic gonadotrophic hormone in the urine or blood.

post-partum haemorrhage
Primary – blood loss in excess of 500 ml from the birth canal during the third stage, and for 24 hours afterwards;

Secondary – bleeding occurring in the interval from 24 hours after delivery until the end of the puerperium.

precipitate labour   Labour of less than 4 hours duration.

pre-eclampsia   Diagnosed when any two of the following signs are present: hypertension (140/90 mmHg or above), generalized oedema, and proteinuria not due to infection or contamination of the urine. Also called proteinuria-hypertension syndrome of pregnancy.

premature infant   One born before 37 completed weeks of gestation, i.e. 259 days (previously, one weighing less than 2,500 g). The incidence of prematurity is 8% and it accounts for 80% of all neonatal deaths.

premature rupture of the membranes   Spontaneous rupture of the membranes before the onset of contractions; usually the membranes rupture at the end of the first stage of labour (this flushes the vagina with sterile fluid before the fetus is born).

presenting part   The part of the fetus felt on vaginal examination.

prolapsed cord   An obstetric emergency where the umbilical cord is delivered before any part of the baby.

proliferative phase of menstrual cycle   The interval after menstruation and up to ovulation during which growth of the endometrium is stimulated by oestrogen from the developing graafian follicle.

prolonged labour   Labour of more than 24 hours duration.

puerperal infection   An infection of the genital tract arising as a complication of childbirth.

puerperium   The period during which the reproductive organs return to their pre-pregnant condition – usually regarded as an interval of 6 weeks after delivery.

quickening   When the patient becomes aware of fetal movements; add 5 calendar months (22 weeks) to calculate the due date.

respiratory distress syndrome in the newborn   Diagnosed in any infant who develops a respiratory rate above 60 per minute, has difficulties in breathing as shown by retraction of the sternum and lower costal margin, has an expiratory grunt and central cyanosis. The incidence is about 3% of neonates, and the mortality is about 20%.

restitution   When the fetal head is born, it is free to undo any twisting caused by internal rotation.

retraction   The quality of uterine muscle whereby permanent shortening occurs after contractions in labour. The uterine fundus thickens and pulls up the dilating cervix like a hood over the presenting part.

rotation of the head

Internal – the occiput rotates to the anterior position, rarely (1–2%) posterior;

External – the head rotates after it is born because the shoulders are turning into the anteroposterior diameter of the pelvic outlet.

secondary powers in labour   Voluntary muscles of the abdominal wall and diaphragm which, by their contraction, increase intra-abdominal pressure in the second stage of labour. Intrauterine pressure rises to 110 mmHg with the combined effect of primary uterine action (35–66 mmHg) and secondary powers (50 mmHg).

secretory phase of menstrual cycle   The interval between ovulation and the succeeding menstrual period during which oestrogen and progesterone from the corpus luteum stimulate growth of the endometrium and glycogen secretion of the glands.

shoulder dystocia   (impacted shoulders) Obstruction to the passage of the shoulders through the bony pelvis, the head having been delivered – the neck fails to appear and the baby's chin burrows into the mother's perineum when the occiput is anterior.

show   A discharge of mucus and blood at the onset of labour when the cervix dilates and the operculum (cervical mucus plug) falls out.

spurious or false labour   Painful uterine contractions without cervical effacement or dilatation.

stages of labour

The first stage is dilatation of the cervix which is finished when the uterine cavity and vagina are no longer separated by a rim of cervix;

The second stage is expulsion of the fetus;

The third stage is expulsion of the placenta and membranes.

stillbirth   An infant born after 24 weeks of pregnancy who did not breathe after birth or show any signs of life.

supine hypotensive syndrome   In late pregnancy 10% of patients experience faintness when lying supine owing to inferior vena caval obstruction causing reduced return and a fall in cardiac output, there being an inadequate collateral circulation via the paravertebral veins.

tachycardia   A fetal heart rate above 160 beats per minute, and a maternal heart rate above 100 beats per minute; in each case indicative of distress.

term   From 37 to 42 completed weeks' gestation (259–293 days) – neither premature delivery (< 37 weeks) nor prolonged pregnancy (> 42 weeks). Full term is 40 weeks – the due date of confinement (often mistakenly referred to as 'term' in contradistinction to the above definition).

third degree tear   A perineal laceration passing through the anal sphincter and laying open the anal canal.

threatened abortion   Any bleeding from the birth canal before 24 weeks gestation, with or without uterine pains, signifies a threat to abort.

umbilical cord   The connecting lifeline between the fetus and placenta; it contains two umbilical arteries and one umbilical vein encased in Wharton's jelly.

uterine inertia   May be primary (inefficient uterine activity) or secondary (uterine exhaustion). Occurs usually in the late first or second stage when uterine action becomes poor or ceases. The most common cause is obstruction due to a tight perineum in a nullipara.

vacuum extraction   Operation to deliver the fetal head by traction on a suction cup placed on the scalp (usually the occipital region).

varicose veins   Dilatation of the veins of the lower half of the body. Usually occur for the first time or worsen in pregnancy.

weight gain   The average weight gain in pregnancy is about 12.5 kg. A weight gain of more than 0.5 kg per week in late pregnancy often precedes generalized oedema and thus pre-eclampsia.

Wharton's jelly   The mucoid connective tissue supporting the umbilical cord vessels.

RADIO COMMUNICATIONS

Each ambulance service operates its own, unique radio communications network. This will consist of a central control room and a number of mobile (ambulance or other vehicle based) radio users, portable (hand-held) radio sets, and fixed users based at ambulance stations, accident and emergency departments and occasionally coronary care units. The control room and all radios operating on the same frequency comprise the *radio net*. The radio frequencies used by an ambulance service, in keeping with other emergency services, are issued under licence by the Department of Trade and Industry Radio Regulatory Department (DTI/RRD) and their use is governed by statutory regulation. Improper use of radio communications may constitute a criminal offence.

It would not be unusual for an ambulance service to have access to more than one frequency (or *channel*). One channel may be used by a service's patient transport vehicles – non-urgent services, outpatient transport or perhaps a doctor's answering service (where the doctors have hand-held radios), while the second channel would be used for all communications by front-line emergency vehicles. A third channel, the emergency reserve channel (ERC) is a common frequency available to all emergency services which can be utilized during major incidents. In addition, an ambulance service may also use other methods of communication including pagers, mobile telephones and of course conventional telephone systems (*land lines*).

THE RADIO NETWORK

Radio communications are central to the functioning of any emergency service, and the control room is the focus of the ambulance service, without which it would be impossible for it to function. The control room is usually based at the ambulance service's headquarters.

An ambulance service radio communication network will consist of the control room itself which is manned 24 hours a day, 365 days a year. Control room staff will receive all requests for ambulances whether via 999 calls, general practitioner requests, or hospital requests for emergency or urgent ambulances. The control room staff will then deploy vehicles and personnel in response to these requests via the radio net. Communication between the control room and users of the radio net must be conducted according to strict *radio procedure* in order to avoid errors and misunderstanding. The potential for errors can be compounded depending on the operating system in use.

Single Frequency Simplex System

In the single frequency system all users, including control, transmit and receive on the same frequency. All users can hear each other and can speak to each other; simultaneous transmission by any two users will therefore result in a garbled transmission. Strict radio procedure via the control is essential when using this operating system.

Two-Frequency Duplex Systems

In the two-frequency system, users transmit on separate frequencies. Each user can communicate with the control only, unless control allows 'talk through' which allows one user to speak directly to another user. When the system is switched to 'talk through', both sides of the conversation can be heard by all users (e.g. one unit giving directions to another). Normally, although control can be heard by all users, the user can only be heard by control. Other users usually hear a pulsed tone when a user transmits to control, which signifies that the channel is busy.

Each radio will be a two-way set capable of communicating with the control room staff on a number of pre-set radio channels. Each unit will be assigned a unique call sign which is used in all transmissions, e.g. Mike Lima One, Medic Three, Quebec Two Zero One. The Oscar One call sign is usually reserved for the chief ambulance officer.

Radio Voice Procedure

The essentials of good radio voice procedure are *clarity, accuracy* and *brevity*. These are important in order to minimize transmission times, as radio networks can be very busy, and while you are speaking to Control no-one else can.

Pay particular attention to the way in which you speak. The *rhythm* should be regular (avoid long pauses between words or running words into each other); the *speed* should be slightly slower than normal conversational speech (words should be pronounced distinctly and at a rate of about 40–60 words per minute); the *volume* should be slightly louder than normal conversational speech (avoid shouting or whispering); the *pitch* is best aimed at that of a female voice which usually appears clearer over the radio; deeper, gruff voices are less clearly heard. Remember 'RSVP':

    R > RHYTHM
    S > SPEED
    V > VOLUME
    P > PITCH

Formulating a Message

Always *listen* before transmitting to ensure that the frequency is clear. Avoid interrupting other transmissions. If a conversation is already taking place and your radio is on an open setting, you will hear the voice of control while the other user conversation may be represented by a beeping tone. Your radio may have a light-emitting diode (LED) e.g. a red light, on the top which flickers when radio transmissions are occurring; look at this to ensure the channel is free before you begin to speak. (On some radios the LED may also serve as a 'battery low' indicator, and will flash at a different rate to normal when the battery is failing). Think through what you are going to say before you transmit a message, and consider whether you really need to transmit at all. Avoid using the radio for trivial conversations or messages that could be better passed by another method or at another time.

If you are inexperienced in using radio procedure, write your message down before transmitting.

Commencing a message
You will need to know:

- Control's call sign (e.g. Leeds Control; Mid-Glamorgan Control; MIDAM Control). Normally, these will be abbreviated in everyday use to a shorter alternative or simply to 'Control'.
- Your own call sign (e.g. Oscar One; Mike Lima One Zero One)
- What you want to say

A typical conversation may be like this:

Oscar One:	Control, from Oscar One, over.
Control:	Oscar One, go ahead, over.
Oscar One:	Oscar One, I have arrived at seventeen, one, seven, Birchgrove, acknowledge, over.

[Always identify yourself at the beginning of each message, giving *your* call sign and not that to which you are speaking. Acknowledge = confirm you have received my message. Give numbers in full, then separately: seventeen, one, seven].

Control:	Control, message received [or Roger], over.
Oscar One:	Oscar One, there are three casualties and I require paramedic support, over.
Control:	Control, Roger, say again number of casualties, over.

['Say again' is used when a message is not received, or the message is not understood. It can be used specifically, as in the above example, or refer to the whole of the preceding message when used alone.]

Oscar One:	Oscar One, I say again three casualties, over.
Control:	Control, message received, three casualties, confirmed, paramedic support is on its way; ETA one zero minutes, out.

[Do not acknowledge a message ending in 'out'. Some controls like to have the last word and 'out' is reserved for their use only. The expression 'over and out' is meaningless and should not be used.]

Oscar One:	Oscar One, there are four casualties, wrong, three casualties, over.

[If you make a mistake, say 'wrong' and give the correct message.]

Radio Check and Signal Strength

When receiving a radio, or assuming responsibility for radio equipment at the start of duty, it is important to check that the equipment is working properly and a good signal strength exists between you and the control. This is established by the *radio check* and involves a brief conversation with control, and an example is given below. It will confirm that you are able to communicate clearly with control and vice versa, or will identify problems in transmission. If it is your first contact with the control room the conversation should also establish and confirm your call sign and present situation. When first contacting control you should establish the following:

- Who you are (e.g. staff coming on duty)
- What your call sign is
- Your present location
- Your present status (e.g. taking charge of a vehicle and ready to respond to an incident if requested)
- Quality of radio reception, by control from you, and by you from control (radio check)

Table C1 Description of radio signal strength

Descriptive terms	Numerical scale
Loud and clear	5 Loud and clear
OK	4 Good but with background noise
Difficult	3 Weak, readable with difficulty
Broken	2 Very weak, rarely readable
Unworkable	1 Unreadable (fading, intermittent, interference)
Nothing heard	

The radio check will establish the signal strength, i.e. the quality of the transmission, which can be described either verbally or using a numbered scale (Table C1).

Numerical scale systems can be misinterpreted, but are still in use. Check the procedure used by your own control room.

Example of radio check procedure

Oscar One:	Control from Oscar One, radio check, over.
Control:	Oscar One from Control, receiving loud and clear (strength five), over.
Oscar One:	Oscar One, receiving loud and clear (strength five), over.
Control:	Control out.

EQUIPMENT

Understand and familiarize yourself with any radio communication equipment you are expected to use. Radios differ in make and type, and it cannot always be taken for granted that the features of operation of one radio will be the same as another. Important features include:

- On/off button
- Volume control
- Channel selection
- Press to talk (PTT) button. This key is used to switch between receive and transmit modes. It normally needs to be pressed in order to transmit, and is otherwise in the receive mode
- LED indicator. May have more than one function, indicating the radio is transmitting, the channel is busy, and may operate as a battery failure indicator
- Special features, e.g. Selcall

Golden Rules of Radio Procedures

Know and follow correct radio procedure at all times:

- Know your control call sign
- Know your own or the radio's call sign
- Keep transmissions as brief as possible
- Think out your message before transmitting
- Do not transmit across others
- Do not speak too quickly, perfect your 'radio voice'
- Where possible, avoid transmitting from noisy areas
- Do not hold the microphone too far from or too close to your mouth
- Remember confidentiality and avoid identifying full patient details, in addition to sensitive clinical information which may be linked to them

Safety precautions:

- Switch off radios when at petrol filling stations, as there is a potential risk of explosion
- Switch off radios when in the vicinity of explosive devices as there is potential for explosion if the devices are radio-controlled

Trouble-Shooting

If the equipment is dead, check:

- Battery – is it (a) connected/fitted, (b) charged?
- Radio — is it switched on?
- Channel selector
- Jack socket, car piece, aerial
- Fuses

If there is background noise, weak sound transmission or distortion, check:

- Channel switch
- Aerial
- Volume control
- Mute control
- Battery
- Location
- Verify problem with use of another set

RADIO TERMINOLOGY

'*Over*' – used to signify the end of a message, and that the speaker is awaiting an immediate reply

'*Out*' – the conversation is finished (normally reserved for use by the control operator, i.e. control always has the last word)

'*Roger*' – message received and understood

'*OK*' – message received and understood

'*Willco*' – message received, understood and will be complied with

'*Wait*' – I am unable to receive your message or reply at this precise moment but will respond within the next 2 minutes.

'*Wait out*' – as '*Wait*', but response may take longer, up to 5 minutes or more

'*Send*' – pass your message, I am ready to receive it

'*Go ahead*' – pass your message, I am ready to receive it

'*Say again*' – repeat what you said (requests caller to repeat all of the last message). This can be qualified; e.g.

'*Say again all after . . . over*'

'*Say again all before . . . over*'

'*Say again name*' '*Say again address*', etc.

'*Acknowledge*' – asks for confirmation that the message has been received

'*Stand by*' – stay alert and on open channel, there is further information to follow. This may be qualified by a time interval; e.g. '*Stand by one*' (1 minute), '*Stand by five*' (5 minutes)

'*Affirmative*' (yes), '*Negative*' (no) – although it is preferable to use simply 'Yes' or 'No', these terms are in common use

'*I spell*' – signifies a word or phrase is to be spelt phonetically

'*Priority, priority*' – (followed by the user's call sign) signifies an emergency situation serious enough to cut in on another transmission. Some radios have alarm buttons which alert the control in the same way

Common abbreviations

* ETA – estimated time of arrival
* ETD – estimated time of departure
* RTA – road traffic accident
* RTB – return to base

Terms to be Avoided

'*Over and out*' – it is either '*Over*' OR '*Out*'

'*Negative*', '*Positive*' – 'Yes' or 'No' will often suffice

'*Roger Dodger*' – slang

'*Ten Four*' – slang

'*Please*', '*Thank you*' – unnecessary

Avoid jargon that may not be understood. The use of obscene language and the passing of gambling information are expressly forbidden under the Radio Telephone Licensing Regulations.

Coded Information

Some ambulance and emergency services operate predesignated codes which are used to signify clinical conditions or types of response. Examples are:

* Respond RED – 999 response requiring lights and sirens
* Respond BLUE – urgent response, but not requiring the use of lights and sirens
* Code 1 – motorway road traffic accident
* Code 2 – other road traffic accident
* Code 5 – chest pain: suspected myocardial infarction
* Code 6 – fire call
* Code 8 – maternity case
* Code 10 – assault

METHODS OF COMMUNICATION

Pagers

A pager is a small radio receiver which when activated can respond in a number of ways depending on the type and model. Functions range from emitting a simple alert tone, usually accompanied by a flashing LED, to sophisticated models with a screen capable of displaying a message in alphanumerical form.

Mobile Telephones

Mobile telephones are increasing in popularity, but have their limitations. In particular, they may be unreliable in certain parts of the country (especially rural areas), and may not always be secure from the point of view of confidentiality. In addition, the mobile telephone network can be subject to system overload when many telephones are in simultaneous use in the same locality. This problem may occur during a major incident, but can be alleviated by using access control overload control (ACCOLC) which denies access to all mobile telephones other than those registered by the Home Office for emergency purposes.

Selcall

Selcall is a signalling system available on some radio networks with appropriate network and radio equipment. It uses a sequence of audible tones to identify individual radios or groups of radios. Selcall allows the pre-programming of radio sets with transmission codes (status codes) that can be signalled to control without having to engage in conversation. This allows transmission of standard information, e.g. 'mobile to incident', 'arrival at incident', 'mobile to hospital' etc., without

Table C2 The phonetic alphabet

Letter	Phonetic Equivalent	Letter	Phonetic Equivalent
A	Alpha	N	November
B	Bravo	O	Oscar
C	Charlie	P	Papa
D	Delta	Q	Quebec
E	Echo	R	Romeo
F	Foxtrot	S	Sierra
G	Golf	T	Tango
H	Hotel	U	Uniform
I	India	V	Victor
J	Juliet	W	Whisky
K	Kilo	X	X-ray
L	Lima	Y	Yankee
M	Mike	Z	Zulu

Table C3 Numbers pronunciation

Number	Pronunciation
0	'ZERO'
1	'WUN' – emphasis on 'N'
2	'TOO' – sharp 'T', long 'OO'
3	'TH-R-EE' – slightly full 'R'
4	'FOUR' – long 'O' as in 'foe'
5	'FIFE' – emphasizing second consonant 'F'
6	'SIX' – emphasizing 'X'
7	'SEV-EN' – two distinct syllables: 'EN' as in 'hen'
8	'ATE' – long 'A' and emphasizing 'T'
9	'NINER' – long 'I' and emphasizing each 'N'

THE NATO PHONETIC ALPHABET

The phonetic alphabet accepted for use by NATO assigns each letter of the alphabet a symbolic word with a distinct sound; these are listed in Table C2. Similarly, there are recommended ways of pronouncing numbers (Table C3).

taking up air time. The message will appear in alphanumeric form on the control operator's control screen, usually with the user's call sign and time of transmission displayed automatically.

TRAUMA SCORING

The principal objective of trauma scoring is to relate a numerical scale of injury severity to the probability of survival. This can be done *prospectively* at the time of injury, when the results may be used by an ambulance officer to decide to which hospital the patient should be transported, or whether the trauma team at the hospital should be alerted in advance. Trauma scoring is also performed *retrospectively* when the patient has been treated in hospital and has died or been discharged, when the scoring may involve complex mathematical calculations. This information is used to review an individual patient's treatment (audit), and to compare the expected outcome with a nationally agreed standard. In general, the retrospective scores will be a more sensitive indicator of probability of survival.

In pre-hospital care the objective of trauma scoring is to identify patients whose cases are 'time-critical', and whose outcome may be adversely affected if they do not receive rapid assessment and treatment at a hospital with appropriate trauma service facilities. Pre-hospital trauma scoring is therefore a triage tool (see Chapter 56). The aim is to deliver *the right patient to the right hospital at the right time*.

METHODS OF TRAUMA SCORING

There are two methods of assessing the severity of injury. One is to relate changes in the patient's physiology to the probability of survival; the other is to directly relate the anatomical injuries to survival.

Physiological Scoring Systems

The first scoring system was physiological, and was introduced by Champion in the USA in 1981 as a triage tool for paramedics. This trauma score has five parameters:

- Systolic blood pressure
- Respiratory rate
- Respiratory effort
- Glasgow coma score
- Capillary return

The maximum score is 16, which indicates 'normal' physiology. A trauma score below 13 indicates a mortality rate of over 10%, and has been used in the USA as an indication to transfer the patient directly to a regional trauma centre. Two problems were encountered with this scoring system:

there is a lack of consistency in the interpretation of respiratory effort

capillary return cannot be reliably measured in the dark or in the cold

In 1989 Champion produced a *revised trauma score* (RTS), which relied solely on systolic blood pressure, respiratory rate and the Glasgow coma scale (GCS) score. He recognized that statistically GCS is more important than respiratory rate. Therefore each parameter is scored out of 4, then multiplied by a weighting coefficient to take account of the parameter's relative importance. The maximum total score is 7.84. It would be impractical to perform such a mathematical calculation at the roadside, and this score is only used as a retrospective audit tool.

What can be used at the roadside is a modification of the RTS known as the *triage revised trauma score* (TRTS) (Table D1). The same three parameters as the RTS are again scored from 0 to 4. The scores are then added, with a maximum score of 12 which is physiologically 'normal'. If there is a fall of 1 point in any one parameter this is considered significant, and in the USA the patient is deemed to require the services of a trauma centre. The probability of survival for each score is shown in Table D.2.

Table D1 Coded values for the triage revised trauma score (and revised trauma score)

Parameter	Score	Coded value
Respiratory rate	10–29	4
(breaths/min)	> 29	3
	6–9	2
	1–5	1
	0	0
Systolic blood pressure	> 89	4
(mmHg)	76–89	3
	50–75	2
	1–49	1
	0	0
Glasgow coma scale	13–15	4
	9–12	3
	6–8	2
	4–5	1
	3	0

Table D2 The relationship of the triage revised trauma score with probability of survival

Triage revised trauma score	Probability of survival (%)
12	99.5
11	96.9
10	87.9
9	76.7
8	66.7
7	63.6
6	63.0
5	45.5
4	33.3
3	30.3
2	28.6
1	25.0
0	3.7

Physiological scoring systems have the following disadvantages:

- The system may overestimate trauma in the very young (a systolic blood pressure of 80 mmHg in an infant is physiologically normal for that age)
- The system may underestimate trauma in the elderly (a systolic blood pressure of 100 mmHg in an 80-year-old is physiologically abnormal for that age)

Anatomical Scoring Systems

Survival can also be retrospectively related to the severity of anatomical injury. The standard method is to use the *abbreviated injury scale* where the body is divided into six regions, and injuries coded from 'mild' (scores 1 point) to 'untreatable' (scores 6 points) within each region. The highest scoring injuries from up to three body regions are taken, squared, and added together to produce the *injury severity score* (ISS), which closely reflects the probability of survival. An 'untreatable' (6 points) injury in any region is automatically awarded the highest total score, which becomes $5^2 + 5^2 + 5^2$ (i.e. 75). The term 'major trauma' is used for casualties who have an ISS greater than 16.

Combined Anatomical and Physiological Scoring Systems

In the UK, the most commonly used audit tool to evaluate trauma care retrospectively is the Triage Revised trauma score and Injury Severity Score (TRISS) methodology. This methodology combines the revised trauma score (physiological score) with the injury severity score (anatomical score), and also takes into account the patient's age and whether the trauma was blunt or penetrating. Results are used nationally to compare a hospital's performance against an agreed norm, and to see how a hospital performs in relation to others (although all other hospitals remain anonymous). This Major Trauma Outcome Survey (MTOS) programme is coordinated nationally in Manchester.

HOW CAN TRAUMA SCORING BE USED IN THE UK?

There is no integrated network of trauma services in the UK. In most areas the ambulance service will take a patient to the nearest hospital, without consideration for the resources of that hospital. A trauma scoring system can be used as a triage tool to allow ambulances to bypass small hospitals, but the following conditions are prerequisites:

- The ambulance service personnel must be taught the system, and the application of the system must be monitored
- The receiving hospitals must understand the system, and the significance of an altered score
- Ambulance officers may require extended protocols (procedures, fluids, and drugs) to sustain a patient over the longer primary road transfers

In the absence of such a trauma system, physiological trauma scoring can still be used in pre-hospital care to identify patients at risk. This information can be used to inform the hospital in advance, and the ambulance crew can then expect to have a suitably trained trauma team waiting in the accident and emergency department to receive the patient.

AC	alternating current
AF	atrial fibrillation
ACLS	advanced cardiac life support
ACTH	adrenocorticotrophic hormone
ADH	anti-diuretic hormone
APH	antepartum haemorrhage
ALS	advanced life support
ARDS	adult respiratory distress syndrome
AST	aspartate amino transferase
ATLS	advanced trauma life support
AVPU	<u>A</u>lert response to <u>V</u>ocal stimulation, response to <u>P</u>ainful stimulation, <u>U</u>nresponsive
BLS	basic life support
BP	blood pressure
BSA	body surface area
CHD	coronary heart disease
CPR	cardiopulmonary resuscitation
CNS	central nervous system
COPD	chronic obstructive pulmonary disease
CRF	chronic renal failure
CSF	cerebrospinal fluid
CT	computerized tomography (a specialized form of X-ray)
CVP	central venous pressure
DC	direct current
DM	diabetes mellitus
DNA	deoxyribonucleic acid
ECG	electrocardiogram
ECT	electroconvulsive therapy
EMD	electromechanical dissociation
ERC	emergency reserve channel
FEV	forced expiratory volume (normally measured over a period of one second)

FHR	fetal heart rate
FVC	forced vital capacity
GCS	Glasgow Coma Score
GTN	glyceryl trinitrate
Hb	haemoglobin
HEMS	helicopter emergency medical service
Hep	one of the forms of viral hepatitis normally followed by a letter such as A, B or C (e.g. Hep B)
HPPF	human plasma protein fraction
IDD	insulin dependent diabetes
IM	intramuscular
IV	intravenous
J	Joule, a unit of energy usually used to measure the amount of electricity discharged from a defibrillator
JVP	jugular venous pulse
LBBB	left bundle branch block (finding on a twelve lead ECG)
LMA	laryngeal mask airway
MAST	military anti shock trousers
MOI	mechanism of injury
MRI	magnetic resonance imaging (a form of imaging of the body)
NIDD	noninsulin dependent diabetes
NSAID	nonsteroidal anti-inflammatory drug
PAC	premature atrial contraction
PASG	pneumatic anti-shock garment
PET	pre-eclamptic toxaemia
PEFR	peak expiratory flow rate
PERLA	pupils equal react to light accommodate
PF	peak flow (same as PEFR)

pH	negative log of hydrogen ions – a measure of the acidity of a fluid
PPH	post partum haemorrhage
PTLA	pharyngeal tracheal lumen airway
PTSD	post traumatic stress disorder
PVC	premature ventricular contraction
RBBB	right bundle branch block
RTA	road traffic accident
RTS	revised trauma score
SaO_2	saturation of a substance with oxygen

SCUBA	self-contained underwater breathing apparatus
SIDS	sudden infant death syndrome
SOCO	scenes of crime officer
SVT	supraventricular tachycardia
TRTS	triage revised trauma score
UKHIS	United Kingdom hazard information system
VF	ventricular fibrillation
VT	ventricular tachycardia

INDEX